Len Oshinski

Len Oshinski

The Art of
LASIK

SECOND EDITION

The Art of
LASIK
SECOND EDITION

Jeffery J. Machat
Stephen G. Slade
Louis E. Probst

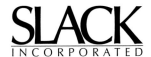
SLACK
INCORPORATED

SLACK Incorporated, 6900 Grove Road, Thorofare, NJ 08086-9447

Publisher: John H. Bond
Editorial Director: Amy E. Drummond
Associate Editor: Jennifer L. Stewart
Cover Design: Linda Baker

The art of LASIK/(edited by) Jeffery J. Machat, Stephen G. Slade, Louis E. Probst. -- 2nd ed.
     p. cm
  Rev. ed. of: Excimer laser refractive surgery. c1996.
  Includes bibliographical references and index.
  ISBN 1-55642-386-1 (alk. paper)
  1. Cornea-Laser surgery.   I. Machat, Jeffery J.,
  II. Probst, Louis. III. Excimer laser refractive surgery.
  [DNLM: 1.Myopia--surgery. 2. Cornea--surgery. 3. Laser surgery--methods
  4. Corneal transplantation--methods. 5. Astigmatism--surgery. WW 320A784 1998}
  RE336.A77 1998
  617.7'55--dc21
  DNLM/DLC
  for Library of Congress   98-22559
                                                        CIP

Printed in the United States of America

Published by: SLACK Incorporated
                   6900 Grove Road
                   Thorofare, NJ 08086-9447 USA
                   Telephone: 609-848-1000
                   Fax: 609-853-5991

Contact SLACK Incorporated for more information about other books in this field or about the availability of our books from distributors outside the United States.

Last digit is print number: 10 9 8 7 6 5 4 3

DEDICATION

Each author dedicates the words he writes to those who make his life complete.
The Art of LASIK is dedicated to my three beautiful children: Justin, age 5; Hayley, age 3; and
Paige, age 1; and to my loving wife Marika, who is now pregnant with our fourth child.
We all know too well what is truly important in our lives,
it is simply that we do not listen to our hearts as often as we should.
Jeffery J. Machat, MD

To my mother, Nell Rowan Slade, for all she has given me and given up for me.
To Rick Baker, John Doane, and Steve Updegraff for teaching me so much.
To Jeff and Elias for sharing their vision with me; and to Leslie,
who gave me everything after all.
Stephen G. Slade, MD

To Jeff, for extending my horizons.
To my parents Louis and Judy, for instilling the values
of honesty and integrity.
To Kate, who provided the love, support,
and understanding that allowed me to complete this project.
Louis E. Probst, MD

We would like to honor the man who was not simply a pioneer, but a visionary.
Jose Barraquer was truly the father of all modern lamellar refractive surgery,
especially LASIK. All of us who practice LASIK owe him an unpayable debt
of gratitude because we are all his students, just as our patients are his too.

CONTENTS

EXPANDED CONTENTS

PREFACE

Excimer Laser Refractive Surgery: Practice and Principles examined the world of refractive surgery as I saw it 3 years ago. It was my first attempt at putting on paper what so many of us have learned through our own clinical experiences with our own patients.

The Art of LASIK represents another chapter in my life of refractive surgery. In the past 2 1/2 years I have learned much as refractive surgery has evolved to a new level. I have now performed over 20,000 refractive procedures including about 15,000 primary and secondary LASIK procedures. I am constantly amazed at how much refinement there can be in such a brief, although life-altering, procedure. This book is important in not only all that it says, but all that it does not. There is still no perfect procedure, no perfect microkeratome, and no perfect laser. There are multiple techniques that work, but all are guided by certain fundamental principles. It is these principles, which I discussed in the first edition that still hold true today.

When writing *The Art of LASIK*, I was overwhelmed at the clinical advancements that had been made in the past 2 years, the greater depth of insight I had acquired, and the maturity that had befallen LASIK. It is clear now the LASIK has become the most dominant refractive procedure in the armamentarium of the refractive surgeon. As Stephen Slade has stated, if one compares refractive surgery to cataract surgery, LASIK has become the "phaco" of refractive surgery.

I have also been overwhelmed by the acceptance of laser refractive surgery by both the medical community and lay public worldwide. Hundreds of thousands of LASIK procedures are performed yearly in countries around the world, and growth continues steadily as word-of-mouth validates LASIK as a safe and effective technique. Equally as important and somewhat distressing is the rise in complications, including those that are preventive. This textbook is a collective effort on the part of all the contributors to share our triumphs and our tragedies in the hopes that all those who read these pages will gain insight into the fundamental and practical principles of LASIK.

In my mind there are three levels of clinical expertise with LASIK. The first level is simply knowing how to utilize the microkeratome and create a corneal flap. The second level is the knowledge and clinical experience that not only helps to perform LASIK on difficult cases, such as those with tight orbits, narrow palpebral fissures, and high brows, but determines the immediate management of a corneal flap complication. The third level is the more complex management of advanced LASIK cases such as those patients who have had previous refractive or ocular surgery, and the management of those advanced complications which include long-standing corneal striae, epithelial ingrowths with stromal melting, aggressive lamellar interface keratitis (Sands), and topographical irregularities. This textbook will attempt to serve as a resource guide to refractive surgeons at all three levels, stressing the refractive surgery principles practiced by all our contributors. As national medical co-directors for TLC The Laser Center, Stephen Slade and myself have tried to teach a healthy respect for LASIK while embracing its virtues. With several hundred accomplished TLC refractive surgeons of varying levels of LASIK experience operating at 48 centers throughout North America, we have learned much ourselves as TLC continues to grow. About 100,000 refractive procedures will be performed this year alone at TLC facilities and our growth will be directly related to not only successful outcomes but a lack of serious complications.

Complications happen to all refractive surgeons, the important issues revolve about proper informed consent, proper technique to avoid preventable complications and adequate knowledge in managing complications when they do occur. It is easy to become overconfident. It is easy to feel that one has mastered LASIK. It is important to remind oneself each surgical day that no one is above complications. Ten months ago, after having performed well over 10,000 LASIK procedures, I had a thin corneal flap on the second eye of a physician from Denver, Colo. I did not lift the flap but allowed the eye to settle for 5 months, which allowed best-corrected vision to be preserved. I then performed repeat LASIK starting my cut 20 microns deeper and temporal to the first. Since I perform 400 to 500 LASIK procedures each month, I was pleased that I had not had another thin flap in the interim, although I had had a buttonholed flap with the Chiron Hansatome just 1 month prior to treating the physician. I was of course becoming increasingly overconfident when 10 months had passed and another thin flap still had not occurred. My current technique utilizing PlanoScan with 9 mm blend zones had significantly reduced qualitative night vision problems and eliminated central islands altogether. My access to the Chiron Hansatome for large flat corneas eliminated my concern for free caps, and other technique modifications for managing corneal flaps reduced my incidence of epithelial ingrowths and striae substantially. Yesterday I had another thin flap and gained respect for LASIK all over again.

In the first edition, my last sentence stated that the final and most important principle of LASIK was simply knowing when to say "no" to a patient, my first principle in this edition is maintaining a true and healthy measure of respect for LASIK.

Jeffery J. Machat, MD

INTRODUCTION

This is one of those rare occasions when something in the not so distant past seems longer ago than it actually was. It was June 1991, and I was about to perform my first LASIK procedure, or excimer laser keratomileusis as we called it then. I had dabbled in lamellar refractive surgery, having made several trips to Houston in the 1980s to visit Ralph Berkeley, Steve Slade, and Lee Nordan, who at that time traveled to Houston to perform MKM on high myopes who were unsuitable candidates for radial keratotomy.

MKM was a wonderful, magical, scary procedure, and most of the time the results were good to remarkable. Lee Nordan made it look easy, and he persuaded me to come to San Diego for one of his MKM courses. In New Orleans, where Werblin, Friedlander, Kaufman and McDonald had done some of the original epikeratophakia work lathing their own lenticles, I was fortunate to have access to one of the Steinway cryolathes.

After taking the course, I gathered several highly myopic candidates together and persuaded Lee to fly to New Orleans and hold my hand during these first MKM cases. I followed with a few more patients who exhausted my backlog of high myopes, as well as my courage. That cryolathe was so intimidating when you had to go it alone!

Luis Ruiz significantly improved the microkeratome; his addition of the automated system instilled more confidence in the surgeon, and ALK was on it's way. Steve Slade and I purchased one of these early units together and I performed my first few procedures, adding ALK to my refractive surgery armamentarium. Steve was quite happy with his freeze MKM results and had perfected this procedure to an art form; he simply wanted a better microkeratome to cut the corneal button.

With the developing technology of the excimer laser, the idea of reshaping the surface of the cornea with a laser was conceived. The ophthalmic use of the excimer, first by Seiler to create arcuate cuts through slits in a metallic mask, followed by McDonald's surface PRK, was groundbreaking work that proved the excimer could be used to accurately remove corneal tissue. Contributions such as the development of early nomograms from many investigators continued to move human clinical studies forward.

Lucio Buratto in Milan, an avid student of refractive surgery, gave birth to the idea of using the excimer to replace the cryolathe. He began his early work in 1989, using the Summit Excimed to "carve" the back of the lenticle for the desired refractive result. Although far from perfect, his superior and more consistent results led to Summit receiving an IDE from the FDA to begin the study of "excimer laser keratomileusis." It was lucky for me to have visited Lucio during this period, putting me in the right place at the right time. I became medical monitor of this Summit study and performed the first LASIK procedure in the United States in June of 1991. It took almost 2 years for that core group of six investigators to compile a series of 60 eyes!

Pallikaris established the idea of creating a hinged flap of corneal tissue and ablating the patient's cornea in situ rather than the stromal side of a free cap, as described by Buratto and used as the technique in the first phase of the Summit study. The advantages to the flap technique quickly became obvious, and LASIK as we know it today was born.

After having performed thousands of LASIK procedures and enjoyed experiencing my patient's happiness with their results, I realized that there was no excuse for not being a patient myself. Although I was a good contact lens wearer, I thought it would be great not to have to think about them anymore. It was also a vote of confidence for a procedure that I knew was excellent in the hands of a good surgeon. On July 2, 1997, I found myself lying under the suction ring of the new Hansatome and hearing it buzz across my cornea. It's been great for me both to enjoy my new freedom and to be able to talk to patients about LASIK from their own point of view. It has made me a better surgeon as well as patient advocate for a procedure that is here to stay for a long time.

Stephen F. Brint, MD, FACS

SECTION ONE
The Fundamentals of LASIK

Options for Refractive Surgery

Louis E. Probst, MD

Refractive surgery continues to evolve rapidly with the refinement of current procedures and the development of new refractive techniques. The indications for these refractive options are also changing as the limitations of each procedure are determined by experience and technology. A comprehensive approach to refractive surgery requires a clear understanding of the current options available to the refractive surgeon.

In 1993, the Casebeer Comprehensive Refractive Surgeon Nomogram was created to summarize the refractive options available at that time.[1] Radial keratotomy (RK), myopic and hyperopic automated lamellar keratoplasty (ALK), photorefractive keratectomy (PRK), and laser in situ keratomileusis (LASIK) were the surgical options described. Since then, the armamentarium of the refractive surgeon has evolved—predominantly due to the widespread use of the excimer laser in the United States for both PRK and LASIK.

The Options for Refractive Surgery diagram has been created to illustrate the refractive options currently available in 1998 (Figure 1-1). The intracorneal ring has emerged as an effective modality for correcting low levels of spherical myopia.[2] In the era of the excimer laser, many of the previous refractive procedures have been supplanted. While RK remains an effective and relatively economical refractive option for up to 4 diopters (D) of myopia in patients of an appropriate age,[3] concerns regarding the long-term instability of the refractive error[4] and the reduction in cornea integrity[5] have lead to a shift in practice patterns towards excimer laser vision correction. Myopic ALK has been shown to effectively treat myopia, yet difficulties with the

second "power" cut and management of the corneal flap resulted in a high loss of best-corrected visual acuity (BCVA).[6] Hyperopic ALK attempted to create a controlled corneal ectasia with a microkeratome cut exceeding 60% of the stromal thickness and a subsequent reduction in hyperopia;[7] however progressive ectasia, myopia, and irregular astigmatism occurred in a number of these eyes. Myopic and hyperopic ALK have been largely superseded by LASIK because of the greater safety and predictability associated with the excimer refractive ablation.[8,9]

> Myopic and hyperopic ALK have been largely superseded by LASIK because of the greater safety and predictability associated with the excimer refractive ablation.

PRK has been shown to be safe and efficacious for the treatment of low to moderate myopia.[10-14] LASIK has also been shown to be effective in this range. LASIK is preferable for high myopia, as it avoids the high incidence of corneal haze and loss of BCVA that can occur after large PRK corrections.[15,16] Greater than 15 D of myopia can be treated with LASIK, however this often requires a multizone excimer ablation to decrease the central corneal ablation depth and preserve adequate posterior corneal stromal tissue (200 to 250 microns) to maintain the corneal integrity. While multizone protocols can reduce the overall depth of ablation, they will also compromise the quality of postoperative vision by decreasing the size of the effective corneal optical zone, which is further decreased by the masking effect of the corneal flap.

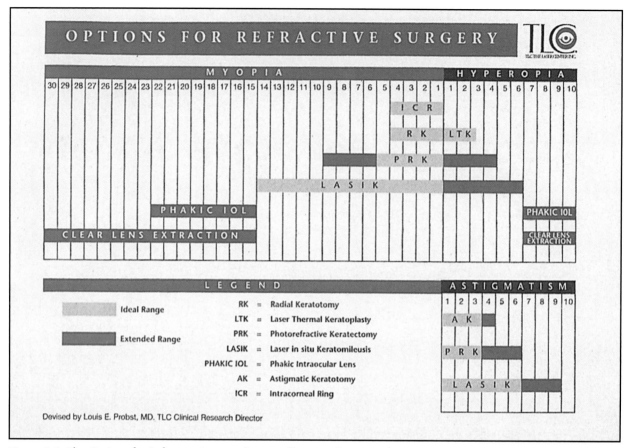

Figure 1-1. The *Options for Refractive Surgery* diagram illustrates the surgical options available for various refractive errors. The recommended ranges are undergoing constant change as each procedure evolves (see Appendix, page 509, for an easy-reference source of this diagram).

> LASIK is preferable for high myopia, as it avoids the high incidence of corneal haze and loss of BCVA that can occur after large PRK corrections.

Laser thermal keratoplasty performed with the Sunrise holmium laser can effectively treat up to 2.5 D of hyperopia.[17] PRK has been used to treat up to 4 D of hyperopia, but concerns about postoperative regression, corneal haze, and loss of BCVA may limit this procedure to the lower degrees of hyperopia.[18] The greatest promise for the surgical treatment of hyperopia is with hyperopic LASIK, which has been reported to be effective to at least 6 D of hyperopia with less regression and little risk of corneal haze.

Less than 3 D of astigmatism can be treated with AK[19] or PRK, however the astigmatism is often undercorrected by the excimer laser.[20] AK is now generally reserved for those eyes with a spherical equivalent near plano. LASIK can be used to treat higher degrees of astigmatism particularly when performed with an astigmatic scanning excimer laser such as the Chiron Technolas Keracor 116.

Phakic intraocular lenses (IOLs) are an investigational refractive option for the correction of both high hyperopia and myopia. Anterior chamber phakic IOLs have been associated with a 12% endothelial cell loss, rendering them unacceptable as a viable refractive option.[21] Posterior chamber phakic IOLs from several manufacturers have achieved positive visual results, however complications such as papillary block glaucoma, anterior subcapsular lens opacities, and decentrations must be minimized before these IOLs can be considered to have an acceptable risk.[22,23] An international clinical trial has been initiated by STARR Surgical for their implantable contact lens, which should provide further information on the viability of this procedure.

Clear lens extraction is another intraocular investigational procedure that has been reported as successful for the treatment of both high myopia and hyperopia.[24,25] The incidence of retinal detachment in two separate series with 4 years of follow-up was 1.9 to 5.4%.[26,27] Capsular tears accompanied by vitreous loss, posterior capsular opacifica-

> The greatest promise for the surgical treatment of hyperopia is with hyperopic LASIK.

accompanied by vitreous loss, posterior capsular opacification requiring YAG capsulotomy, and undercorrection have also been reported as complications associated with clear lens extraction.[25,26,27] Given that the normal lifetime myopia risk of retinal detachment is 2.4%, clear lensectomy could be considered to have an acceptable risk in selected patients.[28]

REFERENCES

1. American Academy of Ophthalmology. Automated lamellar keratoplasty, preliminary procedure assessment. *Ophthalmology.*. 1996;103(5):852-861.

2. Nose W, Neves RA, Burris TE, Schanzlin DJ, Belfort R Jr. Intrastromal corneal ring: 12-month sighted myopic eyes. *Journal of Refractive Surgery.* 1996;12(1):20-28.

3. American Academy of Ophthalmology. Radial keratotomy for myopia, Ophthalmic Procedure Assessment. *Ophthalmology.* 1993;100(7):1103-1115.

4. Waring GO III, Lynn MJ, McDonnell PJ, et al. Results of the prospective evaluation of radial keratotomy (PERK) study 10 years after surgery. *Arch Ophthalmol.* 1994;112:1298-1308.

5. Rashid ER, Waring GO III. Complications of radial and transverse keratotomy. *Surv Ophthalmol.* 1989;34(2):73-105.

6. Lyle WA, Jin GJC. Initial results of automated lamellar keratoplasty for correction of myopia: 1-year follow-up. *J Cataract Refract Surg.* 1996;22:31-43.

7. Manche EE, Judge A, Maloney RK. Lamellar keratoplasty for hyperopia. *Journal of Refractive Surgery.* 1996;12:42-49.

8. Salah T, Waring GO III, Maghraby AE, et al. Excimer laser in situ keratomileusis under a corneal flap for myopia of 2 to 20 diopters. *Am J Ophthalmol.* 1996;121:143-155.

9. Arbelaez M. One year follow-up of hyperopia (LASIK/Planoscan). ISRS 1996 Pre-AAO Conference (abstract), October 24-26, 1996.

10. Epstein D, Fagerholm P, Hamberg-Nystrom H, Tengroth B. Twenty-four-month follow-up of excimer laser photorefractive keratectomy for myopia. Refractive and visual acuity results. *Ophthalmology.* 1994;101:1558-1564.

11. Dutt S, Steinert RF, Raizman MB, Puliafito CA. One-year results of excimer laser photorefractive keratectomy for low to moderate myopia. *Arch Ophthalmol.* 1994;112:1427-1436.

12. McDonald MB, Talamo JH. Myopic photorefractive keratectomy: The experience in the United States with the VISX excimer laser. In: Salz JJ, ed. *Corneal Laser Surgery.* St. Louis, Mo: Mosby; 1995.

13. Alamo S, Shimizu K. Excimer laser photorefractive keratectomy for myopia: 2-year follow-up. *Journal of Refractive Surgery.* 1995;11(suppl):S253-S260.

14. Thompson KP, Steinert RF, Daniel J, Stulting D. Photorefractive keratectomy with the Summit excimer laser: The phase III US. results. In: Salz JJ, ed. *Corneal Laser Surgery.* St. Louis, Mo: Mosby; 1995.

15. Krueger RR, Talamo JH, McDonald MB, et al. Clinical analysis of excimer laser photorefractive keratectomy using a multiple zone technique for severe myopia. *Am J Ophthalmol.* 1995;119:263-274.

16. Pop M, Aras M. Multizone/multipass photorefractive keratectomy: 6-month results. *J Cataract Refract Surg.* 1995;21:633-643.

17. Koch DD, Kohnen T, McDonnell PJ, et al. Hyperopic correction by noncontact holmium: YAG laser thermal keratoplasty, Unites States phase IIA clinical study with 1-year follow-up. *Ophthalmology.* 1996;103:1525-1536.

18. Jackson B, Agapitos PJ, Mintsioulis G, et al. Excimer laser PRK with the VISX STAR for low hyperopia. *VISX Internet Website Physician Study Data*; 1996.

19. Agapitos PJ, Lindstrom RL. Astigmatic Keratotomy. *Ophthalmology Clinics of North America.* 1992;5(4):709-714.

20. Taylor HR, Kelly P, Alpins N. Excimer laser corrections of myopic astigmatism. *J Cataract Refract Surg.* 1994;20(suppl):243-251.

21. Perez-Santonja JJ, Iradier MT, Sanz-Iglesias L, et al. Endothelial changes in phakic eyes with anterior chamber intraocular lenses to correct high myopia. *J Cataract Refract Surg.* 1996;22:1017-1022.

22. Assetto V, Benedetti S, Pesando P. Collamer intraocular contact lens to correct high myopia. *J Cataract Refract Surg.* 1996;22:551-556.

23. Fechner PU, Haigis W, Wichmann W. Posterior chamber myopia lenses in phakic eyes. *J Cataract Refract Surg.* 1996;22:178-182.

24. Siganos DS, Pallikaris IG, Siganos CS. Clear lensectomy and intraocular lens implantation in normally sighted highly hyperopic eyes. Three-year follow-up. *European Journal of Implant and Refractive Surgery.* 1995;7:128-133.

25. Lyle WA, Jin GJC. Clear lens extraction for the correction of high refractive error. *J Cataract Refract Surg.* 1994;20:273-276.

26. Colin J. Robinet A. Clear lensectomy and implantation of a low-power posterior lens for the correction of high myopia. *Ophthalmology.* 1997;104:73-77.

27. Barraquer C, Cavelier C, Mejia LF. Incidence of retinal detachment following clear lens extraction in myopic patients. Retrospective analysis. *Arch Ophthalmol.* 1994;112:321-323.

28. Drews RC. Clear lensectomy and implantation of a low-power posterior lens for the correction of high myopia (discussion). *Ophthalmology.* 1997;104:77-78.

CHAPTER 2

Evolution of Lamellar Refractive Surgery

John F. Doane, MD
Stephen G. Slade, MD

INTRODUCTION

Lamellar corneal surgery for the correction of refractive errors has been evolving for 50 years, albeit much of that time it was in relative obscurity.[1-5] It is through the sheer genius, persistence, and ingenuity of Prof. Jose I. Barraquer that the field of lamellar corneal refractive surgery was born in his dreams in 1948. Many of his concepts remain the foundation of this particular field of ophthalmic surgery.

Fundamentally, refractive lamellar corneal surgery attempts to either remove, add, or modify the corneal stroma so the tear film—anterior corneal interface radius of curvature is altered as desired. For the treatment of myopia, tissue can either be removed centrally (ie, laser in situ keratomileusis [LASIK]) or added peripherally (ie, intracorneal ring or gel injection adjustable keratoplasty) to induce central corneal flattening and a reduction of myopia. For hyperopia, tissue can be added centrally (ie, keratophakia), subtracted peripherally (ie, hyperopic LASIK), or a deep keratectomy with controlled ectasia (automated lamellar keratoplasty [ALK] for hyperopia) can be performed to induce central corneal steepening with a reduction of spherical plus refractive power. The treatment of astigmatism is accomplished by either flattening the steep axis (via removal of tissue) or steepening the flat axis (via removal of tissue) to make the overall cornea spherical.

Many of the instruments currently used in lamellar corneal refractive surgery originate from Barraquer's ideas. Lamellar corneal refractive surgery requires the use of a microkeratome (Figure 2-1), which functions much like a carpenter's plane to perform a planar resection of tissue from the anterior cornea. The microkeratome contains an oscillating blade that incises the tissue at an even depth if the intraocular pressure is maintained at a stable pressure, and the velocity of the instrument as it moves across the cornea is constant.

Lamellar approaches to corneal refractive surgery include no less than 10 distinct techniques listed below in order of evolution:

- Freeze myopic keratomileusis
- Keratomileusis in situ (non-automated)
- Keratophakia
- Barraquer-Krumeich-Swinger technique
- Epikeratoplasty
- Automated lamellar keratoplasty (keratomileusis in situ—automated)
- Buratto-style laser keratomileusis
- LASIK
- Peripheral mass addition techniques of intracorneal ring/segments
- Gel injection adjustable keratoplasty

While all of these approaches strive for the same end result, each have varying degrees of success. As a result of experience with earlier techniques, the field of lamellar refractive surgery has undergone an evolution towards increased simplicity of surgical techniques and greater patient safety, with the end result being improved refractive results and wider surgeon acceptance. Distinct benefits of recent applications of lamellar refractive surgery (ie, ALK and LASIK) include the ability to treat a larger range of refractive errors more effectively, shorter visual rehabilitation time, minimal postoperative discomfort, and a diminished healing response to surgery when compared to other

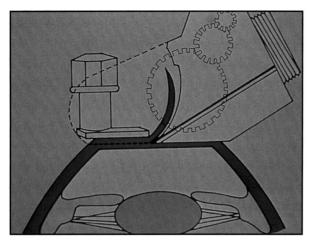

Figure 2-1. Keratome creating a lamellar dissection by applanating the cornea and carving in a similar fashion as a carpenter's plane.

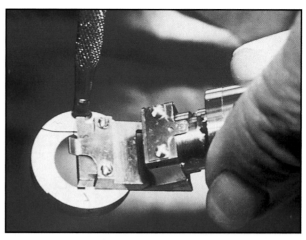

Figure 2-2. Manual Barraquer microkeratome and suction ring.

modalities.[6-19] On the other hand, newer corneal lamellar surgical techniques (specifically LASIK) require advanced technical expertise, large ongoing capital expenditures, and the potential for serious intraoperative complications not observed with less invasive techniques, such as photorefractive keratectomy (PRK), or procedures that spare the central cornea, such as radial keratotomy (RK). Clinical outcomes of lamellar refractive surgery (efficacy, predictability, safety, and stability) are subjects of intense study at this time, and preliminary findings suggest that results are at least comparable to and, in many instances, better than alternative technologies (ie, RK and PRK).

EVOLUTION OF REFRACTIVE CORNEAL SURGERY TECHNIQUES

Corneal lamellar refractive keratoplasty has its roots in the work of Barraquer beginning in 1949 in Bogota, Colombia.[1,3-5] Barraquer developed keratomileusis, which uses the cryolathe to shape the cornea and alter its refractive power, and keratophakia, which entails adding a disc of corneal stroma under a lamellar flap to increase the central corneal curvature. The term keratomileusis is derived from the Greek roots keras (horn-like—cornea) and smileusis (carving).[2] Freeze keratomileusis can be used to treat myopia or hyperopia, but Barraquer had greater success with myopia treatments. The main difficulties with freeze keratomileusis were the learning curve of the keratectomy and the complexity of the cryolathe. A manual keratome driven across the eye by hand is strongly dependent upon the speed of passage to determine the thickness and evenness of the keratectomy (Figure 2-2). Any irregularity in this cut

> Keratomileusis is derived from the Greek roots keras (horn-like—cornea) and smileusis (carving).

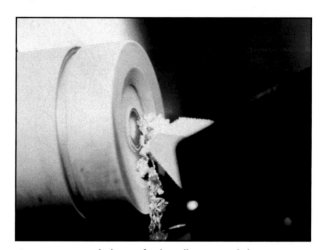

Figure 2-3. Cryolathing of a lamellar corneal disc.

will be exposed as an irregular astigmatism and a subsequent decrease in best-corrected vision in the patient.[2,20-25]

The cryolathe is a difficult instrument to master and maintain (Figures 2-3 and 2-4). Complications with freeze keratomileusis and lamellar keratoplasty include all the normal risks of eye surgery in general, along with specific problems such as epithelial implantation/ingrowth in the stromal interface and possible induction of irregular astigmatism.[2,20-25] Positive results were obtained initially by several investigators, however the technique required substantial surgical skill that did not prove to be transferable to a large number of surgeons.[21,22]

KERATOMILEUSIS IN SITU FOR MYOPIA

The concept of raising a corneal cap and removing central tissue from the bed, keratomileusis in situ, was first conceived by Barraquer. It was also described by Krwawicz[26] in 1964 and subsequently by Pureskin[27] in 1966. Both authors described this technique as central "stromectomy." Barraquer's concept of keratomileusis in situ involved first

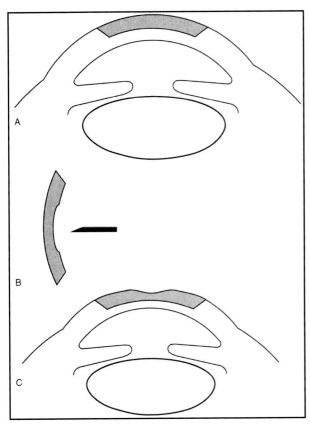

Figure 2-4. Freeze myopic keratomileusis. (A) 300-micron corneal cap created with a microkeratome. (B) Central stroma from the posterior aspect of the cap removed with a cryolathe. (C) Cap replaced and sutured in place with an anti-torque suture. The central cornea was flattened to reduce myopia.

gaining access to the corneal stroma by making a free cap with a manual pass of the microkeratome and then making a second pass across the stromal bed to remove a smaller diameter disc of tissue with a specified thickness depending on the degree of refractive error. The second pass of the microkeratome is, in effect, the refractive part of the procedure. When the tissue disc is removed and the flap or cap is replaced, the anterior corneal curvature is flattened. This effectively decreases the corneal curvature and reduces or eliminates the myopic refractive error (Figure 2-5). Barraquer found greater success using the cryolathe to remove tissue from the posterior aspect of the corneal cap in the freeze keratomileusis technique than he did with keratomileusis in situ so he spent his efforts refining the freeze myopic keratomileusis (MKM) technique.

KERATOPHAKIA

Keratophakia is a tissue addition refractive procedure in which a flap and/or cap is created and a disc of tissue is placed underneath the flap/cap to increase the central corneal curvature, hence the term keratophakia or corneal

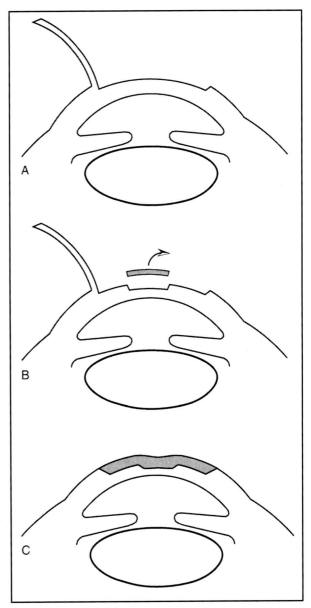

Figure 2-5. Keratomileusis in situ for myopia (manual or automated [automated lamellar keratoplasty]). (A) Creation of a corneal flap with the first pass of the microkeratome. (B) Removal of central stromal tissue from the bed (refractive cut) with the second pass of the microkeratome. (C) Reposit flap. The central cornea was flattened for treatment of myopia.

lens (Figure 2-6). Keratophakia was first developed by Barraquer in the 1960s as a treatment for aphakia after cataract extraction in lieu of the use of cumbersome aphakic spectacles. The added tissue was typically harvested from donor corneal tissue by the microkeratome. Based on the patient's refractive error and target refraction, a specific disc diameter and thickness was planned. With the advent of improved intraocular lens (IOL) technology, keratophakia was relegated to a lesser role since IOLs provided highly accurate refractive results without the induction of significant irregular astigmatism or concern and technical difficul-

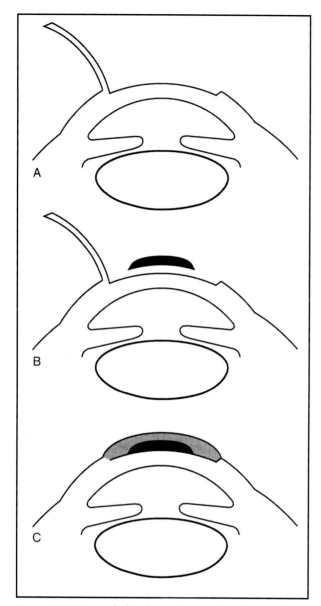

Figure 2-6. Keratophakia (homoplastic allograft or synthetic inlay). (A) Creation of a flap or cap. (B) Graft inlay positioned over the central stromal bed. (C) Flap or cap repositioned. The central corneal power was increased to effectively treat hyperopia or aphakia.

cant irregular astigmatism or concern and technical difficulty in harvesting donor tissue. The future role of keratophakia or corneal inlay techniques in refractive surgery may be with the addition of synthetic tissue/lens material placed under a flap. From the placement of transparent material of differing refractive indexes from the corneal stroma into a stromal pocket, the future may also see the correction of myopia, hyperopia, astigmatism, and presbyopia.

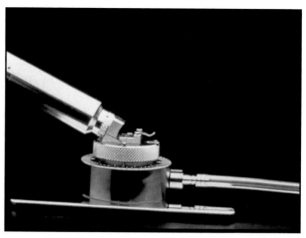

Figure 2-7. Barraquer-Krumeich-Swinger microkeratome and suction platform.

BARRAQUER-KRUMEICH-SWINGER NONFREEZE KERATOMILEUSIS TECHNIQUE

In an attempt to improve results and simplify lamellar surgery, the Barraquer-Krumeich-Swinger (BKS) technique was designed. The BKS technique was developed to avoid the adverse tissue effects of freezing the corneal cap as seen in the freeze keratomileusis technique. Specifically, the technique avoids the loss of fibroblasts during the freeze keratomileusis technique. It also takes advantage of viable epithelium, resulting in a more comfortable postoperative course for the patient.

The BKS technique begins much like the freeze keratomileusis technique in that a 300-micron corneal cap is harvested with the BKS microkeratome (Figure 2-7). The cap is then placed on one of several specific suction dyes for the refractive cut to be made with the microkeratome (Figure 2-8). The suction dye selected will depend on the planned diopter correction of myopia or hyperopia (Figure 2-9). The BKS system does not allow for correction of astigmatism. The most significant benefit the BKS system provides is the tissue is not heavily processed and the epithelium can be maintained in a healthy state; however, significant levels of irregular astigmatism are encountered with this technique.

EPIKERATOPHAKIA

The first Americanized version of a lamellar refractive surgery technique was epikeratophakia/epikeratoplasty as described by Kaufman and Werblin.[28-30] In essence, epikeratoplasty was designed to take the difficult task of using the cryolathe away from the surgeon and providing him or

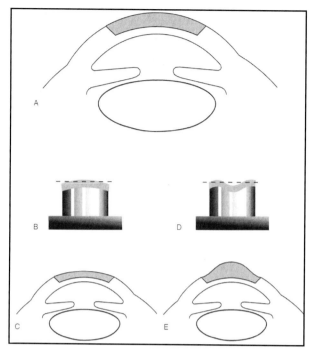

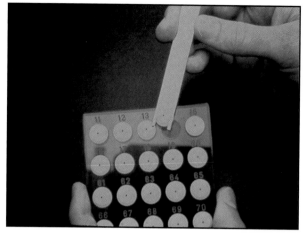

Figure 2-9. Barraquer-Krumeich-Swinger suction dyes.

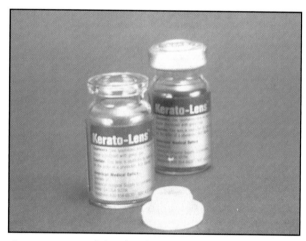

Figure 2-10. Lyophilized epikeratophakia lenticle in a transport bottle labeled with refractive power.

Figure 2-8. Barraquer-Krumeich-Swinger keratomileusis technique. (A) 300-micron cap created with a microkeratome. (B) Cap placed epithelial-side down on suction dye. Stroma removed from the central aspect of the posterior aspect of the cap with a manual microkeratome. (C) Cap reposited with anti-torque sutures. Central cornea flattened to treat myopia. (D) Cap placed epithelial-side down on suction dye. Tissue removed from paracentral stroma of the posterior cap with a manual microkeratome. (E) Cap reposited. Corneal curvature steepened for treatment of hyperopia.

her with a high-quality pre-processed refractive lenticle. This was done by obtaining donor corneal lenticles from a centralized source, freezing and cryolathing specific corrective powers, lyophilizing the lenticle in a sterile bottle (Figure 2-10), and shipping it to the surgeon on demand. Upon its arrival, the surgeon would reconstitute the lenticle with balanced salt solution and suture it onto the eye after host bed preparation (Figure 2-11).

Epikeratoplasty was initially developed for several indications, including the treatment of pediatric and adult aphakia, myopia, hyperopia, keratoconus, keratoglobus, and astigmatism. In reality, what seemed to be a modernization of lamellar surgery was not a viable alternative since surgical results varied, their was poor profitability for the lenticle manufacturers, and better alternative therapies such as IOLs and laser refractive techniques came of age. Additionally, major drawbacks of epikeratoplasty were the many complications that occurred with re-epithelialization of the donor lenticle (delayed healing, interface epithelial ingrowth, and lenticle melting or necrosis).

AUTOMATED LAMELLAR KERATOMILEUSIS IN SITU

The next major advance in the field of lamellar refractive surgery came at the hands of a Colombian surgeon, Dr. Luis Antonio Ruiz, who was Barraquer's protégé. While working in Bogota, Ruiz developed a microkeratome with gears that advanced it across a track in conjunction with an adjustable height suction ring—this defined the technique that is now known as automated lamellar keratoplasty (ALK) (Figure 2-12). The advancement of the motorized microkeratome allowed for a constant passage velocity, which resulted in the resection of a lamellar tissue disc of even thickness and a smoother corneal stromal bed. This substantial instrumentation breakthrough made lamellar corneal surgery more appealing to a larger number of surgeons who had found the manual microkeratome difficult to use.

Certain shortcomings and side effects of surface ablation with excimer laser PRK and predictability shortcom-

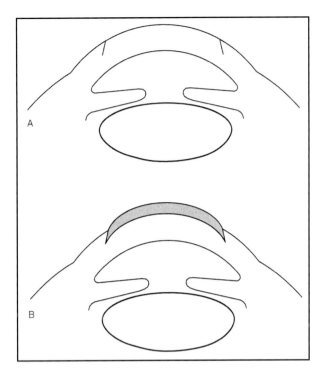

Figure 2-11. Epikeratophakia. (A) Preparing the recipient bed by removing the epithelium and creating a 360° circumferential flange after epithelial removal. (B) A pre-fabricated onlay lenticle is positioned under the flange edge and sutured in place. Depending on the lenticle power, myopic, hyperopic, or aphakic refractive errors can be treated.

ings of ALK gave rise to LASIK—the next evolutionary phase of lamellar refractive surgery.[31-33] Several reports revealed relatively poor predictability, central haze, and regression with PRK for moderate myopia (-6 to -10 diopters [D]) and even more so for high myopia (> -10 D).[6-14,34-50] In addition, relatively wide predictability ranges for myopic ALK prompted researchers to substitute lasers for the keratome in the refractive correction step of the myopic ALK procedure.[31-33,51] It was postulated that the submicron ablation precision of the excimer laser would allow for a much more predictable refractive result that would not depend as heavily upon individual patient healing responses as noted in PRK.[6-19]

Clinically, LASIK offers many attributes that are appreciated by patients and practitioners alike. These include:

- minimal postoperative discomfort;
- early recovery of visual function;
- immediate return to preoperative lifestyle;
- lack of topical steroid usage;
- lack of concern for such healing phenomena as haze formation;
- short postoperative antibiotic regimen;
- less intensive follow-up than PRK; and most importantly,
- increased range of efficacy over PRK for myopia, hyperopia, and astigmatism.

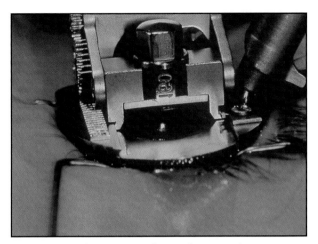

Figure 2-12. The automated microkeratome has a spacer plate set for the desired depth of resection and is engaged in the track for the first pass over the cornea.

RESULTS OF MANUAL MYOPIC KERATOMILEUSIS IN SITU

Despite a relatively long history of lamellar corneal refractive surgery, little published data exists for myopic keratomileusis in-situ. From the available reports that do exist, refractive results appear to be improving. In 1991, Bas and Nano reported on the first large series of myopic keratomileusis in situ and experienced the unpredictable nature of the technique as previously reported by Barraquer 20 years earlier.[52] Arenas-Archila, et al reported that keratomileusis in situ with manual keratomes was not safe, precise, or predictable.[53]

ALK SURGICAL TECHNIQUE

ALK is performed in an outpatient setting under topical anesthesia. As with all refractive surgery, extensive patient education and counseling is required. The patient must have an adequate knowledge of the procedure and realistic expectations. Oral sedation may be used but is not mandatory.

Prior to preparing and draping the patient in a sterile fashion, the conjunctival cul-de-sacs are irrigated to remove debris and eyelid glandular secretions. During the draping, it is important to create a clear path for microkeratome passage. The patient is instructed to look at the microscope light, and an inked marker is used to delineate the optical center, a pararadial line for orientation of the flap, and a 9-mm optical zone circle to center the circular suction ring (Figure 2-13a and 2-13b). A spacer device, or depth plate, is placed in the microkeratome to determine the thickness of the cut. The first keratectomy in the ALK technique typically utilizes a 160-micron depth plate.

An adjustable suction ring is placed on the eye and engaged. The suction ring fixates the globe, provides a geared path for the microkeratome, and raises the intraocu-

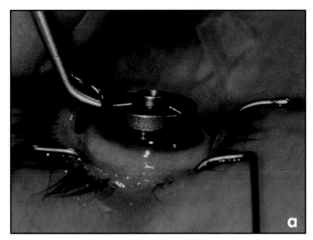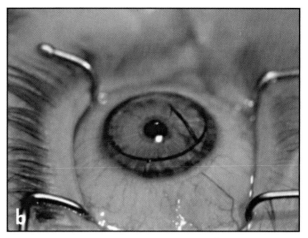

Figure 2-13a and 2-13b. A Ruiz marker is impregnated with ink and used to make a pararadial mark for orientation of the flap and the 9-mm optical zone for proper placement of the suction ring.

lar pressure to present adequate corneal tissue so that a smooth keratectomy of even thickness may be obtained. A stopper device is often used to insure the creation of a hinge in the corneal flap. Just prior to passage of the microkeratome, the intraocular pressure is checked with a hand-held Barraquer tonometer to make certain it is greater than 65 mm Hg. After the first cut, which has a planned diameter of 7.5 to 8 mm, the suction ring is removed.

The adjustable suction ring is then reset to resect a 4.2 mm diameter piece of stromal tissue. A second depth plate is placed corresponding to the planned myopic correction. The suction ring is then replaced and a second cut is made after checking the diameter and intraocular pressure. The flap is then replaced and positioned, usually without sutures. The patient's eye is protected with a clear plastic orbital shield, and the patient is discharged on topical antibiotics. The eye is examined the following day.

> The treatment of hyperopia with ALK is an ectasia procedure.

RESULTS OF ALK

Between 1995 and 1996 several groups reported their ALK results (Table 2-1).[25,54-56] In general, the results showed a moderate degree of accuracy with standard deviation for the procedure between 1 and 2 D. Irregular astigmatism was a significant problem with ALK, and epithelial ingrowth into the keratectomy interface was also noted. Mastering the technical nuances of the procedure created a significant learning curve for the novice lamellar corneal surgeon.

AUTOMATED LAMELLAR KERATOPLASTY FOR HYPEROPIA (ALK-H) SURGICAL TECHNIQUE

The treatment of hyperopia with ALK is an ectasia procedure and may be used to treat up to 6.5 D of intended correction.

This technique with the automated microkeratome was pioneered by Ruiz. Interestingly, in 1949 Barraquer published a preliminary report in four different languages that described an increased central corneal curvature using the controlled ectasia concept.[1] A thick flap is cut to allow the basal stromal bed of the cornea to bow forward and increase the central corneal curvature (Figure 2-14). Typically, this single cut must be at least 60% to 70% of the central corneal thickness. The effect is graded by altering the diameter of the keratectomy. The complications that can occur with this technique are the same as with myopic ALK (centration, epithelium in the interface, and displaced caps, etc).

Hyperopic ALK has also been used in the treatment of consecutive hyperopia after RK. This should be approached with considerable caution. Because an ectasia operation is being used over an existing ectasia operation (eg, incisional keratotomy), a keratoconus-like condition may result.

RESULTS OF ALK-H

Between 1995 and 1996 at least three groups of authors reported results of the ALK for hyperopia technique (Table 2-2).[57-59] Accuracy of approximately ±1 D was reported. In one study,[58] applanation lens diameter and resection depth accounted for 54% of the variability in outcome.

TABLE 2-1.
OUTCOMES OF AUTOMATED KERATOMILEUSIS IN SITU FOR MYOPIA

Reference	Ref #	No of eyes	No of mos follow-up	Preop sphere mean, SD, range	Postop sphere mean, SD, range	% VASC 20/40 (6/12) or better	% ± 1 D from target	% ± .5 D from target	% of 2 or more lines lost BCVA	% of 2 or more lines gained BCVA
ALK study group	25	100	12	-8.89±2.34 (-4 to -16.25)	-.52±2.01 (-3.13 to +10)	75	53	37	2	7
Lyle & Jin 1	54	29	12-19	-6.75±2.45 (-2.5 to -11.25)	-.46±1.71 (-4.25 to +4)	86	72			
2		99	12-19	-7.65±1.87 (-1.75 to -3.75)	-.37±.94 (-3.63 to +2.13)			78		
3		8	12-19	-2.87±.67 (-1.75 to -3.75)	-.58±-.65 (-2 to +1)		63			
Manche, et al	55	136	1-6	-8.3±2.5 (-4.5 to -20.5)		49		25		
Price, et al	56	152	6	-9.3±3.1		75			6	11

VASC = uncorrected visual acuity; BCVA = best-corrected visual acuity; SD = standard deviation; Lyle & Jin 1 = ALK only; Lyle & Jin 2 = ALK with enhancement; Lyle & Jin 3 = ALK for undercorrected radial keratotomy.

TABLE 2-2.
OUTCOMES OF AUTOMATED LAMELLAR KERATOPLASTY FOR HYPEROPIA

Reference	Ref #	No of eyes	No of mos follow-up	Preop sphere mean, SD, range	Postop sphere mean, SD, range	% VASC 20/40 (6/12) or better	% VASC 20/20 (6/6) or better	% of 2 or more lines lost BCVA
Kezirian & Gremilion 1	57	45	1-9	+2.7±1 (1.37 to 5)	+.2±0.9 (-1.25 to +2.5)	76	29	
2		23	1-9	see legend	see legend			
3		17	>5					see legend
Ghiselli, et al	58	38	3	+3.8 (1.5 to 6)	see legend		41	
Manche, et al	59	27	6	+3.6±.9 (+1.75 to +5.25)	see legend			0

VASC = uncorrected visual acuity; BCVA = best-corrected visual acuity; SD= standard deviation. In group 2 of the Kezirian study, the goal was reduction but not elimination of hyperopia, and in group 3 the goal was monovision. Due to the intended goals of groups 2 and 3 the outcome measures of VASC and ± 1 D predictability are not appropriate criteria and the reader should refer to the text and original article. In the Manche study in eyes in which emmetropia was the goal, 13/15 eyes were 20/40 (6/12) or better uncorrected and 8/15 eyes were 20/20 (6/6) or better uncorrected.

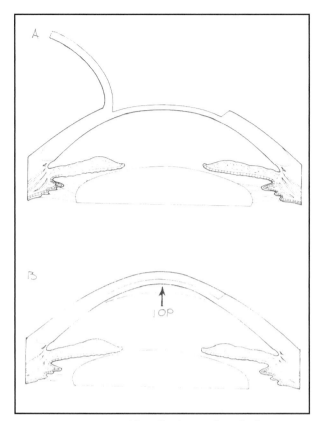

Figure 2-14. Automated lamellar keratoplasty for hyperopia. (A) Seventy percent central corneal thickness keratectomy performed. (B) The flap is reposited. Intracorneal pressure causes ectasia with central corneal steepening.

Nomogram inaccuracies were also reported as a significant problem.[59] Ghiselli, et al[58] reported a mean undercorrection of 1.26 ± .91 D at 3 months postoperatively, whereas Manche, et al[59] reported a mean undercorrection of 1.4 ± .8 D 6 months postoperatively.

PATIENT SELECTION FOR LASIK

The minimum age for LASIK, as for refractive surgery in general, is typically 18 years so that proper informed consent can be given by the patient. More important than age criteria, however, is the refractive stability of the patient. All patients should be selected for LASIK on the basis of how they would do compared with other refractive surgical procedures, such as RK, PRK, intracorneal ring segments, clear lens extraction, or phakic IOL placement. Lastly, thorough patient education and evaluation of the patient's postoperative expectations must be completed along with the informed consent.

LASIK can be performed to correct from .5 to 15 D of myopia, .5 to 6 D of hyperopia, and up to 8 D of astigmatism. These ranges are not absolute, since many surgeons have successfully treated patients beyond these ranges. The above dioptric ranges have been chosen based on prospec-

tive and retrospective evaluations of the predictability (percentage of eyes within a given postoperative target), efficacy (percentage of eyes achieving a certain level of uncorrected visual acuity), safety (percentage of eyes with postoperative loss of best-corrected vision), stability (evaluation of stability of refraction during a certain postoperative interval), and quality of vision issues (incidence of adverse visual phenomena such as halos, glare, or problems with night driving).

PREOPERATIVE EVALUATION FOR LASIK

Prospective LASIK candidates should undergo a complete ocular examination, including visual acuity testing, refraction, pachymetry, computerized videokeratography, slit lamp examination, retinal evaluation, eye dominance testing, and evaluation of monovision when appropriate. Patients who have keratoconus, active corneal or ocular disease, or who are pregnant or lactating should not undergo LASIK.

A history of recurrent erosion syndrome is considered a relative contraindication since an epithelial defect can occur during the keratectomy and lead to poor flap adhesion with subsequent epithelial ingrowth and flap melting.

To ensure success with LASIK, several preoperative measurements are crucial. The refraction of the eye should be compulsively obtained. Manifest refraction with the use of the duochrome test and fogging techniques, as well as cycloplegic refraction, can be utilized. Comparison of the refraction with prior spectacle corrections should be done to assess the stability of refraction for the given eye. Contact lenses should be discontinued to allow the corneal shape to stabilize. Soft lenses should be removed at least 3 days (2 weeks is often preferable) prior to examination, and hard lenses should be removed at least 3 weeks prior. With rigid contact lens wearers, at least two examinations 3 days apart should be obtained. To validate stability, no less than a .25 D difference in refraction should be noted.

Astigmatism should be evaluated with refraction, keratometry, and videokeratography. The axis of the astigmatism noted on refraction should correlate with that found on keratometry and videokeratography. If it does not, lenticular astigmatism should be considered and not treated since corneal ablation will create a crossed cylinder in the eye (induced corneal cylinder in one meridian to neutralize congenital lenticular cylinder in the opposite meridian).

Clinical experience has shown that a 160 μm thick flap affords sufficient safety by minimizing induced irregular astigmatism. A thin stromal bed (less than 200 microns) is postulated to have a greater likelihood of central ectasia with long-term unstable refractive status.

Central corneal thickness is evaluated with ultrasonic pachymetry to assess safe limits of corneal stromal removal with the laser ablation. For each LASIK procedure, three central corneal measurements must be considered:
- the flap thickness,
- the depth of the ablation,
- the residual thickness of the stromal bed after the ablation.

A thin flap is more likely to lead to associated irregular astigmatism and lost lines of best-corrected vision. Clinical experience has shown that a 160 µm thick flap affords sufficient safety by minimizing induced irregular astigmatism. A thin stromal bed (less than 200 microns) is postulated to have a greater likelihood of central ectasia with long-term unstable refractive status.

The recommended maximal amount of tissue removal for a given eye is calculated by subtracting the cap thickness and the suggested residual stromal bed thickness from the central pachymetry reading. For example, if the central corneal reading preoperatively is 560 microns and a 160 micron flap is created, the preablation stromal bed measures 400 microns, of which 200 microns can be ablated. With 200 microns of tissue removal, one can expect 14 D of myopia reduction based on a 6-mm maximal single ablation zone and assuming 14 microns of tissue removal per diopter. The Munnerlyn formula (ablation depth = optical zone^2 x diopters/3) can also be used to predict the amount of stroma removed for a given treatment. If the preoperative central corneal thickness is thinner and the ablation still leaves a 200 micron-thick stromal bed, less refractive error should increase the chance of long-term corneal stability.

The preoperative evaluation of the patient may impact several parameters of the planned ablation. As mentioned previously, 12 to 15 D of myopic correction can be obtained with a single 6 mm ablation zone. Multizone ablations can correct larger amounts of refractive error since less tissue is removed than single zone ablations, but the overall optical zone will be smaller and night vision can be compromised if the scotopic pupil is significantly larger (1 mm or more) than the optical zone of the ablation. With wide area ablation lasers that use an elliptical pattern for astigmatic ablations, there is greater potential for glare since the short axis of the ellipse is even smaller than the standard 6 mm spherical ablation zone. The planned astigmatic ablation should take into consideration the axis, magnitude, and impact of cylinder correction on the spherical component.

Many clinicians feel that a small amount (.5 D) of with-the-rule astigmatism affords better range and depth of vision than spherical or against-the-rule refractive error. This being said, with-the-rule astigmatism (steepest at 90°) should be left slightly undercorrected and against-the-rule (steepest at 180°) slightly overcorrected. Most lasers tend to induce a given amount of hyperopic shift for each diopter of cylinder ablated (typically .2 D of spherical hyperopic shift per diopter of cylinder treated), therefore, this must be taken into consideration when planning the spherical component of the treatment.

As with PRK, the LASIK surgeon must formulate his or her own nomogram. Lasers come with algorithms for treating a specific refractive error. Clinical experience has shown that surgical technique, room conditions (humidity, temperature, air particulate matter), and laser components (quality of optics, gas mixture) directly impact the refractive result. All of the aforementioned factors are laser algorithm independent, but the individual surgeon's nomogram will address these variables.

LASIK SURGICAL TECHNIQUE

At least two different techniques have been utilized in laser myopic keratomileusis. In LASIK, the operation proceeds as in ALK, but once the flap is made, the laser is used to ablate tissue from the bed for the planned correction; both sphere and cylinder depend on the capabilities of the laser (Figures 2-15 through 2-19). Alternatively, the Buratto technique, in which a thick disc of tissue from 300 to 350 microns is completely removed from the eye, can be used. This is placed beneath the laser, stroma side up, and ablated with the excimer laser (Figure 2-20). The disc of tissue, now a lens, is placed on the eye.[28] The Buratto technique is analogous to freeze MKM. The difference is that the excimer laser is substituted for the cryolathe in the refractive step of the procedure. LASIK has become the prevalent technique since it is significantly easier for the surgeon to deal with a sutureless hinged flap than the more cumbersome task of correctly orienting a free cap onto the stromal bed.

Along with the incredible precision of tissue removal, the other distinguishing feature of LASIK in comparison to previous forms of lamellar corneal refractive surgery is its effective treatment of astigmatism. Astigmatism is corrected by differential removal of tissue in the frontal plane of the cornea in one of the two major meridians. Actual tissue removal can occur by flattening the steep axis or steepening the flat axis. Flattening the steep axis (minus cylinder format) can be completed by large area ablation lasers via closing blades (see Figure 2-17), masking systems, or flying spot lasers by passing the spot parallel to the minus cylinder axis or flat axis on keratometry (see Figure 2-18). Steepening the flat axis (plus cylinder format) is probably best treated with scanning spot lasers by removing tissue paracentrally parallel to the minus cylinder axis or flatter axis on keratometry (see Figure 2-19).

One might ask when to treat cylinder in the minus versus plus cylinder format. Clinically, myopic astigmatism is treated effectively with the minus cylinder format since the beam passes over the center of the cornea, flattening not only the steep meridian but also some of the myopia. When treating hyperopic astigmatism in the plus cylinder format, less tissue is removed; thus, steepening the flat meridian has become the preferred technique.

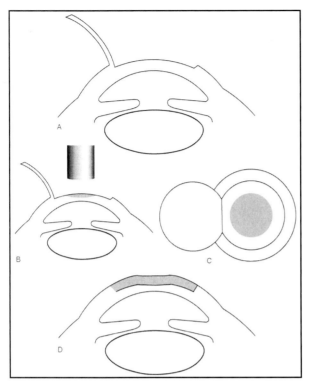

Figure 2-15. Laser in situ keratomileusis for myopia. (A) Creation of the flap. (B) Laser ablation of the stromal bed. Tissue removal (shaded). (C) Top view: shaded area represents the zone of tissue removal. (D) Flap replaced: central cornea flattened.

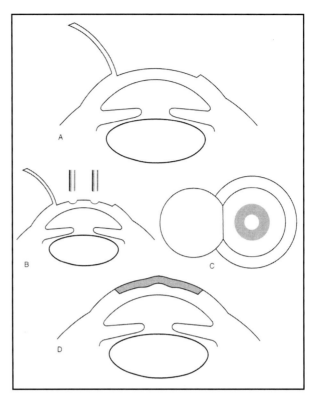

Figure 2-16. Laser in situ keratomileusis for hyperopia. (A) Creation of the flap. (B) Laser ablation of the stromal bed. Paracentral tissue removal (shaded). (C) Top view: shaded area represents the zone of tissue removal. (D) Flap replaced: central cornea steepened.

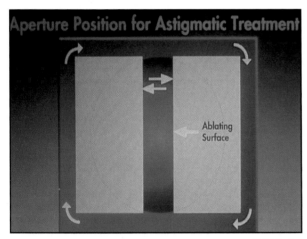

Figure 2-17. VISX Star astigmatic correction. Parallel blades allow preferential ablation parallel to the minus cylinder axis or the flat corneal meridian. This, in effect, flattens the steep corneal axis.

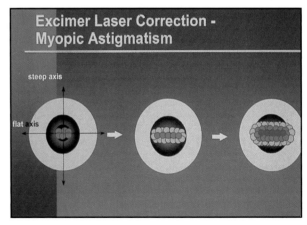

Figure 2-18. Schematic of minus cylinder ablation with a scanning spot laser to flatten the steep corneal meridian.

INSTRUMENT SET-UP

The surgical success of LASIK requires proper cleaning, assembly, and testing of the microkeratome, as well as calibration and set-up of the laser. Each member of the surgical team should be responsible for every aspect of the procedure by doing multiple checks along the way. Appropriate humidity, temperature, and air purification should be present in the laser room at all times. The laser should be turned on and calibrated per the manufacturer's recommendations. Importantly, the laser cutting rate or fluence and the beam quality (homogeneity) should meet acceptable operating standards.

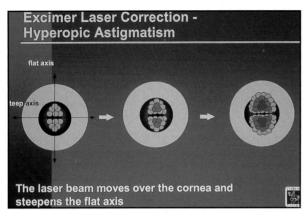

Figure 2-19. Schematic of plus cylinder ablation with a scanning spot laser to steepen the flat axis by removing tissue paracentrally parallel to the minus cylinder axis or the flat axis on keratometry.

PATIENT OPERATIVE PREPARATION

In most cases, oral sedation with 5 to 10 mg of diazepam approximately 45 minutes prior to the procedure is advisable. The patient should be relaxed, but not overly sedated, for the procedure since patient cooperation is, in part, necessary for proper fixation. Standard surgical skin preparation of the eyelids with an iodine-based solution is done before entering the laser suite. An eyewash solution is then irrigated into the conjunctival fornices to remove any meibomian secretions or tear film debris. The patient is positioned in supine position under the laser with the frontal surface of the cornea perpendicular to the laser beam aperture. One to two drops of a mild topical anesthetic such as proparacaine is instilled. Preferably the anesthetic should be preservative-free to help preserve the integrity of the corneal epithelium. The eye lashes are dried with a gauze sponge and a fenestrated drape is placed to keep the eye lashes and redundant peri-ocular tissues out of the surgical field. An eyelid speculum that affords maximal corneal exposure is then placed. No preoperative miotic is used.

PERFORMING THE KERATECTOMY

After the lid speculum is placed, the corneal epithelium should be marked with any commercially available lamellar surgery marker. Markers are useful for proper positioning of a free cap. The LASIK pneumatic suction ring is then placed onto the eye. The LASIK ring provides three useful functions: globe fixation, elevation of intraocular pressure to create an even thickness keratectomy, and a geared track for advancement of the geared microkeratome head. After the vacuum to the pneumatic suction ring has been activated and prior to the passage of the microkeratome, the surgeon must verify that the intraocular pressure is sufficient (greater than 65 mm Hg). This is best achieved with the Barraquer tonometer, which consists of a conical lens with

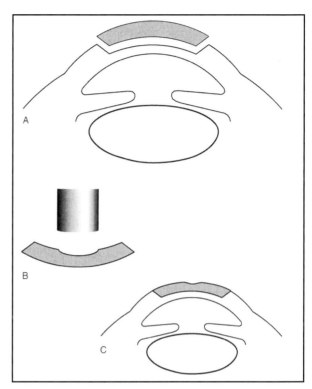

Figure 2-20. Buratto-style laser keratomileusis. (A) A thick (300 micron) free cap is created. (B) The cap is inverted and the laser is used to remove the central cap stroma (shaded area). (C) Reposit the cap in the keratectomy bed. The central cornea is flattened to treat myopia.

a flat undersurface that is marked with a circle and a convex upper surface that acts as a magnifying lens. Some surgeons also find a digital pneumotonometer useful for this step of the procedure.

The lens is held directly over the relatively dry corneal surface, and if the applanated area is smaller than the circle, the intraocular pressure is higher than 65 mm Hg. If the applanated area is larger, the pressure is too low and passage of the microkeratome could result in a thin, irregular keratectomy that is smaller than the desired diameter. Once adequately high intraocular pressure is obtained, the corneal surface is irrigated with balanced salt solution (BSS) to minimize epithelium disruption as the microkeratome is passed. The microkeratome is loaded into the dove-tailed groove on the suction ring and advanced by activation of the surgeon-controlled foot pedal. It is advanced to the stopper mechanism and then reversed. The vacuum is discontinued and the LASIK suction ring is removed.

THE LASER ABLATION

Prior to lifting the flap and beginning the ablation, the surgeon and staff should confirm proper laser settings and position the patient's head so the corneal surface is perpendicular to the ablation beam. The flap is then lifted and folded out of the ablation field. The ablation is centered over the entrance pupil. As the ablation proceeds, the centration should be cautiously monitored. If significant movement occurs, the surgeon should stop the ablation, reorient the patient, and proceed when properly aligned. During the ablation, fluid can accumulate on the corneal surface and should be wiped dry with a single pass of a non-fragmenting cellulose sponge or blunt spatula. As the ablation proceeds to the treatment zones with the largest diameters, the corneal hinge should be covered with a blunt instrument, if necessary, to prevent ablation of the back surface of the corneal flap. If concurrent astigmatism is to be treated, the appropriate axis of treatment should be assured by marking a reference point on the patient's limbus prior to initiating the treatment session. If significant cyclotorsion occurs when placing the patient in the supine position, adjustment should be made to the axis programmed into the laser.

REPOSITIONING THE FLAP

When the ablation is complete, the backside of the flap and the stromal bed are irrigated with BSS using a syringe attached to a small-gauge cannula. The flap is then positioned back onto the stromal bed with a blunt-tipped instrument. The cannula is placed underneath the flap and irrigation is completed to clear any remaining debris from the interface. The flap is inspected to ensure proper position by making certain an equal gutter/keratectomy edge distance is present throughout the circumference. The interface is allowed to dry for several minutes. A striae test is completed by depressing the peripheral cornea with closed blunt-tipped forceps. When striae pass well into the flap, 360° appropriate apposition has been achieved. During the drying phase it is recommended to keep a micro-drop of BSS over the central corneal epithelium to maintain its integrity.

At this point, the case is completed by carefully removing the speculum and drape. The eye is re-examined to make certain the flap is in proper position. Immediately postoperatively, one drop each of antibiotic and nonsteroidal anti-inflammatory agent is instilled. A shield is placed over the orbit, but no pressure patch is applied.

POSTOPERATIVE MANAGEMENT

Typical postoperative care of a patient who underwent LASIK is relatively simple. Generally there is no pain, but there may be some foreign body sensation present immediately after surgery, which dissipates after several hours. On the first postoperative day, the uncorrected visual acuity should be 20/40 or better in the low and moderate myopia treatment ranges. Slit lamp examination should reveal a clear cornea with intact epithelium. Proper flap apposition should be checked and stromal edema or interface debris should be documented. The patient should be placed on top-

ical prophylactic antibiotics four times per day for the first week. Topical preservative-free lubricating drops are helpful in selected patients on an as-needed basis during the first several weeks after surgery. A short course of topical corticosteroids is typically prescribed. Systemic analgesics are rarely necessary with LASIK. The patient can resume regular daily activities after a normal 1-day postoperative examination but should be cautioned to avoid rubbing the cornea and participating in contact sports without wearing proper eye protection. Exposure to potentially contaminated moisture sources such as hot tubs, pools, and fresh water lakes should be avoided for at least 2 weeks. Full visual recovery can take several weeks or more and can be delayed if significant irregular astigmatism exists.

RESULTS OF EXCIMER LASER KERATOMILEUSIS FOR MYOPIA/ASTIGMATISM

Since 1995, several clinical studies of LASIK have been published or reported at major meetings and can be compared with other refractive surgery techniques (Table 2-3).[7,33,40,42,51,60-71] Accuracy appears to be greater in lower degrees of myopia. The Ruiz study[61] showed the greatest degree of precision: standard deviation was ± .3 D. However, in other series, large ranges of residual refractive error were reported with 6 to 10 D ranges not uncommon.[63,65,66] In most of these early clinical series using initial nomograms, as with PRK, refractive predictability declined as the degree of attempted correction increased.[60,62] Significant rates of complications similar to those seen with other forms of lamellar surgery were also noted by many authors.[33,51,60,63,64] One study[60] highlighted that PRK ablation algorithms may not be directly applicable to in situ techniques. The authors noted overcorrection across all levels of myopia treatment attempted, which appeared to be a predictable fixed percentage overcorrection that could be calculated when multiplied with the preoperative refractive error. The authors recommended adjusting for this discrepancy, which varies depending on brands and types of excimer lasers, as well as the individual units themselves and the environmental conditions under which they are operated.

BIOPTIC TECHNIQUE FOR THE TREATMENT OF THE HIGHLY MYOPIC PATIENT

As stated above, the limit to the amount of refractive error that can be treated with LASIK depends on the preoperative central corneal thickness, the ablation algorithm used, and the goal of leaving at least a 200-micron stromal bed after ablation. In myopia treatments on average, the

TABLE 2-3.
OUTCOMES FOR EXCIMER LASER IN SITU KERATOMILEUSIS

Reference 20/20	Ref #	No eyes follow-up	No mos mean, SD, range	Preop sph mean, SD, range	Preop cyl mean, SD, range	Postop sph mean, SD, range	Postop cyl (6/12) or better range	% VASC 20/40 or better (6/7.5) or better	% VASC 20/25 (6/6 or better)	% VASC
Ruiz, et al	61	130	12	3.61±2.95 (-.25 - -18.25)	1.15±1.31 (0 - 8)	-.22±.32 (+1.5 - -2.5)	.35±.4 (0 - 2)	93	85	67
Salah, et al	60	88	5.2	-8.24 (-2 - -20)		+.22 ±1.42		71		36
		40		(-2 to -6)						
		29		(-6 to -12)						
		19		(-12 to -20)						
Guell & Muller	62	43	6	-9.3±1.3 (-7 - -12)		-.8± .79				
				-14.8±1.87 (-12.3 - -18.5)		-1.8±1.29				
Knorz, et al	63	26	1-2	-13.3 (-6.5 - -25)		-1.8 (-8.8 - +2.5)				
		8	4-6	-13.5 (-6.5 - -25)	-2.6 (-7.5 - +2.5)					
		8	4-6	-13.2 (-7 - -25)	-2.6 (-5 - 0)					
		10	1-2	-13.1 (-8.5 - -21)	-2 (-8.8)					
Bas & Onnis	64	88	3	-10.75		-.38		50		
Gomes	65	4	3-12	-15.12 (-12.5to20)	-2.68 (-2.25 - -3)					
		3	4-12	-26.3 (-23 to -30)	-4.3 (-3 - -5)					
		26	1-12	-14.89 (-11 - -18.5)	-.25 (-4.75 - +4.75)					
		9	1-12	-24.5-1.4 (-20.5 - -29)	-1.4 (-3.5 - +3.5)					
Kremer & Dufek	67	31	6	-6.25 (-3.5 - -11.75)	.25to2.75 (-3.5 - +2)	-.5 (.25 - 3.5)	.64	81		
Fiander & Tayfour	66	124	3-11	-7.65 (3.75 - -27)	.88	.27 (-2.75 - +4)	1.24 (0 - 4)	81	50	
Perez-S.	68	143	3	-13.19±2.89 (-8 - 20)	(0 - 2)	.18±1.66		46		
El Danasoury	69	25	12	-4.39±1.74 (-2.25 - 7.25)		-.33±.33 (-1.25 - -.5)	.19±.25 (0 - .75)			76
El	69	62	12	-5.19±2.32 (-2 - -14)	1.19±0.62 (.5 - 3)	-.17±.48 (-1.5 - 1.5)	.32±.3 (0 - 1.25)			55
Pesando	70	46	3-9	-9.4±3.78 (-3.5 - -19.75)		-.75±1.07		85		
Marinho	71	34	6-12	(-10 to -22)	(-3 - 1.5)	-.81±1.71 (-4.75 - 2.25)				33

= total number of eyes; BCVA = best-corrected visual acuity; VASC= uncorrected visual acuity; sphere and cylinder in diopters; SD = standard deviation;* = spherical equivalent.

TABLE 2-3.

OUTCOMES FOR EXCIMER LASER IN SITU KERATOMILEUSIS (CONTINUED)

Reference	% ± -1 D from target	% ± .5 D from target	% 2 or more lines lost BCVA	% 2 or more lines gained BCVA	Laser/ keratome	Nomogram
Ruiz, et al	98	90	0	17.1	Chiron 116/ ACS	Ruiz
Salah, et al	73		3.6*		Summit Omni-med/ACS	PRK or MKM program or Salah excim
	93	63				
LASIK						1993 nomogram for all groups
	65					
	43					
Guell, et al					Chiron 116/ ACS	Personalized modified
Knorz, et al	50		10		Chiron 116/	Single zone 4-5 mm or
	38		13			Multizone 3-6 mm with pretreatment
	38		13			
	60		10			NR
Bas, et al	47				Summit Omni-med/ACS	
Gomes, et al					NR/freehand	4 & 4.5 mm ablations
					NR/freehand	4 & 4.5 mm ablations
					NR/freehand	4.2 & 5 mm ablations
					NR/freehand	4.2 & 5 mm ablations
Kremer, et al	74		0		Custom/ACS	Personalized
Fiander, et al	70	44	0		Summit Omni-med/ACS	PRK modified
Perez-S	60		1.4		VISX 20/20/ ACS	PRK, multizone
El Danasoury	96	68	0		Nidek EC5000/ ACS	Personalized
	91	75	0			
Pesando	78	28			Visx 20/20B/ ACS	
Marinho	67		9	26	Summit Omnimed/ ACS	

*PRK = photorefractive keratectomy; MKM = myopic keratomileusis; NR = not reported; * = 3.6% (three eyes: one with irregular astigmatism, two with myopic maculopathy); ACS = Automatic Corneal Shaper (Chiron Vision Corp, Irvine, Calif).*

error that can be treated with LASIK depends on the preoperative central corneal thickness, the ablation algorithm used, and the goal of leaving at least a 200-micron stromal bed after ablation. In myopia treatments on average, the maximal myopic spherical equivalent attempted with LASIK is -15 D. There are four options above this range: LASIK, clear lens extraction with IOL implant, phakic IOL implantation, and a combination of clear lens extraction with IOL or phakic IOL with LASIK. It is important to note that there are inherent risks with intraocular surgery that are not present with corneal refractive surgery.[72-84]

Alternatively, with highly myopic (greater than -15 D) patients, LASIK alone may not be the best option for every patient because an imbalance between the depth of the ablation and the diameter of the ablation zone comes into play. Ideally, at least 200 microns of stromal bed should be left after ablation. If more is removed, there may be a compromise in structural corneal strength with the potential for long-term central corneal ectasia. One can decrease the depth of the ablation to obtain the same refractive effect by decreasing the maximal size of the ablation zone or using multizone software. Either way, the functional optical zone will be reduced and the patient may have significant unwanted visual symptoms (glare and halos) in scotopic conditions. Instead of performing LASIK or corneal refractive surgery, clear lens extraction with IOL or phakic IOL placement can be considered. Neither technique can treat astigmatism so it would have to be left untreated or managed with another corneal surgical procedure.

With high phakic IOL powers come a compromise in the functional optical zone. The higher the power, the smaller the diameter of the functional optical zone with con-

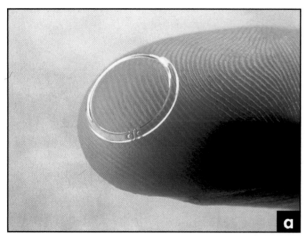
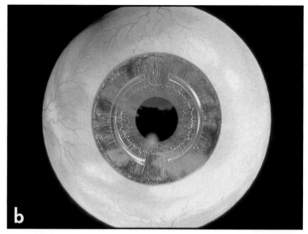

Figure 2-21a and 2-21b. Intracorneal polymethylmethacrylate ring technology (Keravision, Fremont, Calif) can be applied in a continuous ring fashion (a), or segments (b) to affect corneal refractive changes.

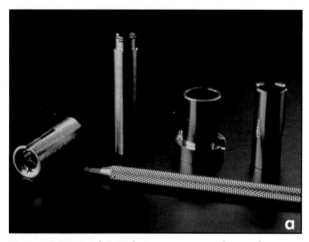
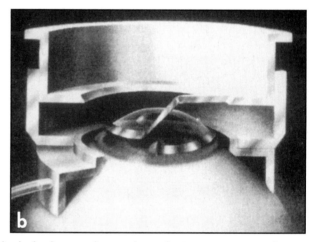

Figures 2-22a and 2-22 b. Instruments used to perform a two-thirds depth corneal stromal tunnel (a). Suction ring on the eye and channel being performed (b).

The limit to the amount of refractive error that can be treated with LASIK depends on the preoperative central corneal thickness, the ablation algorithm used, and the goal of leaving at least a 200-micron stromal bed after ablation.

can be placed with or without lens extraction to reduce spherical myopia, and LASIK can be used to refine the residual spherical refractive error and astigmatism. The bioptic technique (combining IOL and corneal refractive surgery) allows for maximal optical zones to be used with each technique to afford the best possible scotopic vision and also allow for effective treatment of astigmatism. Additional clinical work in the area will clarify the refractive efficacy and patient satisfaction with these techniques.

PERIPHERAL MASS ADDITION TECHNIQUES: INTRACORNEAL RING/SEGMENTS AND GEL INJECTION ADJUSTABLE KERATOPLASTY

INTRACORNEAL STROMAL RING/SEGMENT TECHNIQUE

Intracorneal ring (ICR) technique has been under study for the treatment of myopia since 1978. This technology stems from the innovative work of AE Reynolds, OD and his concept of "Method for Corneal Curvature Adjustment," which was patented in 1984. The collaboration of Reynolds with Joseph Z. Krezanoski, PhD and John C. Petricciani lead to the formation of the Keravision Corporation and subsequent development of this concept.

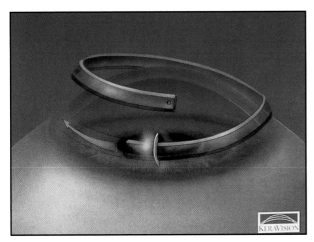

Figure 2-23. Intracorneal ring being fed into the corneal stromal channel.

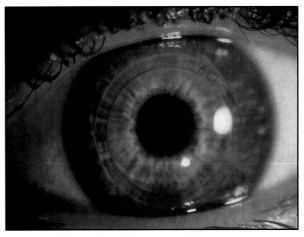

Figures 2-24a. Implanted intracorneal ring.

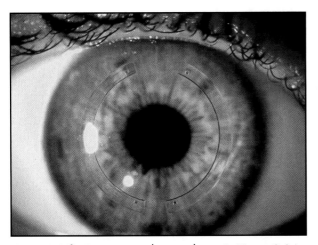

Figure 2-24b. Segments in the eye shown in Figure 2-24a. The central aspect of the ring/segments is the 7-mm optical zone.

ICR technique conceptually adds mass (polymethyl-methacrylate ring or segments) (Figure 2-21a and 2-21b) to the peripheral stroma to affect a central flattening of the cornea and a reduction of myopia. At the present time, it is felt ICR technology for myopia will be restricted to lower levels of myopia (less than 5 D), but current investigation into the treatment of astigmatism and hyperopia is under-way. The perceived advantages of ICR technique are that it is reversible by removing the inserted ring or segments, the central cornea is spared, and there is preservation of the congenital prolate corneal asphericity. ICR technique con-sists of making a channel at two-thirds of the corneal thick-ness at the 7-mm optical zone using special instruments (Figure 2-22a and 2-22b). The channel is initiated through a 2 mm incision and carried circumferentially for 360°. A ring or ring segment is then fed into the channel (Figure 2-23) to affect the final result (Figure 2-24a and 2-24b). The specif-ic ring selected depends on the degree of myopia. Five ring thicknesses ranging from .25 to .45 mm are available. The

entry incision can be closed with a single suture or left to heal without suturing. The technique takes about 15 minutes to perform. Phase III data from the United States Food and Drug Administration (FDA) clinical trial of the ICR for low myopia (-1 to -3.5 D) without astigmatism reported on 244 patients. Eighty-seven percent of the eyes achieved 20/25 or better uncorrected vision and 52% achieved 20/16 or better uncorrected vision. Patients with moderate myopia (-3.5 to –5.0 D) without astigmatism in the Phase II FDA trial achieved 20/40 or better and 20/25 or better unaided vision 98% and 83% of the time respectively. No eyes lost signif-icant levels on contrast sensitivity testing.

ICR technology holds promise as a reversible treatment of lower levels of refractive error, and it should be antici-pated that refractive results will only improve with time. To be a major player in the refractive surgery armamentarium, ICR technique must be able to correct associated astigma-tism and would only help its cause if it could also treat hyperopia and hyperopic astigmatism.

Gel injection adjustable keratoplasty (GIAK) began at Bascom Palmer Eye Institute in Miami, Fla. Gabriel Simon, working in the lab of Jean-Marie Parel in the late 1980s, developed the concept of GIAK. This technique is similar to the ICR technique and is anticipated to be used to correct -1 to - 4 D of myopia. The major difference is that the added mass is an injectable semi-solid. The technique can be titrat-ed by addition or subtraction of the injected material to achieve the desired refractive result over the course of the patient's lifetime. One-year data on non-sighted eyes out-side the United States have revealed no complications. Sighted eye trials outside the United States are currently underway and have shown encouraging results for up to 3 D of myopia (verbal communication, Douglas Koch, MD, December 1997). GIAK is slated to begin FDA trials with Koch as medical monitor in early 1999.

GIAK as a technique is still in its infancy and obstacles seen and unseen will have to be dealt with. At this point in time, the largest obstacle is for the surgeon to identify the exact volume to be injected. Intraoperative refractometry and keratometry may be of some help in determining the refractive endpoint.

FUTURE CONSIDERATIONS

The ultimate goal of refractive surgery might very well be to obtain vision that is quantitatively and qualitatively better than the clinician can obtain with spectacles or contact lenses and is adjustable and reversible. Ideally, as surgeons, the future may see us increasing corneal asphericity to induce a multifocal effect, thereby improving both near and distance unaided vision in the presbyopic population and depth perception in all age groups. However, it is imperative that the technique performed does not compromise scotopic visual function. Complete success is not defined by the patient having 20/20 vision in daylight but severely compromised visual function at night. No peer-reviewed article has been published that reports a technique with either short-term or longitudinal follow-up that can even remotely match the results of spectacles or contact lenses with regard to efficacy for any level of myopia with or without astigmatism.

LASIK is but a step in the continuum of the work initiated by Barraquer nearly 50 years ago. The reports to date are encouraging. Enthusiasm must be tempered by the fact that long-term results are not available. LASIK is still early in development, and there will be continued refinements in microkeratomes, laser delivery systems, software advances, and nomograms that will hopefully only improve the early results. Longer follow-up of current studies in progress and future controlled studies of LASIK, ICR technology, and GIAK will supply long-term data that will define these procedures' efficacy, predictability, safety, and stability, along with outcome reports on patient acceptance and satisfaction.

REFERENCES

1. Barraquer JI. Oueratoplastia refractiva. Estudios Inform Oftal Inst Barraquer. 1949;10:2-21.
2. Bores L. Lamellar refractive surgery. In: Bores L, ed. *Refractive Eye Surgery*. Boston, Mass: Blackwell Scientific Publications; 1993:324-91.
3. Barraquer JI. Keratomileusis. *International Surgery*. 1967;48:103-117.
4. Barraquer JI. Results of myopic keratomileusis. *Journal of Refractive Surgery*. 1987;3:98-101.
5. Barraquer JI. Method for cutting lamellar grafts in frozen corneas: New orientations for refractive surgery. *Arch Soc Am Ophthalmol*. 1958;1:237.
6. Campos M, Cuevas K, Garbus J, et al. Corneal wound healing after excimer laser ablation: effects of nitrogen gas blower. *Ophthalmology*. 1992;99:893-7.
7. Epstein D, Fagerholm P, Hamberg-Nystrom H, Tengroth B. Twenty-four-month follow-up of excimer laser photorefractive keratectomy for myopia. *Ophthalmology*. 1994;101:1558-64.
8. Epstein D, Tengroth B, Fagerholm P, Hamberg-Nystrom H. Excimer retreatment of regression after photorefractive keratectomy. *Am J Ophthalmol*. 1994;117:456-61.
9. Gartry DS, Kerr Muir MG, Marshall J. Excimer laser photorefractive keratectomy. Eighteen-month follow-up. *Ophthalmology*. 1991;99:1209-19.
10. Lohmann C, Gartry D, Kerr Muir M, et al. Corneal haze after excimer laser refractive surgery. Objective measurements and functional implications. *Eur J Ophthalmol*. 1991;1:173-80.
11. Lohmann CP, Fitzke F, O'Bart D, et al. Corneal light scattering and visual performance in myopic individuals with spectacles, contact lenses, or excimer laser photorefractive keratectomy. *Am J Ophthalmol*. 1993;115:444-53.
12. Marshall J, Trokel SL, Rothery S, et al. Long-term healing of the central cornea after photorefractive keratectomy using an excimer laser. *Ophthalmology*. 1988;95:1411-21.
13. Tuft SJ, Zabel RW, Marshall J. Corneal repair following keratectomy. *Invest Ophthalmol Vis Sci*. 1989;30:1769-77.
14. Del Pero RA, Gigstad JE, Roberts AD, et al. A refractive and histopathological study of excimer laser keratectomy in primates. *Am J Ophthalmol*. 1990;109:419-29.
15. Fagerholm P, Hamberg-Nystrom H, Tengroth B. Wound healing and myopic regression following photorefractive keratectomy. *Acta Ophthalmologica*. 1994;72:229-34.
16. Fitzsimmons TD, Fagerholm P, Tengroth B. Steroid treatment of myopic regression. Acute refractive and topographic changes in photorefractive keratectomy patients. *Cornea*. 1993;12:358-61.
17. Gartry DS, Kerr Muir MG, Lohmann CP, Marshall J. The effect of topical corticosteroids on refractive outcome and corneal haze after photorefractive keratectomy. *Arch Ophthalmol*. 1992;110:944-52.
18. O'Brart DPS, Lohmann CP, Klonos G, et al. The effects of topical corticosteroids and plasmin inhibitors on refractive outcome, haze, and visual performance after photorefractive keratectomy. *Ophthalmology*. 1994;101:1565-74.
19. Seiler T, Derse M, Pham T. Repeated excimer laser treatment after photorefractive keratectomy. *Arch Ophthalmol*. 1992;110:1230-3.
20. Maguire LJ, Klyce SD, Sawelson H, et al. Visual distortion after myopic keratomileusis: computer analysis of keratoscope photographs. *Ophthalmic Surg*. 1987;18:352-6.
21. Swinger CA, Barker BA. Prospective evaluation of myopic keratomileusis. *Ophthalmology*. 1984;91:785-92.
22. Nordan LT, Fallor MK. Myopic keratomileusis: 74 consecutive non-amblyopic case with 1 year of follow-up. *Journal of Refractive Surgery*. 1986;2:124-8.
23. Nordan LT. Keratomileusis. *Int Ophthalmol Clin*. 1991;31:7-12.
24. Barraquer C, Guitierrez A, Espinoza A. Myopic keratomileusis: short-term results. *J Refract Corn Surg*. 1989;5:307-13.
25. Slade SG, Doane JF, Dishler JG, et al. A prospective multicenter clinical trial to evaluate automated lamellar keratoplasty for the correction of myopia. Unpublished data.
26. Krwawicz T. Lamellar corneal stromectomy. *Am J Ophthalmol*. 1964;57:828-33.
27. Pureskin N. Weakening ocular refraction by means of partial stromectomy of cornea under experimental conditions. *Vestn Oftalmol*. 1967;80:19-24.
28. Kaufman HE. The correction of aphakia. *Am J Ophthalmol*. 1980;89:1-10.
29. Werblin TP, Kaufman HE, Friedlander MK, et al. A prospective study of the use of hyperopic epikeratophakia grafts for the correction of aphakia in adults. *Ophthalmology*. 1981;88,1137-40.
30. Werblin TP. Epikeratophakia: where did we fail? In: Elander R,

Rich LF, Robin JB, eds. *Principles and Practice of Refractive Surgery*. Philadelphia, Pa: WB Saunders & Co; 1997:391-403.

31. Peyman GA, Badaro RM, Khoobehi B. Corneal ablation in rabbits using an infrared (2.9 microns) erbium: YAG laser. *Ophthalmology*. 1989;96:1160-9.

32. Pallikaris IG, Papatzanaki ME, Stathi EZ, et al. Laser in situ keratomileusis. *Lasers Surg Med*. 1990;10:463-8.

33. Burrato L, Ferrari M, Genisi C. Myopic keratomileusis with the excimer laser: one-year follow-up. *J Refract Corneal Surg*. 1993;9:12-19.

34. Liu JC, McDonald MB, Varnell R, Andrade HA. Myopic excimer laser photorefractive keratectomy: an analysis of clinical correlations. *J Refract Corneal Surg*. 1990;6:321-8.

35. Seiler T, Kahle G, Kriegerowski M. Excimer Laser (193 nM) myopic keratomileusis in sighted and blind human eyes. *J Refract Corneal Surg*. 1990;6:165-73.

36. Seiler T, Wollensak J. Myopic photorefractive keratectomy with the excimer laser. One-year follow-up. *Ophthalmology*. 1991;98:1156-63.

37. Wilson SE. Excimer laser (193) myopic keratomileusis: differential stability in lower and higher myopes. *J Refract Corneal Surg*. 1990;6:383-5.

38. Gartry DS, Kerr Muir MG, Marshall J. Photorefractive keratectomy with an argon fluoride excimer laser: a clinical study. *J Refract Corneal Surg*. 1991;7:420-35.

39. Sher NA, Barak M, Daya S, et al. Excimer laser photorefractive keratectomy in high myopia. *Arch Ophthalmol*. 1992;110:935-43.

40. Sher NA, Hardten DR, Fundingsland B, et al. 193 nM excimer photorefractive keratectomy in high myopia. *Ophthalmology*. 1994;101:1575-82.

41. Heitzmann J, Binder PS, Kassar BS, Nordan LT. The correction of high myopia using the excimer laser. *Arch Ophthalmol*. 1993;111:1627-34.

42. Carson CA, Taylor HR for the Melbourne Excimer Laser and Research Group. Excimer laser photorefractive keratectomy in moderate and high myopia. *Arch Ophthalmol*. 1995;113:431-6.

43. Krueger RR, Talamo JH, McDonald MB, et al. Clinical analysis of excimer laser photorefractive keratectomy using a multiple zone technique for severe myopia. *Am J Ophthalmol*. 1995;119:263-74.

44. Brancato R, Tavola A, Carones F, et al. Excimer laser photorefractive keratectomy for myopia: results in 1165 eyes. *J Refract Corneal Surg*. 1993;9:95-104.

45. Kim JH, Hahn TW, Lee YC, Sah WJ. Clinical experience of two-step photorefractive keratectomy in 19 eyes with high myopia. *J Refract Corneal Surg*. 1993;9(suppl 2):S44-7.

46. Ehlers N, Hjortdal JO. Excimer laser refractive keratectomy for high myopia: 6-month follow-up of patients treated bilaterally. *Acta Ophthalmol*. 1992;70:578-86.

47. Serdarevic O, Vinciguerra P, Bottoni F, Zenoni S, DeMolfetta V. Excimer laser photorefractive keratectomy for high myopia. *Invest Ophthalmol Vis Sci*. 1992;33 (suppl4):763. ARVO abstracts.

48. Ditzen K, Anschuetz T, Shroeder E. Photorefractive keratectomy to treat low, medium and high myopia: a multicenter study. *J Cataract Refract Surg*. 1994;20 (suppl):234-8.

49. Seiler T, Holschbach A, Derse M, et al. Complications of myopic photorefractive keratectomy with the excimer laser. *Ophthalmology*. 1994;101:153-60.

50. Seiler T. Current evaluation of myopia correction with excimer laser. *Ophthalmologe*. 1995;92:379-84.

51. Brint SF, Ostrick DM, Fisher C, et al. Six-month results of the multicenter phase I study of excimer laser myopic keratomileusis. *J Cataract Refract Surg*. 1994;20;610-5.

52. Bas AM, Nano HD. In situ myopic keratomileusis: results in 30 eyes at 15 months. *J Refract Corneal Surg*. 1991;7:223-31.

53. Arenas-Archila E, Sanchez-Thorin JC, Naranjo-Uribe JP, Hernandez-Lozano A. Myopic keratomileusis in situ: a preliminary report. *J Cataract Refract Surg*. 1991;17:424-35.

54. Lyle WA, Jin GJC. Initial results of automated lamellar keratoplasty for correction of myopia: 1-year follow-up. *J Cataract Refract Surg*. 1996;22:31-43.

55. Manche EE, Elkins B, Maloney R. Keratomileusis in situ (ALK) for high myopia. International Society of Refractive Surgery Annual Meeting; October 27, 1995; Atlanta, Ga. Abstract.

56. Price FW, Whitson WE, Gonzales JS et al. Automated lamellar keratomileusis in situ for myopia. *J Refract Surg*. 1996;12:29-35.

57. Kezirian GM, Germillion CM. Automated lamellar keratoplasty for the correction of hyperopia. *J Cataract Refract Surg*. 1995;21:386-92.

58. Ghiselli G, Manche E, Maloney R. Factors that influence the outcome of hyperopic automated lamellar keratoplasty. International Society of Refractive Surgery Annual Meeting; October 27, 1995; Atlanta, Ga. Abstract.

59. Manche EE, Judge A, Maloney RK. Lamellar keratoplasty for hyperopia. *J Refract Surg*. 1996;12:42-9.

60. Salah T, Waring III GO, El Maghraby A, Moadel K, Grimm SB. Excimer laser in situ keratomileusis under a corneal flap for myopia of 2 to 20 diopters. *Am J Ophthalmol*. 1996;121:143-55.

61. Ruiz LA, Slade SG, Updegraff SA, Doane JF, Moreno ML, Murcia A. A single-center study to evaluate the efficacy, safety, and stability of laser in situ keratomileusis for low, moderate, and high myopia with and without astigmatism. Unpublished data.

62. Guell JL, Muller A. Laser in situ keratomileusis (LASIK) for myopia ranging from -7 to -18 diopters. *J Refract Surg*. 1996;12:222-8.

63. Knorz MC, Liermann A, Steiner H, Seiberth V, Lorger CV, Haubrich T. Laser in situ keratomileusis to correct myopia of -6 to -29 diopters. *Journal of Refractive Surgery*. 1996;12:575-84.

64. Bas AM, Onnis R. Excimer laser in situ keratomileusis for myopia. *Journal of Refractive Surgery*. 1995;11(suppl):S229-33.

65. Gomes M. Laser in situ keratomileusis for myopia using manual dissection. *Journal of Refractive Surgery*. 1995;11(suppl):S239-43.

66. Fiander DC, Tayfour F. Excimer laser in situ keratomileusis in 124 myopic eyes. *Journal of Refractive Surgery*. 1995;11(suppl):S234-238.

67. Kremer FB, Dufek M. Excimer laser in situ keratomileusis. *Journal of Refractive Surgery*. 1995;11(suppl):S244-7.

68. Perez-Santonja JJ, Bellot J, Claramonte P, Ismail MM, Alio J. Laser in situ keratomileusis to correct high myopia. *J Cataract Refract Surg*. 1997;23:372-85.

69. El Danasoury MA, Waring GO, El Maghraby A, Mehrez K. Excimer laser in situ keratomileusis to correct compound myopic astigmatism. *Journal of Refractive Surgery*. 1997;13:511-20.

70. Pesando PM, Ghiringhello MP, Tagliavacche P. Excimer laser in situ keratomileusis for myopia. *Journal of Refractive Surgery*. 1997;13:521-7.

71. Marinho A, Pinto MC, Pinto R, Vaz F, Neves MC. LASIK for high myopia: 1-year experience. *Ophthalmic Surgery and Lasers*. 1997; 27:S517-20.

72. Javitt JC. Clear lens extraction for high myopia. *Arch Ophthalmol*. 1994;112:321-3.

73. Barraquer C, Cavelier C, Mejia LF. Incidence of retinal detachment following clear lens extraction in myopic patients. *Arch Ophthalmol*. 1994;112:36-9.

74. Coonan P, Fung WE, Webster RG Jr, et al. The incidence of retinal detachment following extracapsular cataract extraction: a 10-year study. *Ophthalmology*. 1985;92:1096-1101.

75. Lindstrom RL, Lindquist TD, Huldin J, Rubenstein JB. Retinal detachment in axial myopia following extracapsular cataract surgery. *Transactions of the New Orleans Academy of Ophthalmology*. 1988;36:253-68.

76. Goldberg MF. Clear lens extraction for axial myopia. *Ophthalmology*. 1987;94:571-82.

77. Rodriquez A, Gutierrez E, Alvira G. Complications of clear lens extraction in axial myopia. *Arch Ophthalmol*. 1987;105:1522-3.

78. Jaffe N, Clayman H, Jaffe M. Retinal detachments in myopic eyes after intracapsular and extracapsular cataract extraction. *Am J Ophthalmol*. 1984;97:48-52.

79. McPherson A, O'Malley R, Bravo J. Retinal detachment following late posterior capsulotomy. *Am J Ophthalmol*. 1983;95:593-7.

80. Alio JL, Ruiz-Moreno JM, Artola A. Retinal detachment as a potential hazard in surgical correction of severe myopia with phakic anterior chamber lenses. *Am J Ophthalmol*. 1993;115:145-8.

81. Javitt JC, Street DA, Steinberg EP, Cataract Patient Outcomes Research Team. National outcomes of cataract extraction: retinal detachment and endophthalmitis following outpatient cataract extraction. *Ophthalmology*. 1994;101:100-5.

82. Steinert RF, Puliafito CA, Kumar SR, et al. Cystoid macular edema, retinal detachment, and glaucoma after nd:YAG laser posterior capsulotomy. *Am J Ophthalmol*. 1991;112:373-380.

83. Javitt JC, Tielsch JM, Canner JK, et al. National outcomes of cataract extraction: increased risk of retinal complications associated with nd:YAG laser capsulotomy. *Ophthalmology*. 1992;99:1487-98.

84. Jaffe NS, Clayman HM, Jaffe MS. Retinal detachment in myopic eyes after intracapsular and extracapsular cataract extraction: a 10-year study. *Am J Ophthalmol*. 1984;97:48-52.

Fundamental Concepts and Principles of the Excimer Laser and LASIK

Jeffery J. Machat, MD

INTRODUCTION

More than 100 years of lamellar surgery and 50 years of lamellar refractive surgery has provided the background for the development of laser in situ keratomileusis (LASIK), which combines the precision of photorefractive keratectomy (PRK) with the superior healing characteristics of lamellar surgery. The primary limitation of PRK is the delayed healing response, which can require topical corticosteroids to modulate and may result in corneal haze. With LASIK, by performing the excimer ablation within the relatively inert stromal bed, the visual rehabilitation is dramatically faster, there is less postoperative pain, less susceptibility to infection, and virtually no risk of stromal haze formation. However, the creation of the corneal flap during LASIK can be associated with a new set of complications that can potentially be more serious.

While there is no procedure that is ideal for every patient, LASIK represents the most refined and all-encompassing procedure at present. Requiring greater technical skill than PRK, LASIK represents a more complex procedure for altering the refractive properties of the cornea while utilizing the excimer laser. LASIK is still evolving both in the technology, technique, and peri-operative patient management. Even over the last 2 years, major advancements have been made in the refinement of LASIK.

> While there is no procedure that is ideal for every patient, LASIK represents the most refined and all-encompassing procedure at present.

The long history of lamellar surgery has provided an abundance of fundamental principles upon which the lamellar aspects of LASIK should evolve. The ablation parameters are different for LASIK because of the unique factors related to the intrastromal ablation, including altered mid-stromal wound healing and greater mid-stromal hydration. The greater proximity to the endothelium must be considered, as endothelial changes and corneal instability may be caused by excessive ablations. The greatest areas of evolution for LASIK have been in the microkeratome design, the improvement of the excimer laser hardware, and laser software design.

ROLE OF LASIK IN REFRACTIVE SURGERY

Refractive surgery can be categorized by the method of action:

- Bending of tissue = radial keratotomy (RK), astigmatic keratotomy (AK), intracorneal rings, and Holmium: YAG laser thermokeratoplasty (LTK)
- Addition of tissue = keratophakia, intracorneal inlays, intracorneal rings, intraocular lens
- Subtraction of tissue = LASIK, PRK, phototherapeutic keratectomy (PTK), automated lamellar keratoplasty (ALK)

INCISIONAL SURGERY

Incisional techniques include both AK and RK. In the

1890s, Leendert Jan Lans performed the first systematic study of incisional surgery for the management of astigmatism. In 1943, Tutomu Sato performed the first human keratotomy, utilizing an anteroposterior keratotomy approach, as the importance of the endothelium was not adequately appreciated at that time.[1] Unfortunately, this resulted in corneal decompensation in the majority of cases.[2] In 1960, Fyodorov[3-4] pioneered modern RK with an anterior keratotomy approach, which was introduced to the United States in 1978 by Leo Bores.[5]

There have been a number of significant advances in improving RK both in technology and technique. The introduction of diamond and biphasic blades, ultrasonic pachymetry, microscopes, nomogram developments, and technique alterations in the number and length of incisions have enhanced RK with respect to both safety and efficacy. Publication of the 10-year Prospective Evaluation of Radial Keratotomy (PERK) study,[6] conducted by George Waring III, MD, demonstrated reasonably good safety and efficacy but reduced predictability and stability compared to current RK techniques. In the PERK study, only 38% of eyes were within .5 diopters (D) of emmetropia, and 60% of eyes were within 1 D emmetropia. The most disconcerting information provided by the PERK study, however, was the hyperopic shift that occurred in a progressive manner at an average rate of +.21 D per year, which caused 43% of the RK eyes to have a hyperopic shift of greater than 1 D between the 6-month and 10-year follow-up visits. The PERK study remains one of the best prospective evaluations of any medical procedure to date.

Charles Casebeer, MD revolutionized RK in the early 1990s by creating a systematic approach to RK and RK enhancements with the development of conservative age- and gender-based nomograms and instructional courses. Richard Lindstrom, MD defined the parameters for AK with the ARC-T multicenter trials. Current nomograms and RK techniques utilize biphasic blades and have been developed by both Casebeer and Kerry Assil, MD. Studies with low to moderate myopia have found that the Casebeer system of RK achieved 20/20 uncorrected visual acuity (UCVA) or better in 52% to 54% of eyes and 20/40 or better UCVA was achieved in 93% to 99% of eyes.[7-9] The hyperopic shift has again been identified as a potential long-term concern with +.6 D shift over 3-year follow-up.[10] Recognition of this corneal instability resulting in progressive hyperopia from the initial RK techniques have led to the mini-RK concept and technique, which was pioneered by Lindstrom.[11]

EVOLUTION OF PRK

In 1983, Trokel, et al first described the removal of corneal tissue with an excimer laser for refractive surgery.[12] Srinivasan, et al coined the term photoablative decomposition, or photoablation, to describe the photochemical process by which far ultraviolet light energy produces tissue

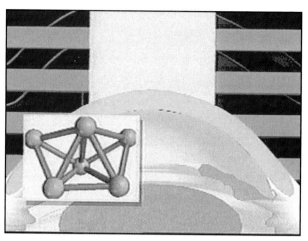

Figure 3-1. Graphic illustration of PRK photoablation. The excimer laser utilizes a 193-nm ultraviolet wavelength, which acts upon carbon-carbon molecular bonds to achieve photoablation.

removal through the breakdown of molecular bonds. The process of photoablation is unlike any other ophthalmic laser interaction. Each pulse of ultraviolet light energy possesses 6.4 eV, more than double that of any other ophthalmic laser and more than adequate to cleave 3.5 eV carbon-carbon bonds (Figure 3-1). On the other hand, photocoagulation with an argon laser utilizes heat, and photodisruption with the YAG laser is dependent upon explosive shockwaves to produce its results. The effects of photoablation are related to direct breakdown of molecular bonds.

Excimer lasers can produce ultraviolet light energy at various wavelengths depending on the gas elements utilized. Ultraviolet light energy of 248 nm not only results in potentially mutagenic behavior as evidenced by unscheduled DNA synthesis, but requires a higher energy density to achieve similar ablative effects as 193 nm and produces greater collateral damage. Similarly, ultraviolet light energy of a 308-nm wavelength is associated with an increased risk of cataract formation. Ultraviolet light energy of a 193-nm wavelength is associated with smoother ablation effects at lower energy densities and does not exhibit mutagenic or cataractogenic behavior.

Excimer laser PRK utilizes controlled pulses of 193 nm ultraviolet light energy to ablate stromal tissue producing a refractive excision pattern. The term excimer is derived from "excited dimer," which consists of an inert gas and a halide, specifically argon and fluoride gaseous elements, which are excited to a higher energy state by thousands of volts of electricity. Dimer is actually a misnomer, as it applies to two of the same element. The argon and fluoride elements are in very small concentrations in a helium mixture known as premix. The elements combine to form an unstable compound that rapidly dissociates and releases the ultraviolet light energy.

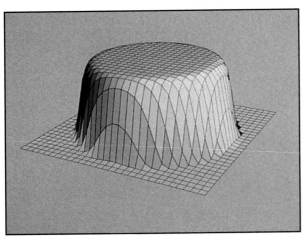

Figure 3-2. Homogeneous (flat) energy beam profile of Coherent-Schwind Keratom laser system.

EXCIMER LASER CONCEPTS AND PRINCIPLES

FUNDAMENTAL ELEMENTS OF LASER REFRACTIVE SURGERY

The first two fundamental elements governing the limitations and capabilities of the excimer laser concern fluence and beam homogeneity. Fluence is defined as the amount of energy applied to the ablative zone, whereas homogeneity is defined as the pattern of energy distribution within the exposed area. Homogeneity can be subdefined into microhomogeneity and macrohomogeneity. The term microhomogeneity defines localized variability in energy beam density, that is, "hot" and "cold" areas within the beam. The hot areas represent the highest energy density areas or peaks; conversely, the cold areas represent the areas of lowest energy density or valleys. Microhomogeneity is best represented by the peak-to-valley ratio. The term macrohomogeneity, rather than defining localized energy patterns, tends to refer to the overall energy beam profile of a specific excimer laser system.

FLUENCE AND HOMOGENEITY

Each excimer laser system has a characteristic energy beam profile, which may be homogeneous, gaussian, or reverse gaussian. A homogeneous or flat beam profile indicates an overall equal distribution of energy density. A gaussian energy beam profile, which is bell-curved in nature, indicates that there is a greater energy density centrally within the beam, while reverse gaussian implies less energy density centrally. The importance of the energy beam profile is that it affects the clinical profile, determining clinical factors such as refractive predictability and stability as well as the incidence of certain complications, such as central island formation. The simplest way to envision the energy beam profile (Figure 3-2) is to imagine the shape

of a single pulse being delivered to the surface of the cornea. In actuality, it is a composite of many pulses. A homogeneous energy beam profile would look like a top hat with equal amounts of energy centrally and peripherally. Each part of the beam would therefore remove identical amounts of tissue from the corneal surface. A gaussian beam is hotter centrally (having more energy centrally than peripherally), thereby removing more tissue centrally than peripherally with each pulse.

Fluence, defined as energy applied to a given area, is expressed in units of millijoules per square centimeter (mJ/cm^2) and varies from approximately 100 to 250 mJ/cm^2 depending on the specific excimer laser system discussed, for example:

- VISX: 160 mJ/cm^2
- Summit: 180 to 200 mJ/cm^2
- Technolas: 130 mJ/cm^2
- Nidek: 130 mJ/cm^2

A simple way to understand the importance of fluence is that it is the primary determinant of the amount of tissue ablated with each pulse. Fluence determines the ablation rate, whereas the computer algorithm is merely programmed to apply a given number of pulses in a given manner for any given refractive error. The precise amount of energy delivered per pulse will help determine outcome predictability. With fluence below 50 mJ/cm^2, there is minimal ablative effect, and at 120 mJ/cm^2, the ablative effect appears to level off. As one increases fluence, the pulse-to-pulse variability decreases, improving overall beam quality. However, the improvement in beam homogeneity from increased fluence is accompanied by increased thermal energy effect, increased optic degradation, and increased acoustic shockwave effect.

ENERGY OUTPUT

Excimer lasers should not be viewed merely as black boxes. The excimer must be understood not only to achieve superior refractive results but to avoid complications. The laser head is at the heart of the black box and consists of the laser cavity and electrodes. The two primary determinants of energy output, or fluence, are the freshness of the laser gas and the voltage. The laser gas becomes consumed as pulses are produced. When the fluence is low, the voltage within the cavity can be increased. Once maximal voltage is obtained, a gas exchange must be performed, putting fresh gas within the cavity. Higher voltages also have the benefit of producing improved beam homogeneity; therefore, one can maintain high voltage within the laser cavity as well as filter or attenuate beam energy later within the optical pathway to control fluence. To further complicate our developing insight into excimer lasers, the energy output from each laser varies, thus frequent recalibration is vital. The importance of recalibration to assess beam output, not only quantitatively but qualitatively, cannot be overstated.

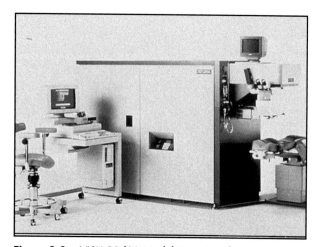

Figure 3-3a. VISX 20/20 Model B excimer laser system.

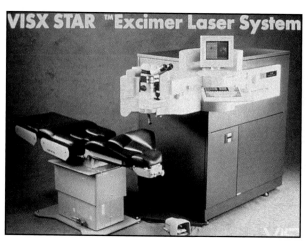

Figure 3-3b. VISX Star excimer laser system with a substantially smaller footplate.

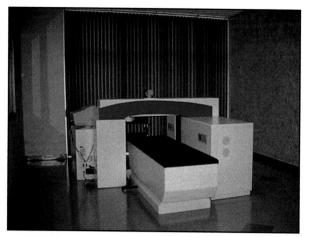

Figure 3-4a. Chiron Technolas Keracor 116 excimer laser system.

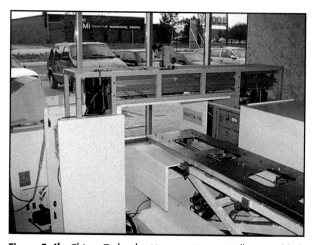

Figure 3-4b. Chiron Technolas Keracor 116 partially assembled.

Fundamental to understanding the excimer is the fact that energy output from this laser is inherently nonhomogeneous and therefore requires sophisticated optical delivery systems to render it usable. Importantly, it is much more difficult to produce and maintain a homogeneous beam of large diameter making wide-area surface ablation more challenging.

There are two basic laser delivery systems: broad beam (wide field ablation) and scanning. Broad beam delivery systems, such as the Summit Excimed, OmniMed, Apex systems, the VISX 20/20 (Figure 3-3a) and Star (Figure 3-3b), and the original Chiron Technolas Keracor 116 system (Figures 3-4a and 3-4b), utilize a computer-controlled variable iris diaphragm for myopic correction (Figures 3-5a and 3-5b), whereas the Coherent-Schwind Keratom broad beam system (Figure 3-6a) utilizes a series of round or elliptical apertures to produce the desired ablation pattern (Figure 3-6b). The beam is delivered at the maximal optical zone, but the diaphragm controls the area of the cornea exposed for each pulse. Scanning delivery systems such as the Aesculap-Meditec MEL 60 (Figure 3-7) and Nidek EC-5000 utilize a scanning slit to alter the corneal curvature, whereas the CIBA–Autonomous Technologies Corporation Tracker-PRK, LaserSight Compak-200, LaserScan 2000, and LSX excimer lasers use a flying spot. The advantage of scanning systems is that they manipulate a small beam, typically .8 to 2 mm in diameter, which can be made highly homogeneous much more easily.

The energy output of an excimer laser system is actually rectangular initially and manipulated through a series of lenses, prisms, and spatial integrators to improve beam quality (Figure 3-8). A tremendous amount of energy is lost through the optical pathway. It is important to recognize that these lasers are sensitive to optic misalignment and degradation, which can dramatically alter beam quality. Understanding that larger beams are more at risk for beam abnormalities is important for developing a realistic understanding of the limitations of broad beam excimer lasers.

TABLE 3-2. (CONTINUED)
PHOTOREFRACTIVE DELIVERY SYSTEMS

Scanning	
Slit	**Spot**
1. Intermediate energy output requirements 2. Improved beam uniformity 3. No central islands 4. Reduced acoustic shockwave 5. Smoother ablative surfaces 6. No optical zone limitations for PRK/PTK	1. Small energy output requirements 2. More complex ablation patterns possible, including hyperopic and asymmetric astigmatism 3. Lower beam homogeneity requirements 4. Lowest maintenance and fewest optics 5. No optical zone limitations for PRK/PTK 6. Reduced acoustic shockwave 7. No central islands
1. Eye tracker more important 2. Eye mask awkward 3. Slower procedure	1. Eye tracker necessary 2. Slowest procedure 3. Higher repetition rate necessary 4. Unknown/evolving algorithms

Aesculap-Meditec MEL 60	Nidek EC-5000	Autonomous Technologies Corp Tracker-PRK	LaserSight LSX	Chiron Technolas Keracor 117c and 217	Novatec LightBlade (nonexcimer)
250	130	180	160 to 300	130	100
20	30 [46]	100	100	20 to 50	> 200
1.5 x 10 mm	2 x 7 mm, optical zone 7.5 mm maximum, TZ 9 mm maximum	< 1 mm	< 1 mm	1 to 2 mm	< .3 mm
Rotating eye mask	Iris diaphragm, scanning slit rotates 120°/pass	Spiral scanning program	Rotating linear scanning spot	Spiral/random scanning spot	Spiral scanning spot
Rotating (variable) eye mask	Rotatable scanning slit beam	Meridional scanning	Meridional scanning	Meridional scanning	Elliptical scanning spot
Rotating (inverse) eye mask	Annular scanning slit beam	Annular scanning spot	Annular scanning spot	Annular scanning spot	Annular scanning spot
None	Passive	Active dual axis	Active	Active	Active
		Laser radar = LADAR eye tracking	ScanLink topography-assisted software	TopoLink topography-assisted software	Solid-state tunable titanium sapphire

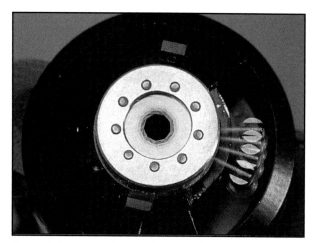

Figure 3-24a. Aesculap-Meditec metallic rotatable mask for myopia.

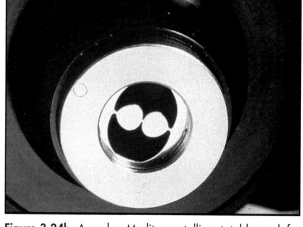

Figure 3-24b. Aesculap-Meditec metallic rotatable mask for hyperopia.

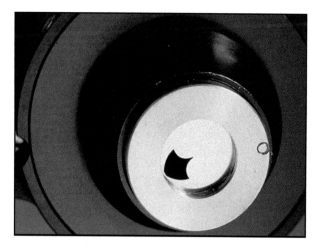

Figure 3-24c. Aesculap-Meditec metallic rotatable mask for presbyopia.

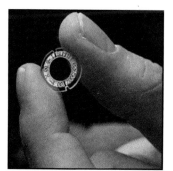

Figure 3-25a. Summit SVS Apex Plus Emphasis erodible mask.

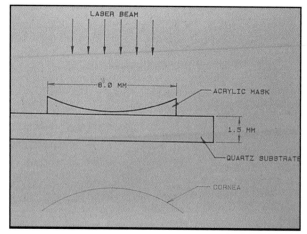

Figure 3-25b. Schematic of Emphasis erodible mask composed of PMMA supported on quartz substrate. Erodible mask acts as a template for shape transfer process.

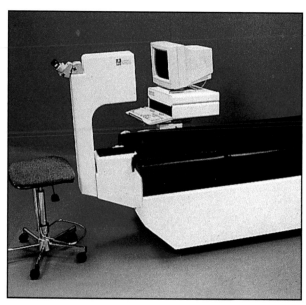

Figure 3-26. CIBA Autonomous Technologies Corporation laser system.

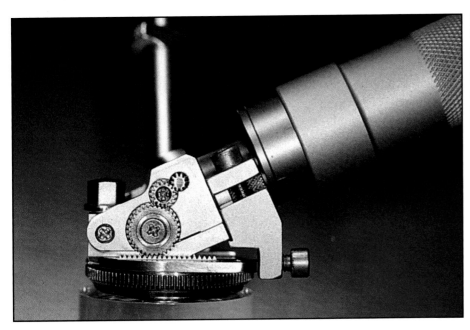

Figure 3-36. Chiron Corneal Shaper with adjustable three-piece suction ring for automated lamellar keratoplasty and LASIK. A smaller single-piece suction ring is used for LASIK alone (courtesy of Stephen Slade, MD).

smoothness, blending, and beam homogeneity observed with newer laser delivery systems are of limited clinical significance with LASIK.

LASIK still requires multizone or aspheric ablation patterns to limit the depth of ablation while maximizing the effective optical zone. It is important to monitor the depth of ablation to not only protect the endothelium, but to maintain long-term corneal stability. The residual corneal tissue pachymetry should ideally exceed 380 microns and allow for a 160-micron flap and 220-micron stromal bed. While it is possible to utilize a 130-micron corneal flap and leave a 200-micron bed, it is always safest to avoid pressing the limits of any refractive procedure. Similarly, smaller treatment areas of 4.2 to 5 mm were initially used to treat high myopia with LASIK in order to limit the amount of tissue ablated, however, visual quality under low levels of illumination was often compromised, sometimes severely. Typically, a 6-mm area of ablation is utilized to provide adequate night vision quality, although this limits the maximal treatment to about -12 D unless multizone or aspheric programs are used. A patient with limited corneal thickness should be left undercorrected but with an adequate optical zone rather than fully corrected with an inadequate optical zone or inadequate residual corneal thickness.

LASIK creates a spherical or toric lenticular pattern with tapered edges, whereas ALK creates a plano lamellar excision pattern with sharp margins. The induced topographical change on videokeratography with respect to the effective optical zone generated is markedly different between ALK and LASIK. The resected lenticle in ALK is only 4.2 mm, however, the corneal flap blends the plano excision pattern to create a 5- to 5.5-mm effective optical zone (Figures 3-36 through 3-37c). In direct contrast, the effective optical zone is smaller than the treatment zone with LASIK. The tapered wound edge profile of LASIK is masked by both the corneal flap and the increased stromal hydration of the deeper stroma.

Like PRK, LASIK is subject to the development of central islands when larger optical zones of 6 mm or greater are utilized with broad beam excimer lasers. In fact, the risk of central island formation is likely greater with LASIK because of the increased hydration status of the deeper stroma and absence of epithelial remodeling. Alterations in the technique or ablation profile are required to compensate for the central undercorrection anticipated with larger optical zones. Modifications in technique include drying the central stroma with a surgical spear, air, or wiping with a blunt spatula.

Ablation profile compensation utilizes a pretreatment approach; that is, the application of additional pulses centrally beyond what is required for the refractive correction. Conversely, a scanning excimer laser may be used to avoid central island formation altogether.

Original ablation nomograms for LASIK were based on ALK concepts. Later nomograms were tailored after PRK, but LASIK requires a combination approach. PRK central treatment and blending combined with ALK wound margin profile means that a large transition zone is not mandatory with LASIK as it is with PRK. The central 3 mm of the ablation zone is responsible for daytime qualitative vision, whereas the peripheral 5 to 7 mm is responsible for nighttime qualitative vision. Most ablation nomograms are designed with respect to dioptric correction and are essentially meaningless to the cornea. Ablation profiles must be designed with respect to micron depth and corneal contour produced. Each zone must have a minimum depth to be effective in producing a change in contour, overcoming the masking effects of the corneal flap, and deeper stromal hydration. Each zone must also have a maximum depth to avoid steep contours, promote blending, and reduce the overall depth of ablation.

Figure 3-37a. Schematic illustration of ALK demonstrating the lamellar excision pattern of the refractive pass with steep wound margins.

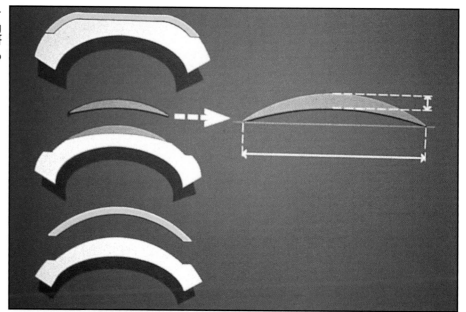

Figure 3-37b. Clinical intraoperative view of ALK, performed by Stephen G. Slade, MD, demonstrating steep 4.2 mm wound margins.

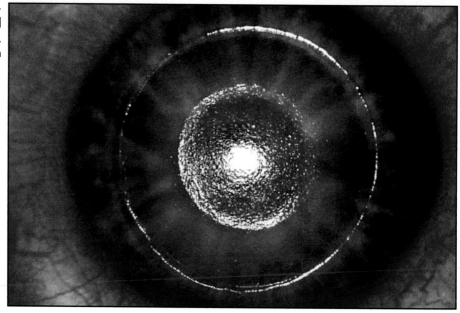

> LASIK nomogram refinement must have two guiding principles: corneal safety and visual quality.

> The corneal epithelium has emerged as the crucial component of the LASIK procedure.

ADVANCEMENTS IN LASIK

In order to improve quality of vision following LASIK, it was necessary to increase the amount of refractive correction performed at the larger optical zones. According to the Munnerlyn formula, this increased the ablation depth for a given myopic correction. The multizone nomogram, which is described in Chapter 5, is now used by most surgeons for LASIK. Because of the greater ablation depth per diopter with this nomogram, the maximum correction possible with LASIK has been reduced. While corrections of greater than 20 D of myopia are possible with small treatment zones or excessive blending, night visual disturbances are too often encountered. The maximum correction possible with conservative multizone ablation patterns is approximately 15 D.[16] The corneal thickness must be measured in each eye prior to LASIK to determine the tissue available for ablation so that adequate posterior corneal stroma remains following LASIK to maintain the long-term corneal integrity. Therefore, LASIK nomogram refinement must have two guiding principles: corneal safety and visual quality.

The corneal epithelium has emerged as the crucial com-

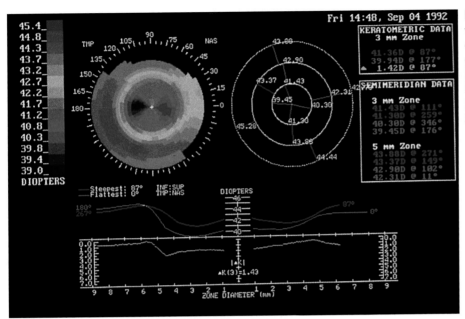

Figure 3-37c. Postoperative videokeratography of ALK demonstrating enlarged 5.5-mm effective optical zone due to bending of corneal flap noted from topographical profile (courtesy of Stephen G. Slade, MD).

ponent of the LASIK procedure. Epithelial defects found at the time of surgery greatly increase the risk of postoperative discomfort and epithelial ingrowth. Preoperative anesthesia must be minimized both in dosage and duration of activity prior to LASIK. If excessive topical anesthesia is used or the topical anesthesia is applied too long before LASIK, the epithelium will be attenuated, which could result in epithelial defects. The amount of gentian violet used for the preoperative corneal markings must also be minimized, as this has some epithelial toxicity. When the microkeratome cut is made, the cornea must be thoroughly covered with balanced salt solution to ensure that the passage of the microkeratome is as atraumatic as possible. Patients are given ocular lubricants after LASIK and told to rest for the evening in order to encourage the epithelium to heal.

Methods to deal with stromal hydration during LASIK have been simplified with the improved technology of the scanning lasers. With the Chiron Technolas 116 excimer laser and some other broad beam systems, excessive central corneal hydration was removed with compressed air or by wiping with a blunt spatula or surgical spear. This introduced another variable into the predictability of the procedure and may have been responsible for some of the initial hyperopic shift of the postoperative refractions in the first few weeks following LASIK. With the Chiron Technolas 117 and 217 excimer laser systems utilizing PlanoScan flying spot software, compressed air is not required, so there are less surgical variables. During our first year of experience with this laser software and delivery system, we noted greater refractive predictability and stability following LASIK.

Most surgeons include irrigation under the corneal flap as a crucial and accepted step of LASIK. When LASIK was first performed, the flap was replaced without irrigation of the interface. This allowed for a very quick and strong adhe-

sion of the flap to the stromal bed. Unfortunately, interface debris was recognized frequently postoperatively when this technique was used. While this did not have any detrimental effects on the final visual outcome or the comfort of the eye, the appearance of these particles under the flap was quite disturbing for both the surgeon and the co-managing doctors. Irrigation of the flap interface following flap replacement greatly improves integrity of the flap interface following LASIK. Interface debris has been virtually eliminated with this technique. Furthermore, irrigation under the flap allows the flap to be "floated" back into its natural position and allows the stromal side of the flap to mold itself onto the new curvature of the ablated stromal bed. This ensures optimal alignment of the flap following LASIK. Unfortunately, interface irrigation does have one disadvantage—a reduction in the initial adhesion of the flap to the stromal bed. When interface irrigation is used, it is important to wait a few minutes after the flap is replaced to ensure good flap adhesion prior to removing the lid speculum.

Microkeratome technology has also evolved. The introduction of the pivoting Chiron Hansatome and disposable microkeratomes, such as the Ruiz Automated Disposable Keratome distributed by LaserSight, will increase the acceptance and safety of LASIK because of the lower cost and less intensive maintenance requirements. The emergence of scanning lasers with peripheral blend zones that extend out beyond 8.5 mm for myopic corrections and beyond 9 mm for hyperopic correction have necessitated the creation of flaps larger than the average 8.5 mm flap of the Chiron ACS microkeratome. The Chiron Hansatome creates 9.5 mm corneal flaps that are hinged superiorly and may offer further benefits in terms of flap stability. Due to the wide acceptance of the classical Chiron ACS microkeratome, changes in the use of microkeratomes for LASIK may be gradual.

Finally, postoperative care of the LASIK patient has changed. Topical NSAIDs are now recommended sparingly to LASIK patients both immediately preoperatively and postoperatively to improve their comfort. Excessive or prolonged use of topical NSAIDs with both PRK and LASIK postoperatively may have contributed to stromal melting in some cases. Lubrication has been strongly encouraged in all patients during the acute recovery period. Currently, patients are given Tobradex (Tobramycin .3%-Dexamethasone .1%, Alcon), Ciloxan (ciprofloxacin .3%, Alcon), and Voltaren (Diclofenac sodium .1%, CIBA) both immediately preoperatively and postoperatively. Postoperatively, LASIK patients are maintained on Tobradex to be used four times a day for 4 days and Genteal (hydroxypropyl methylcellulose, CIBA) used frequently during the first few weeks following LASIK.

REFERENCES

1. Sato T, Akiyama K, Shibita H. A new surgical approach to myopia. *Am J Ophthalmol.* 1953;36:823.
2. Akiyama K, et al. Problems arising from Sato's radial keratotomy procedures in Japan. *CLAO J.* 1984;10:79.
3. Fyodorov SN, Durnev VV. Operation dosaged dissection of the corneal circular ligament in cases of myopia of a mild degree. *Am J Ophthalmol.* 1979;11:1885.
4. Fyodorov SN, Durnev VV. Surgical correction of complicated myopic astigmatism by means of dissection of circular ligament of cornea. *Annals of Ophthalmology.* 1981;13:115.
5. Bores LD, Myers, et al. Radial keratotomy: An analysis of the American experience. *Annals of Ophthalmology.* 1981;88:79.
6. Waring GO III, Lynn MJ, McDonnell PJ. Results of the prospective evaluation of radial keratotomy (PERK) study 10 years after surgery. *Arch Ophthalmol.* 1994;112(10):1298-1308.
7. Werblin TP, Stafford GM. The Casebeer system for predictable keratorefractive surgery. One-year evaluation of 205 consecutive eyes. *Ophthalmology.* 1993;100(7):1095-1102.
8. Waring GO II, Casebeer JC, Dru RM. One-year results of a prospective multicenter study of the Casebeer system of refractive keratotomy. Casebeer Chiron Study Group. *Ophthalmology.* 1996;103(9):1337-1347.
9. Werblin TP, Stafford GM. Three year results of refractive keratotomy using the Casebeer system. *J Cataract Refract Surg.* 1996;22(8):1023-1029.
10. Werblin TP, Stafford GM. Hyperopic shift after refractive keratotomy using the Casebeer system. *J Cataract Refract Surg.* 1996;22(8):1030-1036.
11. Lindstrom RL. Minimally invasive radial keratotomy: mini-RK. *J Cataract Refract Surg.* 1995;21(1):27-34.
12. Trokel SL, Srinivasan R, Braren B. Excimer laser surgery on the cornea. *Am J Ophthalmol.* 1983;96:404.
13. Munnerlyn CR, Koons SJ, Marshall J. Photorefractive keratectomy: a technique for laser refractive surgery. *J Refract Surg.* 1988;14:46-52.
14. Seiler T, Kahle G, Kriegerowski M. Excimer laser (193 nm) myopic keratomileusis in sighted and blind human eyes. *J Refract Corneal Surg.* 1990;3:97-100.
15. McDonald MB, Frantz JM, Klyce SD, et al. One-year refractive results of photorefractive keratotomy for myopia in nonhuman primate cornea. *Arch Ophthalmol.* 1990;108:40-47.
16. Probst LE, Machat JJ. The mathematics of LASIK for high myopia. *J Cataract Refract Surg.* In press.

LASIK Mathematics

Louis E. Probst, MD
Jeffery J. Machat, MD

All excimer laser refractive procedures modify the refracting power of the cornea by altering the anterior corneal curvature by the process of photoablation. The correction of myopia involves the relative flattening of the central cornea compared to the peripheral cornea, which reduces the anterior corneal curvature and hence reduces the refractive power of the treated area. Because the maximal corneal stromal tissue will be photoablated from the central cornea, the thickness of the central cornea becomes important when LASIK is performed for high refractive errors with large ablation depths.

> Because the maximal corneal stromal tissue will be photoablated from the central cornea, the thickness of the central cornea becomes important when LASIK is performed for high refractive errors with large ablation depths.

SINGLE AND MULTIZONE ABLATION PROTOCOLS

The PRK excimer ablation technique has evolved. The initial single zone techniques increased from 4 to 6 mm,[1,2] to improve the quality of postoperative vision and reduce the incidence of halos and regression. The multipass multizone technique was developed by Mihai Pop, MD for the VISX excimer laser,[3] and the multi-multizone technique was developed by Jeffery J. Machat, MD for the Chiron Technolas excimer laser.[4]

These multizone techniques divide the myopic treatment into multiple zones, which decrease the ablation depth and create a smoother ablation surface. This blending and smoothing effect of the multizone protocols has helped to reduce the incidence of post-PRK regression and haze particularly for the treatment of high myopia.[5]

PRETREATMENT PROTOCOLS

Pretreatment protocols have been added to the ablation profiles of the broad beam excimer lasers such as the VISX Star, Summit Omnimed, and Chiron Technolas Keracor 116 to reduce the incidence of postoperative central islands.[6] The VISX Star pretreatment is automatically calculated by the central island factor (CIF) 4.01 software and incorporated into the excimer ablation protocol. Approximately 1 micron per diopter of spherical correction plus an additional 2 microns is added to each ablation protocol and performed at 2.5 mm. The Chiron Technolas Keracor 116 pretreatment is surgeon programmable. Generally, 1 micron per diopter plus 2 to 4 microns is added to each ablation protocol and performed at 3 mm.[7] The Summit Omnimed excimer laser has a gaussian beam distribution for which a relatively greater amount of laser energy is produced in the center of the ablation circle, so less pretreatment is required. A pretreatment of 1 micron per diopter is generally performed using the patient training "A" mode with an optical zone of 2.6 to 2.8 mm.

TABLE 4-1.
EXCIMER LASER ABLATION PER DIOPTER

Excimer laser	Zone size	Ablation protocol	Ablation per diopter
Chiron Technolas	6.6 mm	Single zone (1 to 2 D) pretreatment	20 microns
VISX Star	6 mm	Standard cards (1 to 2 D) single zone pretreatment	17 microns
Chiron Technolas	6.6 mm	Single zone (>3 D) pretreatment	17 microns
VISX Star	6 mm	Standard cards (>3 D) single zone pretreatment	15 microns
Summit Omnimed	6 mm	All levels of myopia single zone pretreatment	13 to 14 microns
VISX Star	6 mm	International cards multipass multizone pretreatment	12.5 microns
Chiron Technolas	6.6 mm	Surgeon programmable partial multi-multizone pretreatment	12.5 microns
Chiron Technolas	6.6 mm	Surgeon programmable full multi-multizone pretreatment	10 microns

ABLATION DEPTH PER DIOPTER

Each excimer laser ablates a different amount of stromal tissue per diopter of refractive correction because of the differences in the ablation zone diameters, amount of pretreatment, and the ablation protocols (Table 4-1). The Munnerlyn formula[8] (depth of ablation = diopters of correction x ablation diameter^2 ÷ 3) indicates that each spherical equivalent (SE) diopter of myopic correction performed at a 6 mm single zone will ablate 12 microns of tissue.

Pretreatment protocols added to the ablation profile of broad beam excimer lasers such as the VISX Star and Chiron Technolas Keracor 116 will increase the depth per SE diopter to 17 to 20 microns for low corrections (1 to 2 diopters [D]) and 15 to 17 microns for higher corrections (3 D or more). The Summit Omnimed will ablate 13 to 14 microns per SE diopter for all levels of myopia with pretreatment.

The multipass multizone ablation technique used with VISX Star "international cards" has an average stromal ablation of 12.5 microns per SE diopter. The full multi-multizone ablation technique with the ablation pattern distributed between 3.6 and 6.2 mm reduces the average stromal ablation to approximately 10 microns per SE diopter.[9] While the full multi-multizone protocol significantly reduces ablation depth, it should only be used for LASIK when necessitated by a thin cornea associated with high myopia because of the compromised quality of postoperative night vision.

With the Chiron Technolas 116 excimer laser, the ideal zone depth for each step of the multizone PRK ablation was determined to be 15 to 20 µm to create the smoothest blended multizone ablation. For LASIK, however, Machat has found that the size of the ablation zones should be increased so that most of the treatment is performed at a 5.5 mm or

larger ablation zone. This increases the depth of ablation to 30 to 40 µm per zone in the partial multi-multizone protocol, which accounts for the hydration effects of the deeper stroma and the masking effect of the corneal flap. By increasing the size and depth of ablation of each zone to 30 to 40 µm and decreasing the number of zones, the effective postoperative optical zone on videokeratography can be increased and night vision difficulties minimized. This partial multi-multizone ablation that we now use for LASIK ablations removes 12.5 microns of stroma per SE diopter. With the Chiron 217 PlanoScan program, we utilize a 6 mm treatment zone with an 8.2 to 9.2 mm blend, which ablates 17 to 23 microns per diopter.

BASIC TENETS OF LASIK

There are four critical values or dimensions that must be considered when performing LASIK. They are the flap thickness, the amount of residual corneal stroma, the diameter of the excimer ablation, and the depth of the excimer ablation. These values determine the key concepts of LASIK—safety of the procedure, stability of the procedure, quality of the laser correction, and quantity of the laser correction. (Doane JF, Nordan LT, Baker RN, Slade SG. Basic tenets of lamellar refractive surgery. Unpublished data) (Figure 4-1).

The flap thickness must be sufficient to prevent irregular astigmatism, but at the same time not so excessive as to remove stroma potentially available for ablation. We gener-

The flap thickness must be sufficient to prevent irregular astigmatism, but at the same time not so excessive as to remove stroma potentially available for ablation.

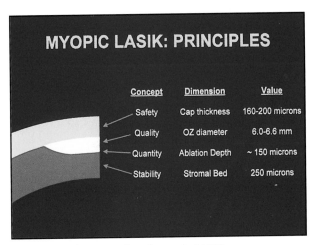

Figure 4-1. The principles of myopic LASIK.

ally use a 160 μm flap for thin corneas or large refractive corrections (> 10 D), a 180 μm flap for average corneas and moderate corrections (> 6 D), and a 200 μm flap for thick corneas and small corrections (< 6 D). Sufficient residual central posterior stromal tissue (CPST) must be left after the LASIK procedure to avoid a decrease of the corneal integrity and the subsequent development of corneal ectasia. The diameter of the excimer ablation should be at least 6 mm to create a functional postoperative optical zone of at least 4 mm, which will allow for sufficient quality of vision. Finally, the depth of the excimer ablation determines the quantity of myopia that can be safely treated while preserving adequate residual corneal stroma.

> Sufficient residual central posterior stromal tissue must be left after the LASIK procedure to avoid a decrease of the corneal integrity and the subsequent development of corneal ectasia.

The distribution of the central stromal thinning is different following ALK and LASIK. With ALK, a 4.2-mm lamellar disc is removed from the center of the visual axis, creating uniform thinning over the entire area where the tissue was removed. With LASIK, however, the excimer ablation by either the single zone or the multizone techniques results in a gradient of thinning maximal only in the very central region of the ablation zone, with the remaining CPST maintaining substantially more thickness. Therefore, corneal integrity should be better preserved following LASIK when compared to ALK for an equal refractive correction.

ALK has provided the most extensive experience with lamellar surgery prior to LASIK, and as refractive surgeons, we must make every effort not to compromise the long-term integrity of the cornea. The Ruiz nomogram for hyperopic ALK[10] suggests a 300-micron cut in corneas that ranged in thickness from 490 to 575 microns will produce a 1 D myopic shift from the subsequent "controlled" corneal ecta-

sia. Ruiz and coworkers[11] have also noted that microkeratome cuts greater than 60% of the central corneal thickness can produce uncontrolled corneal ectasia. Similarly, Gris and coworkers have stated that a microkeratome cut greater than 350 microns can produce corneal ectasia.[12] Since the average corneal thickness is approximately 540.5 + 38.5 microns,[13] subtraction tells us that corneal ectasia with ALK is produced with 180 to 275 microns of CPST.

Iatrogenic keratoconus has been reported after LASIK for high myopia, although the amount of tissue in the posterior stromal bed was not recorded.[14] Given this information from the experience with ALK, the authors believe that a careful and conservative approach, which ideally preserves 250 microns of posterior stromal bed after LASIK, represents the best current guideline and should be used until further research or experience indicates that corneal integrity is preserved with less posterior tissue.

> Iatrogenic keratoconus has been reported after LASIK for high myopia.

> Probst and Machat believe in a careful and conservative approach, which ideally preserves 250 microns of posterior stromal bed after LASIK.

MATHEMATICS FOR PRIMARY LASIK

The average central cornea thickness is approximately 550 ± 100 μm. Since the flap thickness during the LASIK procedure is generally 160 μm, the average cornea will have 390 μm of posterior stromal bed left after the flap creation. Therefore, the maximal myopic correction that should be performed on a patient with a 550 μm cornea using a full multi-multizone technique is generally less than 14 D, while leaving a residual posterior stromal bed of 250 microns.

> Maximal Myopic Correction with Chiron Full Multizone LASIK Technique #1:
>
> [550 μm - 160 μm (flap) - 250 μm (bed)]/10 μm per D = 14 D

A simpler and less mathematically complex way of calculating the safe maximal correction is to always leave at least 400 μm of total stromal tissue following LASIK. With an average flap thickness of 160 μm, approximately 240 μm of CPST would be left to maintain the integrity of the cornea. For the average cornea of 550 μm, this would allow a maximal myopic correction of 15 D.

With a VISX single zone LASIK technique, the ablation per diopter would be increased to 15 μm and would allow the maximal correction of between 9.3 D and 10 D.

The Summit Excimed excimer laser will ablate at least

Maximal Myopic Correction with Chiron Full Multizone LASIK Technique #2:

[550 μm - 400 μm (flap & bed)]/10 μm per D = 15 D

Maximal Myopic Correction with VISX Single Zone LASIK Technique #1:

(550 μm - 160 μm - 250 μm)/15 μm per D = 9.3 D

or

Maximal Myopic Correction with Visx Single Zone LASIK Technique #2:

(550 μm - 400 μm)/15 μm per D = 10 D

13 microns per diopter for single zone LASIK with pretreatment. This will allow between 10.8 and 11.5 D of myopic correction of a cornea of average thickness (depending on the calculation method used).

Maximal Myopic Correction with Summit Single Zone LASIK Technique #1:

(550 μm - 160 μm - 250 μm)/ 13 μm per D = 10.8 D

or

Maximal Myopic Correction with Summit Single Zone LASIK Technique #2:

(550 μm - 400 μm)/ 13 μm per D = 11.5 D

Modified Chiron Technolas 116 partial multi-multizone LASIK algorithms with increased zone depths of 30 to 40 μm and the multipass multizone ablation of the VISX Star with an international card result in an ablation of 12.5 μm per diopter and allow a maximal correction of up to 12 D.

Maximal Myopic Correction with Partial Multi-multizone LASIK Technique #1:

(550 μm - 160 μm - 250 μm)/12.5 μm per D = 11.2 D

or

Maximal Myopic Correction with Partial Multi-multizone LASIK Technique #2:

(550 μm - 400 μm)/ 12.5 μm per D = 12 D

Some surgeons have recommend that the depth of the stromal ablation not exceed more than 50% of the preoperative pachymetry value. Using this method, the average 550 μm cornea with a 160 μm flap would have 115 μm available for ablation for a correction of 11.5 D and 275 μm of remaining CPST.

Maximal Myopic Correction with Chiron Full Multizone LASIK Technique #3:

[550 μm / 2 - 160 μm (flap)]/ 10 μm per D = 11.5 D

MATHEMATICS FOR LASIK ENHANCEMENTS

While these calculations are crucial for preoperative planning and patient counseling for the original LASIK procedure, they are no less important during the LASIK enhancement procedure. All patients must have preoperative pachymetry prior to the enhancement procedure to determine whether an adequate amount of CPST remains to allow for an enhancement procedure to be performed.

During an enhancement procedure, we always leave at least 200 μm of CPST, but ideally 240 μm.

During an enhancement procedure, we always leave at least 200 μm of CPST but ideally 240 μm. Since enhancement ablations are generally performed for small refractive errors with a single 6 to 6.5 mm pretreatment ablation zone, up to 20 μm of stromal tissue is ablated per diopter of correction. Therefore, a post-LASIK patient with pre-enhancement pachymetry readings of 440 μm would have the absolute maximal amount of tissue to allow a 2 D correction if the flap thickness was 160 μm.

Maximal Myopic Correction with LASIK Enhancement Example #1:

[440 μm - 160 μm (flap) - 240 μm (bed)]/20 μm per D = 2 D

We have lifted corneal flaps for LASIK enhancements up to 14 months after the primary LASIK. This is our preferred technique if the original LASIK was difficult due to a small palpebral opening or a deep orbit, as well as when CPST must be preserved in a thin cornea. However, for routine LASIK enhancements 6 or more months after the primary procedure, we generally recommend recutting the corneal flap because of the difficulty associated with lifting a corneal flap and the subsequent trauma that can be caused to it and the surrounding epithelium. When performing a LASIK enhancement by this technique, special consideration must be given to the centrally flattened corneas that are typically found following LASIK. The same consideration must be given when LASIK is being planned for virgin eyes with flat central keratometry or post-PRK and post-RK. The

The flattest central corneal keratometry is generally less than 40 D for these eyes; consequently, there is a greater risk of creating a perforated or free cap.

Maximal Myopic Correction with LASIK Enhancement
Example #2:

$$[440\ \mu m - 200\ \mu m\ (flap) - 240\ \mu m\ (bed)]/20\ \mu m\ per\ D = 0\ D$$

flattest central corneal keratometry is generally less than 40 D for these eyes; consequently, there is a greater risk of creating a perforated or free cap.

To minimize the risk of these potential problems, we routinely increase our keratectomy depth to 200 μm for safety in cases with the flattest central keratometry measurement less than 40 D. Because this requires more corneal stroma to be allocated to the corneal flap, there is less CPST available for safe ablation without compromising the corneal integrity and causing corneal ectasia. In this case, a post-LASIK patient with pre-enhancement pachymetry readings of 440 μm would have inadequate tissue available to perform an enhancement.

In general, we do not recommend enhancing eyes with less than 400 μm of total remaining corneal tissue. It is also important to recognize that epithelial hyperplasia occurs following high myopia correction and that the actual stromal tissue remaining may be less than calculated. In general, it is always safer to leave a patient mildly myopic than to aggressively treat both primary and repeat LASIK patients.

Clinical Note

A 35-year-old healthy female was seen in consultation for LASIK. Her SE refraction was -10 D OD and -9.75 D OS. The corneal pachymetry measurements averaged 571 OD and 554 OS. Serial corneal topographies indicated a stable astigmatic pattern. The flattest corneal curvature was 44.25 OD and 44 OS. The patient's pupils were dilated to 5 to 6 mm in dim illumination.

Given the adequate corneal curvature and relatively high level of myopia, a 160 micron plate was selected for the Chiron ACS microkeratome. The partial multizone ablation with the Chiron Technolas 116 was selected to provide the best quantity of daytime vision and best quality of night vision. The depth of the ablation OD would be approximately 125 microns (-10 D x 12.5 microns/D) and OS 121.9 microns (-9.75 D x 12.5 microns/D). This would leave residual CPST of 286 microns OD and 272.1 microns OS. Given the adequate CPST, the procedure was completed after preoperative counseling and consent.

Three months later, the patient returned for evaluation. Refractive examination found -.50 + -.50 x 90 OD and -2 OS. The patient indicated that the left eye had regressed over the first preoperative 2 months. Previous postoperative refractions indicated that the left eye was now stable. Corneal pachymetry was 451 OD and 458 OS. Since the

original LASIK procedure was only 3 months prior, the technique of lifting the corneal flap was selected. The original corneal flap was 160 microns, so the CPST was 298 microns (458 microns to 160 microns). For a -2 D correction with the Chiron Technolas 116 excimer laser using a 6.6 mm ablation zone, approximately 40 microns of CPST were ablated (-2 D x 20 microns/D). Therefore, a total of 258 microns of CPST were left OS after the enhancement procedure. This amount of CPST should be more than adequate to preserve the long-term corneal integrity.

REFRACTIVE CONSIDERATIONS FOR EXTREME MYOPIA

Greater then 15 D of myopia can be treated with LASIK, however this often requires a multizone excimer ablation to decrease the central corneal ablation depth and preserve adequate CPST tissue (200 to 250 microns) to maintain the corneal integrity. While multizone protocols can reduce the overall depth of ablation, they will also compromise the quality of postoperative vision by decreasing the size of the effective corneal optical zone, which is further decreased by the masking effect of the corneal flap.

With careful attention to the thickness of the cornea and adherence to the basic tenets of LASIK, the refractive surgeon should be able to successfully and safely treat most high myopes without compromising the corneal integrity and still provide better qualitative vision.

REFERENCES

1. Gartry DS, Kerr Muir MG, Marshall J. Photorefractive keratectomy with an argon fluoride excimer laser: a clinical study. *J Refract Corneal Surg.* 1991;7:420-435.

2. Talley AR, Hardten DR, Sher NA, et al. Results 1 year after using the 193-nm excimer laser for photorefractive keratectomy in mild to moderate myopia. *Am J Ophthalmol.* 1994;118:304-311.

3. Pop M, Aras M. Multizone/multipass photorefractive keratectomy: 6-month results. *J Cataract Refract Surg.* 1995;21:633-643.

4. Machat JJ. PRK procedure. In: Machat JJ (ed). *Excimer Laser Refractive Surgery.* SLACK Incorporated: Thorofare, NJ; 1996.

5. Pop M. The Multipass/multizone PRK technique to correct myopia and astigmatism. In: Machat JJ (ed). *Excimer Laser Refractive Surgery.* SLACK Incorporated: Thorofare, NJ; 1996.

6. Machat JJ. PRK complications and their management. In: Machat JJ (ed). *Excimer Laser Refractive Surgery.* SLACK Incorporated: Thorofare, NJ; 1996.

7. Machat JJ. LASIK procedure. In: Machat JJ (ed). *Excimer Laser Refractive Surgery.* SLACK Incorporated: Thorofare, NJ; 1996.

8. Munnerlyn CR, Koons SJ, Marshall J. Photorefractive keratectomy: a technique for laser refractive surgery. *Journal of Refractive Surgery.* 1988;14:46-52.

9. Machat JJ LASIK procedure: Chiron Technolas PRK and LASIK nomogram. In: Machat JJ (ed). *Excimer Laser Refractive Surgery.* SLACK Incorporated: Thorofare, NJ; 1996.

10. Kezirian GM, Gremillion CM. Automated lamellar keratoplasty for the correction of hyperopia. *J Cataract Refract Surg*. 1995;21:386-392.

11. American Academy of Ophthalmology. Automated lamellar keratoplasty. Preliminary procedure assessment. *Ophthalmology*. 1996;103(5):852-861.

12. Gris O, Güell JL, Muller A. Keratomileusis update. *J Cataract Refract Surg*. 1996;22:620-623.

13. Emara B, Probst LE. Correlation of intraocular pressure and corneal thickness before and after LASIK. *J Cataract Refract Surg*. Submitted.

14. Baikoff G. Induced pseudo-keratoconus after LASIK. Presented at the Symposium on Cataract, IOL, and Refractive Surgery; American Society of Cataract and Refractive Surgery Meeting; April 1997; Boston, Mass.

CHAPTER 5

Predictive Formulas for LASIK

Louis E. Probst, MD
Jonathan Woolfson, MD
Michiel Kritzinger, MD

INTRODUCTION

The predictive formulas for laser in situ keratomileusis (LASIK) have two components: the excimer laser ablation nomogram and the adjustment factors.

The excimer laser ablation nomogram controls the relative distribution of the refraction correction into one or more zones. In some of the newer excimer lasers, such as the VISX Star, the excimer ablation nomogram is controlled by the laser's computer, while in other excimer lasers, such as the Chiron Technolas 116, the ablation nomogram is fully programmable by the surgeon.

The adjustment factors allow surgeons to refine the treatment protocol to reflect their particular refractive situation. In order for these formulas to be predictive, a high level of consistency must be achieved in the application of both the ablation nomograms and adjustment factors. Other extraneous variables such as the methods of preoperative refraction, room temperature and humidity, room air quality and flow, surgical technique and time, and postoperative medications must be tightly controlled to avoid deviations from the intended correction.

It is crucial to remember that the predictive formulas, including both the excimer laser ablation nomogram and the adjustment factors, must be individualized for each surgeon. Direct extrapolations from the experience of one surgeon or one center will likely lead to an unexpected deviation of the surgical results from emmetropia. Since it is impossible to control every aspect of surgery, each surgeon must develop his or her own predictive formulas once his or her technique has become standardized and the postoperative results can be analyzed. For the beginning LASIK surgeon, conservative corrections are preferable, as enhancements are easy to perform while overcorrections can be much more challenging.

> The predictive formulas for LASIK have two components: the excimer laser ablation nomogram and the adjustment factors.

> Direct extrapolations from the experience of one surgeon or one center will likely lead to an unexpected deviation of the surgical results from emmetropia.

Once the excimer ablation nomogram and adjustment factors have been standardized and individualized for each excimer laser surgeon, LASIK's final uncontrolled variable is the healing pattern of the cornea. While there is a clear tendency for greater amounts of regression for higher levels of myopia, often the degree of regression after LASIK is unpredictable. Younger patients (< 25 years) often demonstrate significant regression, while older patients (> 50 years) may not regress at all. We have often observed regression of 1 to 2 D in one eye and no regression in the other eye after bilateral simultaneous LASIK in which the excimer nomogram, adjustment factors, surgical technique, and extraneous variables were all exactly the same for the correction of both eyes. This unpredictable healing pattern of the cornea represents the limitation of corneal refractive surgery. In order to avoid LASIK overcorrections,

TABLE 5-1.

MELBOURNE EXCIMER LASER GROUP MULTIZONE PRK TREATMENT ALGORITHM

Diopters at Corneal Plane

Ablation zone (mm)	-3	-4	-5	-6	-7	-8	-9	-10	-11	-12	-13	-14	-15	-16	-17	-18
4.5	-	-	-	-	-	-	-	-	-3.67	-4	-4.33	-4.67	-5	-5.33	-5.67	-6
5	-	-	-	-3	-3.5	-4	-4.5	-5	-3.67	-4	-4.33	-4.67	-5	-5.33	-5.67	-6
6	-3	-4	-5	-3	-3.5	-4	-4.5	-5	-3.67	-4	-4.33	-4.67	-5	-5.33	-5.67	-6

> This unpredictable healing pattern of the cornea represents the limitation of corneal refractive surgery.

it is best to plan for a 10% to 20 % enhancement rate for lower myopes and even higher rates with high myopes, which will allow retreatment for those patients who regress.

EXCIMER LASER ABLATION NOMOGRAMS FOR PHOTOREFRACTIVE KERATECTOMY

The excimer laser nomograms for LASIK have been developed from the excimer LASIK experience with photorefractive keratectomy (PRK). The concepts of laser pretreatment to prevent central islands as well as multizone ablations to decrease ablation depth and smooth the laser contour evolved as the worldwide PRK experience. In addition, the technological capabilities of excimer lasers increased.

PRETREATMENT PROTOCOLS

Pretreatment protocols have been added to the ablation profiles of the broad beam excimer lasers such as the VISX Star, Summit Omnimed, and Chiron Technolas Keracor 116 to reduce the incidence of postoperative central islands.[1] The VISX Star pretreatment is automatically calculated by the central island factor (CIF) 4.01 software and incorporated into the excimer ablation protocol. Approximately 1 micron per diopter of spherical correction plus an additional 2 microns is added to each ablation protocol and is performed at 2.5 mm. The Chiron Technolas Keracor 116 pretreatment is surgeon programmable. Generally, 1 micron per diopter plus 2 to 4 microns is added to each ablation protocol and is performed at 3 mm.[2] The Summit Omnimed excimer laser has a gaussian beam distribution for which a relatively greater amount of laser energy is produced in the center of the ablation circle, so less pretreatment is required. A pretreatment of 1 to 2 microns per diopter is generally performed using the patient training "A" mode with an optical zone of 2.6 to 2.8 mm. The newer scanning excimer laser systems such as the Chiron Technolas 217 excimer

> Pretreatment protocols have been added to the ablation profiles of the broad beam excimer lasers such as the VISX Star, Summit Omnimed, and Chiron Technolas Keracor 116 to reduce the incidence of postoperative central islands.

laser do not need pretreatment protocols as this phenomena of undertreatment of the central cornea is avoided with these scanning laser systems.

SINGLE AND MULTIZONE ABLATION PROTOCOLS

All excimer laser refractive procedures modify the refracting power of the cornea by altering the anterior corneal curvature by the process of photoablation. The correction of myopia involves the relative flattening of the central cornea compared to the peripheral cornea, which reduces the anterior corneal curvature and hence reduces the refractive power of the treated area. Because the maximal corneal stromal tissue will be photoablated from the central cornea, the thickness of the central cornea becomes important when LASIK is performed for high refractive errors with large ablation depths.

The excimer ablation techniques have evolved. The initial single zone techniques increased from 4 to 6 mm,[3,4] to improve the quality of the postoperative vision and reduce the incidence of halos and regression. The multipass multizone technique was developed by Mihai Pop, MD for the VISX excimer laser[5,6] and the multi-multizone technique was developed by Jeffery J. Machat, MD for the Chiron Technolas excimer laser.[1] These multizone techniques divide the myopic treatment into multiple zones, which decreases the ablation depth and creates a smoother ablation surface. This blending and smoothing effect of the multizone protocols has helped to reduce the incidence of post-PRK regression and haze particularly for the treatment of high myopia.[6]

> This blending and smoothing effect of the multizone protocols has helped to reduce the incidence of post-PRK regression and haze particularly for the treatment of high myopia.

TABLE 5-6.
TLC THE LASER CENTER CHIRON NOMOGRAM

Correction	Pretreat	%	Zone diameter	Ablation	Total
0-3.5		100	6.5		
-3.51-5.5		54.5	6.1		
		45.5	6.6		
-5.75	3.1@3	60	5.5	41.25	
		40	6.6	42	91
-6	-3.15@ 3	60	5.5	43.25	
		40	6.6	43.75	97
-6.5	-3.35@ 3	60	5.5	46.75	
		40	6.6	47.25	104.25
7-	3.5@3	41	5.5	34.5	
		32	6.1	34	
		27	6.6	34.5	114
-7.5	-3.65@3	41	5.5	37	
		32	6.1	36.5	
		27	6.6	36.75	121.75
8-	3.85@3	41	5.5	39.25	
		32	6.1	38.75	
		27	6.6	39.5	129.5
-8.5	-4@3	41	5.5	41.75	
		32	6.1	41.25	
		27	6.6	41.75	137.25
		45	5	37	
		30	6.1	38.25	
		25	6.6	38.75	127
		48	4.5	31.25	
		31	5.5	31.5	
		21	6.5	31.25	106.5
-9	-4.15@3	41	5.5	44.25	
		32	6.1	43.75	
		27	6.6	44.25	145.25
		45	5	39.25	
		30	6.1	41	
		25	6.6	41	134.25
		48	4.5	33.25	
		31	5.5	33.5	
		21	6.5	33.25	113
-9.5	4.25@3	41	5.5	46.75	
		32	6.1	46	
		27	6.6	46.75	153
		45	5	41.75	
		30	6.1	43.25	
		25	6.6	43.25	141.5
		48	4.5	35	
		31	5.5	35.25	
		21	6.5	35.25	119
-10	-4.45@3	45	5	43.5	
		30	6.1	45.5	
		25	6.6	45.5	148.5
		48	4.5	36.75	
		31	5.5	37.25	
		21	6.5	37	125

vision is improved with these new algorithms, the depth of ablation per diopter must increase with the corresponding increase in zone size. This limits the quantity of myopia that can be safely corrected to approximately 15 D in an eye with an average corneal thickness.

Early in our LASIK experience with the Chiron

TABLE 5-6.
TLC THE LASER CENTER CHIRON NOMOGRAM (CONTINUED)

Correction	Pretreat	%	Zone diameter	Ablation	Total
-10.5	-4.6@3	48	4.5	38.75	
		31	5.5	39	
		21	6.5	38.75	131
		40	4	25	
		25	5	25.5	
		19	6.1	30.5	
		16	6.6	30.75	126.25
-11	-4.75@3	48	4.5	40.5	
		31	5.5	41	
		21	6.5	40.75	137.25
		40	4	26	
		25	5	26.75	
		19	6.1	31.75	
		16	6.6	32	131.5
11.5	4.9@3	48	4.5	42.25	
		31	5.5	42.75	
		21	6.5	42.5	143
		40	4	27.25	
		25	5	28	
		19	6.1	33.25	
		16	6.6	33.5	137.5
-12	-4.75@3	48	4.5	44.25	
		31	5.5	44.5	
		21	6.5	44.25	148
		40	4	28.5	
		25	5	29	
		19	6.1	34.75	
		16	6.6	35	142.25
13	-5.1@3	48	4.5	47.75	
		31	5.5	48.25	
		21	6.5	48	160
		40	4	30.75	
		25	5	31.5	
		19	6.1	27.5	
		16	6.6	38	153.75

Technolas 116, we experienced undercorrections. For PRK we used the vertex corrected refraction, however for LASIK we found that the non-vertex corrected refraction produced more accurate results. The surgical technique was modified to allow treatment of the central corneal hydration. Filtered compressed air is applied to the central stroma during pretreatment and for the first 3 seconds of each zone. An additional 3 seconds are applied during the middle of the last zone. By adhering to the partial multizone ablation nomogram and applying these techniques consistently, we have achieved very predictable results.

CHIRON TECHNOLAS 217: PREDICTIVE FORMULAS FOR LASIK

THE KRITZINGER NOMOGRAM

In addition to the nomogram, other factors affect the success of excellent postoperative visual results, such as:
- environmental factors in the operating room (tempera-

ture, humidity, and drafts in the air)
- surgical technique of the surgeon
- preoperative refraction of the patient
- postoperative medication to the patient
- type and make of the laser in use (broad beam/scanning)

General Rules
- Room temperature: 16° to 18°C
- Room humidity: 45% to 50%
- Exact superimposition of red and green HeNe beam is critical to avoid undercorrections.
- Use 6x magnification. Anything larger will cause the surgeon to loose orientation of the visual axis
- Correctly align the patient prior to lifting the flap in order to limit exposure time of stroma before the treatment starts. This will give the surgeon more accurate and consistent visual results.
- Lift the flap with a Colibri. Do not use a balanced salt solution cannula as this may introduce moisture to the bed. Do not use a spatula since foreign material (eg, epithelium) may be introduced into the interface.
- Commence laser treatment and let the assistant press the "enter" key to give continuous treatment without breaks. This will allow the surgeon to make the treatment time and stromal exposure time as short as possible.
- Avoid contact with the stromal bed. Do not wipe while lasering the stroma. This is totally contraindicated because it will give overcorrections with the 217 laser.
- The minimum residual cornea after ablation is 250 microns (excluding flap thickness).
- The ideal treatment zone is 4 to 6 mm.
- It is advisable not to use a zone diameter smaller than 4 mm (night vision glaze) and a zone diameter larger than 6 mm (unnecessary vertex ablation and overcorrections will result).

Kritzinger Nomograms

Myopia
- For treatment of -1 to -13 SE diopters.
- Use *subjective* spectacle correction for minus spheres.
- Add 10% to the sphere and cylinder.
- Subtract or add the calculated cylindrical correction to the calculated spherical correction because -20% *hyperopic* coupling shift with *negative* cylinders on the spherical diopters and -10% *myopic* coupling shift with *plus* cylinders on the spherical diopters.

Hyperopia
- For treatment of +1 to +3 (rarely up to +4) SE diopters.
- Selection of the treatment program of the laser (hyperopia/myopia) is dependent on the sphere and not the cylinder.

- Use subjective spectacle correction.
- Add 15% to sphere and 10% to the cylinder.
- Subtract or add the calculated cylindrical correction to the calculated spherical correction because -20% hyperopic coupling shift with negative cylinders on the spherical diopters and -10% myopic coupling shift with plus cylinders on the spherical diopters.

Information
- Hyperopic treatments regress more than myopic treatments.
- If one has a high plus sphere and any strength minus cylinder, one should do a transposition to a plus cylinder (less tissue ablation, shorter treatment time, less gas consumption).
- Most plus spheres are treated in the plus cylinder prescription, therefore a transposition is often required.

Transposition Method
- If a plus sphere with a minus cylinder transpose, change the axis by 90° (eg, 180° to 90°). The new sphere after transposition is the difference between the sphere and cylinder of the original spectacle correction (eg, +2/-1 x 180° = +1/+1 x 90°).

ADJUSTMENT FACTORS FOR THE REFRACTIVE CORRECTION OF LASIK

Aside from the altitude of the refractive center, patient age is the other commonly considered adjustment factor. Patient age has been used in the past predominantly for radial keratotomy (RK) and astigmatic keratotomy nomograms.[12] Age adjustments have been less consistently applied for LASIK. Since a refractive stability is achieved with LASIK by 3 to 6 months postoperatively, the hyperopic drift that occurs with RK is not a concern with LASIK. Slight overcorrection of .5 D is preferable in patients under the age of 25 years, as the vision will be excellent and a small buffer is created against a future regression of effect. Middle-aged patients (between 25 and 50 years) are best treated with the full refractive correction unless monovision is planned in the nondominant eye. Older patients (< 50 years) are usually best undercorrected by .5 D, as they tend to have a greater response to the excimer ablation and are less tolerant of overcorrections. J. Charles Casebeer, MD has described his nomogram for LASIK based on the dry climate of Arizona[13] (Table 5-7).

SUMMARY

LASIK is a procedure in evolution. While LASIK surgeons originally performed corrections over 20 D,[14] we now limit our corrections to much lower levels of myopia to preserve the integrity of the cornea and the quality of postoperative vision. As

TABLE 5-7.
THE CASEBEER LASIK PERSONAL CALIBRATION NOMOGRAM BASED ON ARIZONA'S DRY CLIMATE

The VISX Star excimer laser was used on patients with myopia and astigmatism. Pretreatment was per the laser program, ablation took place on a dry stromal bed, and there was no intraoperative wiping.

Refraction	20 to 25	26 to 30	31 to 35	36 to 40	>40
-1	-1	-.98	-.95-	.9	-.85
-1.5	-1.5	-1.46	-1.43	-1.35	-1.28
-2	-2	-1.95	-1.9	-1.8	-1.7
-2.0	-2.5	-2.44	-2.38	-2.25	-2.13
-3	-3	-2.93	-2.85	2.7	-2.55
-3.5	-3.33	-3.24	-3.15	-2.98	-2.8
-4	-3.8	-3.7	-3.6	-3.4	-3.2
-4.5	-4.28	-4.16	-4.05	-3.83	-3.6
-5	-4.75	-4.63	-4.5	-4.25	-4
-5.5	-5.23	-5.09	-4.95	-4.68	-4.4
-6	-5.7	-5.55	-5.4	-5.1	-4.8
-6.5	-5.85	-5.69	-5.53	-5.2	-4.88
-7	-6.3	-6.13	-5.95	-5.6	-5.25
-7.5	-6.75	-6.56	-6.38	-6.4	-6
-8.5	-7.65	-7.44	-7.23	-6.8	-6.38
-9	-8.1	-7.88	-7.65	-7.2	-6.75
-9.5	-8.08	-7.84	-7.6	-7.13	-6.65
-10	-8.5	-8.25	-8	-7.5	-7
-10.5	-8.93	-8.66	-8.4	-7.88	-7.35
-11	-9.35	-9.08	-8.8	-8.25	-7.7
-11.5	-9.78	-9.49	-9.2	-8.63	-8.05
-12	-10.2	-9.9	-9.6	-9	-8.4
-12.5	-10.63	-10.31	-10	-9.38	-8.75
-13	-11.05	-10.73	-10.4	-9.75	-9.1
-13.5	-11.48	-11.14	-10.8	-10.13	-9.45
-14	-11.9	-11.55	-11.2	-10.5	-9.8
-14.5	-12.33	-11.96	-11.6	-10.88	-10.15

worldwide LASIK experience increases, the variables affecting our results are being controlled and minimized. However, each year new excimer laser are becoming available that have different ablation nomograms and will, therefore, have some variation in their predictive formulas. A slow conservative initial approach to these innovations will lead to the best results for our patients.

REFERENCES

1. Machat JJ. PRK complications and their management. In: Machat JJ (ed). *Excimer Laser Refractive Surgery.* SLACK Incorporated: Thorofare, NJ; 1996.

2. Machat JJ. LASIK procedure. In: Machat JJ (ed). *Excimer Laser Refractive Surgery.* SLACK Incorporated: Thorofare, NJ; 1996.

3. Gartry DS, Kerr Muir MG, Marshall J. Photorefractive keratectomy with an argon fluoride excimer laser: a clinical study. *J Refract Corneal Surg.* 1991;7:420-435.

4. Talley AR, Hardten DR, Sher NA, et al. Results 1 year after using the 193-nm excimer laser for photorefractive keratectomy in mild to moderate myopia. *Am J Ophthalmol.* 1994;118:304-311.

5. Pop M, Aras M. Multizone/multipass photorefractive keratectomy: 6-month results. *J Cataract Refract Surg.* 1995;21:633-643.

6. Pop M. The multipass/multizone PRK technique to correct myopia and astigmatism. In: Machat JJ (ed). *Excimer Laser Refractive Surgery.* SLACK Incorporated: Thorofare, NJ; 1996.

7. Alpins NA, Taylor HR, Kent DG, Lu Y, et al. Three Multizone photorefractive keratectomy algorithms for myopia. *J Refract Surg.* 1997;13:535-544.

8. Munnerlyn CR, Koons SJ, Marshall J. Photorefractive keratectomy: a technique for laser refractive surgery. *Journal of Refractive Surgery.* 1988;14:46-52.

9. Emara B, Probst LE, Tingey D, et al. Correlation of intraocular pressure and corneal thickness in normal myopic eyes and following LASIK. *J Cataract Refract Surg.* 1997. In press.

10. Probst LE, Machat JJ. The mathematics of LASIK for high myopia. *J Cataract Refract Surg.* 1997. In press.

11. Probst LE, Machat JJ. LASIK enhancements techniques and results. In: Buratto L (ed). *LASIK Principles and Techniques.* SLACK Incorporated: Thorofare, NJ; 1997:325-338.

12. Committee on Ophthalmic Procedures Assessment. American Academy of Ophthalmology. Radial keratotomy for myopia. *Ophthalmology.* 1993;100(7):1103-1115.

13. Casebeer JC. A systemized approach to LASIK. In: Buratto L (ed). *LASIK Principles and Techniques.* SLACK Incorporated: Thorofare, NJ; 1997:225-228.

14. Salah T, Waring GO III, Maghraby AE, Moadel K, Grimm SB. Excimer laser in situ keratomileusis under the flap for myopia of 2 to 20 diopters. *Am J Ophthalmol.* 1996;121:143-155.

Personalized LASIK Nomogram Development

John F. Doane, MD

The impetus of this chapter is to describe to the beginning surgeon, and possibly the experienced laser refractive surgeon, the importance of understanding the specific laser and software in use, the laser room environment, and the surgeon's technique, because this will determine the refractive success and the patient's postoperative satisfaction. It is the hope of the author that experience from surgical results of six different excimer laser manufacturers, nine different laser models, and innumerable software versions for the treatment of myopia, hyperopia, astigmatism, presbyopia, asymmetric ablations, and customized specialty ablations will engender respect for the vast complexity of available systems as well as the understanding to provide the beginning laser/laser in situ keratomileusis (LASIK) practitioner with a basis for rational surgical decision-making.

INTRAOCULAR LENS "A-CONSTANT" VERSUS EXCIMER LASER ALGORITHM

As ophthalmic surgeons practicing at the turn of a new millennium, we are extremely fortunate to be able to use advanced intraocular lens (IOL) formulas for performing small-incision phacoemulsification and IOL placement. In a typical case, excellent refractive results can be obtained by a either a novice or an experienced surgeon. How is this possible? Doesn't experience matter? Yes experience matters, but at this point, lens implantation procedures are highly mature because well-defined "A-constants" for each commercially available lens have been determined. Once the A-constant is obtained, all other things being equal, the expe-

rience of and better yet the individual surgeon is taken out of the equation. (At this point, the highly experienced and opinionated surgeon may say, "hearsay," and move on to the next chapter of this text. I encourage you to read on for an explanation.)

Let us propose that the average patient with average keratometry values and axial length measurements is examined by an expert technician who will share his or her findings with an experienced and novice surgeon. If the technician obtains high quality, repeatable keratometry and axial length values and subsequently enters this data into a modern IOL formula to be used by the two surgeons, the lens calculated for emmetropia would be identical. If we then assume a standard cataract procedure is performed with IOL placement in the capsular bag after uncomplicated continuous curvilinear capsulorhexis, the refractive effect should be identical for the two surgeons. Why is this? The same IOL placed in the given eye will achieve identical results since it is a fixed optic placed at the same location (within the capsular bag) by both surgeons. With IOL placement in small-incision cataract surgery wound healing is not a major factor in surgical results. Hence, the A-constant is an invaluable reference number to provide transferable refractive predictability and accuracy to any surgeon who selects a given lens model. We will see with laser refractive surgery (photorefractive keratectomy [PRK] or LASIK) that an A-constant or laser algorithm does not necessarily predict excellent refractive results.

Excimer lasers are not manufactured or shipped with an A-constant per se, but they are built and tested with a manufacturer-supplied algorithm. An algorithm is similar, but not synonymous, to a tool familiar to radial keratotomy surgeons—the nomogram. In incisional keratotomy surgery, the surgical plan (number, length, and depth of incisions) is based on the patient's age, degree of ametropia, sex, and other factors. The original design of excimer laser algorithms dictated that a given degree of refractive error with a specified number of pulses at selected ablation diameters would be applied to the cornea. The algorithm is provided to the laser as a software package that is typically encoded on the central processing unit's hard drive or, less commonly, by an optical reader. The algorithm is unique to a given laser model from the specific manufacturer. The algorithm can be different for the same model from a manufacturer if different software versions are downloaded onto the hard drive.

If we are dealing with a singular patient with, for example, 4 diopters (D) of spherical myopia, why then would the algorithm between laser models or manufacturers have to be different? There are two main reasons: the beam delivery system and the beam fluence. There is a wide variation in beam delivery systems available for use. Large area ablation single-zone systems are available that have different maximum treatment zones from 4.5, 5, 5.5, 6, 6.5, 7 mm. All systems with maximal treatment zones below 6 mm have been discontinued due to significant visual symptoms, such as halos, glare, starbursts, and difficulty with nighttime driving.

With varying maximal treatment zone diameters there will obviously be a different number of pulses required for any given refractive error. Multizone software for large area ablation lasers is also available for use. For a given refractive error using the same laser, multizone software will dictate fewer pulses than single zone software since the purpose of multizone software, in theory, is to remove less corneal tissue. As with single zone software, when the maximal ablation diameter is altered, the overall number of pulses will vary. The functional optical zone obtained generally tends to be smaller for multizone software than single zone software. This becomes important when treating highly myopic refractive errors, since scotopic visual function will be hindered by unwanted optical effects like halos and glare because the functional optical zone will be a smaller diameter than that tolerated by the larger scotopic entrance pupil.

With scanning laser technology (spot or slit), a completely different approach is taken to achieve the same refractive result. With a smaller area of tissue exposed to the incident beam per pulse, a significantly larger number of pulses would have to be applied to the corneal surface for the aforementioned 4 D myopic eye. As with the two previous examples, the maximal ablation zone diameter can be changed and commensurate adjustments of the number of pulses applied will have to be made.

To this point, only spherical myopia has been discussed. With the treatment of myopic astigmatism, hyperopia, hyperopic astigmatism, bifocal presbyopic ablations, and asymmetric ablations, the variance in pulse number, laser beam aperture size, and orientation becomes exponential.

Excimer laser beam fluence is defined as the amount of energy per pulse that is distributed over a defined area (mJoules/cm^2). The laser fluence will determine the overall number of pulses for removing a specific micron thickness of tissue to affect a given refractive error. Two different beam profile characteristics (Guassian [greater energy density centrally than peripherally] versus table top [relatively even energy distribution across the ablation zone diameter]) have been described for excimer lasers. It should also be realized that excimer lasers are not static instruments but ever-fluctuating energy sources. This fact requires frequent calibration so the laser energy is released in a controlled fashion. If different fluences exist between lasers, then differing amounts of tissue will be removed per pulse. It is then clear that with differing fluence between lasers (Table 6-1)[1] the algorithms for specific refractive errors will be quite different.

It is clear that production of excimer lasers and software design can be highly variable among different manufacturers. There are additional variables that need to be considered when evaluating the overall performance of a given laser. These include inter-model performance variation, laser room environment, geographic profile of the laser center, and surgeon technique.

The performance comparison of lasers within the same manufacturer model number is not always identical. To the beginning surgeon this is probably another confusing and confounding factor. Why would a laser within the same model not perform the same as a colleague's? There may be true variation among lasers of the same model despite the engineer's and design team's best efforts and consistent instrument set-up and calibration. This variation should not be overly concerning since, as discussed later, the surgeon must define the laser performance to obtain the best surgical outcomes.

> **The performance comparison of lasers within the same manufacturer model number is not always identical.**

Maintenance of the laser room environment is critical for laser refractive surgery success. It is critical not only for performing surgery but also for proper laser maintenance. All laser manufacturers recommend that certain conditions be maintained for optimal laser performance. The laser room should be a closed environment rather than a multipurpose room with open access. Temperature should be controlled between 18° to 24°C, humidity maintained between 30% to 50%, and low particulate matter filtration should be maintained 24 hours per day, 7 days per week. This is done to provide each treatment session with a consistent environment since laser ablation rates are highly dependent on atmosphere from the optical train to the corneal surface. Additionally, maintaining these variables creates the most favorable environment to increase the longevity of the optics within the laser. For instance, if high particulate matter is present in the laser room it can coat the lenses within the optical train. When the laser is used next, the particulate matter can be "burned" into the lens as an imperfection, which will subsequently decrease the homogeneity (pattern of energy distribution across the ablation zone) of the laser ablation. If this becomes a chronic situation, the life span of individual optics will be reduced leading to increased laser operation costs. Even more importantly, it could lead to a poor ablation pattern on the cornea with possible visual morbidity. Perfumes, deodorants, scents, alcohol, and other combustible liquid vapors should be prohibited in the laser room since they will coat the lens and potentially effect the same change as particulate matter.

Geography also plays a role in laser performance. The relative humidity and altitude will cause variation in laser performance. On average, a high humidity, sea-level locale will realize less refractive effect than the same treatment entered into the laser at a low humidity, high altitude locale.

Temperature should be controlled between 18° to 24°C, humidity maintained between 30% to 50%, and low particulate matter filtration should be maintained 24 hours per day, 7 days per week.

BUILDING THE NOMOGRAM

Success with LASIK is intimately dependent on two important factors: obtaining an excellent keratectomy and performing an accurate ablation. It has been quoted that LASIK is 90% keratectomy and 10% laser. I have termed this the "novice surgeon mentality." It has also been my observation that there is a patient viewpoint on this topic. A patient is interested in 100% keratectomy success followed by a 100% successful laser ablation. With experience, I believe that the surgeon's viewpoint also changes. As he or she becomes comfortable performing the keratectomy, about 5% of his or her time is spent contemplating and performing the keratectomy, and 95% of the effort is spent making certain the laser is operating properly and no human errors have been made by the surgical team. The experienced surgeon's success then comes from having a highly predictable nomogram that has been customized to the laser environment and surgical technique. Without a surgeon's customized approach to a LASIK nomogram, haphazard surgery will likely be performed with less than excellent outcomes. One would perform equally well if this approach is taken doing haphazard incisional keratotomy, or automated lamellar keratoplasty (ALK) or any refractive surgical technique. With this being conceptually understood, this section will describe the process by which a surgical team

TABLE 6-1.
EXCIMER LASER FLUENCE LEVELS

Laser manufacturer	Fluence (energy distribution)
VISX Star	160
Summit SVS Apex Plus	180
Technolas 217	120
Schwind Keratom	< 250
Nidek EC-5000	130
Aesculap-Meditec MEL 60	250
Laser Sight Compak 200	160-300
Autonomous	130
Kera Technology IsoBeam	150
Novatec LightBlade (nonexcimer)	150

approaches the task of delivering accurate and reproducible results.

The process of developing a LASIK nomogram requires four steps: obtaining patient data, formulating an initial nomogram, entering data into the laser's computer and evaluating data and outcomes, and making adjustments based on this information. At first glance, obtaining patient refractive data seems mundane and not necessarily where the action is. This is a grave error in refractive surgery, especially LASIK. LASIK is incredibly powerful. The laser will ablate whatever is entered into the treatment plan. If inaccurate refractive data is entered, the difference between true refraction and that obtained will be the residual refractive error.

The process of developing a LASIK nomogram requires four steps: obtaining patient data, formulating an initial nomogram, entering data into the laser's computer and evaluating data and outcomes, and making adjustments based on this information.

It is very important to complete several basic refraction principles. For eyes with greater than 5 D of refractive error, it is important to have proper vertexing to the spectacle plane (12.5 mm) if this is the convention entered into the laser. This can be completed with trial frame glasses. Significant error in refraction outcome can be realized if patients with large refractive errors are refracted at a spectacle plane vertex distance and data is entered at the corneal plane. Fogging techniques should be completed so the least amount of myopia to see the best spectacle-corrected line of vision is the refractive endpoint. This minimizes iatrogenic causes for overcorrection. Cycloplegic refraction can also be done to confirm the fogged manifest refraction. Comparison to past or recent refractions should be noted. If large discrepancies are noted, concern for examination error or refraction instability should be considered. For patients wearing contact lenses, special consideration should be given in obtaining this data. Soft contacts should be removed at least 3 days prior to examination, and computerized videokeratography should be obtained to rule out corneal warpage. Rigid contact lenses should be removed at least 3 weeks prior to examination, and stability should be noted from two separate examinations 3 days apart. Likewise, topography should be obtained to rule out abnormalities.

The initial nomogram used should be based upon available data and not a "shot in the dark" approach. The novice surgeon should utilize all available information to decide on his or her initial surgeon factor adjustments to the laser algorithm. Knowledge of the specific laser's performance with PRK should be taken into consideration. If the laser is overcorrecting long-term with PRK, one can anticipate it doing the same with LASIK. If the laser is undercorrecting long-term with PRK, it can also be assumed that undercorrection will be obtained with LASIK. The difference between what is entered into the laser and that obtained is typically a set percentage difference at all levels of refractive error. Therefore, the individual surgeon should increase or decrease the planned treatment by a set percentage from the manufacturers' algorithm to achieve the target postoperative refraction.

Entering data into the computer ostensibly seems to be the easiest step in laser refractive procedures, but this is not always the case. Typing errors on the computer keyboard, incorrect cylinder convention or vertex distance entry, and incorrect cylinder axis entry are just a few potential errors that can lead to poor outcomes. Calculation of the treatment to be entered into the laser should be checked multiple times by more than one member of the surgical team. If the treatment entered differs from the manifest refraction, and certainly if a percentage difference must be made for the treatment entered, simple math errors can occur with even the most competent person. Hence, multiple calculations and checks should be made for each entry. Is the correct patient chart being used for the next patient to be treated? Is data for the correct eye being entered? Is monovision being treated for the eye? These are but a few of the questions that need to be answered for each data entry. The convention by which data is obtained and entered into the laser should be consistent (Table 6-2). For example, if refractions are done in plus cylinder convention they should be entered in plus cylinder. Transposition errors can occur, so if the surgical team can completely avoid this step, it is advisable. It is extremely important to check the axis and the cylinder convention on each case. Minus cylinder can be entered when the patient was actually refracted in plus cylinder; subsequently, the surgeon will induce cylinder on the patient's cornea. Proper vertex distance entry should also be made. When treating myopia, if the patient is refracted at a 12.5-mm vertex distance and the data is entered at corneal plane, a percentile overcorrection will occur or vice versa. This will be more significant the higher the refractive error treated and may lead to visual morbidity in some cases. In summary, it is extremely important to use a single cylinder con-

---

TABLE 6-2.
TREATMENT CALCULATIONS

Line 1:	Refraction	-6 D
Line 2:	Target	-1 D
Line 3:	Line 1 - 2	-6 - -1 = -5
Line 4:	Multiply surgeon factor* by line 3 and add or subtract as indicated by the specific laser used	-6 – (.1 x –6) = -6 - -.6 = -5.4 D
Line 5:	Number entered as treatment	-5.4 D

Addition or subtraction will depend on if the specific laser is undercorrecting or overcorrecting in relation to what the algorithm suggests. In the above example, the laser is overcorrecting compared to the algorithm, so a set percentage is taken away from the spherical treatment.

---

vention and enter data the same every time at the same vertex distance. Multiple checks of the calculated entry should be made by more than one person on the surgical team. No member of the refractive surgery team should feel intimidated to announce they have noted an error that can be corrected prior to patient treatment at whatever stage of the process the error is found. Overbearing egos should be avoided in the treatment of refractive surgery patients. They will be a hindrance to the patient's best care as well as to the correction of avoidable human errors.

TECHNIQUE CONSIDERATIONS

After the keratectomy is completed, the actual ablation becomes the key factor and the surgeon's defining act in determining the treatment nomogram. The time it takes to initiate and complete the ablation and the management of the stromal bed during the ablation will determine the amount of dry stroma removed to affect refractive change. The drier the bed during the ablation, the more dry weight corneal stromal tissue that will be removed.[2] Ablation technique can encompass anything from initiating the ablation and completing the pulse count without interruption to stopping at selected intervals to dry the stromal bed with a cellulose sponge or metal spatula, or alternatively wiping the stromal bed only on the appearance of condensation on the stromal bed surface.

How does this affect refractive outcomes and dry corneal tissue removal? The drier the stroma, the more dry weight tissue that will be removed for the same number of pulses, and likewise, the wetter the stromal bed, less dry weight tissue will be removed for the same number of pulses. Therefore, on average, less refractive change than with

The drier the bed during the ablation, the more dry weight corneal stromal tissue that will be removed.

"dry ablation" will be obtained. This technique nuance is the reason each surgeon must define his or her own nomogram since surgeons using the same laser but markedly different technique will obtain completely different surgical outcomes if they enter the same treatment plan for an identical preoperative refraction. For each individual surgeon, the lesson to be learned from this discussion is consistency in technique. Consistent time to lift, initiate and complete a case should be a goal, as should the frequency of wiping (every 50 or 100 pulses, etc). If one elects to have forced air passed over the stromal bed during the ablation, be sure it is done consistently. Two surgeons using the same laser but markedly different ablation techniques can achieve equal results as long as they both understand the tissue effects of their technique and employ their technique in a consistent fashion.

LASIK NOMOGRAM REFINEMENT

LASIK nomogram refinement begins immediately in the postoperative course. Refraction data should be obtained at each postoperative visit. Quality improvement requires evaluation of the postoperative data with adjustment of the nomogram based on this data. Not obtaining and utilizing postoperative data for improving the individual surgeon's results is as logical as not obtaining a refraction or topography prior to surgery. It is a necessity for the surgeon to provide optimal care and refractive outcomes. Refractive and topographic stability is obtained by virtually every patient by the 3-month examination. It is this data that should guide precise refinement of the individual surgeon's nomogram. The surgeon's nomogram becomes more powerful with the more eyes treated at any given level of ametropia and with the more postoperative data that is obtained.

SPHERICAL EFFECTS OF ASTIGMATIC ABLATION

It is important to recognize possible spherical refractive effects of astigmatic correction with the particular laser a surgeon uses. Most excimer lasers, when treating myopic astigmatism, operate under minus cylinder convention. The author has noted in all systems used to date (large area ablation or scanning spot lasers) that for each diopter of cylinder ablated, approximately .1 D to .2 D of overall central corneal flattening will occur, which leads to small amounts of hyperopia. If this is not accounted for by reduction of the spherical ablation plan, unwanted hyperopia may be noted postoperatively. Postoperative refractive data will help the surgeon identify this possibility and be a basis to identify the exact correction for each diopter of cylinder ablated.

In conclusion, LASIK nomogram development is an individual process in which every surgeon is, in essence, an island. There are three important elements in the equation: the laser, the laser room environment, and the surgeon's technique. The excimer laser beam is not a static force but an ever-changing one. Likewise, laser refractive surgery is not a static process and requires the practitioner to be an active flexible participant in the process. The process requires ongoing data acquisition, assimilation, and refinement to provide the highest quality postoperative vision that patients are entitled to and demand in this era of laser refractive surgery.

REFERENCES

1. McDonald MB, Doubrava MW. New developments in excimer laser. In: Pallikaris IG and Siganos DS, eds. *LASIK*. SLACK Incorporated: Thorofare, NJ; 1997:8-11.
2. Dougherty PJ, Wellish KL, Maloney RK. Excimer laser ablation rate and corneal hydration. *Am J Ophthalmol*. 1994;118:169-76.

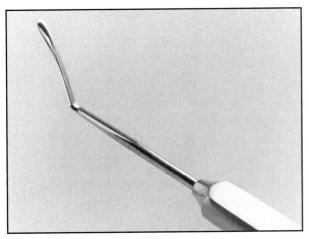

Figure 7-11. Slade retreatment spatula (ASICO AE-2832).

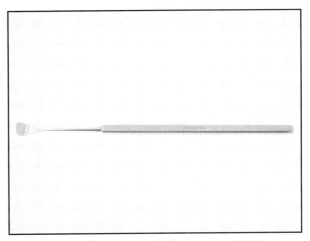

Figure 7-12. Probst tape spatula (ASICO AE-2565).

Excimer lasers such as the Chiron Technolas 116 scan outside the ablation zone during the treatment of the astigmatism, necessitating protection of the flap during this phase of the ablation.

protection of the flap during this phase of the ablation.

Machat has designed the Machat Retreatment Spatula (Figure 7-10) that has a semi-sharp angulated tip at one end to lift the LASIK flap edge along the cut edge of Bowman's layer. The short, fine tip of this instrument allows for a localized dissection along Bowman's layer without excessive insertion of the instrument underneath the flap, which could result in displacement of epithelial cells and postoperative epithelial ingrowth. A fine spatula at the other end will allow dissection of any central interface adhesions as well as allow easy repositioning of the flap. The Slade retreatment spatula (Figure 7-11) has semi-sharp edges to effectively lift the flap and separate the epithelium.

Probst has designed the Probst tape spatula (Figure 7-12) to tuck the surgical drape/tape painlessly into the fornices so that there is maximum exposure of the globe along with isolation of the intrapalpebral opening from the eyelashes and the meibomian gland orifices.

LASIK IRRIGATION CANNULAS

These irrigation devices are used to irrigate under the flap after the excimer ablation to remove any interface debris and refloat the corneal flap into the correct location. If this step is not performed, interface debris will frequently be observed underneath the corneal flap. The debris does not affect the visual performance of the eye, however it greatly diminishes the slit lamp appearance of the post-LASIK cornea, which can cause concern for co-managing doctors. Perfect repositioning of the flap is almost always possible by refloating the flap after LASIK. Surgeons

should be aware, however, that excessive irrigation (greater than 10 seconds) under the flap will decrease the flap adherence and increase the chances of flap movement or dislocation after LASIK. The irrigation cannula can be attached to a filter, such as the 0.22-Micron Hydrophilic Sterile Filter (Oasis), so that any foreign material is filtered prior to irrigation under the flap.

Kritzinger has developed an irrigating needle (Storz) that contains multiple openings on its tip to direct the irrigating fluid diffusely underneath the cap. The Slade LASIK cannula (ASICO) is a 26-gauge cannula with a spatulated tip to allow easy insertion beneath the flap so that irrigation is performed in a closed system. The Buratto LASIK cannula (ASICO) has a 25-gauge flat tip to allow for easy entry under the flap. Three exit ports at the front, left, and right sides of the tip allow for effective diffuse irrigation under the flap. The Ku irrigation cannula is designed to be connected to the balanced salt solution (BSS) bottle and provide controlled continuous flow beneath the flap.

Irrigation devices are used to irrigate under the flap after the excimer ablation to remove any interface debris and refloat the corneal flap into the correct location.

OTHER INSTRUMENTS

An antidesiccation chamber (Figure 7-13) should be available in order to address the potential complication of a free flap. The free flap or cap should be placed epithelial side down on a few drops of BSS solution to preserve the integrity of the epithelium. No BSS solution should be placed on the stromal side of the free flap, as this will result in stromal hydration and make adhesion to the stromal bed extremely difficult. Since the occurrence of a free flap is no longer a planned event with LASIK, the surgeon must decide whether the situation is appropriate to continue with

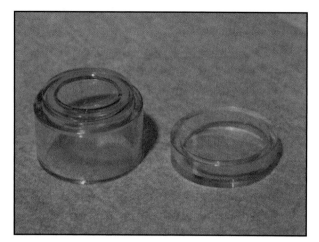

Figure 7-13. An antidesiccation chamber.

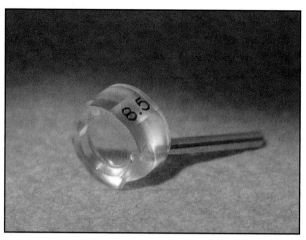

Figure 7-14. Applanation lens used to measure 8.5 mm.

the excimer laser ablation. If there is any doubt about the integrity of the flap, it is best replaced without any correction and the refractive procedure repeated in 3 months.

With the development of a single-piece LASIK suction ring to give a maximal diameter flap, it is no longer necessary to use an applanation lens (Figure 7-14), as one is assured of obtaining the largest possible flap. This can be useful, on rare occasions, to allow the surgeon to estimate the size of the flap that will be produced.

> If there is any doubt about the integrity of the flap, the flap is best replaced without any correction and the refractive procedure repeated in 3 months.

CHAPTER 8

Microkeratomes

John F. Doane, MD
Stephen G. Slade, MD

With the introduction of laser in situ keratomileusis (LASIK) there has been tremendous interest on the part of surgeons and other industry professionals to bring forth a microkeratome that offers the highest quality, predictability, repeatability, and ease of use. In theory, a microkeratome designed for LASIK should give the surgeon access to the corneal stroma in order to apply laser energy to remove corneal tissue and effect a refractive change. There are many variations on this theme. In fact, laser technology has taken this idea one step further to completely do away with microkeratomes by creating a corneal flap using intrastromal lasers. Since necessity is the mother of invention, one is led to believe that with the tremendous activity in the microkeratome industry, a better product can be designed. This chapter will describe the early history of microkeratome development, discuss goals of microkeratome design and evaluation, and list technical attributes of individual devices.

HISTORY

Corneal lamellar refractive keratoplasty has its roots in the work of Dr. Jose Ignacio Barraquer beginning in 1949 in Bogota, Colombia.[1-5] Barraquer developed freeze keratomileusis, which used two instruments he designed—a manually driven microkeratome (Figure 8-1) and the cryolathe (Figure 8-2)—to reshape the cornea and alter its refractive power. Barraquer's technique involved resecting a 300 micron lamellar disc of corneal tissue, staining it with Chiton green dye for easier handling (Figure 8-3), placing it on the cryolathe freezing block, sculpting or reshaping the stromal surface with dictates entered into the computer (Figures 8-4 and 8-5), and then suturing it back into position (Figure 8-6). This technique did not prove to be applicable to a large number of surgeons due to the difficulty in mastering the manual microkeratome and the complexity of the cryolathe.[6,7]

In an attempt to avoid the side effects of tissue processing seen with the cryolathe, the Barraquer-Krumeich-Swinger (BKS) nonfreezing system was developed. In this technique, after a keratectomy was performed to obtain a corneal disc of tissue, the corneal cap was inverted (epithelial side down) over a formed suction die (Figure 8-7). Once in place, a second pass of the microkeratome was made to remove tissue centrally for myopia and peripherally for hyperopia[8] (Figures 8-8 and 8-9). This technique did not gain widespread acceptance because of the complexity of the system as well as the inaccurate results of a manual keratectomy by the majority of surgeons attempting the procedure. It did, however, lead researchers to investigate the damage present in corneal tissue after freezing and to demonstrate the clinical advantage of rapid healing when corneal tissue is not heavily processed.[9-12]

The next advance in microkeratome development again occurred in Bogota, Colombia. Barraquer and Luis Antonio Ruiz felt the next direction to explore was keratomileusis in situ. This technique involved two passes of the microkeratome over the cornea: the first to remove a planar cap of tissue and the second to perform the refractive cut, which was based on the planned correction. Importantly, there was no processing of tissue so these unwanted effects could be avoided. Initially, they used a manual microkeratome, as did

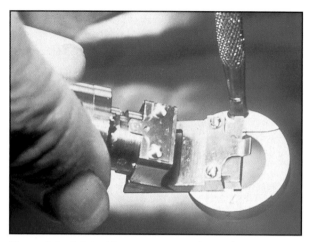

Figure 8-1. Original Barraquer manual microkeratome on a suction ring.

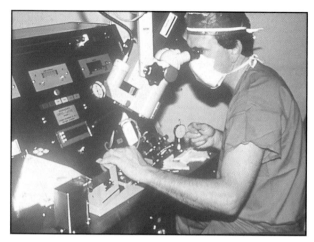

Figure 8-2. Cryolathe used in freeze myopic keratomileusis.

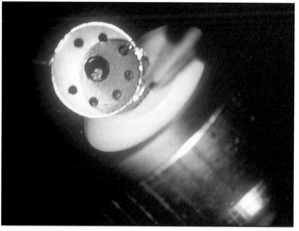

Figure 8-3. Chiton green stained corneal disc being transferred to the cryolathe cutting block on a corneal spatula.

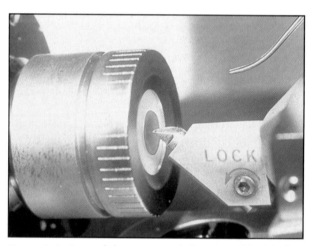

Figure 8-4. Corneal disc on a cryolathe cutting block before shaping.

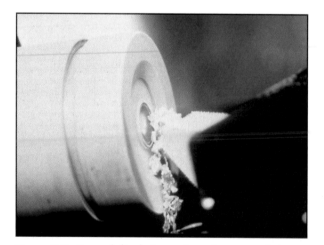

Figure 8-5. Corneal disc being reshaped on a cryolathe.

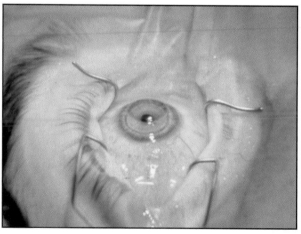

Figure 8-6. Disc reposited to the corneal bed in preparation for suturing.

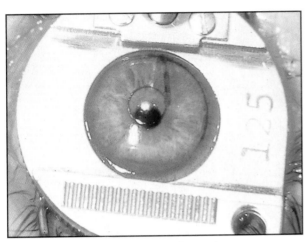

Figure 8-12. Automated Corneal Shaper three-piece suction ring over an ink-marked cornea. Note the geared track on the suction ring that accepts gearing on the microkeratome body for automated advancement of the keratome.

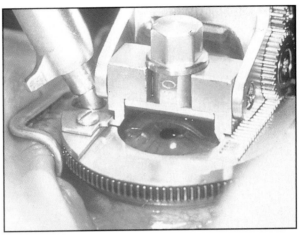

Figure 8-13. Automated Corneal Shaper microkeratome head advancing over the suction ring, which has been applied to the corneal surface.

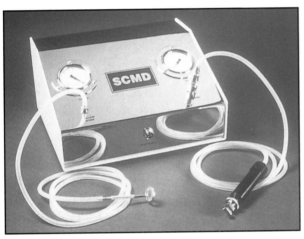

Figure 8-14. TurboKeratome by Visionaerie, Inc, includes a microkeratome, suction ring, and module.

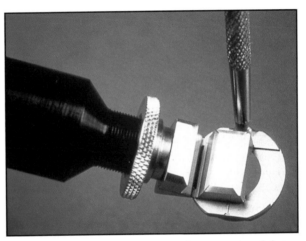

Figure 8-15. TurboKeratome microkeratome head being inserted into the suction ring.

ed one-piece head that can be ordered to obtain a variety of flap thicknesses. It utilizes a bifaceted metal blade with a 22.5° angulation that oscillates at 14,000 cycles per minute via a nitrogen gas turbine. The unit comes with multiple suction rings depending on the diameter of keratectomy desired, which ranges from 6 to 10 mm. The keratome is advanced manually across the cornea by the surgeon, who does not have direct view of the operating field. The orientation of the hinge can be varied by the surgeon's placement of the suction ring. The system is sterilizable.

MICROPRECISION MICROLAMELLAR KERATOMILEUSIS SYSTEM

This device is distributed by Eye Technology, Inc of Saint Paul, Minn, USA (Figure 8-17 and 8-18). The system features a patented adjustable plate that allows for a range of lamellar resections from 0 to 466 microns in 1 micron

increments. A micrometer handle is attached to the adjustable plate and provides for calibration and verification of desired thickness. This unit also comes with multiple suction rings that allow for varying diameter flaps (7.5 to 8.5). The manufacturer also has an adjustable ring under development. The suction rings and microkeratome head have dual dove-tail rail systems, which the manufacturer states causes less jumping and chatter marks in the stroma, leading to a smoother keratectomy bed surface (Figures 8-19a and 8-19b). The unit includes a "stop pin" system, which helps create a hinged flap. The hinge can be oriented in any direction. A bifaceted steel blade is used and angulated 9°. The blade drive moves sideways with 20,000 oscillations per minute. The blade drive is powered by a pneumatic turbine, which the manufacturer states has six times the torque of electric motors. The microkeratome has no gears and is manually advanced by the surgeon. The system is sterilizable.

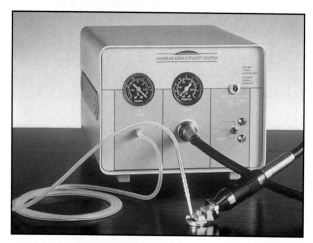

Figure 8-16. Lamellar keratoplasty system (Plancon/Moria) displaying a power module, suction ring, and microkeratome head on a handpiece.

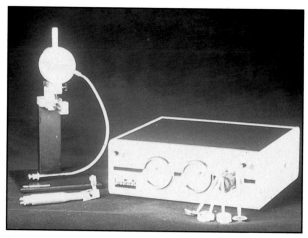

Figure 8-17. MicroPrecision's microlamellar keratome system tissue thickness gauge, microkeratome, power source, applanation lenses, and suction rings.

UNIVERSAL KERATOME

This unit is manufactured and distributed by Phoenix Keratek, Inc of Scottsdale, Ariz, USA (Figure 8-20). This microkeratome comes as a single unit with no handled suction rings (Figure 8-21). The system is unique in that it has customized polymethylmethacrylate optical inserts (Figure 8-22) that can be used to achieve a planar disc of tissue with subsequent ablation with an excimer laser with the LASIK technique. Lenticular inserts can also be used for a lenticular resection of tissue in the keratomileusis in situ—automated technique. The manufacturer asserts that with the lenticular inserts myopia, hyperopia, and astigmatism can be treated with this mechanical device. A unifaceted metal blade is used and oscillates at 14,000 cycles per minute and has 0° angulation. The device can be calibrated to create a hinge in the flap. Flap thickness is typically set at 160 microns for LASIK, but it can be set from 1 to 500 microns thick. The flap diameter can be varied from 3 to 10 mm. The surgeon has direct view of the surgical field through the optical inserts but is unable to check the intraocular pressure (IOP) immediately before the passage of the blade. This device is automatically advanced with an electrical motor drive at a rate of .75 mm/second. The microkeratome can not be sterilized, but the blade and optical inserts can be autoclaved or chemically sterilized.

FLAPMAKER DISPOSABLE MICROKERATOME

This unit was first displayed in October 1996 by Refractive Technologies of Cleveland, Ohio, USA. This device is completely disposable and requires no assembly; it is also sterilizable and no cleaning or maintenance is necessary. The unit is gearless. It is driven by flexible shafts powered from a control module that reportedly provides uniform motion of the microkeratome with blade oscillation at 12,500 cycles per minute. The unit is made of clear acrylic and enables the surgeon to directly visualize the

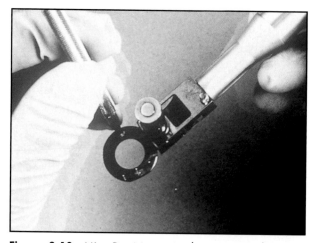

Figure 8-18. MicroPrecision microkeratome and suction ring. Note the thumb screw on top of the microkeratome that can be adjusted to determine lamellar resection thickness.

operation (per the manufacturer). The FLAPmaker is purchased with a fixed preset resection depth, but a variety of choices are available to the surgeon. The surgeon is able to control flap diameter from 9.5 to 10.5 mm and can adjust for hinge creation.

SCHWIND MICROKERATOM

This device is made by Herbert Schwind Gimble & Co of Germany. It comes as a single microkeratome unit (Figure 8-23) with an accompanying power module (Figure 8-24) and foot controls. This device has an electric motor system with drive cables that connect to the microkeratome head for advance and return of the cutting blade. The vacuum system consists of two suction rings. One is for stabilizing the microkeratome to the globe and the other is for stabilizing the cap/flap during the incision (Figure 8-25). The surgeon has a direct view of the procedure through an optically flat quartz window. The system is unique in that it has

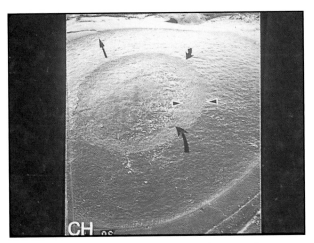

Figure 8-19a. Comparative scanning electron microscopy. Chiron Vision, Inc Automatic Corneal Shaper immediately following ALK for a myopia procedure of a donor eye showing a primary keratectomy border (straight solid arrow) and a second keratectomy border (solid curved arrow) at 25x.

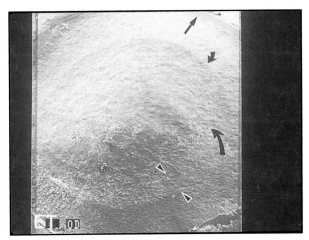

Figure 8-19b. Eye Technology, Inc microlamellar keratome system on a donor eye showing a primary keratectomy border (straight solid arrow) and a secondary keratectomy border (solid curved arrow) at 25x.

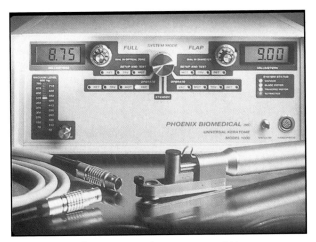

Figure 8-20. Phoenix Keratek, Inc Universal Keratome.

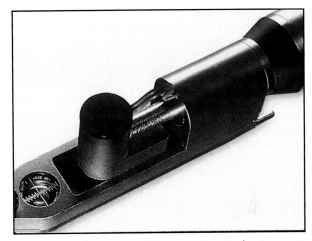

Figure 8-21. The Universal Keratome is a single-piece unit. Note the optical insert with a calibrated surface.

a sapphire blade that can be reused for several hundred cases (Figure 8-26). The blade cuts parallel to the quartz window to a fixed 150-micron depth with an oscillation rate of up to 4000 cycles per minute. The translation rate is 1.3 mm/second in the forward direction and 3 mm/second in the return direction. The keratectomy is made at 0° angulation. A shallow cavity that is precisely 9 mm in diameter is provided around the upper suction ring, and the upper surface of the cornea is sucked into it. No disassembly or reassembly of the eye module is required between cases. An automatic cleaning procedure allows thorough cleaning of the assembly between cases before sterilization. The entire assembly may be steam sterilized or autoclaved.

CLEAR CORNEAL MOLDER MICROKERATOME

Drs. Ednei Nascimento and Ricardo Guimaraes of Brazil developed this device for use in LASIK. The patent

rights for this device have been transferred to the Loktal Company of Brazil. Reportedly, the surgeon has wide-ranging control of flap diameter and incision depth. Surgeon visualization is permitted through a clear plastic platform. The drive source can be manual or automated. Blade angulation is set at 0°. In addition to being used in the LASIK technique, the system's cutting mechanism enables surgeons to perform convex or concave keratectomies of any dimension, so keratomileusis in situ—manual or automated—can be performed.

BARRAQUER/CARRIAZO MICROKERATOME

Dr. Cesar Carriazo, working at the Barraquer Institute of America in Bogota, Colombia with recommendations from Barraquer himself, has developed a yet-to-be-released geared automated microkeratome. The microkeratome head is slightly smaller than the Ruiz-designed microkeratome,

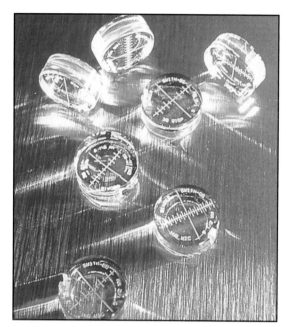

Figure 8-22. Universal Keratome polymethylmethacrylate optical inserts.

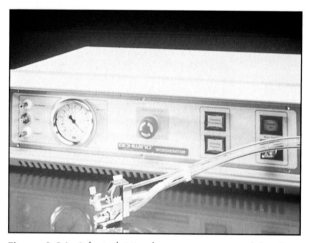

Figure 8-24. Schwind Microkeratom power module, drive cables, and microkeratome head.

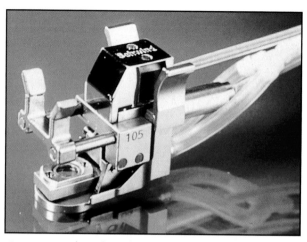

Figure 8-23. The Schwind Microkeratom is a single unit with a double suction ring.

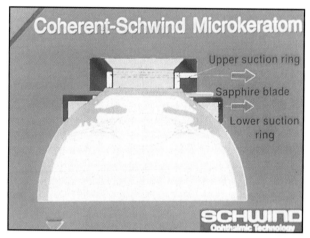

Figure 8-25. Animated view depicting the double suction ring apparatus of the Schwind Microkeratom.

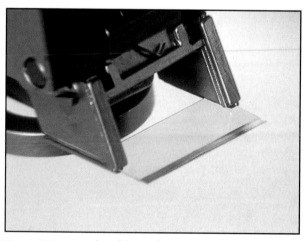

Figure 8-26. Sapphire blade of the Schwind Microkeratom.

which will potentially allow for greater maneuverability in performing keratectomies at any orientation (ie, superior hinges). The microkeratome comes with four different suction rings. One of these rings is for use by novice lamellar surgeons, in which the microkeratome can be preplaced on a platform and the entire unit can be engaged over the operative eye. Therefore, the surgeon does not have to load the microkeratome after the suction is activated. The remaining rings are of variable sagittal heights and diameters to accommodate different eye dimensions. The geared advance mechanism is located underneath the microkeratome (although still to the lateral aspect) and reportedly results in less torque of the head as it is advanced. The microkeratome comes with a fixed rotatable triangular depth plate that can be oriented to achieve 130, 160, and 220

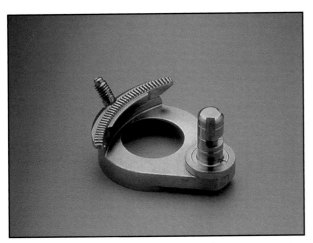

Figure 8-27. Hansatome suction ring with a pivot post that accepts an outrigger adapter and includes a geared track that is positioned nasally away from the speculum blades and lid tissue.

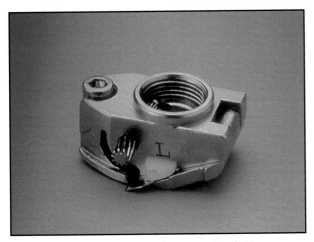

Figure 8-29. Hansatome microkeratome head. Note patented plastic blade holder and the leading edge of the blade in the blade receptacle.

micron flap thicknesses as desired. A metal blade is used and oscillates at 8000 cycles per minute side-to-side. The microkeratome comes with a stop to allow for hinge formation and has an automated reverse of the microkeratome head as soon as the stop is reached.

HANSATOME

The Hansatome is designed and manufactured by Hansa Research and Development of Miami, Fla, USA and is distributed by Chiron Vision Corporation (Irvine, Calif, USA). This automated microkeratome has a completely new design that is touted as being easier for the novice surgeon

This automated microkeratome has a completely new design that is touted as being easier for the novice surgeon to master.

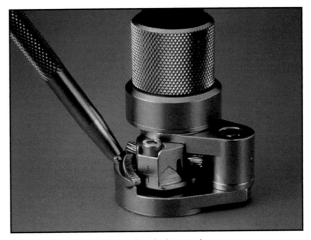

Figure 8-28. Hansatome loaded onto the suction ring.

to master. The microkeratome is loaded onto a pivot post on the suction ring (Figure 8-27) unlike the dovetail track of its predecessors. The manufacturer claims it is ergonomically easier to load the microkeratome onto the pivot post than older systems (Figure 8-28). This system is designed for superior hinge formation, which is felt, but not scientifically proven, to be more physiologic with superior to inferior lid blinking. The suction ring has an elevated geared track that is anatomically distant (see Figure 8-27) from the speculum or lid, which avoids blockage. Assembly is quite simple and includes loading the disposable blade into the microkeratome head (Figure 8-29), followed by placement of the outrigger adapter (Figure 8-30), and then the motor. The new power supply includes several safety features including internal diagnostics to ensure system integrity prior to each procedure. The cutting motion will not start until the appropriate vacuum level is reached and will stop if the vacuum level drops below the threshold. Constant motor speed is delivered to the microkeratome head by electronic compensation via the new internal power supply design. The high output vacuum has a back-up power supply. 160 or 180 micron microkeratome heads are available. The bifaceted steel blade oscillates sideways. The blade oscillation is faster and the translation slower for the Hansatome in comparison to the Automatic Corneal Shaper, resulting in a smoother keratectomy surface. The unit can be heat sterilized between each case.

INNOVATOME

This instrument is manufactured by Innovative Optics of Albuquerque, NM, USA, as a lightweight (12 grams) microkeratome head (Figure 8-31) for use in creating a flap for the LASIK technique. The suction apparatus is integrated into the microkeratome head. The head has a sapphire applanation plate that allows direct visualization of the keratectomy. The manufacturer states that this affords protection from "donut" keratectomies seen with conventional microkeratomes due to a phenomenon it terms as elastohy-

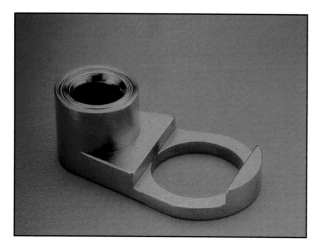

Figure 8-30. Hansatome outrigger adapter.

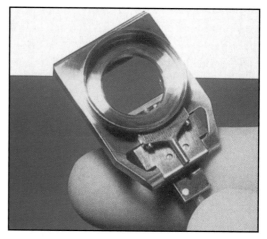

Figure 8-31. InnovoTome microkeratome head.

drodynamic entrapment. This process apparently occurs when a fluid meniscus comes between the applanation plate and corneal surface in conventional microkeratome designs. Flap diameter is adjustable by a thumb screw from 8 to 10 mm, and keratectomy depth is preset to 160 microns. A disposable 50-micron thick steel blade that measures 1 mm from the front cutting surface to the distal edge oscillates 12,000 to 15,000 times per minute sideways with an angulation of 6°. The blade has a chiseled edge. The blade translates at 4 mm/second, and the total forward travel time is 2.5 seconds. The mechanism for blade translation and oscillation is unique in this unit. The blade and blade holder are cable driven. The blade has a conventional stroke (side-to-side movement) of .9 mm. An electrically powered cable shaft drives a pair of eccentric masses in rotation. Acceleration of the eccentric masses in the cutting plane produces a periodic force on the blade holder that results in reciprocation. The eccentric masses are mounted on a countershaft, which is supported in the blade holder by a pair of ball bearings. Axial thrust of the rotating cable's flexible shaft moves the blade in translation. The unit comes with a 15-pound console with internal diagnostics that continually monitor the IOP by transducer during the operation. The hinge can be oriented in any direction depending on the surgeon's desire. The microkeratome head can be heat sterilized.

AUTOMATED DISPOSABLE KERATOME

This microkeratome is distributed by LaserSight Technologies, Inc (Figure 8-32). The device was designed by Ruiz, who also designed the Automatic Corneal Shaper. The keratome is manufactured in an injection molding technique with either 130 or 160 micron cutting depths. The keratome features a "positive traction" dual drive mechanism to prevent binding. The gear drive mechanism is completely covered, which reportedly prevents tissue or eyelashes from interfering with the cut or translation of the keratome. A stainless steel blade oscillates at 10,000 cycles per minute

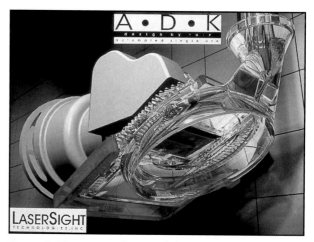

Figure 8-32. Animated view of the Automated Disposable Keratome on the suction ring.

and advances at a rate of 3.6 mm/second. Flap diameter can be varied up to 10 mm. The suction ring has a narrow profile, which helps with deep-set eyes. The unit comes with an electric power console featuring an internal alarm that alerts the surgeon to inadequate suction. The motorized drive mechanism can be attached directly to the keratome or remotely situated with an external drive cable. After use, the entire microkeratome assembly is discarded. The nondisposable portion is purchased separately from the manufacturer.

MICRA KERATOME

This manual microkeratome is manufactured by Micro Specialties, Inc. The manufacturer states the system uses a free-floating stainless steel blade with 25° angulation. A vented nitrogen gas turbine powers the unit to 15,000 oscillations/minute. An electric powered version is also supposed to be available in the future. Two suction rings help to achieve globe fixation. Flap diameters of up to 10 mm are possible. Flap thickness of 130, 160, or 200 microns can be

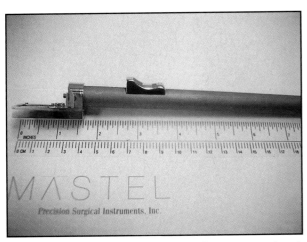

Figure 8-33. Mastel diamond lamellar keratome: a "hand-held surgical instrument."

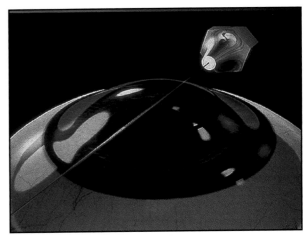

Figure 8-34. Animated view of the Hydroblade performing a refractive cut after a free cap has been created. This instrument is being developed to create flaps for the LASIK technique.

achieved by various blade configurations. The power console has a digital read-out that monitors blade speed and suction. An audible alarm sounds if suction is lost or inadequate. A viewing area allows the surgeon to visualize the surgery.

KRUMEICH-BARRAQUER MICROKERATOME

This device was designed by Jorg Krumeich, MD, PhD and Barraquer and is manufactured by Eye Tech Ltd Of Balzars, Switzerland. This system allows for full visualization of the cut through a transparent plate and features an automatic safety stop. The system is manually advanced and has a blade oscillation rate of 14,000 cycles per minute. The blade is a natural diamond 14 mm in length with an angulation of 26°. Keratectomy diameters of up to 9 mm are possible. Cutting depth is standard at 160 microns, although other depths can be ordered.

KRUMEICH MICROKERATOME

Krumeich designed this unit as a fully automatic system in which the advance rate and blade oscillation rate are adjustable and controlled by a microprocessor in an external power unit. The system is manufactured by Eye Tech Ltd. All vital information is displayed on a computer screen. It uses the same head as the Krumeich-Barraquer microkeratome, which affords intraoperative visualization. An automatic safety stop allows the surgeon to preset the hinge location. The advance rate is adjustable up to 2 mm/second. The blade is an 11-mm natural diamond. It is angulated at 26°, and the typical keratectomy depth is 160 microns. Flap diameters up to 9 mm are possible.

BUZARD-BARRAQUER LASER DIAMOND KERATOME

This instrument was designed by Mastel Precision Surgical Instruments, Inc of Rapid City, SD, USA. The sys-

tem features all titanium and stainless steel construction and weighs less than 40 grams (Figure 8-33). The microkeratome head is 15 mm in width and houses a synthetic yellow-colored diamond that can be inspected under a conventional calibration microscope. All phases of the operation can be viewed by the surgeon through a transparent sapphire applanation plate. Resection depth can be varied according to the surgeon's preference and is determined by adjustable applanation surfaces. The principle of operation is to first incise the outer rim of a flap with a diamond-bladed trephine followed by lamellar dissection with the microkeratome of the previously defined flap outline. The flap has a hinge parallel to the eyebrow. The unit will be available with suction as an option. The manufacturer does note that this product is a "hand-held surgical instrument" and not a motorized machine. The diamond blade can be inspected under a calibration microscope and is easily cleaned and sterilized.

WATER SCALPELS

Two high-pressure water incising instruments are currently under design and development. Medjet, Inc (Edison, NJ, USA) has been developing the Hydroblade (Figure 8-34) to avoid what its developers perceive as fundamental deficiencies in oscillating metal, diamond, or sapphire blade microkeratomes. Among these deficiencies are the necessity to establish high IOP (65 mm Hg) and the potential for irregular keratectomies or intraocular entry and collagen fibril shearing caused by a blade. David Dillman, MD, first reported on the waterjet concept for lamellar surgery at the *Ocular Surgery News* Third Annual Meeting in New York City, October 1994. The Hydroblade (Medjet, Inc has been issued a basic patent for the method and the device) uses a circular parallel beam of sterile, highly filtered balanced salt solution moving in a rectilinear motion at supersonic speed.

Beam diameters from 10 to 100 microns are used depending on the application. The velocity of the beam depends on the stagnation pressure (ie, the water pressure before it issues from the orifice, which is a specially shaped ruby with a circular hole). The emerging beam looks like a fine monofilament (fish line) in the homogenous region and breaks into a fine mist beyond the fish line. The length of the fish line depends on the orifice shape and diameter, the orifice holder design, and the stagnation pressure.

For lamellar surgery, the beam parameters are not especially critical. Typical settings are stagnation pressure of 20,000 psi or 1360 atmospheres, beam diameter of 33 microns, and velocity of more than 400 meters/second. The fish line length is a few centimeters. The water flow rate is about one-third of a millimeter per second, and the beam carries a continuous power of about 30 watts. The globe is kept at normal IOP. The beam is mechanically scanned in a direction perpendicular to its length, defining a cutting plane. The cut within the plane across 8 mm of the cornea takes several tenths of one second compared to 2 seconds for a scalpel cut and requires a few hundred microliters of sterile water. No tissue is lost during the cut; the cut is demonstrably a perfect blunt dissection. Only fibrils interconnecting lamellae are bisected. No lamellae or associated fibrils are cut or damaged. The short time for the cut and a force on the cornea of only a few grams (compared to tens of grams for a conventional scalpel cut) insure the precision of the cut. Even an unsupported cornea at normal IOP does not visibly move or compress when it is cut by the Hydroblade.

The emerging beam beyond the cutting region is barely changed in appearance since only the surface of the beam is in contact with the tissue. There is no hydration since the water moves only parallel to the surface of the cut tissue, not into the tissue. Absence of hydration is proven by the absence of aeration in the tissue since the beam's water contains substantial air. There is virtually no heating of the tissue. There are no shock waves. In fact, there are no known physical or chemical mechanisms, other than the minimal mechanical forces, that might impact the safety of the procedure.

The nature and shape of the incised tissue is defined by the shape of the anterior surface of the cornea during the planar cut. The anterior shape during the cut is established by a suction template since dissection by a waterjet requires that the tissue not be under significant compression. The shape of the template depends on the requirements. For example, a flat template produces a parallel lamellar flap of predetermined thickness. A hinge of predetermined width may be produced by stopping or blocking the jet during the scan. A slightly spherical template allows removal of a plano convex lenticle of predetermined refraction. Lenticles with positive, negative, or astigmatic refraction may be removed. It is observed in parallel flap cuts, for example,

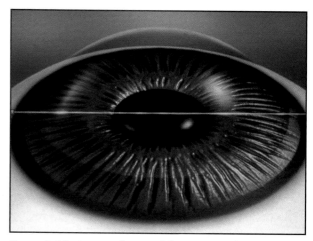

Figure 8-35. Animated view of the Visijet Hydrokeratome.

that the new stromal surface is strictly a lamellar surface such as would be expected with an ideal blunt dissection. On a microscopic level, it is not smooth since the ideal lamellar surface is not smooth. A visibly smooth surface would be a damaged surface. Classical microkeratomes shear lamellae while the Hydroblade cuts the few collagen fibrils linking vertically adjacent lamellae.

Surgijet is developing the Visijet Hydrokeratome (Figure 8-35). This instrument uses a water beam size of 36 to 50 microns operating at 6000 to 12,000 psi. The manufacturer reports good lamellar incisions with no collateral damage. Since the procedure only lasts 2 seconds, when incising the cornea the manufacturer speculates that significant stromal hydration will be unlikely. Possible treatments include myopia, hyperopia, and astigmatism with either direct reshaping of the surface or flap creation with removal of stromal tissue. In the last application, the Hydrokeratome would perform functions of both the microkeratome and an excimer laser. The manufacturer reports that flaps from 3 to 9 mm in diameter will be possible.

Laser Keratomes

Several lasers capable of intrastromal ablation through an intact corneal surface are currently being tested to create a corneal flap. These lasers will simultaneously remove corneal stromal tissue to affect a refractive change.

Escalon Laser Microkeratome

Escalon Medical, Inc (Skillman, NJ, USA) is developing a laser microkeratome with the use of a picosecond infrared laser to create a corneal flap of any dimension and to eventually also perform tissue removal in the stromal bed for the refractive correction (Figures 8-36a and 8-36b).

Novatec Laser Microkeratome

Novatec, Inc (Carlsbad, Calif, USA) is developing as laser to perform lamellar surgery using two different surgi-

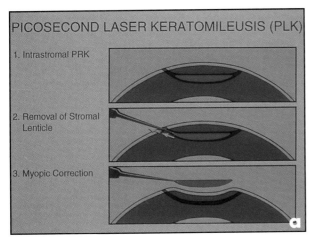
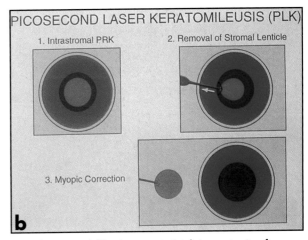

Figure 8-36a. and 8-36b. Animated view of picosecond laser keratomileusis (a: [left] side view; B: [right] top view) to first create keratectomy and then refractive lenticle. The lenticle is subsequently removed with forceps, resulting in a flattened central cornea in the treatment of myopia.

cal approaches. The laser can either be focused to create a lamellar flap or focused to create intrastromal cavitation. In the latter approach, as the cavitation bubbles collapse, the refractive correction occurs. In either technique, an active eye tracking system is important for proper beam delivery.

MICROKERATOME SELECTION

Historically, microkeratomes for corneal refractive surgery have been difficult instruments to master. Regardless of what device a surgeon elects to use, he or she must come to master all aspects of its design, cleaning, maintenance, operation, limitations, potential side effects, and complications. There are several salient features that can be discussed to champion one microkeratome over another. These include:

1. visibility of the cornea during the creation of the keratectomy;
2. automated systems that control the rate of the microkeratome pass;
3. blade angulation and its impact on adherence of the keratectomy and secondary epithelial ingrowth;
4. blade oscillation rate;
5. blade oscillation rate to keratome advancement rate;
6. torque delivered to the cutting blade;
7. suction to create a lamellar corneal flap and ability to check the IOP intraoperatively; and
8. case after case dependability, repeatability, and durability.

With all the above stated, creation of a flap of corneal tissue for LASIK is still surgery and conveys a certain amount of risk. Is there a perfect system? Not yet, and possibly never. After the surgeon compulsively studies the various attributes of the available microkeratomes and purchases a unit for clinical use, he or she then must begin an integral and tremendously important educational process.

The surgeon and staff should become intimately familiar with the microkeratome's design, maintenance, operation, limitations, and complication management. Potentially, the most important recommendation would be for the surgeon to perform a large number of dry runs and cadaver practice eyes to perfect his or her understanding and operation of the microkeratome before proceeding to the first live case. To this end, the safest and most reliable application of microkeratome technology for patient care will be achieved.

> The surgeon and staff should become intimately familiar with the microkeratome's design, maintenance, operation, limitations, and complication management.

REFERENCES

1. Barraquer JI. Oueratoplastia refractiva. *Estudios Inform Oftal Inst Barraquer.* 1949;10:2-21.
2. Barraquer JI. Keratomileusis. *Int Surg.* 1967;48:103-117.
3. Barraquer JI. Results of myopic keratomileusis. *Journal of Refractive Surgery.* 1987;3:98-101.
4. Barraquer JI. Method for cutting lamellar grafts in frozen corneas: new orientations for refractive surgery. *Archives of the Society of American Ophthalmology.* 1958;1:237.
5. Bores L. Lamellar refractive surgery. In: Bores L, ed: *Refractive Eye Surgery.* Blackwell Scientific Publications: Boston, Mass; 1993:324-91.
6. Slade SG, Updegraff SA. Advances in Lamellar Refractive Surgery. *Int Ophthalmol Clin.* 1994:147-62.
7. Nordan LT, Maxwell WA. Keratomileusis. In: Schwab IR, ed. *Refractive Keratoplasty.* Churchill Livingstone: New York, NY; 1987: 41-68.
8. Swinger CA, Krumeich J, Cassiday D. Planar lamellar refractive keratoplasty. *J Refract Surg.* 1986;2:17-24.
9. Binder PS. What we have learned about corneal wound healing

from refractive surgery. *J Refract Corneal Surg.* 1989;5:98-120.

10. Binder PS, Zavala EY, Baumgartner SD, et al. Combined morphological effects of cryolathing and lyophilization on epikeratoplasty lenticles. *Arch Ophthalmol.* 1986;104:671-9.

11. Zavala EY, Krumeich J, Binder PS. Laboratory evaluation of freeze vs. nonfreeze lamellar refractive keratoplasty. *Arch Ophthalmol.* 1987;105:1125-1128.

12. Buratto L, Ferrari M. Retrospective comparison of freeze and non-freeze myopic epikeratophakia. *J Refract Corneal Surg.* 1989;5:94-7.

13. Arenas-Archila E., Sanchez-Thorin JC, et al. Myopic keratomileusis in-situ: a preliminary report. *J Cataract Refract Surg.* 1991;17:424-35.

14. Bas AM, Nano HD. In-situ myopic keratomileusis results in 30 eyes at 15 months. *J Refract Corneal Surg.* 1991;7:223-231.

Down-up LASIK with the Chiron Hansatome

Lucio Buratto, MD

INTRODUCTION

Down-up laser in situ keratomileusis (LASIK) (superior-hinge LASIK, top-hinge LASIK) with the new Chiron Hansatome is similar to the classical LASIK technique with the standard Chiron Automated Corneal Shaper (ACS). The difference between these two techniques lies in one very important detail: the cut is performed from the bottom upwards. This means that a "superior hinge" is created, which is a more natural position for the flap hinge.

THE COMPONENTS OF CHIRON'S HANSATOME

Like all other microkeratomes, the Chiron Hansatome has three distinct parts:

1. a motor
2. a head fitted with a blade
3. a suction ring

While the Hansatome appears to be just like the other Chiron microkeratomes, it is actually completely different. Aesthetically, the instrument differs from other designs as it is developed vertically with the motor applied above the suction ring, which is above the eye (Figures 9-1 and 9-2).

The cutting action is also different. While other microkeratomes have manual or automated progression from the temporal to the nasal side, the cut with the Hansatome is performed by the rotation of the head around a pin located in the lower portion. The cut is performed from the inferior aspect of the cornea upward. The true innovation of this instrument is its ability to create superior hinges. The use of the instrument is also different, as it is much simpler, safer, and more precise to use. It performs high quality cuts of a large diameter with an exact, preset thickness.

SUCTION RING

The suction ring consists of two parts: the handle, which is connected to the vacuum pump by a tube; and the suction ring itself (Figures 9-3 and 9-4). It has a concave part on its inferior aspect that comes into contact with the conjunctiva and the sclera. There is just one suction orifice, however this is sufficient to allow the ring to adhere tightly to the bulb. Because the ring is specifically designed to provide good contact when suction is activated, there is strong adhesion. This is important in order to obtain good quality cuts and to avoid the risks of complication through inadequate or insufficient suction.

The upper part of the ring differs from other microkeratomes because it does not have tracks. Near the suction handle, the ring has an arch-shaped toothed path, which engages with a rolling gear in the terminal part of the head to perform the cut. Anterior to the toothed path and slightly below the ring, there is an arch-shaped protrusion that blocks the microkeratome's cutting action (the stop). Distal to the suction handle there is a pin (Figure 9-5). The head is inserted vertically onto this pin and can rotate around it. This pin has two notches, which ensure the correct position of the microkeratome. By rotating the head on the pin, the microkeratome will drop down at a specific point and rest onto the inferior surface of the ring, which is the operating plane. This is the only position that allows the automated

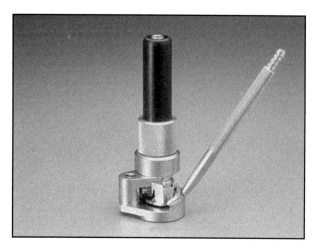

Figure 9-1. The Chiron microkeratome complete with suction ring, motor, and head.

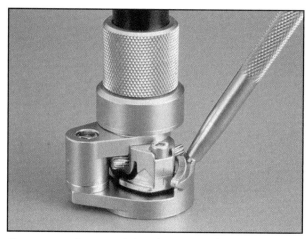

Figure 9-2. Close-up of the Chiron microkeratome: suction ring, motor, and head.

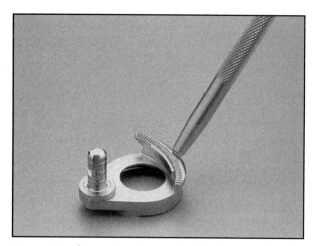

Figure 9-3. The suction ring: on the left, the pin where the head of the microkeratome is inserted; the microkeratome rotates around this pin. On the right, the handle, toothed arch-shaped track, and below it the stop mechanism. The suction ring plane has no grooves.

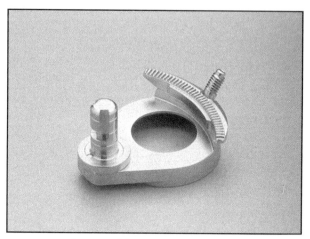

Figure 9-4. Close-up of the suction ring: on the bottom of the arch-shaped toothed track the stop mechanism can be seen.

mechanism of the head to come in contact with the toothed gear of the ring to perform the cut. Therefore, the rolling gear of the head can be engaged in the toothed mechanism of the suction ring only when the head has been positioned correctly.

Because the head is locked on the pin, it maintains a constant relationship with the suction ring. This ensures that the cutting plane is uniform and reduces the opportunity for human error by performing the cut only when the head and its blade have reached the correct position.

THE MOTOR

The motor is similar to those of the other microkeratomes. It has an eccentric gear that rotates and activates the blade. It also moves the head of the microkeratome along the toothed wheel of the suction ring. The automation is visible through the screw hole in the head of the microkeratome.

THE HEAD

The head is a single-piece unit unlike the Chiron ACS, which is composed of many component parts that must be cleaned and assembled before use. The upper part of the head has an opening for screwing in the motor (Figures 9-6 and 9-7). The central part has a slot for the insertion of the blade (Figure 9-8). Anterior to this, there is another curved opening that receives the lamellar tissue during the microkeratome cut.

The head includes a depth plate that determines the thickness of the cut, which is 150 microns. This plate is fixed and is an integral part of the head. It is never removed except for periodic maintenance when it can be unscrewed with the appropriate screwdriver. This fixed plate is an important safety feature, as it prevents the most serious potential complication of LASIK—perforation of the cornea. This has been reported with the ACS microkeratome

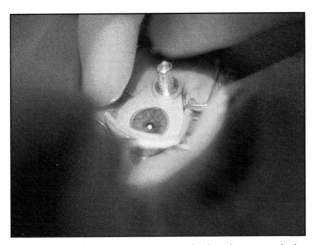

Figure 9-13. The suction ring is applied to the eye with the handle nasally; the foot pedal is pushed to activate the aspiration.

APPLICATION OF THE SPECULUM

The Buratto-Machat speculum (ASICO) is carefully applied by placing it under the eyelids and opening the aperture gently and gradually. The palpebral opening should be sufficient to allow the suction ring to be applied and the microkeratome to be inserted. Any barrier must be removed (pieces of plastic from the drape, an eyelash, etc) before proceeding. The cornea and conjunctival sac are washed with balanced salt solution (BSS), and then the conjunctival sac is carefully dried with Merocel sponges to remove any secretions, eyelashes, or other debris. This procedure is also useful for removing any residual fluid in the conjunctival sac that could otherwise be aspirated by the suction ring and interfere with the adhesion of the ring to the globe.

CORNEAL MARKING

The corneal marker must reach the peripheral cornea to guide the exact replacement of the corneal flap. I use the Buratto marker (ASICO). The instrument tip is first stained with methylene blue and then firmly applied to the dry cornea. Three radii are produced on the cornea (inferior, superior, and temporal). These markings are important guides to allow the surgeon to replace the flap in its original site in the event of free cap (an extremely rare occurrence with the new Chiron Hansatome).

TRANSFER OF THE SUCTION RING

The assistant is generally positioned in front and left of the laser and instruments. The instruments should be handed to the surgeon in the correct position for immediate use. If the right eye is being operated on, the suction ring must be placed in the surgeon's left hand, and the suction tube must pass in front of the surgeon. The handle of the ring must be in the nasal position. For right eye LASIK, the microkeratome is held in the right hand.

With left eye LASIK, the aspiration tube will pass

behind the surgeon above the right shoulder. It is held in the right hand with the handle positioned nasally. For left eye LASIK, the microkeratome is held in the left hand.

APPLICATION OF THE SUCTION RING

Before the suction ring is applied, the patient is reassured that LASIK is proceeding smoothly. Prior to applying the ring on the flap, I check that the speculum has created sufficient space for the insertion and positioning of the ring. The intrapalpebral space can be increased by rotating the screws on the instrument. With the handle placed nasally, the suction ring is gently placed on the globe (Figure 9-13). The cornea and pupil centration is checked, and when it has been confirmed to be appropriate, downward pressure is placed on the suction ring. I activate the suction and wait a few seconds until the vacuum is sufficient to provide good adhesion.

When the vacuum is activated, there is a slight increase in the diameter of the pupil. This is a good sign, meaning the intraocular pressure (IOP) has increased and the ring has adhered correctly to the globe. Then I control the exact centering of the ring on the cornea and pupil. Since this microkeratome creates large flaps (9 to 9.5 mm diameter), good centering of the cut is a less important factor than when the resection is performed with smaller rings. Nevertheless, good centering of the cut is important because it will reduce the risk of bleeding from the perilimbal corneal vessels. A final check is then performed to ensure that there are no obstructions in the operating field.

TONOMETRY

Prior to proceeding with the cut, the IOP is always checked with the Barraquer tonometer by ensuring that the flattening of the cornea induced by the tonometer lies inside the circle drawn on the surface of the tip of the tonometer, which confirms that the pressure is about 65 mm Hg. For this measurement, the cornea must be only somewhat dry. If the cornea is wet, the meniscus of fluid will provide a flattened area that is wider than the real one, suggesting a falsely low IOP reading. If the cornea is dry, it will provide a smaller applanated area, which suggests that the pressure is higher than the real value.

WETTING THE CORNEA

Following tonometry, with a small cannula mounted on a syringe, 2 to 3 drops of BSS are applied to the cornea. This will make the microkeratome run along the cornea much smoother, which minimizes epithelial defects and enhances the quality of the microkeratome cut.

GRASP OF THE MICROKERATOME

For right eyes, the microkeratome is held with the right hand, and for left eyes the microkeratome is held with the left hand. The microkeratome is initially slid onto the pin on

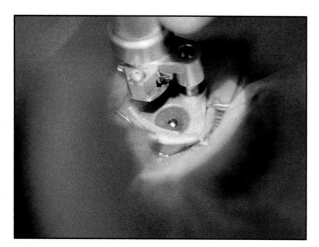

Figure 9-14. The lateral orifice of the head of the microkeratome is slipped over the pin of the suction ring.

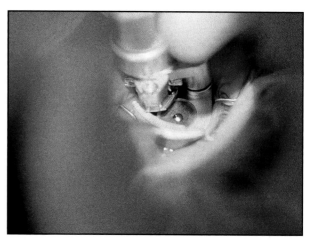

Figure 9-15. The head of the microkeratome is rotated in the direction of the toothed track on the suction ring; in this way the microkeratome can drop further down the pin and position itself on the cutting plane of the suction ring. At this point, the gear located laterally on the head of the microkeratome can come into contact with the toothed track of the suction ring.

the suction ring and rotated gently until it clicks into position. The microkeratome moves about halfway down the pin (Figure 9-14). By rotating it further, it will move down and come into contact with the ring's cutting plane. At the same time, the toothed mechanism of the head comes into contact with the toothed run of the suction ring (Figure 9-15). The instrument is now ready to perform the cut. At this stage, the patient is informed that the sensation of eye pressure will increase but without causing any great discomfort.

ENGAGING THE MICROKERATOME TO THE TEETH OF THE RING

I activate the pedal (and therefore the progression) of the microkeratome until the toothed wheel of the instrument moves between the first and second tooth on the surface of the suction ring. The microkeratome advancement is then arrested to make a final check prior to the critical cutting phase to ensure that the path of the microkeratome is free from any impediments.

PERFORMANCE OF THE CUT

The performance of the cut is the most important and delicate phase of the operation. I push the pedal ("go"), and for about 6 to 7 seconds the microkeratome follows the toothed path of the suction ring until it can go no further because of the stop (Figures 9-16 through 9-18). I then push the pedal in the opposite direction ("go back"), and the microkeratome returns to the original position (this takes another 6 to 7 seconds) (Figure 9-19). The microkeratome progresses gently at a uniform speed in both directions. The cut is performed from down upward, and the hinge is formed at the 12 o'clock position (Figure 9-20). The most difficult aspect of the procedure has now been completed (Figures 9-21 through 9-26).

When the microkeratome is active:

- The teeth of the microkeratome must lock in with those of the suction ring. If this does not happen, the progres-

sion of the microkeratome will not occur. In this situation, I reverse the direction of the gears of the microkeratome and repeat the forward gear movement until I have the teeth correctly locked.
- I try not to exert downward or upward pressure on the microkeratome because this could make the progression more difficult. Gentle support on the connecting cable allows the instrument to progress smoothly.
- Any debris on the ring guides will make the progression of the microkeratome difficult or impossible, therefore the toothed guides must be carefully checked to ensure that nothing obstructs the microkeratome path.
- Suction must always be active during the cut. If suction is interrupted, the suction will be incomplete and the operation will have to be interrupted.
- The microkeratome must reach the stop; if it stops earlier, the cut will be incomplete.
- The progression of the microkeratome must occur with no obstructions (speculum, drapes, eyelashes, etc).

REMOVAL OF THE RING AND MICROKERATOME

When the microkeratome has returned to the starting position, I stop the suction by pushing on the pedal, and the ring (along with the microkeratome) is removed from the surface of the eye. The two instruments are handed to my assistant, who will attend to dismantling, cleaning, and sterilizing them for the next operation.

Within possible limits, I try to keep the period of time between the beginning and end of suction to under 1 minute in order to avoid any compromise of the internal vascular structures of the eye caused by the high IOP. When the procedure is completed according to plan, the suction time is reduced to less than 30 seconds.

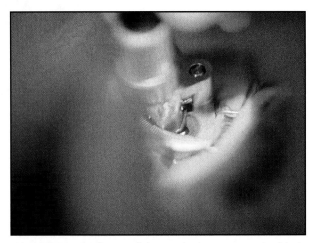

Figure 9-16. The foot pedal is pushed to activate the blade and the automation of the microkeratome. The instrument progresses, rotating around the pin of the suction ring.

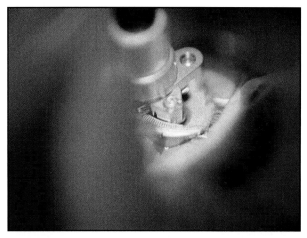

Figure 9-17. The microkeratome has already completed a large portion of the cut.

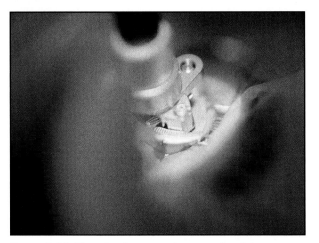

Figure 9-18. The microkeratome has completed the cut.

CENTERING THE LASER AND REPOSITIONING THE PATIENT

Often during the microkeratome cut, the patient's head and eye will move from the original position. Both should be returned to the correct position with the patient's chin on the same level as the forehead. An imaginary straight line must pass through the nose and through the middle of the two feet; the eye must be directly below the fixing target, and the two targets of the Chiron Technolas excimer laser must be well focused on the cornea above the pupillary center. The patient is then asked to stare at the fixation light and continue staring at it for a few minutes even if it appears to be out of focus.

I use special toothless Buratto forceps for raising the flap (ASICO) (See Figure 9-26). I use them to catch the flap at the lower edge, taking care not to damage the epithelium. The flap is placed superiorly and held back with a flap speculum (ASICO).

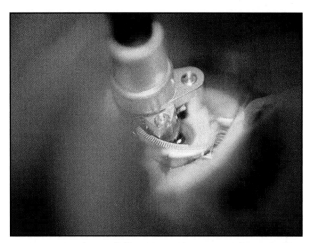

Figure 9-19. The pedal is activated to return the microkeratome to its starting position. The suction ring and microkeratome are removed.

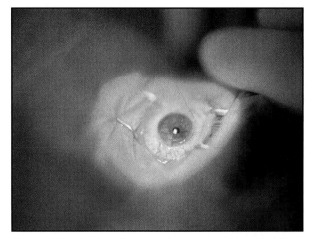

Figure 9-20. The lamellar cut with a superior hinge has been completed. Now it is sufficient to raise the flap and perform the ablation with the Chiron Technolas excimer laser and replace the corneal flap without sutures.

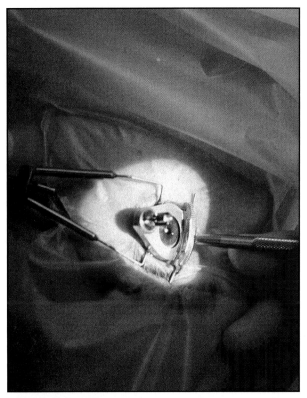

Figure 9-21. ASICO speculum and suction ring in position.

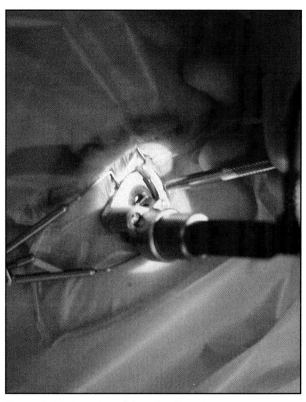

Figure 9-22. Insertion of the microkeratome.

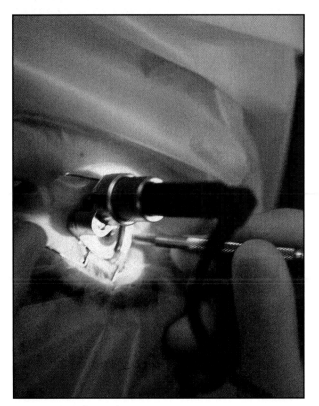

Figure 9-23. The cut begins.

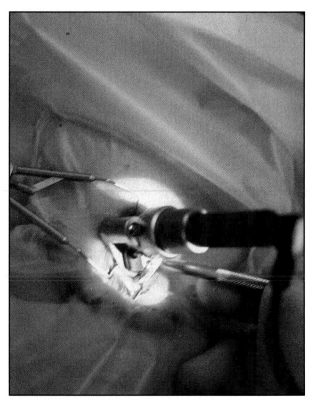

Figure 9-24. The cut is completed.

Disposable Keratomes

Sheraz M. Daya, MD, FACP, FACS, FRCS (Ed)
Marcela Espinosa, MD

Precision and attention to detail are factors that are mentioned over and over again in discussions about laser in situ keratomileusis (LASIK). To attain the goal of a perfect result, ensuring reproducibility of the procedure by minimizing variables is essential. As the majority of LASIK difficulties arise from creation of the flap, simplification of instrument assembly and design has been a focus for many microkeratome manufacturers. Many approaches are being considered, from adaptation of current keratomes and use of diamond technology, to the novel use of high-pressure water jets. Another approach to minimizing variability has been the development of disposable microkeratomes.

The advantages and disadvantages of disposable keratomes, as well as early experience with two recently manufactured keratomes—the FLAPmaker (Refractive Technologies, Inc) and the Ruiz Automated Disposable Keratome (ADK) (Lasersight Technologies, Inc)—will be described.

> As the majority of LASIK difficulties arise from creation of the flap, simplification of instrument assembly and design has been a focus for many microkeratome manufacturers.

WHY DISPOSABLE KERATOMES?

The main advantages of disposable microkeratomes can be broadly approached by the improvements in their ease of use, safety, and cost implications, although it must be stated that newer nondisposable microkeratomes appear to be working toward similar goals. Specific advantages can be found in the area of quality control, implications on learning, and the impact on cost. Indeed disposable keratomes may well provide a gateway for surgeons considering the procedure.

QUALITY AND REPRODUCIBILITY

There are considerable theoretical advantages with disposable keratomes that make the concept quite attractive. Disposability eliminates the requirement for meticulous care, assembly, cleaning, and sterilization; hence it "disposes" of the need for a dedicated microkeratome technician. Responsibility for quality control lies with the manufacturer, and the potential for keratome "wear and tear" and resultant complications is eliminated. Disposable keratomes eliminate this potential problem. The possibility of breakdown, with consequences and implications on down time, are also minimized. Many surgeons have been in a situation in which a large list of patients were scheduled for surgery and had to be canceled and rescheduled because of microkeratome problems.

The disposable keratome blade is incorporated in the device, and there is no handling thereafter. This eliminates the possibility of inadvertent blade damage, which is another factor that can hinder the production of a good quality flap.

> Disposability eliminates the requirement for meticulous care, assembly, cleaning, and sterilization; hence it "disposes" of the need for a dedicated microkeratome technician.

Further keratome refinements can be made and implemented by users without the need to send the instrument to its manufacturer for expensive modification.

Another clear benefit with disposable keratome technology is that further keratome refinements can be made and implemented by users without the need to send the instrument to its manufacturer for expensive modification.

EASE OF USE AND IMPLICATIONS ON LEARNING

The greatest number of complications appear to arise during the learning phase of the LASIK procedure.[1,2] This is a result of several factors including poor familiarity with instrumentation, novelty of the procedure, and lack of similarity with many other ophthalmic surgical procedures. Removal of the need for complex assembly eliminates a major component of the learning curve among beginners, allowing them to concentrate on the creation and handling of the flap. Prefixing the microkeratome head to the suction ring further improves the ease of use and enhances safety by eliminating the error that sometimes occurs as a result of faulty insertion in older microkeratome systems. The incorporation of a fixed depth plate, a converging concept with all keratome manufacturers, is a reassurance against the worst complication—a corneal perforation.

Removal of the need for complex assembly eliminates a major component of the learning curve among beginners.

These design modifications make the procedure less daunting and improve the margin of safety. That is not to say the need for familiarization with the concepts and principles of instrumentation can be done away with; these are still vital to get the maximum benefit from the instrument, as with any instrument-dependent surgical procedure. The importance of prior training, practice, and familiarity cannot be overemphasized.

COST

Another considerable advantage is the reduction in instrument start-up costs. Since disposable keratome manufacturers are able to continuously create revenue from disposable components, they are motivated to make the base drive units highly affordable, thus reducing the start-up costs for performing LASIK by transferring the expense to a "pay as you earn" basis. This has obvious benefits with regard to cash flow and business planning especially in the early stages of starting a refractive surgical center. The improvement in surgical throughput also has a tremendous cost implication.

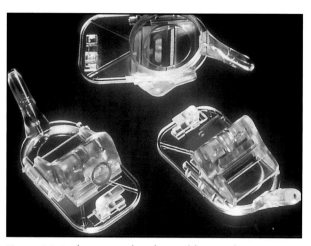

Figure 10-1. The FLAPmaker disposable microkeratome. It is a cable-driven device with an independently controlled blade oscillation mechanism (courtesy of Refractive Technologies).

Disposable keratome manufacturers are able to continuously create revenue from disposable components, they are motivated to make the base drive units highly affordable.

IMPROVED SURGICAL THROUGHPUT

One of the disposable keratome's areas of greatest impact is the improvement in surgical throughput. There is no need to clean and prepare instrumentation prior to the next case, nor is there a need to have a second device. In the authors' experience, surgical room turn-over can be less than 5 minutes, so more patients can be scheduled with comfort. Maximizing use of surgical time has numerous obvious cost-saving implications.

THE FLAPMAKER

The FLAPmaker is a new disposable microkeratome developed by Alexander Dybbs, PhD of Refractive Technologies, Inc (Ohio, USA). Under the supervision of clinical director Jeffrey B. Robin, MD, the FLAPmaker has been used on a monitored basis at numerous sites throughout the world, including the Centre for Sight at the Queen Victoria Hospital in England.

COMPONENTS

The FLAPmaker consists of a control console that provides three attachments to the disposable microkeratome: disposable tubing for suction, a drive cable for the keratome head, and a rotating cable that drives the blade mechanism. There are two foot pedals: one for initiating suction and the other for advancing and retracting the microkeratome head. The microkeratome head and suction plate are fabricated from transparent, injection-molded polycarbonate (Figure 10-1). Each keratome comes individually sterile packed.

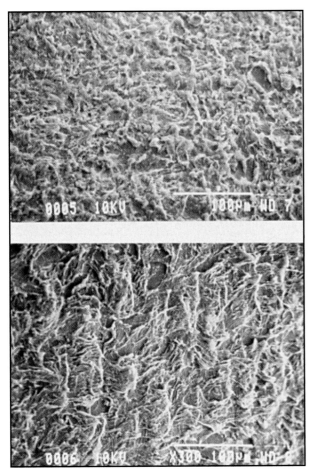

Figure 10-2. Scanning electron microscopy (SEM) (300x) comparing the FLAPmaker (top) to the more commonly used Automated Corneal Shaper (bottom). SEMs are at the center of the corneal stromal bed on mate eye bank eyes with the same IOP (courtesy of Refractive Technologies).

FEATURES

The transparency of the device permits greater visualization, which, in turn, improves centration, ease of use, and safety. The overall design is similar to that of other Barraquer-style devices and prefixes the keratome head with its preloaded blade into the suction ring. The blade angle is set at 26°. The depth plate is set to 160 microns, and two models are presently available that produce two different size lamellar flaps—8.5 mm for myopia and 10.5 mm for hyperopia. More recently, a 200-micron keratome has been designed specifically for retreatments.

The suction ring size is 18 mm and connected by disposable tubing to the control console. The adequacy of suction is indicated by a dial gauge, and there is a feedback mechanism that arrests blade oscillation in the event suction is lost. This is a remarkable safety feature that will eliminate the possibility of "funny flaps" with comet-shaped tails (usually in the visual axis) that occur when suction is lost during flap creation with the Automatic Corneal Shaper (ACS) (Chiron, USA). When suction is switched off, it is

gradually reduced by the control console and can only be released when the pressure gauge reads 5 inches Hg. This feature certainly appears safer for the eye.

The blade oscillates when the microkeratome moves forward, and on the reverse translation, the microkeratome head moves back without blade oscillation (a further contribution to safety). Additionally, if for any reason the procedure is stopped in the forward translation, the microkeratome head cannot be further advanced. Pressing the forward pedal makes the head retract without blade oscillation, in effect abandoning the procedure. Advancement after a temporary stop could produce an irregular surface or, even worse, cut a free short flap.

The cable drive mechanism provides considerable advantages over gear mechanisms. The flexible drive cable attaches to the middle of the microkeratome head and is advanced by the base drive unit with a force of more than 300 pounds. The forward pass is smooth and regular, and the central position of the cable ensures there is no torque or instrument jam as occasionally described with the single lateral drive mechanism in the ACS. Uncovered gear systems also have the potential for debris and lash interference, which may result in irregular beds.

Distinctly different from other microkeratomes, the disposable unit has no bulky motor handpiece. The cable driving the blade is flexible and powered from the control console extending out at the same rate as the head drive cable. The cable is attached directly to the head with a small pin inserted into the blade holder. The blade oscillation rate at 12,500 revolutions per minute (RPM) produces a significantly smoother cut confirmed by scanning electron microscopy (Figure 10-2).

> The transparency of the device permits greater visualization, which, in turn, improves centration, ease of use, and safety.

EXPERIENCE WITH THE FLAPMAKER

One of the authors of this chapter has had considerable prior experience with the Chiron ACS, and in this report is understandably prone to making a comparison.

Assembly

Since the FLAPmaker is constructed of plastic, it is extremely light in weight. The simplicity of use is the first observation made by the surgeon. Attachment of the suction tube provides a way to hold the device, and it is simple to perform. The drive cable is then attached after advancing the cable a short distance. A T-shaped bar slides into a slot on the microkeratome head, and the outer casing of the cable attaches to the base of the suction ring, providing two points of fixation. The third attachment is the blade oscillation cable, which has a pin that slots into the blade holder and is locked into the microkeratome by turning an outer

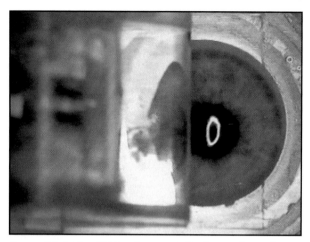

Figure 10-3. The FLAPmaker ready for forward translation. Transparency of the device greatly improves visibility.

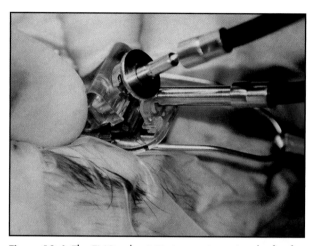

Figure 10-4. The FLAPmaker initiating suction using the forefinger and thumb at 6 and 12 o'clock to push the ring posteriorly.

ring in a similar manner to a Luer lock. The microkeratome head is then retracted and a forward translation is initiated to ensure that the microkeratome functions properly with a smooth translation. The head is then retracted again and the FLAPmaker is ready for use.

Surgical Procedure

Following typical preparation of the eye, the microkeratome is placed on the eye. Centration is easy to obtain and greatly assisted by the transparency of the device (Figure 10-3). Irrigating the limbus with balanced salt solution (BSS) helps to obtain suction. The suction pedal is depressed, and to ensure attachment of the ring to the globe, the thumb and forefinger are used to push on either side of the ring at the 12 and 6 o'clock positions (Figure 10-4). Suction is confirmed by the suction gauge as well as auditory feedback (the tone of the suction pump changes when vacuum is present). Once the gauge reading rises to an appropriate level as advised by the manufacturer, the microkeratome head can be advanced. As a precautionary measure, I prefer to digitally check that the pressure is adequately high. Additionally, BSS fluid is placed in the grooves of the keratome ring and on the cornea, providing a hydrating and lubricating effect. The forward pass produces a loud buzzing sound and vibration to the face (as related by a patient), which can cause the patient to jump if not forewarned. Retraction of the keratome head is, by contrast, silent and the flap can be seen as it is replaced onto the bed on the return.

A striking difference from the ACS is the quality of the bed when the flap is elevated. It is extremely smooth—almost shiny. The edges of the flap are also regular with no real difference from the ACS. Initial experience with the FLAPmaker was with the large flap microkeratome. This consistently produced diameters of 10.5 mm vertically and 10 mm horizontally with an approximate 5.5-mm hinge. Because of the large diameter, there were instances of

> A striking difference from the ACS is the quality of the bed when the flap is elevated. It is extremely smooth—almost shiny.

bleeding, often in the superior and inferior quadrants, especially in those subjects who had previously worn contact lenses. Control of bleeding was simple with the use of cut strips of a minimally moistened instrument sponge wipe (Visitec, Fla, USA) placed at the edge of the incision. Lack of familiarity with large flaps initially made replacement a little difficult; however, after four cases, this was no longer a problem because of reassurance that the flap was well positioned. The newer 8.5 mm microkeratome produces smaller flaps and does not produce the problem of bleeding edges.

The development of the FLAPmaker was to improve the ease of use and, more importantly, improve the safety of the LASIK procedure. Like all keratomes, problems and complications do occur when attention to details are compromised (Table 10-1). The current option of two keratome sizes rather than one is attractive, as there is no necessity in creating large flaps for myopic correction. Encouragingly, further refinements are planned with modifications to suit the desires of individual surgeons.

THE RUIZ AUTOMATED DISPOSABLE KERATOME (ADK)

This new disposable microkeratome (Figure 10-5), developed by Luis A. Ruiz, MD and engineer Sergio Lenchig of Bogota, Columbia, is manufactured and distributed by Lasersight Technologies, Inc (Orlando, Fla). It is an automated device much like the ACS, however it incorporates several new features that eliminate many of the ACS's problems.

TABLE 10-1. **FLAPMAKER COMPLICATIONS** *Marvin Kwitko, MD* As with all microkeratomes, problems and complications occur when attention to details are compromised. **Ergonomics** • difficulty placing keratome • speculum interference • partial cut • cable weight torquing • slippage off foot pedal—control with stocking foot **Suction/Pressure (low)** • case should not begin without adequate suction • thin flaps • buttonholes **Improper Set-up** • instruction manual should be known by heart • blade oscillation cable • blade stoppage/skipping • keratome translation cable • keratome stoppage **Large flaps** • bleeding—controlled before case completed • debris—inadequate irrigation

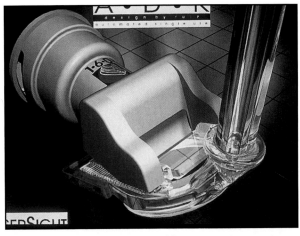

Figure 10-5. Automatic Disposable Keratome—Ruiz (courtesy of Lasersight Technologies, Inc).

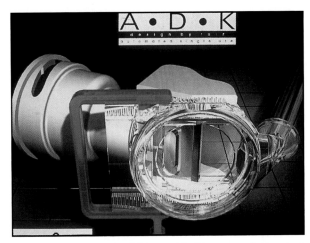

Figure 10-6. Automated Disposable Keratome demonstrating transparent applanation plate and suction ring safety ridge (courtesy of Lasersight Technologies, Inc).

COMPONENTS

Much like the FLAPmaker, the ADK is preassembled with the blade inside a microkeratome head, which is pre-attached to the suction ring. While the device is also made of a plastic polymer, the only transparent components are the suction ring and the applanation plate. The control console provides an attachment for suction, a wire cable for the motor handpiece, and two foot pedals for forward and reverse control.

FEATURES

For present ACS users, the ADK can be used on the ACS control console through the use of an adapter cable and motor handpiece. There are several advantages, however, touting the ADK console. Designed in a similar style to complement the Laserscan LSX excimer laser, the console inspires the image of high technology.

The ADK, like the FLAPmaker, is also a single-use device that is individually packed as a preassembled keratome and comes in two models preset to either 130 or 160 microns. The transparent ring and applanation plate permit greater visibility, which aids in centration of the device on the eye. Like the ACS, the ADK has a gear drive mechanism on both sides of the ring. This tandem gear mechanism eliminates the effect of torque seen in the ACS. Additionally, the gears on either side are covered to minimize the chance of lash and lid entrapment. The microker-

atome and ring are preassembled and held in place by a red head retaining clip (Figure 10-6). Prior to use on the eye, this red clip is removed, which allows the microkeratome head to come off the ring on the reverse pass of the procedure. This allows the suction ring to be used for fixation during the laser ablation component of the procedure.

The control console has a button for suction, however a foot pedal is an option. Two levels of suction are possible: "high" for the keratome pass and "low" to enable the suction ring to be used for fixation during ablation. Suction level is a major determinant of safety in the procedure and is monitored by the console, which provides auditory and visual feedback if there is a drop in suction. Additionally, the microkeratome head will not drive if the machine is not in the high suction setting. To prevent false occlusion, the suction ring has been designed with what Lasersight terms as a "vacuum safety ridge" that creates dual vacuum chambers.

The motor handpiece drives both the microkeratome

and the blade. Unlike the FLAPmaker, the blade continues to oscillate on the reverse pass. To improve smoothness of the cut, the blade oscillation rate is 10,000 RPM, which is higher than that of the ACS.

EXPERIENCE WITH THE ADK

At the time of writing this book, the ADK is in clinical investigation. Analysis of results is available on procedures performed by Ruiz comparing the ADK to the ACS. Table 10-2 provides 6 months of clinical visual data comparing the ACS to the ADK for eyes treated with similar range and mean preoperative myopia.

Overall, eyes treated with the ADK tended to provide more predictable outcomes with 64.4% of eyes achieving final refraction within .5 D and 83.1% within 1 D compared with 55.9% and 70.6% respectively using the ACS. The eyes treated with the ADK obtained uncorrected visual acuity of 20/20 more often—61% compared with 44.1% using the ACS.

The ADK has several new features that are welcome additions and enhancements to the ACS. The ability to use the control console of the ACS is desirable and certainly makes the ADK attractive as a replacement, if not a useful back-up device in the event of microkeratome breakdown.

> Overall, eyes treated with the ADK tended to provide more predictable outcomes with 64.4% of eyes achieving final refraction within .5 D and 83.1% within 1 D compared with 55.9% and 70.6% respectively using the ACS.

SUMMARY

The advent of disposable microkeratomes is extremely exciting and permits further enhancements and refinements of keratomes in the future. Minimizing start-up cost, simplifying portions of the learning curve, incorporating safety features and feedback mechanisms, as well as improving ease of use are major steps forward in the challenge to make LASIK more safe, reliable, and predictable. In spite of standardization

TABLE 10-2.
COMPARISON OF THE ACS AND ADK

Results at 6 mos	ACS*	ADK**
N	39	81
Preop mean SE	-5.92	-5.07
	(-12.63 D to -1 D)	(-12.63 D to -1 D)
UCVA		
20/20 or >	44.1%	61%
20/40 or >	79%	81.4%
BCVA		
20/20 or >	88.2%	81.4%
20/40 or >	100%	100%
Lost lines of BCVA		
1 line	0%	6.8%
2 lines	0%	0%
Diopters within target		
± .5 D	55.9%	64.4%
± 1 D	70.6%	83.1%

*ACS = Automated Corneal Shaper; **ADK = Automated Disposable Keratome (courtesy of Lasersight Technologies, Inc)*

and simplification, one must not forget that the cornea is biological tissue with the potential to behave unpredictably. Knowledge of the behavior of the cornea combined with skillful execution of the procedure are components that ensure that for the moment LASIK remains an art.

REFERENCES

1. Gimble HV, Basti S, Kaye GB, et al. Experience during the learning curve of laser in situ keratomileusis. *J Cataract Refract Surg.* 1996;22:42-550.
2. Bas AM, Onnis R. Excimer laser in situ keratomileusis. *J Cataract Refract Surg.* 1995;11(suppl):S229-S233.

Proprietary interest statement: The authors have no proprietary or financial interest in any of the products described. Dr. Marcela Espinosa is a paid employee of Lasersight Technologies, Inc.

The Hydroblade Microkeratome for LASIK and Corneal Lamellar Surgery

Barbara Parolini, MD
Ronald R. Krueger, MD, MSE
Eugene I. Gordon, PhD

The use of a high-speed waterjet is not a new concept. It has been used in nonmedical application for more than 100 years, primarily for cleaning, mining, and cutting. It is now used extensively for cleaning surfaces and food preparation.

Medical applications at an experimental level are also reported.[1] Recently, the waterjet has been revealed to be a promising new instrument in the field of corneal surgery.[2,3]

HOW THE MICROJET WORKS IN SURGICAL APPLICATIONS

TISSUE SEPARATION MECHANISMS

Cutting of soft, relatively rigid material by a microjet is accomplished by a process of erosion. As the material is fatigued by the impact of the microjet, structural bonds break and material is washed away. As we described elsewhere,[3,4] in understanding cutting of nonrigid tissue, the classic text by Eisner is fundamental.[5] Eisner described cutting, cleaving, and eroding as the fundamental tissue separation options. The sectility of the tissue is essential to the choice of the tissue separation mechanism. In the case of low sectility material, cutting with a blade of rigid material is optimal since the sharp edge of the blade stretches and fatigues the tissue, bonds are broken, and the tissue separates under the blade edge. Moving blades enhance the tissue separation since fatigue is increased. However, cutting with metal and sapphire blades is necessarily damaging since there is a tearing and shredding component associated with blade friction. Damage associated with blade cutting is exceptionally high in the cornea and highly undesirable. Moreover, the blade forces on the tissue are high and compress, stretch, or displace the tissue to compromise the accuracy of the cut.

Erosion (ablation) produces tissue damage and loss of tissue, which should be avoided in lamellar surgery except when shaping is desired. The cornea is highly sectile in a direction roughly parallel to the lamellar interface. The collagen bonds between lamellae are weak. Tissue that is highly sectile favors cleaving as the separation mechanism, which limits tissue damage. In a cleaving mode, only the bonds between lamellae are broken, preserving the basic integrity of the lamellae and keratocytes. Hence, it follows that lamellar surgery is best done in a cleaving mode. The microjet can operate in a cleaving mode, and is therefore an ideal tool for lamellar surgery.

In particular, it has been shown in extensive unpublished experiments by the authors that a microjet, scanned in an approximately lamellar direction perpendicular to the

> Cutting with metal and sapphire blades is necessarily damaging since there is a tearing and shredding component associated with blade friction.

> In a cleaving mode, only the bonds between lamellae are broken, preserving the basic integrity of the lamellae and keratocytes.

TABLE 11-1.
SPECIFICATION OF THE
WATER-JET MICROKERATOME

Stagnation pressure	20,000 psi (1360 atm)
Beam diameter	33 μm
Fish line length	5 cm
Water flow rate	367 μl/sec
Beam speed	450 m/sec
Kinetic power of the beam	35 watts (95 joules/ml)
Scanning speed	10 mm/sec
Cleaving time	.8 seconds
Cleaving fluid	294 μl
Force exerted on the cornea during the cut	1 to 2 gr wt
Temperature rise in the tissue during the cut	No more than 1° - 2°C

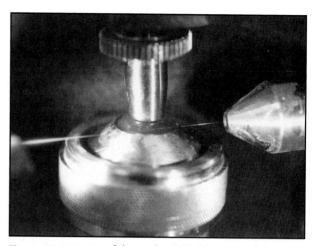

Figure 11-1. Beam of the HydroBlade keratome: the emerging beam near the orifice looks like a fine monofilament (fish line). An enucleated eye is held in an eye-check; only the cornea is protruding.

direction of the water flow, operates in a cleaving mode only if the tissue is not under compression. When the tissue is under compression it separates by erosion. Hence, whenever corneal tissue is to be cleaved by a microjet, it must be under slight tension in a direction perpendicular to the anterior surface. In contrast, when tissue is to be removed, such as in epithelial removal or in refractive surgery, erosion is appropriate and the tissue should be under compression. Careful attention must be given to the means for applanation, which depends on the objective of the surgery.[3]

Another characteristic of the microjet is its ability to cut, cleave, or erode certain tissue when the water speed is above a threshold value but not when it is below. The threshold value depends on the tissue and is typically different for each tissue in a heterogeneous structure. The water speed may be set above the threshold value for cutting the tissue of interest, but below the threshold value for damage to adjacent material. Hence, the microjet is capable of anisotropic tissue separation or removal when the beam speed is chosen properly. Therefore, it is possible to totally erode away the epithelium in a prescribed area with no loss or damage to the Bowman's layer.[2]

It might be instructive to think of the microjet as a circular cylindrical wedge—a needle. It exerts radial outward forces on tissue by virtue of collisions of water molecules moving at the surface of the beam. The slight inward deflection of water molecules toward the inner part of the beam produces a reactive outward force on the tissue. By virtue of the extremely high speed of the water, the available forces are much greater than can be applied by a solid needle of the same diameter. Solid material blades have limits on the accelerations they can sustain. An oscillating blade in a microkeratome moves at a maximum speed of a few meters per second. The microjet, in the microkeratome application, moves at a speed of approximately 450 mm per second. In other words, the microjet may be thought of as a rapidly moving, unidirectional needle of enormous rigidity.

MICROKERATOME DESIGN

The results described in Table 11-1 were obtained on a laboratory microkeratome utilizing computer controlled X-Y linear position drives for scanning and positioning with 1 micron placement accuracy, a filtering system for the sterilized water with .1 micron pores, and water pressure capability up to 20,000 pounds per square inch (psi). The beam-forming orifice is a ruby jewel with a specially shaped aperture (36 μm diameter) and shaped nozzle. The resulting beam diameter is typically about .9 times the orifice diameter (~33 μm). Other orifice diameters, ranging from 10 μm to 100 μm, are used depending on the application.

BEAM CHARACTERISTICS

The microjet microkeratome (the HydroBlade) is implemented by using a circular, parallel beam of sterile, highly filtered water (other fluids are possible) moving at supersonic speed. The speed of the beam depends on the stagnation pressure (ie, the hydrostatic water pressure before the beam gains speed, passes through and issues from the orifice). For an appropriately designed and constructed orifice, the emerging homogeneous beam (Figure 11-1) near the orifice looks like a fine monofilament (fish line). The fish line region of the beam is capable of sustaining radial oscillations, but the amplitude in an appropriately formed beam is too low to be visible. The perimeter of the beam interacts with the surrounding air or other media. Gradually, the homogeneity of the beam is compromised and micron-sized droplets form. It becomes unstable at some distance from the orifice. Once the beam loses its homogeneity, it quickly slows down and breaks into a fine mist beyond the fish line region (the incoherent region). The length of the fish line region depends on the orifice shape and diameter, the nozzle or orifice holder design, and the stagnation pressure. The achieved fish line lengths are typically more than adequate

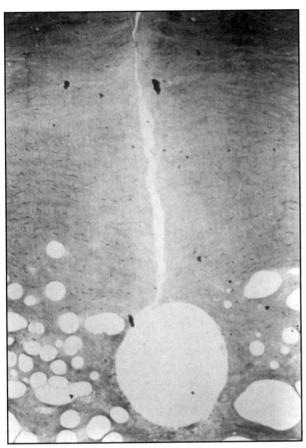

Figure 11-2. TEM (1500x). Cross section of a cornea after a blunt dissection performed with a waterjet intentionally directed into the tissue to produce hydration. Hydration is revealed by aeration.

for the applications described here. Although friction of the beam as it travels through the air does slow down, loss of speed is negligible in the homogeneous region.

For lamellar surgery, the typical settings are as follows: the stagnation pressure is 20,000 psi (1360 atmospheres) and beam diameter is 33 μm. This produces a fish line length of about 5 cm. The measured water flow rate in the beam is about 367 microliters per second. The average beam speed, as established by experimental measurements, is ~450 m/s. From the flow rate and average speed, we calculate that the beam carries a continuous kinetic power of approximately 35 watts (95 joules per milliliter). The measured temperature rise of the spent beam in a calorimeter is at most 23°C, but in cutting the tissue, temperature rise is negligible. The globe is kept at normal intraocular pressure (IOP), which increases by no more than 15% during the cut (as measured by a needle tonometer). The beam is mechanically scanned in a direction perpendicular to its length,

> For lamellar surgery, the typical settings are as follows: the stagnation pressure is 20,000 psi (1360 atmospheres) and beam diameter is 33 μm.

defining a cutting plane. During a cleave, the exiting beam force, as measured on the force transducer, is reduced by only 1.5 gram weight for the longest cleave dimension (8 mm). This force deficiency represents the maximum force exerted on the cornea by the beam.

The cleave, within the plane across 8 mm of cornea at a scan speed of 10 mm per second, takes .8 seconds (compared to 2 seconds for a scalpel cut) and requires no more than 294 μl of sterile water. The short time for the cleave and the negligible force on the cornea during the process insures the precision of the cut. Even an unsupported cornea at normal IOP does not visibly move or compress when it is cut by a microjet. In this case, the microjet can shave off layers as thin as a few microns.

Beam contact with the tissue along its path takes place for only about 18 μsec, and the water moves only parallel to the surface of the cut tissue, and not into the tissue; hence there is no hydration. Absence of hydration is verified by the complete absence of aeration in the tissue, which would be expected if there was hydration since the water in the beam contains air in a concentration well above the normal concentration at atmospheric pressure. When hydration is intentionally produced, as by directing the beam into the tissue, there is substantial aeration. This is further confirmed by transmission electron microscope observation of the cross section after a blunt dissection (Figure 11-2).[3]

There are no shock waves, although a low background acoustic spectrum might be generated based on microjet studies on hard materials (HY Li, International Waterjet Conference, Scotland, 1993). In fact, there are no known physical or chemical mechanisms other than the mechanical force at the level of 1 gram that might impact the safety of the procedure or the condition of the tissue. As noted, the magnitude of the mechanical force is substantially lower than that associated with scalpel cuts.

THE MICROJET AS A MICROKERATOME

INTER-LAMELLAR CLEAVING

The physical explanation for how the HydroBlade cleaves is fairly complex, but a simple way to understand the physics is to consider that water molecules or micron-sized droplets at the boundary of the beam collide with tissue as the beam begins to come into contact with the tissue. The boundary water mass is deflected and changes its transverse momentum component from virtually zero to some finite value directed inward into the beam. This is equivalent to providing an outward reactive force on the tissue from the beam. The beam behaves much like a dull circular wedge of enormous rigidity not available from normal materials. It cleaves along the easiest path, sacrificing beam energy and scattering as it goes. The stagnation pressure and beam velocity are made large enough that the cleave is completely through the tissue for the chosen scan speed, which is typically about 10 to 20 mm per second. The emerging beam shows relatively little degradation.[3]

Across Lamellae Cutting

When necessary, the microjet beam is perfectly capable of cutting like a blade across lamellae as in producing a shaped lenticle. However, cutting across a lamella and breaking all the fibrils within it takes substantially more energy than an interlamellar cleave in which only a few fibrils need to be cut. Thus, the scan rate is chosen to be lower for producing a shaped lenticle in which lamellae must be cut.

The Shape of the Cut

The nature and shape of the incised tissue is defined by the shape of the anterior surface of the cornea during the planar microjet cut. The anterior shape during the cut is established by a suction template since incision by a microjet without erosion requires that the tissue not be under significant compression. A suction template deforms the tissue by pulling it toward and into the template rather than by compression applanating the tissue.

A flat suction template, spaced at a predetermined distance away from the plane of the cut, produces a parallel lamellar flap of thickness equal to the distance. A hinge of predetermined width may be produced by blocking the jet during the scan so that it does not cut all the way from side to side. A slightly concave template allows removal of a plano convex lenticle of predetermined refraction. Lenticles with positive, negative, or astigmatic refraction may be removed. The position of the hinge can be chosen wherever desired by establishing the scan direction.

The design features of the actual template (Figure 11-3) are complex and include a micro-roughened surface that grips the anterior corneal surface and insures the stability of the cornea during the cleave. This minimizes corneal oscillations, thereby ensuring achievement of the desired thickness of the lenticle and the accuracy of position of the cleaved boundary region. In producing a flap, the template design includes a circular cylindrical trephine as its boundary. A small circular gap between the template and inner wall of the trephine provides a vacuum suction ring that converts the template surface into a vacuum chuck. The trephine is used to create a well-defined shallow gutter region surrounding a central corneal plateau. The jet, therefore, enters the lamellar structure without the need to cut through lamellar layers.

Experimental Results of Lamellar Resections (Cleaving versus Cutting)

Pairs of cadaver eyes from the same donor, 48 hours after enucleation, were mounted in holders. A flap was created in one eye using a Chiron ACS keratome. The Medjet

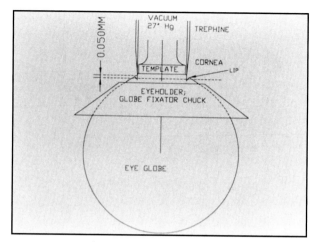

Figure 11-3. Schematic representation of the template. In producing a flap, the template design consists of a cylindrical trephine in which the circular template is located. A small circular gap between the template and the inner wall of the trephine provides a vacuum suction ring that converts the template surface into a vacuum chuck.

microjet microkeratome was used to produce an 8 mm diameter, 150 μm-thick flap in the other eye. Samples were immediately fixed in Karnovsky's solution (2.5% glutaraldehyde and 2% paraformaldehyde) and then processed for scanning electron microscopy.

Parallel cleaving with a HydroBlade to generate a corneal flap produces a new stromal (lamellar) surface such as would be expected with an ideal blunt dissection. The removed cap is without wedge. The cadaver eye cap shown in Figure 11-4a is 8 mm in diameter and about 150 microns thick. The top untouched surface and the underside cleaved surface are essentially indistinguishable. The associated surface of the stromal bed is seen in Figure 11-4b without a tear film.

> Parallel cleaving with a HydroBlade to generate a corneal flap produces a new stromal (lamellar) surface such as would be expected with an ideal blunt dissection.

It can be seen in Figure 11-5a through 11-5c that the mechanical microkeratome pulls and rips tissue (the white areas are the ends of cut lamellae) while the HydroBlade (Figure 11-5d through 11-5f) cuts only the few collagen fibrils linking vertically adjacent lamellae (the white spots in the figure are the bulbous ends of cut interconnecting fibrils). The white spots appear in all images of the surface and can be observed even under low magnification. Figure 11-6 illustrates that the keratocytes are not removed in the process of HydroBlade cleaving.

Resection of nonparallel lenticules (cutting through the lamellae) takes more energy from the beam. The trajectory of the cut is along the interlamellar boundary and then quickly across the lamella, then along the boundary again.

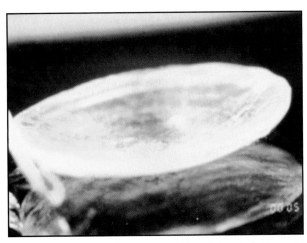

Figure 11-4a. Corneal cap cut with the HydroBlade 8 mm in diameter and approximately 150 μm thick.

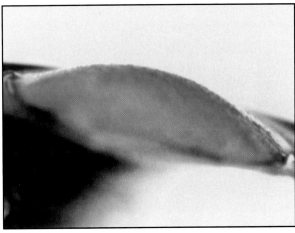

Figure 11-4b. Surface of the stromal bed associated with the cap.

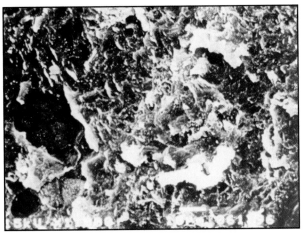

Figure 11-5a. Scanning electron microscope (1000x). Human corneal surface after creating a flap with a Chiron ACS keratome. The mechanical microkeratome pulls and rips tissue (the white areas are the ends of cut lamellae).

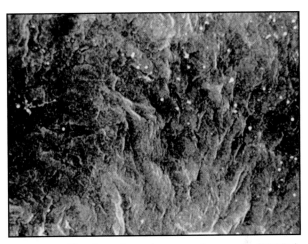

Figure 11-5b. Scanning electron microscope (1000x). Human corneal surface after creating a flap with the HydroBlade. Only the few collagen fibrils linking vertically adjacent lamellae are cut (the white spots in the figure are the bulbous ends of cut interconnecting fibrils).

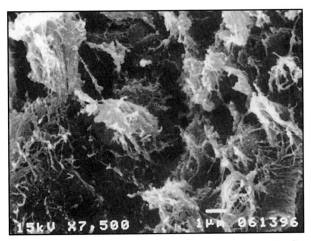

Figure 11-5c. Scanning electron microscope (7500x). The same image at higher magnification.

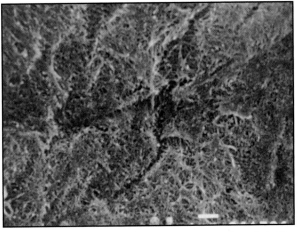

Figure 11-5d. Scanning electron microscope (7500x). The same image at higher magnification.

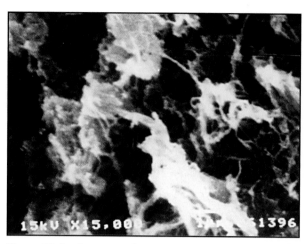

Figure 11-5e. Scanning electron microscope (15,000x). The same image at higher magnification.

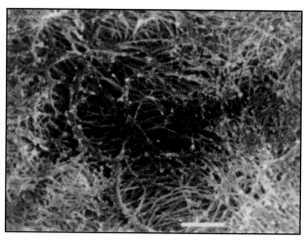

Figure 11-5f. Scanning electron microscope (15,000x). The same image at higher magnification.

The transit across the lamellae requires cutting many more fibrils than in an interlamellar cleave. The locus of the across-the-lamella transit is generally a narrow circular ring, it was anticipated that this would be the site of haze in the post surgical live cornea because the fibril spacing is increased at the position of the cut, and increased spacing allows backscatter. Elimination of optical back scattering, or haze, depends critically on maintaining the normal spacing of fibrils. In contrast, no haze was expected in the interlamellar cut region. It was, in fact, observed experimentally in rabbits that low level haze occurs only where the cut is across the lamella. It does not occur along the cleaved interlamellar boundary. Thus, the haze in Dutch belted rabbits was observed in the form of a bull's eye pattern and was generally low level and gone in less than 15 weeks (Figure 11-7). (The experimental details and results on a 20-rabbit study will be reported in a separate publication.)

Waterjet-only Procedures

The HydroBlade keratome can be used for therapeutic surgery and refractive surgery.

Therapeutic Surgery: Hydro-therapeutic Keratoplasty

The HydroBlade keratome is intended to be used for lamellar keratoplasty. Lamellar keratoplasty is currently performed with a blade-based device and involves the removal of a disc of diseased tissue from the patient's cornea, the separation of a corneal disc of equal diameter and depth from a donor cornea, and the application of the donor's corneal disc onto the patient's corneal bed.

Lamellar keratoplasty is the ideal method of surgery for corneal diseases because it attacks the stroma (the internal part of the cornea) and leaves the endothelium (the posterior part of the cornea) intact. The reason why lamellar keratoplasty is preferred over penetrating (full thickness) keratoplasty is safety. The main cause for corneal graft rejec-

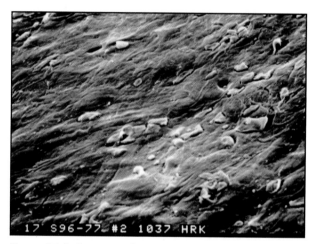

Figure 11-6. Scanning electron microscope (400x). Human corneal surface after creating a flap with the HydroBlade. The keratocytes are not removed in the cleaving process.

tion is the endothelium. By leaving the endothelium of the patient in place, we can expect to reduce the rate of rejection. While the epithelium (the anterior layer) regrows in a few days if removed, the endothelium has no mitosis ability and does not regrow if damaged. With lamellar keratoplasty, the risk of endothelium damage is avoided. Furthermore, with lamellar keratoplasty there is no penetration of the globe, thus there is no risk of endophthalmitis, secondary glaucoma, or secondary cataract.

In past decades, lamellar keratoplasty was frequently performed. Later it was abandoned and substituted with penetrating (full thickness) keratoplasty, due to the difficulties in performing the lamellar procedure with the available devices (blade microkeratome). It was difficult, in fact, to separate the donor's corneal disc and prepare a smooth corneal bed in the recipient's cornea with a blade. This often led to scarring, irregularities, and haze at the donor/recipient interface, resulting in postoperative visual acuity rarely better than 20/40.

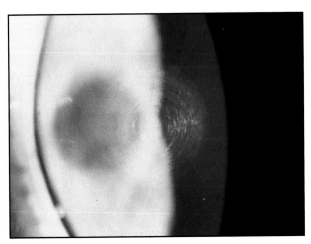

Figure 11-7. Rabbit cornea as seen using slit lamp biomicroscopy after across-lamellae cutting. A low level haze in the form of a bull's eye pattern occurs only where the cut is across the lamellae. It does not occur along the cleaved interlamellar boundary.

These difficulties were overcome by separating the donor's and recipient's corneas with a waterjet-based device due to the high sectility properties of the cornea and cleaving ability of the waterjet.

The surgical procedure with the HydroBlade keratome is exactly as described for lamellar keratoplasty; the only difference is that the procedure would be performed with a waterjet cutting device instead of a blade-based cutting device.

With the HydroBlade keratome, corneal discs for partial thickness transplants can be taken at death from donors who are over 65 years of age. This is not possible for conventional full-thickness transplants in which donors are required to be under 65 years of age because of age-related degradation of the endothelium. Furthermore, by providing a smoother surface and thus a smoother donor/recipient corneal interface, less scarring should occur.

Currently, penetrating keratoplasty involves removing and exchanging a full disc from the donor and patient corneas. Approximately 45,000 penetrating keratoplasty procedures are performed annually in the United States. It is estimated that 5000 to 6000 of those procedures could be lamellar keratoplasty based on the corneal pathology.

Refractive Surgery: Hydro-refractive Keratoplasty

The Hydroblade keratome is a microkeratome capable of performing refractive surgery using four different procedures: hydro-refractive keratectomy (HRK), hydro-lamellar keratoplasty (HLK), hydro-lenticuloplasty (HLP), and waterjet in situ keratomileusis (WISK).

Hydro-refractive Keratomectomy

During HRK Figure 11-8, a determined amount of

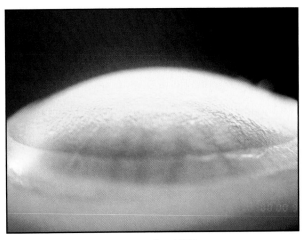

Figure 11-8. Human cornea after HRK.

epithelium, Bowman's membrane, and stroma are removed to produce a refractive change. The shape of the removed tissue resembles the shape of the tissue removed during PRK. It has been shown by topography studies on human corneas that Medjet can calculate the shape of special templates used in the procedure that precisely determine the refractive power of the tissue removed, and these can be provided to the surgeon for HRK. Thus, it was shown that the accuracy of the final refraction was determined by mechanical templates. The surface of the stromal bed is so smooth that it can be readily observed topographically (Figure 11-9a and 11-9b) (Gordon EI. ISRS Meeting. San Francisco, Calif; 1997).

Based on animal studies we anticipate that HRK will heal with a low level of haze (See Figure 11-7). It should be less traumatic than PRK because of the benign nature of the microjet cut.

> During HRK, a determined amount of epithelium, Bowman's membrane, and stroma are removed to produce a refractive change.

Hydro-Lamellar Keratoplasty

HLK (Figures 11-10a and 11-10b) with the microjet is akin to keratomileusis in situ with a knife blade (ALK) to correct myopia. The differences are that the blade is replaced by a microjet and the shaping of the tissue removal from the stromal bed is done with a stationary template and with less trauma. Another difference is that the removed tissue in the second cut has the prerequisite shape to produce the desired refractive change accurately enough to treat myopia, hyperopia, and astigmatism (Gordon EI. ISRS Meeting. San Francisco, Calif; 1997).

> HLK with the microjet is akin to keratomileusis in situ with a knife blade (ALK) to correct myopia.

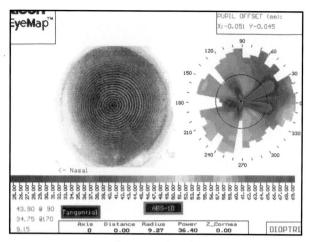

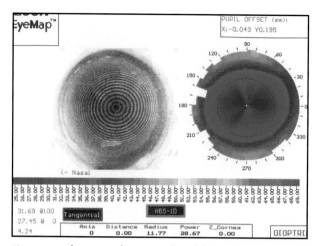

Figure 11-9a. Corneal topography of a human cadaver eye.

Figure 11-9b. Corneal topography of the stromal bed of the same eye after HRK. Note the regularity of the Placido rings.

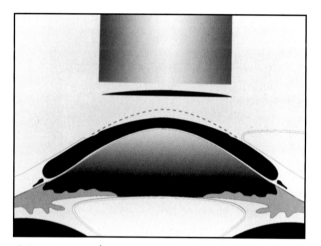

Figure11-10a. Schematic representation of HLK.

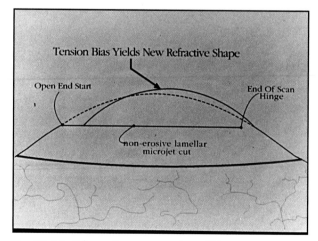

Figure 11-10b. Cornea of a human cadaver eye after HLK.

Hydro-lenticuloplasty

Because of the difficulty of doing meaningful experiments on enucleated eyes. A technique known as HLP (Figure 11-11) is similar to one-pass ALK for hyperopia. Limited experimental data is presented.

The basic idea is that the eye globe resembles a lightly inflated rubber ball with tension in the surface. It is possible to make localized changes in the shape of the anterior surface for refractive correction of myopia, hyperopia, and astigmatism by one or more judicious, shallow incisions approximately parallel to the surface. A specially shaped lenticular hinged flap is created, which then assumes a new shape by virtue of a new local distribution of mechanical tensions and is left to heal in place. No material is removed. The surface layer is preserved. Because the cuts are being shallow, they do not threaten the integrity or stability of the globe. The flaps that are made by this technique are similar to the hinged lamellar flaps used in LASIK except for their special nonlamellar shape, which is determined by the choice of template (Gordon EI. ISRS Meeting. San Francisco, Calif; 1997).

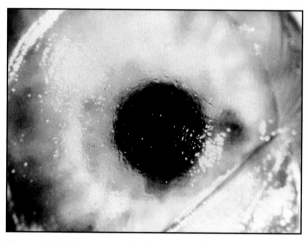

Fig. 11-11. Schematic representation of HLP.

Hydro-lenticuloplasty is similar to one-pass ALK for hyperopia.

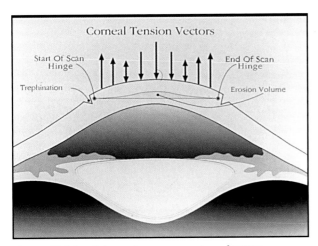

Figure 11-12a. Schematic representation of WISK.

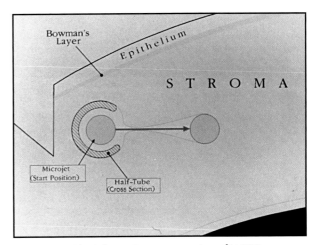

Figure 11-12b. Schematic representation of WISK.

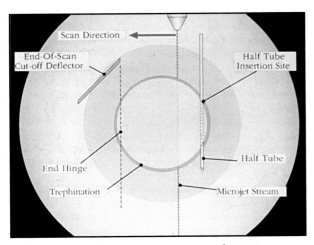

Figure 11-12c. Schematic representation of WISK.

Waterjet in situ keratomileusis

WISK is a new and unique approach to lamellar surgery that is possible with only a waterjet device (not a laser or a scalpel) (Figure 11-12a through 11-12c). WISK is an intrastromal procedure under a fixed double-hinged flap. A lamellar cut (at normal IOP) parallel to, but under the surface of, the cornea is made instantaneously and simultaneously producing a tissue flap that is held in place by two narrow opposing tissue hinges. The flap is never removed; it stays in its normal position and cannot come off the cornea. It need not be positioned by the surgeon because it does not move. However, by judiciously applying compression or torsion locally to the cornea with shaped templates, the extent of erosion or cleaving of the tissue under the flap is controlled during which the cut produces the flap. The erosion leads to shaping of the anterior surface because tissue is removed. Thus, in less than 1 second and with one drop of saline solution, the space under the surface is shaped. The necessary tissue to be removed is eroded and washed away, and the original preserved surface assumes a new shape and new refractive power. Correction of myopia by flattening the cornea was demonstrated with topography

> Waterjet in situ keratomileusis is an intrastromal procedure under a fixed double-hinged flap.

studies on human corneas (Gordon EI. ISRS Meeting. San Francisco, Calif; 1997).

The basic idea rests in Medjet's discovery that the microjet cuts corneal tissue by cleaving or erosion. Cleaving occurs when the tissue is under slight tension perpendicular to the plane defined by the direction of scan and direction of the beam.

Erosion occurs when the tissue is under compression perpendicular to the plane defined by the direction of scan and direction of the beam. The degree of erosion is controlled by compression. Since the degree and extent of local compression or tension can be controlled by a shaped template placed on the anterior surface of the cornea with or without suction, it is possible to remove a shaped volume of tissue intrastromally while the surface is in place and never removed. The surface would be a large diameter with an opposing hinged flap.

In effect, one can do a procedure like keratomileusis in situ in a single scan step, leaving a double-hinged flap in place that is never moved from its customary position. There is no hydration or aeration since the beam passes completely through the tissue. So far, we have done a myopic correction simply by pressing on the apex of the cornea with a flat template while cutting at normal IOP. However, hyperopic and astigmatic corrections are also possible and have been demonstrated (Gordon EI. Unpublished material).

CONCLUSION

A new surgical instrument—a microkeratome with multiple possible applications was presented. Although Medjet's HydroBlade keratome will be presented in the near future to the ophthalmology community as an alternative to

> First used in flap-making for LASIK, we believe that the future of refractive surgery will be waterjet-only procedures.

the current microkeratomes and will probably be first used in flap-making for LASIK, we believe that the future of refractive surgery will be waterjet-only procedures.

REFERENCES

1. Baer HU, Metzger A, Barras JP, Mettler D, Wheatley AM, Czerniak A. Laparoscopic liver resection in the large white pig—a comparison between waterjet dissector and ultrasound dissector. *Endosc Surg Allied Technol.* 1994;2(3-4):189-93.

2. Parolini B, Turdiu P, Abelson M, Zarbin M, Gordon EI. Hydro-epithelial keratectomy performed with the HydroBrush. *Journal of Refractive Surgery.* In press.

3. Gordon EI, Parolini B, Abelson M. The HydroBlade and the HydroBrush™ keratomes. Principles and microscopic confirmation of surface quality. *Journal of Refractive Surgery.* In press.

4. Krueger RR, Parolini B, Gordon EI, Juhasz T. Nonmechanical microkeratomes using laser and waterjet technology. In: Pallikaris IR, Siganos DS, eds. *LASIK.* SLACK Incorporated: Thorofare, NJ; 1998:81-105.

5. Eisner G. Eye Surgery, An Introduction to Operative Technique. Springer-Verlag: Berlin, Germany; 1990:64.

SECTION THREE
Preoperative LASIK Evaluation

Preoperative Myopic and Hyperopic LASIK Evaluation

Jeffery J. Machat, MD

CONSULTATIVE PROCESS

The consultative process for all refractive procedures is similar in concept. The risks, benefits, limitations, and reasonable expectations of the procedure are reviewed with each potential candidate. Although laser in situ keratomileusis (LASIK) may offer candidates the ability to correct mild to severe degrees of myopia, hyperopia, and astigmatism with rapid visual rehabilitation; the intraoperative risks must be discussed.

The ability to successfully manage each patient both intraoperatively and postoperatively is facilitated, as well as the medical-legal responsibilities fulfilled, when a conservative and direct approach is taken with each patient. Managing patient expectations is the pivotal element to creating happy refractive patients.

When the outcome is successful, the preoperative informed consent process has very little meaning; however, if a poor result is obtained, the preoperative consent is indispensable. A surgeon who never has a complication is one who never performs surgery. Complications are an inherent part of any surgical procedure. Visual complications are emotionally traumatic, as the patient is reminded of the poor outcome during every waking hour. It is because the world is so visual that refractive surgery has the ability to dramat-

> When the outcome is successful, the preoperative informed consent process has very little meaning; however, if a poor result is obtained, the preoperative consent is indispensable.

ically improve the quality of a patient's life. Conversely, complications can be just as detrimental. Legal blindness has now been reported with photorefractive keratectomy (PRK) and LASIK, therefore the potential for LASIK to produce real and irreversible harm to an eye cannot be overstated.

LASIK offers rapid visual recovery without the discomfort commonly associated with PRK and without the loss of corneal stability associated with RK. LASIK also enjoys the greater refractive predictability associated with PRK but without significant risk of subepithelial haze formation. Therefore, LASIK can offer the best characteristic of both PRK and RK without many of their disadvantages.

In explaining to patients the LASIK procedure as compared to PRK, we state that both procedures are designed to change the curve of their eye to match that of their prescription, be it in glasses or contacts. It is not important whether the laser changes the curve on the surface of the eye or in the deeper layers, so long as the curve is changed. The surface of the eye is more sensitive and more reactive, requiring a longer healing time and more eye drops. Therefore, if we are performing a lot of surgery to correct moderate or high myopia, we prefer to treat the deeper layers with LASIK rather than superficially with PRK. PRK is associated with greater risk of infection, in the range of 1/1000 to 1/2000 compared to 1/5000 to 1/10,000 with LASIK. PRK is also associated with more risk of pain, approximately 1/10 compared to 1/50 following LASIK. It is best never to state LASIK is completely painless as any epithelial defect will be associated with some discomfort. The risk of haze or scarring after PRK is only 1% or less for

Figure 12-1. Dense confluent haze following attempted PRK correction of -10.5 D myopia.

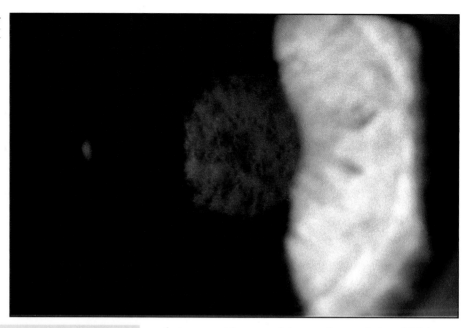

	PRK	LASIK
Pain	1/10	1/50
Infection	1/1000	1/5000
Scarring	1-5/100	1/1000
Steroid drops	1 - 6 months	4 - 7 days
Visual recovery	1 - 4 weeks	1 - 4 days

low degrees of correction, but as high as 5% to 8% for higher degrees (Figure 12-1). The risk of scarring with LASIK is likely in the order of .1% for all degrees of correction but is rarely observed with low corrections. Steroid drops are typically needed for only 4 to 7 days with LASIK compared to 1 to 6 months with PRK. Visual recovery typically requires 1 to 4 weeks for PRK, compared to 1 to 4 days with LASIK.

The main disadvantage for LASIK is that a lamellar cut is involved, which adds a new element of risk—that of serious corneal flap complications, including corneal perforation. Incredibly, corneal perforation has also been reported after multiple enhancement procedures with PRK.

When discussing LASIK with our patients, we explain the LASIK procedure and instrumentation by describing the microkeratome as being analogous to a carpenter's plane, which is used to create a protective corneal flap. We describe the cornea as a book consisting of approximately 550 pages. LASIK involves the creation of a corneal flap consisting of typically 160 to 180 pages, then removing approximately 17 to 170 pages. The final step is closing the book, which when closed, looks virtually unchanged. This is in direct contrast to PRK, which involves removing the protective surface epithelium, or book cover, and Bowman's layer, or important first chapter. Alternatively, the typical corneal thickness is approximately 11 hairs thick, with the corneal flap being about three hairs thick; we further explain

that we must leave a minimum of seven hairs of thickness, but ideally eight hairs (400 microns) for long-term corneal stability. This concept is especially useful when treating very high degrees of myopia or when considering enhancement of high myopes. We continue to state that when a complication does occur, it is more serious with LASIK. We place LASIK in the context that we consider it to be the best overall refractive procedure, but that all procedures have to be considered in terms of their risk-to-benefit ratio for each patient. As clinical experience develops, refractive surgeons will offer LASIK for virtually all degrees of myopia, hyperopia, and astigmatism, but until adequate experience is gathered, LASIK should be reserved for moderate to high myopia. For low degrees of myopia, the predictability of PRK has been extremely high, and the risk of serious complication extremely low. Since the final uncorrected visual results of PRK and LASIK are similar for the lower end of the myopic spectrum, the selection of the refractive procedure should be based on the experience and skill level of the surgeon and the risk potential for flap complications. That is, it is much more difficult to justify both to a patient and to the courts having a serious flap complication when attempting LASIK for low myopia correction when little experience has been achieved. The risk-benefit ratio concept for LASIK must take surgeon experience into account.

The most important factors for patients contemplating LASIK have been the speed of recovery and the lack of pain. It appears that most patients, even those with more moderate and severe degrees of myopia, still wish to have a procedure that disrupts their life as little as possible. Additionally, most people find it difficult to proceed with any procedure that produces pain, even if they place significant long-term value on a procedure associated with short-term discomfort. Fear of pain and discomfort from eye surgery may keep the majority of myopes from considering

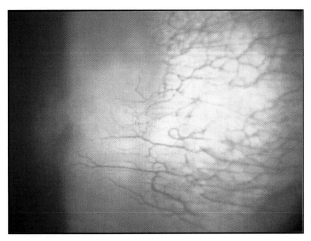

Figure 12-2. Corneal neovascularization can result in postoperative bleeding if the vessels are cut during LASIK.

refractive surgery. As a general rule, female patients tolerate eye procedures better than male patients do. Young male patients are generally extremely anxious and often require additional preoperative sedation prior to LASIK. All patients considering refractive surgery are fearful of losing their eyesight, which is why most patients, regardless of how motivated or affluent they are, will not proceed with any procedure. We believe that only 5% to 10% of myopes will ever seriously contemplate any refractive procedure, and only 1% to 2% of myopes will eventually undergo PRK or LASIK.

CANDIDATE SELECTION

LASIK is capable of treating up to 15 D of myopia. The lower refractive limit for which LASIK is the preferred procedure is variable and somewhat controversial, primarily because of the variability in surgeon comfort and skill level with LASIK. With PRK's excellent clinical results and safety profile for mild and moderate myopia, the benefits of LASIK for these patients mainly consist of the convenience of the postoperative course. As stated, some surgeons perform LASIK for all refractive procedures, even for corrections as low as -.5 D, while others reserve LASIK for patients with more than -10 D. The general consensus appears to be that the distinct clinical advantage of LASIK over PRK occurs over -4 D, with significant benefits occurring above -6 D. A reasonable range for the experienced LASIK surgeon extends from -.75 D or -1 D to -15 D with the upper limit depending upon the corneal thickness.

PRK astigmatic ablations greater than 3 D and myopic ablations greater than 6 D are associated with a higher degree of clinically significant haze, in the range of 2% to 5%, even with the best techniques. Although clinically significant haze is treatable, prolonged visual recovery and multiple procedures are required. LASIK is rapidly replacing PRK as the preferred procedure for not only moderate to high myopia but moderate to high cylinder. Toric ablations may be performed with LASIK within the stromal bed for the correction of several diopters of cylinder. Similarly, hyperopic ablation patterns are more likely to be associated with haze and regression of effect; therefore, LASIK is recommended for hyperopia correction, hyperopic astigmatism correction, and mixed astigmatism correction.

Candidate selection must also include other elements independent of refractive error, specifically orbit configuration, as well as ocular and general health considerations. Candidates with small or deep-set orbits should be avoided or forewarned that the procedure may have to be aborted if the microkeratome ring cannot be well-positioned. Once surgical experience is adequate, these cases may be attempted, but they are initially discouraged altogether. Similarly, narrow palpebral fissures may complicate placement of the suction ring and may interfere with passage of the microkeratome. If there are concerns about the ability to place the suction in a small orbit, a preplacement attempt can be made to evaluate the potential LASIK candidate. Any obstacles to smooth passage of the microkeratome will undoubtedly compromise the success of obtaining a good corneal flap and result in a higher complication rate. Patients with small orbits or narrow palpebral openings may experience increased discomfort intraoperatively and should be counseled appropriately. In general, it is advisable to openly discuss any difficulties that may be encountered with each candidate as patients rarely elect not to proceed and are far more understanding of intraoperative complications. Surgical techniques to deal with these patients will be discussed later.

Corneal neovascularization or macropannus should be identified preoperatively, as this may result in intraoperative bleeding following the lamellar cut (Figure 12-2). Although LASIK in these patients is not contraindicated, measures (discussed later) may be taken to reduce intraoperative difficulties. Similarly, a patient with a flat cornea (mean keratometry of $\leq$ 41 D) treated with the classic Chiron Corneal Shaper will have a small corneal flap and an increased risk of developing a free cap. The antidesiccation chamber should be on-hand while a thicker corneal flap and hinge is fashioned. Pachymetry should be performed on all patients to ensure an adequate stromal bed thickness exists for the planned treatment (Figure 12-3). Progressive corneal ectasia may be observed with a residual total corneal thickness of 300 microns with PRK or a residual stromal bed thickness of less than 200 microns with LASIK. An absolute minimum total corneal thickness of 360 microns, ideally 380 to 400 microns, should remain postoperatively. Since the corneal flap thickness may vary, it is the stromal bed thickness that is most important, with the absolute minimum stromal bed thickness of 200 microns required to ensure long-term corneal stability. Alternatively, the most conservative approach states that no greater than 50% of the corneal thickness should be penetrated to ensure long-term

Figure 12-3. Preoperative ultrasonic corneal pachymetry is performed for all patients prior to LASIK to ensure adequate corneal thickness.

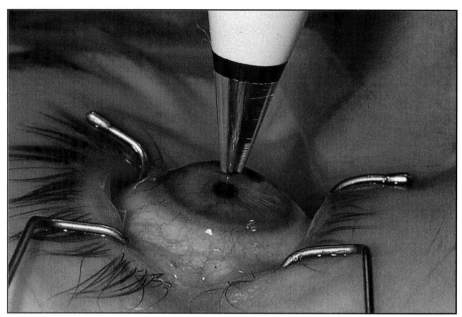

corneal stability. For example, with a 540-micron cornea and 160-micron flap, the maximum ablation depth is 110 microns of the initial 380-micron stromal bed, which will leave 50% or 270 microns. Patients with a history of prior ocular surgery, including vitreoretinal and cataract surgery, should be approached cautiously, as it is often difficult to achieve adequate suction pressure throughout the microkeratome cut, and an irregular thin flap may be obtained. It may also be more difficult to maintain adequate suction in eyes with conjunctival scarring arising from infection, trauma, or prior surgery such as strabismus surgery.

PRK may be preferable to LASIK in cases of recurrent corneal erosion syndrome, anterior basement membrane dystrophies, or superficial corneal scarring, in that surface photoablation offers these patients some specific benefits in improving epithelial adhesion or eliminating visual opacification. Furthermore, poor epithelial adherence complicates lamellar surgery, dramatically increasing the incidence of epithelial ingrowth and prolonging the LASIK visual rehabilitation timeline. Any active inflammation, infection or other ocular pathology are contraindications for LASIK.

LASIK and RK should be considered preferable to PRK for any patient who requires rapid visual rehabilitation, although newer PRK techniques such as transepithelial ablations and scanning lasers have reduced recovery time to as little as 1 week for driving vision for many patients. LASIK should be considered and perhaps even be indicated in cases in which proper wound healing is critical or may be impaired, such as with keloid formers. PRK is absolutely contraindicated for autoimmune diseases and collagen vascular diseases, as the risk of stromal melt with an exposed stromal surface is significantly elevated. In LASIK, since the epithelium remains intact and the stroma only exposed intraoperatively, the concerns for precipitating a stromal melt are unclear but likely minimal. The authors have per-

formed LASIK on patients with rheumatoid arthritis antibodies with lupus antibodies without active disease without experiencing any recovery problems or ocular sequelae. There have, however, been other anecdotal reports of patients with early rheumatoid arthritis and lupus being treated successfully, but caution must be exercised. The authors have treated active scleroderma and fibromyalgia without sequelae, but these conditions pose little risk for stromal melting. Active or severe vasculitic conditions should always be avoided for any refractive surgery procedure, as refractive procedures are elective. Other inactive or resolved conditions that have been treated successfully without healing or surgical sequelae include multiple sclerosis, Graves and Hashimoto's thyroiditis, and Crohn's disease.

Another subset of patients who are better treated with LASIK rather than PRK are those who exhibit medication intolerance or noncompliance. Specifically, steroid responders observed from PRK treatment of the first eye or those with a strong family history of glaucoma may do better with LASIK, since a steroid-induced pressure rise may seriously complicate the postoperative course or result in visual field loss. Patients with glaucomatous field loss should ideally be avoided, as the brief intraoperative rise in intraocular pressure (IOP) from the suction may theoretically damage the optic nerve and cause further field loss. Of sufficient clinical importance is the fact that IOP is underestimated following laser refractive surgery, making follow-up cases more difficult. Glaucoma, however, is considered by many to be a relative contraindication and must be assessed on a case-by-case basis. The fear with many of these progressive conditions is that any progression of the underlying disease may be attributed to the refractive procedure. Similarly, some neuro-ophthalmologists have suggested that patients with optic nerve disease should be fully evaluated prior to

TABLE 12-1.
LASIK

Indicated	Caution	Relative contraindications	Absolute contraindications
Up to 15 D of myopia	Flat corneas	Endothelial dystrophies (cell count < 1500)	
Low to moderate hyperopia			
Low to high astigmatism	Small orbits	Monocular patients	
Keloid formers			Herpes zoster
Long rigid gas permeable contact lens history		Abnormal eyelid closure	ophthalmicus (HZO)
		Anterior basement membrane dystrophy	
Forme fruste keratoconus (adequate corneal thickness)	Post-RK	Active collagen vascular disease	
Medication intolerance or noncompliance	Post-PKP	Systemic vasculitis	
Steroid responders	Endothelial dystrophies (cell count > 1500)		Keratoconus (KC)
Rapid visual recovery desired		Thin corneas	

LASIK. Patients who live far away or may be traveling in the near future may also be better served with LASIK, as less follow-up is required (Table 12-1).

RELATIVE AND ABSOLUTE CONTRAINDICATIONS

There are far fewer contraindications to LASIK than to PRK because of the dramatically reduced wound-healing requirements. Systemic contraindications, as outlined earlier in the chapter, are almost nonexistent, with only a few ocular contraindications. Monocular patients are always contraindicated for elective refractive surgery in our opinion. Clinical keratoconus is a specific absolute contraindication for LASIK, and forme fruste keratoconus is a relative contraindication because the results are less predictable and the stromal ablation may lead to further loss of corneal stability. Autoimmune and collagen vascular disorders, as described above, are not absolutely contraindicated with intrastromal ablation techniques, but caution is always advised and it is best to avoid any patients with active disease.

> There are far fewer contraindications to LASIK than to PRK because of the dramatically reduced wound-healing requirements.

Although undercorrected RK is not a contraindication to LASIK, there is a risk that the corneal flap will fragment, especially in patients with greater than eight radial incisions. Prior lamellar surgery or even PRK are also not contraindications. Patients with prior penetrating keratoplasty should be approached cautiously because of graft dehiscence and rejection, however LASIK after penetrating keratoplasty has been performed successfully throughout the world (see

Chapter 28). Corneal scars usually do not present difficulties in LASIK but must be evaluated carefully to determine that they are well-healed and not more amenable to surface ablation. Corneal scarring from Herpes simplex is more complex and remains a relative contraindication as reactivation may occur and antiviral prophylaxis is indicated. Surgeons should ideally avoid all refractive procedures in herpetic eyes with reduced corneal sensation, a significant history of keratouveitic disease, recent or multiple recurrences, or a history of Herpes zoster ophthalmicus. A history of retinal detachment or retinal tears is not a contraindication for LASIK. Caution should be exercised and proper counseling initiated in patients with lacquer cracks and other significant retinal pathology. Retinitis pigmentosa is a relative contraindication, as the increased IOP may have an amplified effect due to the attenuated vasculature, optic nerve, and retinal changes. Most importantly, refractive surgery may further compromise night vision. Diabetes mellitus types I and II are not contraindicated, but the presence of diabetic retinopathy indicates that caution should be exercised and thorough preoperative counseling documented, as progression of disease is to be expected.

Reduced best-corrected visual acuity (BCVA) of less than 20/50 in one eye essentially creates a functionally monocular patient because any visual compromise in the better vision eye may prevent the patient from legally driving. Patients with 20/30 or 20/40 BCVA in one or both eyes should be carefully counseled and ideally treated in only one eye at a time to ensure that best-corrected vision is maintained. The most important aspect in counseling these patients is to maintain a conservative and honest approach while painting a clear picture of the worst case scenario, as even the loss of one line of best-corrected vision may be functionally devastating to these patients. High myopes not

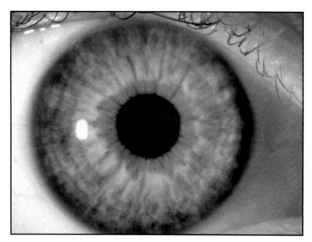

Figure 12-4a. Bilateral LASIK correction of residual myopia following RK in the right eye. A LASIK procedure was performed after 1 year to allow for full refractive stabilization and improved corneal integrity.

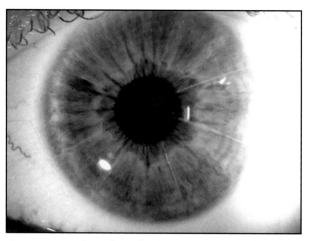

Figure 12-4b. Bilateral LASIK correction of residual myopia following RK in the left eye. A LASIK procedure was performed after 1 year to allow for full refractive stabilization and improved corneal integrity.

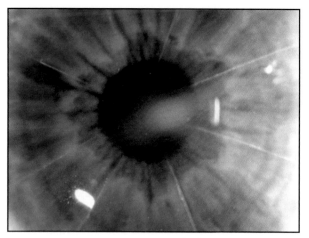

Figure 12-4c. Biomicroscope slit lamp clinical photo demonstrating small corneal flap misalignment under high magnification.

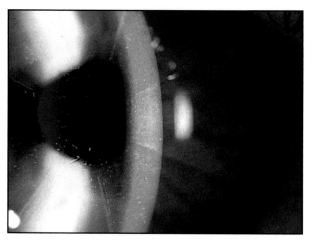

Figure 12-4d. Biomicroscope slit lamp clinical photo demonstrating small corneal flap misalignment under optical slit section.

only commonly have reduced best-corrected vision, but also night glare, and it is important to evaluate these candidates carefully, taking into account the corneal thickness, pupil size, and planned optical zone when counseling them.

Patients with anterior basement dystrophy and epithelial adherence problems should avoid LASIK whenever possible. If the epithelial surface becomes partially or fully denuded due to the microkeratome pass, an increased risk of epithelial ingrowth is observed and slower visual recovery noted. Prior procedures that have significantly altered the conjunctiva may interfere with the ability to obtain and maintain adequate suction during the lamellar cut, increasing the risk of a thin or perforated corneal flap. Similarly, any condition that results in significant vitreous syneresis, including pathological myopia or procedures such as vitrectomy, may result in inadequate suction pressure intraoperatively. An experienced lamellar surgeon may attempt these

more challenging cases, but complication rates are expectedly higher. The suction ring profile of the Chiron Hansatome is preferred in these cases.

LASIK AFTER RK

LASIK is the procedure of choice for retreatment of RK patients. Although 93% of our post-RK patients treated with PRK achieved 20/40 or better with one or more procedures and were stable at 1 year postoperatively, others developed dense haze that remained problematic after multiple procedures.

It appears that the poorest post-RK enhancement results occur in patients with the greatest number of incisions and the smallest optical zones.

Results with LASIK in undercorrected RK patients are excellent and stable, and unlike with PRK, the patients are not at risk for developing haze (Figures 12-4a to 12-4d). The visual recovery is rapid and the patient has little if any discomfort, which is similar to their RK experience and definitely preferred over the PRK experience.

It appears that the poorest post-RK enhancement results occur in patients with the greatest number of incisions and the smallest optical zones. Consequently, we shy away from treating patients with greater than eight radial incisions, although we have successfully treated many patients with 16 radial RK incisions. The over-riding concern in these patients is the risk of corneal flap fragmentation. The risk of flap fragmentation is increased in RK patients with a high number of incisions, astigmatic keratotomy (AK) incisions that bisect a radial incision, an optical zone smaller than 3 mm, or a history of peripheral redeepening or macroperforation (especially if they are exhibiting large diurnal fluctuations in their refractive error). Epithelial inclusions within RK incisions increase the risk of epithelial ingrowth and possibly fragmentation. Furthermore, RK patients should wait at least 1 year before undergoing LASIK retreatment, and preferably 2 years if a lack of incision scarring is evident.

Results in patients with consecutive hyperopia following RK are quite good but less predictable, especially when associated with cylinder. In cases of post-RK hyperopia, there are two important considerations: first, whether the hyperopia represents a true overcorrection or hyperopic creep that has been progressive over time indicating corneal instability; second, whether the hyperopia is associated with reduced BCVA, indicating that the hyperopia may simply be related to irregular astigmatism and not a true overcorrection amenable to hyperopic LASIK. Patients with spherical hyperopic overcorrections or with small degrees of hyperopic cylinder that have been documented as stable and have preserved best-corrected vision appear to do best.

RK often induces corneal instability that is exacerbated by PRK and LASIK. Post-RK patients to be wary of include those with:
- Poorly healed incisions
- Large epithelial cysts
- Very small optical zones (in the range of 2.5 mm or less)
- 16 or more incisions
- Large diurnal fluctuations
- Reduced BCVA of two or more lines
- Documented hyperopic shift

To date, I've been extremely pleased with the clinical results using LASIK to treat both consecutive myopia and hyperopia following RK. My preference is to use a 200-micron depth plate and target slight myopia based on a morning cycloplegic refraction. In general, post-RK patients should be treated one eye at a time with a high possibility of being treated on consecutive days. Alignment of the corneal flap is important because the number of incisions will appear to double if the incisions are not aligned. A surgeon should consider treating these patients only after he or she has performed at least 50, and preferably 100, LASIK procedures because management of the corneal flap is definitely more demanding. If there is a need to retreat again, the flap should be recut after several months—not lifted—to avoid fragmentation. I have successfully lifted LASIK flaps in RK patients within 1 week of the primary enhancement procedure when predictability was very poor. This concept works on the principle that flap adhesion is still minimal and less than the RK incision strength. In these cases, I typically float the flap to elevate it using a 27-gauge cannula and BSS, avoiding overhydration.

PREOPERATIVE EXAMINATION

VISUAL ACUITY

Just as with all refractive procedures, documentation of UCVA and BCVA must be made. Severe and extreme myopia is associated with reduced BCVA, which may differ between spectacle correction and contact lens correction. Higher myopes and astigmats may enjoy a level of visual acuity in rigid gas permeable contact lenses that may be impossible to replicate with refractive surgery. Documentation and discussion of these more challenging cases is important both medically in assessing postoperative outcomes and in achieving high levels of patient satisfaction. Patients with reduced best-corrected vision in one eye may not be suitable candidates, as complications in the good eye may preclude driving.

REFRACTION

A careful manifest and cycloplegic refraction must be performed with attention given to true vertex distance in cases of high myopia. Higher myopes are often overcorrected in their spectacle correction in an attempt to improve their quality of vision. In cases of extreme myopia, it may be necessary to fit the patient with a disposable contact lens for -8 D or -9 D and over-refract the patient.

ANTERIOR SEGMENT EXAMINATION

In order to anticipate difficulties, the orbit configuration, palpebral aperture, corneal diameter, corneal endothelial appearance, and presence of corneal neovascularization should be studied when evaluating each LASIK candidate. Clinical keratoconus is contraindicated and ultrasonic pachymetry should be performed on all patients to assess the amount of obtainable correction. Endothelial changes should be assessed, as Fuchs' endothelial dystrophy, traumatic breaks in Descemet's membrane, and other causes of endothelial dysfunction may preclude intrastromal ablation.

POSTERIOR SEGMENT EXAMINATION

Dilated retinal evaluation is of particular importance in high myopia, and any retinal tears or pathology requiring treatment should be referred preoperatively for management. Documentation of myopic macular degeneration and posterior staphylomas is important because postoperative deterioration of vision may be independent of the procedure.

CORNEAL TOPOGRAPHY

Corneal topography is important in assessing not only the target correction to be programmed but the corneal curvature. Most importantly, cylinder axis and magnitude must be compared to that obtained with both the manifest and cycloplegic refractions. In fact, the corneal map findings should be used to guide the refractions, as toric ablations are more successful if a high degree of correspondence is noted between the map and refraction. Excessively flat corneas with mean keratometry below 41 D produce smaller corneal flaps unless associated with a small corneal diameter with the Chiron ACS unit. The surgeon must anticipate that the presence of a flat cornea may result in a free corneal cap. Furthermore, it is harder to flatten a flat cornea, so the patient should be counseled with respect to a higher incidence of myopic regression and enhancement. Additionally, the combination of myopia and a flat cornea indicates axial myopia; therefore, night glare may be more prevalent in these cases. Appropriate counseling is indicated.

Patients with a long history of rigid gas permeable contact lens wear are best treated with LASIK, but it requires 1 to 6 months of hard contact lens abstention for the natural contour to return. In general, soft contact lenses need only be removed 3 to 7 days prior to LASIK, but longer in cases of extended wear with overnight use. A reasonable rule of thumb recommends rigid gas permeable lenses must be removed for approximately 4 weeks for each decade of use, and polymethylmethacrylate (PMMA) lenses 6 weeks for each decade of use. Corneal videokeratography must then be evaluated looking for areas of persistent corneal flattening, warpage, irregularity, and contour stability.

Corneal asymmetry or forme fruste keratoconus must be carefully evaluated and distinguished from true clinical keratoconus. Corneal pachymetry values must be assessed centrally and compared to those obtained over the cone apex. The age of the patient must be taken into account, along with the contact lens history, which may be indicative of warpage; reduced best-corrected vision, which may be indicative of irregular astigmatism; and the refractive error, which may demonstrate significant myopic astigmatism. Clinical examination of the cornea must be carefully evaluated for any signs of clinical keratoconus. Even the retinoscopic reflex should be assessed for scissoring. Some corneal videokeratographic systems have indices that measure the degree of asymmetry and irregular astigmatism, and detect keratoconus. While patients with undiagnosed or unrecognized clinical keratoconus will experience progressive corneal ectasia, even forme fruste variants may experience a greater prevalence of asymmetric healing, slow visual recovery, loss of BCVA, induced astigmatism, and a higher enhancement rate. These patients are often seen in consultation for refractive surgery, as they may be displeased by the quality of vision they perceive with glasses and even contact lenses. Careful counseling and documentation is mandatory, including the possible need for corneal transplantation should the corneal asymmetry represent a true disease state. In many cases of atypical maps, it is often best to avoid surgery altogether because the clinical results are often less predictable and the healing pattern irregular and prolonged.

THE MONOVISION OPTION

During the preoperative consultation process, all patients who are over 40 years of age should have the option of monovision discussed. Many of these patients have already experienced monovision with their contact lenses, therefore they are very familiar with the advantages and disadvantages of this refractive arrangement. Many patients, particularly those who are pre-presbyopic or hyperopic LASIK candidates and are spectacle corrected, have not experienced monovision and require detailed preoperative counseling. Discussions regarding their expectations and motivations for LASIK are essential, as is an appreciation of their work requirements and leisure activities, to determine if they are good candidates for monovision.

> During the preoperative consultation process, all patients who are over 40 years of age should have the option of monovision discussed.

Monovision represents a compromise in which the dominant eye is fully corrected for distance vision and the nondominant eye is undercorrected. We generally leave 40- to 50-year-old patients with a -.5 D to -1.25 D undercorrection and patients over 50 years of age with a -1 to -1.75 D undercorrection in the nondominant eye. Some surgeons prefer to make the near eye the dominant eye if a great deal of near work is performed. Another consideration would be if the patient has been fitted with monovision contact lenses in this manner, with the dominant eye adjusted for near tasks, and is tolerating this approach well. In general, patients who play a great deal of golf or tennis, or who drive a great deal at night or in unfamiliar situations, typically prefer no monovision. In addition, patients who appear to be perfectionists or with precise personalities, such as engineers, are poor candidates for monovision. Even those patients who do tremendous reading will usually require reading glasses, preferring to utilize both eyes for improved detail vision. Other patients who should avoid monovision include those with reduced best-corrected vision in one eye and selected high myopes who are more likely to complain of night glare due to residual myopia in even one eye.

For most patients, monovision is a difficult concept to understand. Our patients are told that monovision represents a compromise that will increase their "functional" vision both at near and far while somewhat decreasing the overall "sharpness" of their distance vision. Patients are told that monovision will give them the ability to read things such as their watch or a menu, but will not enable them to read a book or newspaper for prolonged periods without reading glasses. Patients are told that their dependency on reading glasses will be reduced, but not eliminated, and those reading abilities will come at the expense of distance acuity. With monovision, light prescription glasses may be required while driving at night to improve the distance vision and reduce night glare in the undercorrected eye.

Monovision in the hyperope is somewhat different than in the myope considering refractive surgery in that we are performing a planned overcorrection of the hyperope and a planned undercorrection of the myope. Reversal of monovision is much easier to facilitate in the case of the myope, as it simply involves lifting the corneal flap after at least a 6-week adjustment period and further ablating the residual myopia. In the case of the hyperope, a higher initial correction requires additional healing and an increased incidence of irregular astigmatism, especially in cases of more severe degrees of hyperopia. Reversal of monovision involves placing a myopic ablation pattern over a hyperopic ablation pattern, which may once again increase the potential for irregular astigmatism. Also, the corneal flap alignment in these cases may demonstrate a residual gap along the flap edge that can potentially invite epithelial ingrowth. Monovision in the hyperope is usually better tolerated and appreciated than in the myope, as the hyperope could never see close and therefore sees it as an improvement, whereas the myope always could, and desires better distance acuity.

In summary, good candidates for monovision are patients with daily visual needs at both near and far that are not exacting. Nurses, school teachers, and homemakers are usually good candidates for monovision. Poor candidates for monovision are patients who have precise, demanding visual needs at near or far. Truck drivers, computer programmers, accountants, pilots, and especially golfers are generally not good candidates for monovision.

HYPEROPIC LASIK EVALUATION

I've been working on hyperopia correction for approximately 3 years but have only been pleased with the results since I started using the Chiron Technolas 117 50 Hz (TLC Toronto) and the 217 (TLC Windsor). Both excimers are equipped with PlanoScan, which uses a 2 mm flying spot that ablates at 50 pulses per second. A distinguishing feature of the 217 is the eye tracker. The most sophisticated tracker available, it features an infrared camera that locks onto the

---

The Option of Monovision

Candidates
- Greater than 40 years of age
- Desire to avoid reading glasses
- Visual needs at near and far
- No precise, exacting visual demands

Advantages
- Functional reading ability
- Able to do most tasks without glasses
- Enhancement possible if monovision not accepted

Compromises
- Decreased distance visual acuity
- Increased night glare
- Loss of depth perception that can be restored with corrective eyewear
- Will still need reading glasses for some tasks

---

eye position and sends messages back to the laser's computer. It works equally well for PRK and LASIK, and is especially important in hyperopic LASIK treatments.

The upper limit for hyperopia correction appears to be about +6 D. The increased curvature of the stromal bed created by the hyperopic ablation pattern limits our ability to realign the corneal flap when treating higher degrees of correction. While it is possible to treat low degrees of hyperopia with PRK, hyperopic LASIK is the preferred treatment for two reasons: the stability of the hyperopic ablation pattern beneath the corneal flap; and faster recovery time. Regardless of the degree of hyperopic correction, LASIK is the only treatment I use.

> The increased curvature of the stromal bed created by the hyperopic ablation pattern limits our ability to realign the corneal flap when treating higher degrees of correction.

PLUS CYLINDER TRANSPOSITION

Hyperopic candidates must be evaluated in the plus cylinder format. Therefore, a patient who is +4 - 2 x 170 should be transposed into the plus cylinder format for evaluation by:
1. Axis changed by 90° to 80°
2. Reverse sign on cylinder (but amount unchanged) +2
3. New sphere is the algebraic sum of old sphere and cylinder +4 - 2 = +2.

> Therefore +4 - 2 x 170 in plus cylinder format is +2 + 2 x 80

TABLE 12-2.
HYPEROPIA TREATMENT CHART

Likelihood of being within .75 D of plano sphere or .75 D of plano cylinder

Sphere	Cylinder	One procedure	Two procedures	Bilateral
+1 D to +3 D	< 1 D	92%	98%	Yes
+3 D to +6 D	< 1 D	74%	95%	Yes
+1 D to +3 D	+1 D to +4 D	66%	89%	Yes
+3 D to +6 D	+1 D to +4 D	46%	77%	Yes
Plano	+1 D to +4 D	73% plano cyl	91%	Yes
	Mixed	70% mixed	91%	
	Previous surgery (ie, RK)	50% - 75%	75%	No

CLINICAL RESULTS FOR SPHERICAL HYPEROPES UP TO +6 D (< 1 D CYLINDER)

The hyperopic treatment chart (Table 12-2) shows our success rates in treating patients at various levels of hyperopia and hyperopic astigmatism with one or more procedures. A successful treatment is defined as one in which the patient is within .75 D of residual refractive error. As you can see, our success rates to date are quite good, particularly with hyperopes < +3.

Here are some important points to consider when counseling hyperopic patients:

- Since many patients (particularly younger patients) with lower degrees of hyperopia can see 20/40 uncorrected, it is best when speaking to them to talk about final refractive results.
- For patients with more severe degrees of hyperopia, one should discuss the treatment in terms of a reduction in the degree of hyperopia. The goal is to have less than 1 D of residual hyperopia remaining postoperatively after an enhancement.
- Enhancements are typically performed earlier than with myopic patients, usually 6 weeks following the primary procedure.
- It is also important to note that patients have a multifocal cornea postoperatively and often see better than one would expect—near and distance.
- Furthermore, we can often produce monovision, creating 1 D of myopia typically in the nondominant eye, so long as the total degree of hyperopia treated does not exceed +6 D spherical equivalent.

CLINICAL RESULTS FOR HYPEROPIC CYLINDER

The correction of hyperopic cylinder is even more challenging than correcting myopic cylinder, which is more challenging than correcting myopia. While the results are impressive, the enhancement rate is higher. The number of patients achieving near emmetropia with two procedures is excellent (70% to 92% depending on the degree of hyperopic cylinder and the absolute spherical equivalent), with an enhancement rate of 30% to 48%. Both distance and near vision are improved following the primary procedure. Consequently, these patients are extremely happy after their first procedure, as any reduction in their hyperopia reduces their accommodative demand.

Enhancements can be performed at 6 weeks, allowing adequate time for regression and stabilization. Patients, especially those with higher, more complex prescriptions, often have reduced best-corrected vision during the first 1 to 4 weeks, which recovers during this period.

The maximum amount of hyperopic cylinder we are currently treating is +4 D. Patients who have between +3 D and +6 D of hyperopic sphere and between +1 D and +4 D of hyperopic cylinder were initially treated one eye at a time because of their complexity and are still encouraged to consider this more conservative approach. Patients with lower degrees of hyperopic sphere and cylinder may be candidates for bilateral surgery, while spherical hyperopes of all degrees are routinely being treated bilaterally.

HYPEROPIC SPHERICAL EQUIVALENT < +3 D WITH < +4 D CYLINDER

Generally, patients who have a hyperopic spherical equivalent of +1 D to +3 D with +1 D to +4 D of associated hyperopic cylinder achieve results similar to those with severe spherical hyperopia in the +3 D to +6 D range. That is, 66% of patients achieve a refractive endpoint near plano with less than 1 D of cylinder and less than 1 D sphere after one procedure. Almost 90% of patients achieve this refractive target with two procedures.

HYPEROPIC SPHERICAL EQUIVALENT > +3 D WITH < +4 D CYLINDER

Patients who fall into the most severe hyperopic sphere and cylinder range should be told that this is a two-step procedure. There is a 77% chance that we will be able to reduce them to the point in which they may not need any distance correction. They also should be told that the enhancement rate is 50%.

The goal is to dramatically reduce their degree of hyperopia sphere and cylinder. Patients with severe hyperopic astigmatism have been extremely pleased with the improvement they have achieved in their distance vision, which often is dramatic. Some even note improvement in near vision.

Remember that treating hyperopia is twice as difficult as treating myopia. This is true even with the advancements in laser technology available with the Chiron 217. It simply is not always possible to achieve the desired endpoint, especially in cases of severe hyperopic astigmatism.

HYPEROPIC PLANOCYLINDRICAL CORRECTIONS

Hyperopic planocylindrical corrections are a little bit trickier. For example, while it is possible to treat someone with Plano +2 x 180 and our results have been good, they have not been as good as for hyperopic sphere or compound hyperopic cylinder. As with myopia, it is easier to treat a patient with +4 D sphere or +2 + 2 x 180 rather than plano +2 x 180. Once again, it does not mean that these patients are not candidates. It means that they have a higher enhancement rate. For patients with hyperopic planocylindrical correction up to +4 D, there is a 73% chance that we can reduce their cylinder to less than 1 D with one procedure and a 91% chance that we can achieve that correction with two procedures.

MIXED ASTIGMATISM

Mixed astigmatism, such as -2 + 3 x 90, continues to be a challenge for us, as it is for surgeons worldwide. The reason for this is that we are trying to make one meridian steeper while flattening another. Our initial results with the Chiron 217 laser have been very promising. When correcting mixed patterns, it is often necessary to decrease the myopic spherical correction by about one-third of the plus cylinder in order to avoid myopic overcorrections with postoperative hyperopia. For the example above, a correction of -1 + 3 x 90 would likely give an emmetropic outcome.

COMPLEX CASES: PATIENTS WITH A HISTORY OF PRIOR REFRACTIVE SURGERY

It is important to know that patients with consecutive hyperopia following previous refractive surgery (RK, ALK, PRK, or LASIK) are less predictable in their results. This is true either because they continue to have the same healing problems as they experienced after the original surgery or as a result of performing two different types of refractive surgery or ablation patterns on the same eye.

In my experience, a patient who is overcorrected with a truly complex case has a 50/50 chance of being able to achieve acceptable results with one procedure. Chances are much better (75/25) if the enhancement is straightforward. In other words, someone who has had PRK or LASIK and is overcorrected, but whose BCVA is preserved, has a success ratio of 75% for 20/30 or better unaided or to be within .75 D of emmetropia. This is in sharp contrast to a patient with significant hyperopic cylinder postoperatively with a loss of BCVA and previous ALK or RK surgery, who only has a 50% chance of achieving this same excellent visual and refractive outcome.

BILATERAL SIMULTANEOUS SURGERY

The patients that seek LASIK are generally successful, active professionals who are interested in a simple, painless procedure with quick visual recovery. Bilateral simultaneous LASIK is extremely convenient for these patients because it allows the surgery to be performed only once, the eyes can heal together, the time away from work is minimized, and the difficulties with postoperative anisometropia and contact lenses in one eye are eliminated. At TLC, we have performed thousands of bilateral simultaneous LASIK procedures with very successful results. While every patient is counseled regarding the risks of bilateral procedures, and a consent form specifically deals with this aspect of the surgery, well over 90% of our patients elect to have bilateral simultaneous LASIK.

Some surgeons have expressed concern about the performance of bilateral simultaneous LASIK, which they have summarized in *EyeWorld* (March 1998). These authors have referenced cases of bilateral LASIK infections, interface opacities, iatrogenic keratoconus, retinal hemorrhages, and retinal detachments as examples of the risks of bilateral surgery, which have been presented at refractive surgery conferences. Concerns were also expressed about the predictability of LASIK and the inability to utilize the result in one eye to adjust the LASIK correction in the second eye. Finally, the issue of larger malpractice awards for cases of bilateral visual loss was cited as another factor to support sequential rather than simultaneous surgery.

When bilateral simultaneous surgery is performed, the risks associated with the LASIK procedure in each eye is combined so that they occur together rather than individually for each eye. The incidence of most of these risks is not altered when simultaneous surgery is performed. The only risk that could potentially be increased is infection, which can be transferred from one eye to the other; however, this is rare following LASIK, with an incidence of approximately 1/5000 to 1/10,000. At TLC, all patients are placed on topical antibiotics and followed until all epithelial defects have healed. Using this protocol, we have never experienced a case of bilateral LASIK infection with an overall experience of more than 25,000 procedures.

The relationship of the LASIK procedure to the bilateral retinal complications is suspect. High myopes have a significant lifetime risk of both macular hemorrhages and retinal detachment, and a causal relationship to these complications in either unilateral or bilateral situations has not been substantiated by our clinical experience. Even treating patients on subsequent days or a week apart would not eliminate this risk entirely. The iatrogenic keratoconus caused by bilateral keratectomies at 360 microns would be an error detected on the first eye by a refractive surgeon with proper LASIK training and adequate experience. Therefore, we agree that bilateral LASIK not be performed until a reasonable comfort level with the technique and nomogram have been developed. The other bilateral complications could occur with both simultaneous and sequential LASIK surgery, and the management of these problems would be the same in either case. The Emory group has presented and published its results of bilateral and simultaneous LASIK in this textbook. In its series, there was no difference in the results or the complications for patients undergoing bilateral simultaneous LASIK versus bilateral sequential LASIK.

After performing more than 10,000 LASIK procedures at our center alone, we have found that the operative procedure on the second eye is rarely altered based on the operative experience of one eye. With the success of both hyperopic and myopic LASIK, both under and overcorrections can be treated with enhancement surgery without difficulty. For unilateral or bilateral LASIK, corrections should always aim to be conservative as undercorrections, are easier to treat and more corneal tissue can be preserved.

It should also be recognized that bilateral simultaneous LASIK truly represents rapid sequential surgery. In this regard, bilateral surgery with LASIK is safer than with PRK, as 95% of the complications with LASIK occur intraoperatively (flap complications), compared to 95% of the PRK complications occurring postoperatively (haze). Therefore, when the LASIK procedure has been completed, a good level of comfort has already been achieved prior to the fellow eye being treated, which is in direct contrast to bilateral PRK. However, bilateral PRK has also been widely and successfully performed throughout the world.

The safety of bilateral LASIK compared to unilateral surgery is completely dependent on the surgeon's ability to recognize operative complications. With proper surgeon training and good surgical technique, we feel bilateral LASIK does not place our patients at increased risk. We routinely perform bilateral LASIK and have achieved excellent results without any visually significant bilateral complications. Many refractive surgeons themselves have elected to undergo bilateral rapid sequential LASIK, which suggests that it does represent the practice of conscientious refractive surgery.

> Many refractive surgeons themselves have elected to undergo bilateral rapid sequential LASIK, which suggests that it does represent the practice of conscientious refractive surgery.

CANDIDATE PREPARATION

There is little difference in candidate preparation between surface photoablation and intrastromal ablation. Each patient not only requires a detailed understanding of the risks and benefits of each procedure but also what to expect at each stage of the procedure and postoperative recovery.

As discussed earlier in this chapter, contact lenses must be removed in advance with a re-establishment of the preoperative natural topography. LASIK is the preferred procedure if corneal warpage persists for months or the patient is a long-time rigid gas permeable or PMMA hard lens wearer.

The immediate postoperative examination schedule is far simpler, with only one visit required the following day, as the epithelium typically remains intact. In fact, a baseline visual acuity and refraction can be performed. Fellow eyes are treated within days if bilateral surgery is not performed the same day and can be tentatively scheduled as such. Repeat examination should then be scheduled at 1 week and 4 weeks, at which time assessment for enhancement surgery can be made.

SECTION FOUR
Personal LASIK Techniques

Personal LASIK Technique

Jeffery J. Machat, MD
Louis E. Probst, MD

OVERVIEW

Laser in situ keratomileusis (LASIK) involves the use of a microkeratome to create a 160-micron flap, approximately one-third the depth of the cornea. A suction ring is used to both fixate the globe and increase the intraocular pressure (IOP) to a minimum of 65 or 70 mm Hg, which is necessary for a proper lamellar incision. Small and deep-set eyes are generally avoided until sufficient surgical experience is obtained, as exposure is needed for the suction ring and microkeratome. An attachment is typically left nasally to "hinge" the flap and secure it in position during the immediate postoperative period. The photoablation is made in the stromal bed. The high IOP blurs the patient's view intraoperatively. The corneal flap is then laid back down, ensuring proper alignment. In experienced hands, the entire procedure takes approximately 5 minutes to perform. The steps of our current LASIK technique with the Chiron ACS are summarized in Table 13-1 and Figures 13-1 through 13-18.

PATIENT PREPARATION

The fornices may be cleaned or irrigated preoperatively in order to help maintain a clean interface. There is a tremendous amount of debris and sebaceous secretions within the fornices and tear film of some patients. Lid hygiene is also of great importance to reduce the risk of potential infections and immune reactions postoperatively. Lid scrubs should be used immediately before LASIK, however antibiotic ointments are contraindicated, as they may contaminate the stromal interface postoperatively. An anti-septic scrub is effective for sterilizing the peri-orbital skin prior to LASIK.

PREOPERATIVE MEDICATIONS

Preoperatively, each patient receives a topical anesthetic, topical antibiotics, and preoperative sedation. In general, it is wise not to pharmacologically manipulate the pupil preoperatively. Miotics may induce a superonasal shift, although they tend to reduce patient discomfort due to the microscope light glare. A topical nonsteroidal anti-inflammatory (NSAID) drop, such as Voltaren (diclofenac sodium .1%, CIBA), may be instilled preoperatively to help reduce any discomfort or inflammatory reaction.

Various topical anesthetics can be used; however, it is best not to use excessive amounts of topical anesthesia since it will disturb the surface epithelium. Proparacaine .5% or lidocaine 2% are probably preferable to tetracaine, which has a greater epitheliotoxicity. Some surgeons alternate the use of proparacaine and tetracaine to achieve better anesthesia, as one is an amide and the other an ester derivative. Typically, in bilaterally treated eyes during the same session, the second eye will experience greater sensation, this is commonly referred to as second eye syndrome. There appears to be multiple factors for increased sensitivity, including a heightened awareness of what will transpire and tachyphylaxis of the eye to repeated application of proparacaine. Therefore, it is best in bilaterally treated patients to apply the topical anesthesia to each eye only immediately before treatment. Application of topical anesthesia with a soaked surgical spear to the upper and lower fornices is highly recommended (Figure 13-19), as this is where most

TABLE 13-1.
OPERATIVE STEPS OF LASIK

1. Calibrate and program the excimer laser system.
2. Assemble and test the microkeratome.
3. Prepare the eye with topical anesthesia, antibiotics, and nonsteroidal drops.
4. Prepare the patient with the proper sedation.
5. Clean the eyelashes and fornices.
6. Drape the eye, covering over eyelid margins.
7. Place a locking eyelid speculum.
8. Obtain adequate exposure.
9. Center the eye in the operative field by adjusting head position.
10. Place alignment markings.
11. Apply the pneumatic suction ring, seat firmly, and activate vacuum pressure.
12. Check for adequate pressure with a Barraquer tonometer.
13. Insert the microkeratome and advance it into the starting position.
14. Check the operative field for obstacles.
15. Depress the forward pedal until the hinge stop is reached.
16. Reverse the microkeratome and remove the microkeratome head alone or with the suction ring.
17. Open the corneal flap with a spatula or blunt forceps.
18. Ablate the stroma bed with the programmed refraction.
19. Protect the undersurface of the flap during the excimer ablation.
20. Control stromal hydration with air or wiping between laser steps.
21. Place drops of BSS on the flap to lubricate it when the ablation is complete.
22. Close the flap with a flap spatula or forceps.
23. Irrigate beneath the flap to remove debris and float it into position.
24. Wipe the corneal flap with a wet surgical spear.
25. Check corneal alignment markings to ensure correct positioning.
26. Dry the fornices of excess fluid.
27. Wait 2 to 3 minutes for flap adhesion.
28. Insert an antibiotic-steroid combination and ocular lubricant.
29. Carefully remove the eyelid speculum without touching the cornea.
30. Recheck the flap alignment after the patient has blinked.
31. Recheck the flap alignment again 20 to 30 minutes following the procedure.

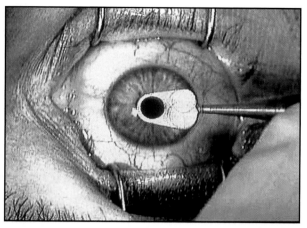

Figure 13-1. Surgeon's view of the placement of the corneal alignment marks using the Machat LASIK corneal marker with two circles of different sizes prior to performing the keratectomy.

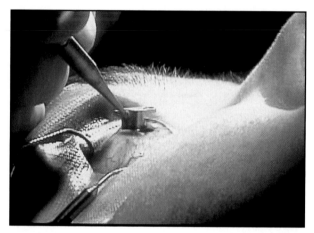

Figure 13-2. Side view of the placement of the corneal alignment marks using the Machat LASIK corneal marker with two circles of different sizes prior to performing the keratectomy.

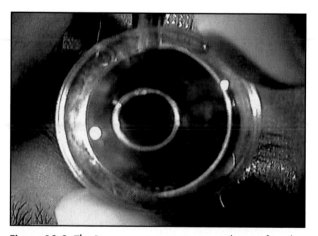

Figure 13-3. The Barraquer tonometer is used to confirm that the IOP is at least 65 mm Hg. The pressure should be checked on a dry cornea to avoid a false meniscus.

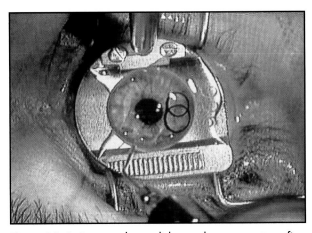

Figure 13-4. Depress the eyelid speculum to create a firm globe and taut conjuctiva prior to applying the suction ring. This technique creates a firm seal and avoids pseudosuction.

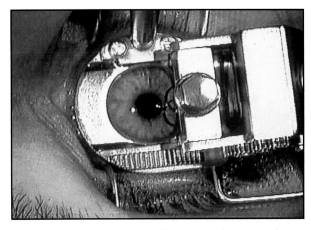

Figure 13-5. Insertion of the Chiron microkeratome shaper head into the suction ring tract. The microkeratome pass should always be performed on a wet cornea. The rule of thumb is to apply suction, check the pressure, then wet the cornea, and cut.

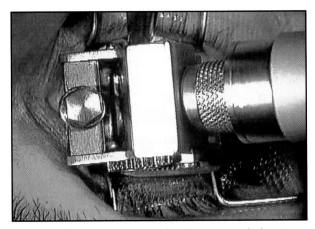

Figure 13-6. Once the shaper head is engaged, the microkeratome is advanced to create the flap.

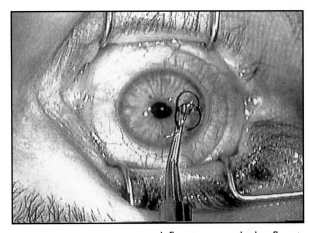

Figure 13-7. Once a corneal flap is created, the flap is reflected nasally using nontoothed forceps or a flap spatula to reveal the stromal bed.

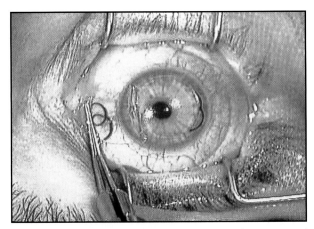

Figure 13-8. The flap is folded onto the nasal conjunctival surface.

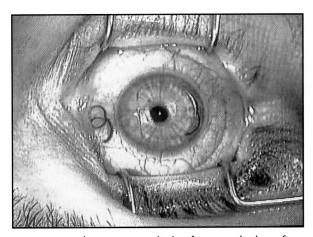

Figure 13-9. The patient is asked to fixate on the laser fixation beam as the laser alignment beam is centered and the excimer laser ablation is performed.

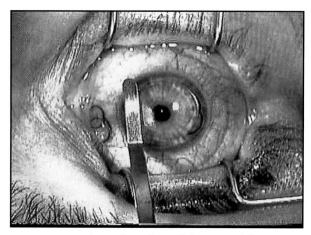

Figure 13-10. The undersurface of the corneal flap is protected from the excimer ablation with the Slade flap protector.

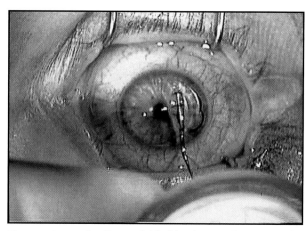

Figure 13-11. The flap is folded back into place using the irrigation cannula tip.

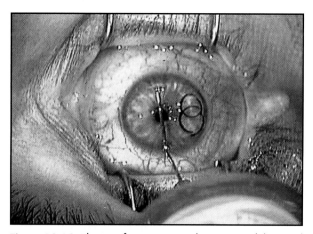

Figure 13-12. The interface is irrigated to remove debris and any implanted epithelial cells.

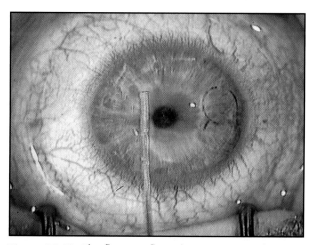

Figure 13-13. The flap is refloated into its correct location, which is verified by the realignment of the corneal alignment marks. Irrigation should take less than 10 seconds to avoid overhydrating the corneal flap and prolonging flap adhesion.

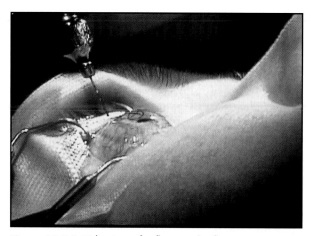

Figure 13-14. Side view of refloating the flap into its correct location.

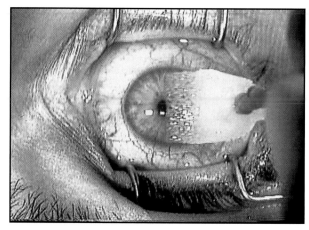

Figure 13-15. The flap is gently wiped with a wet Merocel spear to smooth the surface and remove any excess fluid in the interface.

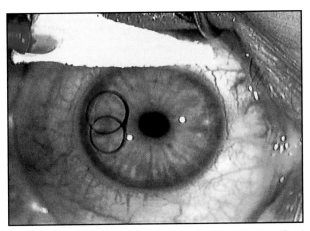

Figure 13-16. The fornices are dried of any excess fluid using a dry sponge to encourage dehydration of the corneal flap and promote adhesion.

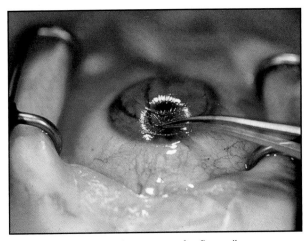

Figure 13-17. The Slade striae test for flap adhesion.

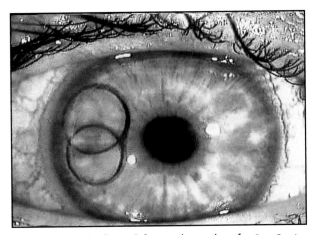

Figure 13-18. The flap is left to seal into place for 2 to 3 minutes. Note the clarity of the cornea immediately following LASIK and the accurate alignment of the corneal marks.

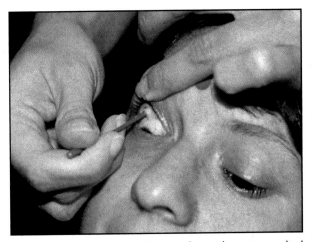

Figure 13-19. Lidocaine 4% topical anesthesia is applied directly to the superior fornix with a soaked surgical spear preoperatively to avoid direct epithelial toxicity of ophthalmic drops.

of the discomfort from LASIK occurs (in relation to the eyelid speculum). The lamellar incision itself is virtually painless, and the vacuum from the suction ring creates a well-tolerated mild pressure sensation. Therefore, by anesthetizing the fornices well, especially the upper fornix, patient comfort and cooperation are greatly enhanced. Apply anesthesia immediately preoperatively to reduce epithelial toxicity. Patients should also keep their eyes closed once anesthetized, as the blink reflex is diminished and the corneal surface will by further damaged by the drying effect of the opened eye.

A topical antibiotic and Betadine or other antiseptic preparations are utilized preoperatively to reduce the bacterial load in the conjunctiva. The choice of antibiotics is far less important than with PRK, as the risk of infection is greatly reduced. The epithelial toxicity of the antibiotic must once again be considered. Topical gentamycin is quite epitheliotoxic and therefore should be avoided. We current-

ly use a combination of Tobradex (tobramycin .3%-dexamethasone .1%, Alcon) and Ciloxan (ciprofloxacin .3%, Alcon) successfully. Fluoroquinolones are not epitheliotoxic and provide excellent broad spectrum bacterial coverage and penetration; however, some surgeons have questioned their association with precipitates and interface opacities in some cases of LASIK. At TLC, we have used Tobradex alone, Ocuflox (ofloxacin 0.3%, Allergan) alone, and currently recommend Ciloxan immediately preoperatively and postoperatively, but provide 4 days of prophylaxis postoperatively with Tobradex alone, which has been well-tolerated and the single combination agent has enhanced compliance.

Preoperative sedation with a short-acting benzodiazepine such as lorazepam 1 to 2 mg sublingual is recommended, which can be doubled for very agitated patients. Fixation may be ensured with the use of the suction ring, even without application of vacuum pressure, so that temporary sedation should not affect centration, although this is usually unnecessary. Many surgeons prefer to utilize diazepam, in a range of 5 to 10 mg orally, which typically produces a more intense sedation with a more prolonged action. Versed (Madazolam .3 to .5 mg/kg) has also been used effectively to alleviate anxiety peri-operatively and also providing an amnesic effect. Preoperative sedation for LASIK tends to lower the tension level of all patients and all the benzodiazapines have some amnestic effect. This makes the LASIK experience much more pleasant for the patient. Once the adrenaline associated with anxiety prior to LASIK has subsided after the procedure, the preoperative sedation takes full effect and patients often become somewhat unstable on their feet and even drowsy, so care should be taken. Sedation allows the LASIK flap to heal adequately and probably provides the ideal postoperative environment of sleep for the postoperative LASIK eye.

LASER CALIBRATION AND TESTING

There is no difference in the laser calibration technique required for LASIK compared to that for PRK. The only important differences lie in the software utilized and target correction attempted. In response to less wound healing than anticipated, some lasers require that a lower correction be targeted to avoid significant overcorrection, while others require additional correction to compensate for the increased stromal hydration of the deeper stroma. The VISX Star excimer laser requires a reduction in the programmed correction of 10% to 20% depending on the surgeon's technique, excimer laser suite environment, and the altitude of the laser center itself (see Chapter 5).

Most other lasers require the use of the spectacle plane refraction and may even add an additional diopter to the attempted correction because of the mid-stroma hydration factor, which may produce significant undercorrections. It is not important which nomogram is used, simply that the nomogram is conservative since undercorrections are far more easily managed than overcorrections. Some surgeons leave the stroma naturally hydrated throughout the procedure, which may improve corneal interface clarity. Other surgeons apply a fan across the entire surgical field, while some use a blunt spatula to wipe excessive stromal fluid away or a surgical spear to dehydrate the stroma. With the VISX Star excimer laser, the suction nozzle is typically retracted during the LASIK cut and then replaced during the LASIK procedure. Most surgeons who use the VISX Star will remove the central accumulation of fluid with a dry Merocel spear, which commonly occurs during larger myopic corrections. Another technique utilized to control the hydration status of the deeper stroma and the ablation rate is to utilize a 23-gauge cannula that applies 3 liters of air per minute to the stromal bed for 2 seconds between each zone of ablation. In general, excessive dehydration should be avoided, as it is best to keep the cornea in a more physi-

ological state during the procedure so excessive dehydration does not result in an increased incidence of overcorrections, interface haze, fibrosis, and epithelial ingrowth.

The increased hydration status of the mid-stroma is also responsible for an increased incidence of central island formation when optical zones greater than 5 mm are used with all broad beam lasers. Therefore, either a pretreatment step can be added prior to the refractive treatment (patient training A with Summit Omnimed) or within the ablation algorithm itself (VISX Star), or an aspheric ablation pattern can be used (Summit Omnimed multizone international program), which concentrates the treatment within a small area of 4.5 mm with a 6-mm transition zone. Although night glare may be more apparent with the aspheric pattern compared to single zone techniques, central islands are almost nonexistent. Pretreatment can be applied with both single or multizone ablation patterns (see Chapter 5).

Although wound contour and edge profile are far less important with LASIK than PRK, optical zone size and depth of ablation become critical factors to consider in the correction of severe myopia. Specifically, optical zones of at least 6 mm are required to avoid significant glare. It is impossible to use single zone techniques for severe myopes greater than -10 D because of the significant depth of ablation required. Therefore, it is best to use multizone or aspheric techniques to reduce depth of ablation without sacrificing optical zone size. A pretreatment is necessary to avoid central island formation with broad beam lasers unless it is incorporated into the laser algorithm by the manufacturer, the amount of which varies with the particular laser system. Larger optical zones also help to reduce regression and night glare.

OPERATIVE STEPS AND SURGICAL PRINCIPLES

The first step in the LASIK procedure, following fluence testing and programming of the laser, is the microkeratome evaluation. Preparation and care of the instrumentation is the most important element for a successful outcome (Figure 13-20). Staff training and expertise are also of paramount importance—equally significant to surgeon training.

Five specific checks should be made prior to each procedure (Figure 13-21):
1. The first test involves listening to the microkeratome unit while in both forward and reverse motion. Each unit has a particular sound or pitch that is often altered when the unit is not functioning correctly. The unit should always be checked to ensure that the sound of the microkeratome motor has not changed. A lower or irregular microkeratome pitch often indicates a microkeratome malfunction, and a service check should be made prior to the performance of further procedures.
2. The number and position of the microkeratome depth

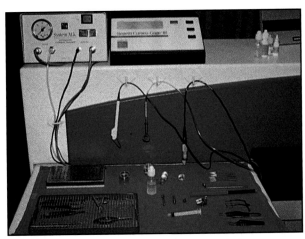

Figure 13-20. LASIK operative set-up including Corneo-gauge ultrasonic pachymeter, Chiron suction pump, Chiron Corneal Shaper, and additional fine instruments (courtesy of Stephen Slade, MD).

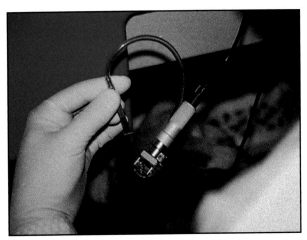

Figure 13-21. Preoperative testing of the Chiron-Steinway microkeratome. Prior to each lamellar procedure, the unit must be examined for proper assembly and function. The formalized concept of a preflight checklist was advanced by J. Charles Casebeer, MD, to avoid potential serious lamellar complications due to microkeratome malfunction.

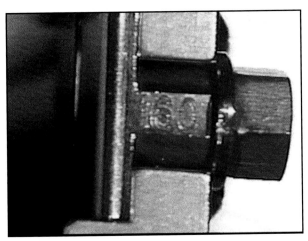

Figure 13-22a. Preoperative testing of the Chiron Corneal Shaper demonstrating a 160-μm depth plate in proper position to prevent corneal perforation and control corneal flap thickness. A gap between the depth plate and blade must be assessed to ensure no debris has inadvertently been introduced and is blocking the flap passage.

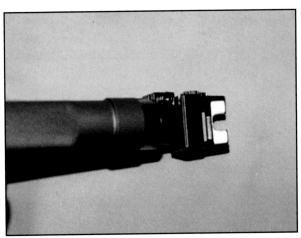

Figure 13-22b. The microkeratome with the depth plate in position should be compared with the appearance of the unit without the depth plate inserted (seen here).

plate should be checked carefully (Figures 13-22a and 13-22b). The 160- or 180-micron plates are used routinely with the Chiron ACS unit depending on the degree of myopia. The 160-micron plate is used for high myopes to preserve stromal tissue, while the 180-micron plate is used for lower myopes to improve the integrity of the flap and minimize postoperative flap striae. An even thicker flap may smooth any irregularities, but the 240-micron plate may mask the ablative effect and is more difficult to manipulate. The 130 plate should generally not be used, as the incidence of postoperative flap striae is higher and flap manipulation far more difficult. Most importantly, the plate must be in place. Failure to insert the depth plate will result in a cut depth of

900 microns, perforating the cornea and risking expulsion of the ocular contents with potential postoperative blindness. The plate must also be fully inserted and flush with the end of the unit, with no gap visible above the blade edge, as sight-threatening complications may also result. The plate screw must be firmly inserted to ensure that the plate is not displaced during the handling of the microkeratome.

3. The blade must then be checked under the microscope for any blade edge irregularities. Blade oscillation is then checked to ensure smooth back-and-forth motion. The gap between the plate and the blade should be clear of any debris or plastic filings (Figure 13-23a).

4. The safety hinge must then be examined to ensure that it

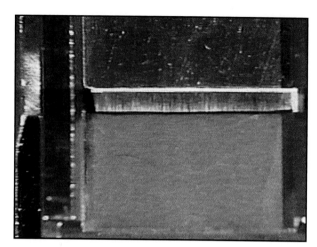

Figure 13-23a. Preoperative testing of the Chiron Corneal Shaper evaluating blade quality and demonstrating movement of the blade. The blade can be stationary if the blade block is assembled incorrectly or blocked with debris.

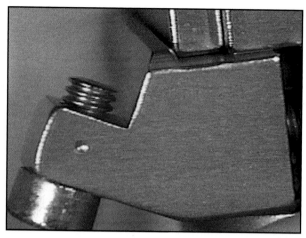

Figure 13-23b. Preoperative evaluation of the Chiron Corneal Shaper hinge stop setting. The adjustable screw setting can be varied for controlling corneal flap and hinge size based on preoperative keratometry.

is attached and that the hinge screw is set accordingly if the stopper is not fixed into the unit (Figure 13-23b and 13-23c). If the microkeratome is used without the stopper in the correct position, a free cap may be produced.

5. The microkeratome is then inserted into the suction ring and the gears engaged. The foot pedal is depressed in the forward and reverse direction to ensure a smooth procession. Any difficulty engaging the microkeratome or lack of smoothness requires additional cleaning of the microkeratome and suction ring tract. The microkeratome should never be used unless the passage is smooth. The microkeratome head should literally glide along the tract (Figure 13-24).

The entire testing process requires less than 30 seconds when the unit is cleaned, prepared, and functioning properly.

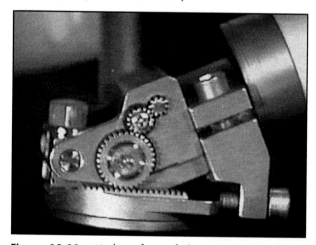

Figure 13-23c. Undersurface of the suction ring during microkeratome passage demonstrating oscillation of the blade.

SURGICAL PREPARATION OF THE OPERATIVE EYE

The patient is properly aligned with centration on the pupil, which is preferred over the visual axis to avoid postoperative night glare. If a large angle kappa exists, I routinely shift toward the midpoint. The fellow eye is taped closed to prevent cross fixation and maintain corneal hydration of the fellow eye epithelium. Taping the fellow eye closed is helpful in preventing any drying effects of the epithelium.

An additional application of anesthesia immediately preoperatively is often effective, as well as comforting, to the patient and is done by soaking a surgical spear with topical proparacaine .5% and placing it firmly on the bulbar conjunctiva in the upper and lower fornices. Many surgeons apply topical anesthesia at this point and not before in order to minimize the time of potential epitheliotoxicity. The eyelids are then dried and the eyelashes removed from the surgical field with surgical draping of the surgeon's preference.

I have personally used surgical micropore tape with great effectiveness. Steri-strips or foam strips can also be used. The objective is to clear the eyelashes from the surgical field and microkeratome gears, while covering the meibomian orifices of the lid margin.

OBTAINING ADEQUATE EXPOSURE

The ideal speculum is an adjustable wire speculum to provide maximum exposure, rather than that of a solid blade variety. A titanium Lieberman speculum or the Machat locking wire speculum (ASICO) provides excellent exposure (see Chapter 7) (Figure 13-25a). I ensure that the draping is folded into the fornices so as to cover the upper and lower lid margins (Figure 13-25b). If one looks carefully, an oily film is sometimes evident in the tear film from the meibomian secretions; therefore, covering these orifices is important.

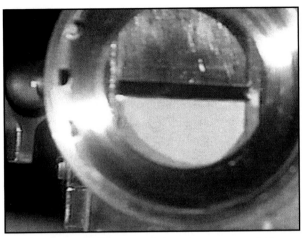

Figure 13-24. Profile view of the Chiron Corneal Shaper head during preoperative testing denoting action of the hinge stop, which prevents further advancement of the unit. The hinge stop is set to create the size of hinge desired but must take into account the preoperative keratometry.

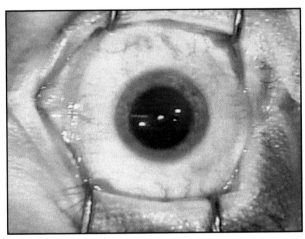

Figure 13-25b. Preparation of the operative field for LASIK with a wire eyelid speculum for maximal ocular exposure and draping of the eyelashes and lid margins to reduce surgical field contamination. It is important to properly position the head to obtain the best centration, with equal amounts of sclera visible superiorly and inferiorly.

For deep-set orbits or high brows, it is important to elevate the chin by hyperextending the neck position. Furthermore, for small orbits or narrow palpebral fissures, turning the face away from the eye being treated will shift the eye temporally within the orbit, allowing the surgeon to avoid the most narrow nasal portion of the orbit for both suction placement and microkeratome passage. The head should be properly positioned for the ablation once the corneal flap has been fashioned.

ALIGNMENT MARKINGS

Alignment markings are then placed on the corneal surface. There are two reasons for the markings: first for align-

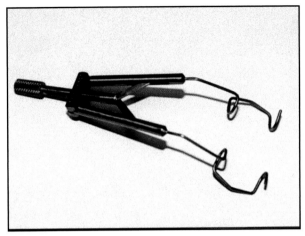

Figure 13-25a. Lieberman design adjustable wire eyelid speculum.

ment with an intact hinge and second for alignment with an inadvertent free cap. The alignment marks should be placed so that the correct orientation of a free cap is assured with the epithelial side up. The classic alignment markings consist of a central 3-mm circular mark with a concentric 10-mm circular mark and a paraxial line radiating between the circles temporally (Figure 13-26). However, there are two problems with this alignment system: the central marking disturbs the central epithelium and the paraxial marking only provides a single point of alignment. I utilize two circular markings of 3.25 and 3.75 mm. The Machat LASIK marker (ASICO) serves as a template for these circular marks. The circles are marked with gentian violet and placed peripherally and temporally (Figure 13-27). The circles extend from the limbus to leave the central 3 mm of epithelium untouched, improving the visual recovery rate. Additionally, the circles provide four-point alignment with the different sized circles, preventing any chance that a free cap may be placed epithelial-side down. The size of the flap varies from 7.2 to 9 mm, with a mean cap diameter of 8.5 mm, which is dependent on the preoperative corneal curvature, corneal diameter, and suction pressure achieved. Smaller diameter corneas act like steeper corneas and produce relatively larger corneal flaps. The diameter of the cornea also varies greatly between patients; therefore, the advantage of the circles is that they encompass the flap to a variable degree in all cases. There are a number of simplified LASIK alignment markers currently available that provide both radial and pararadial lines.

CENTRATION OF THE SUCTION RING

The excimer LASIK ring, which is a nonadjustable suction ring, is then placed on the eye with the flat portion temporal (Figure 13-28). To obtain adequate exposure readily and safely, the lid speculum can be depressed to proptose the eye and allow for better apposition of the suction ring. Proper placement of the suction ring is one of the most piv-

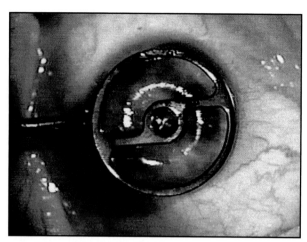

Figure 13-26. Ruiz marker for lamellar surgery creating central and peripheral circular markings connected by a pararadial mark. The handle must be held temporally to correctly orient the pararadial mark.

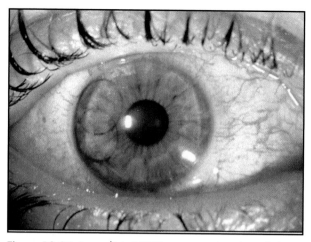

Figure 13-27. Immediate LASIK postoperative clinical photograph demonstrating Machat alignment markings with slight conjunctival infection and eyelid edema.

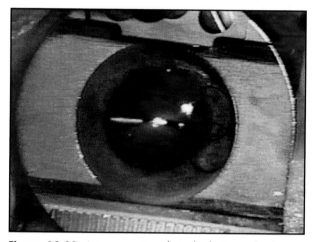

Figure 13-28. Intraoperative clinical photograph demonstrating application of the suction ring on the right eye. Note the enlargement of the pupil upon activation of suction pressure and slight inferior decentration to avoid pronounced superior neovascularization from contact lens wear.

otal steps in achieving consistency in corneal flap quality. Although suction ring placement only takes a few seconds, one can divide the maneuver into three steps:

1. The eyelid speculum is depressed and the patient forewarned that he or she will experience an increase in pressure. At this point, the eye is proptosed, the globe firm, and the conjunctiva taut.

2. After a brief pause, the suction ring is firmly applied to create a complete seal.

3. After another brief pause, the suction pressure is activated and the patient warned that he or she may lose the fixation light, as vision will become dark.

In this manner, pseudosuction of the conjunctiva is avoided, the firmness of the eye and improved exposure simplifies ring placement, and the suction ring is elevated above the plane of the speculum and draping. The suction is only activated once the suction ring is precisely positioned and seated firmly in place. If the suction is first initiated and then lowered into position, two complications may occur: the centration may not engage as anticipated, and the conjunctiva may be pulled into the ring creating pseudosuction and interfering with obtaining or maintaining adequate suction pressure. That is, the globe may feel firm with pseudosuction and may even measure an adequate IOP, but the pressure associated with the passage of the microkeratome often results in a thin or button-holed corneal flap. The suction ring should be lightly supported and maintained in a plane slightly above the speculum once activated so that microkeratome passage remains unobstructed. This maneuver of suction ring placement is essential in small, deep-set orbits or in cases of narrow palpebral apertures.

The centration of the suction ring is another essential step, but far more so for automated lamellar keratoplasty (ALK) than for LASIK. With ALK, centration of the ring over the cornea for the initial or access pass in creating the lamellar flap is essential to allow for centration of the second refractive pass. With LASIK, however, centration of the flap is not essential for centration of the ablation within the stromal bed. There is actually an advantage to slight nasal decentration of 1 mm or less. Slight nasal decentration allows the ablation to be centered without concern that the ablation will ablate the undersurface of the flap, which would result in doubling of the refractive effect along the hinge. Excessive decentration may, however, compromise smooth passage of the microkeratome. Inferior decentration is indicated in cases of severe superior corneal neovascularization, commonly associated with contact lens wear. The incision of these vessels intraoperatively may complicate the surgery, as bleeding along the peripheral flap edge may interfere with the laser application and may remain in the interface.

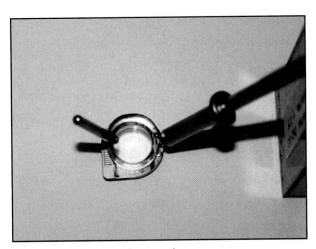

Figure 13-29a. An applanation lens.

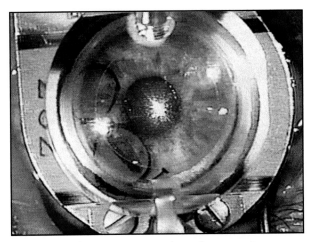

Figure 13-29b. Intraoperative photo demonstrating assessment of corneal flap size with an 8.5-mm applanation lens. Meniscus exceeds the 8.5-mm demarcated ring, indicating that the corneal flap will be slightly larger. The applanation lens mimics the microkeratome head, demonstrating the corneal tissue that will be presented to the advancing corneal shaper head.

DETERMINING CAP DIAMETER

The ring is held perpendicularly and lightly to avoid breaking suction (Figures 13-29a and 13-29b). A stable surgical chair with armrests is recommended. The diameter of the corneal flap to be fashioned is then ensured to be adequate by inserting the 8.5-mm applanation lens. It is important that the corneal surface is relatively dry for both diameter and pressure measurements, as excessive moisture will create a false meniscus. When measuring the diameter, a meniscus is visible to the surgeon (Figure 13-30) and should be centered and symmetrical. Within the applanation lens a ring is visible, indicating the 8.5 mm diameter. The applanation lens acts like a transparent microkeratome, allowing the surgeon to visualize what will be presented to the microkeratome. Therefore, one can judge the anticipated diameter of the cap as well as centration.

Most surgeons, including the authors, no longer check the cap diameter with the standardized Chiron ACS, as the corneal flap size cannot be adjusted and additional manipulation may only serve to break suction. The experienced LASIK surgeon can preoperatively predict the size of the corneal flap based on the curvature and diameter of the cornea. In rare cases it may be useful to check the cap diameter prior to LASIK if the keratometry readings are very flat and there are concerns about creating a free cap.

DETERMINING IOP OBTAINED

When measuring IOP, the Barraquer tonometer is suspended by the ring vertically and perpendicularly over the pupil center, allowing the tonometer tip to applanate the corneal surface. Pressure is defined simply as force over area. The weight of the Barraquer tonometer applies a given force that applanates a variable area depending on the pressure within the eye (Figure 13-31). If the eye is very soft, the area will be great, as the force is capable of compressing a larger surface area. If the pressure within the eye is very high, the force will not be able to compress the eye very much, which will generate a small meniscus. The surgeon

visualizes a ring within the tonometer, the diameter of which signifies 65 mm Hg. If the meniscus observed is larger, the pressure within the eye is less than 65 mm Hg; if the meniscus is smaller, the pressure is greater than the minimum acceptable IOP of 65 mm Hg. The smaller the meniscus, the higher the IOP, the safer the procedure, and the better the quality and thickness of the flap. In general, IOP is usually in the range of 100 mm Hg, well in excess of the 65 mm Hg minimum. Under no circumstances should a surgeon ever attempt to perform a microkeratome pass without adequate pressure, as the integrity of the flap will be extremely poor with a thin, torn, or perforated flap. The management of such complications will be discussed later. Excessive surface moisture of the cornea will increase the size of the meniscus applanated and indicate a falsely low IOP. Therefore, it is important not to rehydrate the epithelium immediately prior to checking the IOP and to dry the epithelium and re-applanate if a large meniscus is observed.

Some very experienced LASIK surgeons do not check the IOP with applanation, but either digitally or not at all, as they feel proper technique and visual clues such as dilation of the pupil can ensure that adequate LASIK IOP is present. However, unless the surgeon is extremely experienced with LASIK, it is recommended that the IOP be checked routinely in each procedure to avoid thin and perforated flaps. In complicated cases such as with flat corneas, post-retinal detachment, or small orbits, it may be wise to applanate, as the potential for inadequate suction or suction loss is greater. It is also useful to very gently digitally applanate the cornea to become familiar with the feel of adequate IOP before using digital palpation alone, remembering that all manipulations should be performed prior to the tonometer reading. The tonometer measurement should always be the

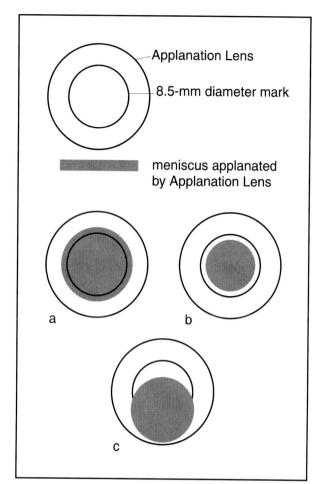

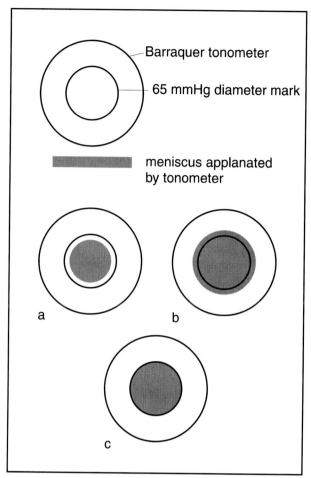

Figure 13-30. *Excellent/acceptable* (a): Proceed to IOP measurement. Meniscus larger then 8.5 mm indicates that a large corneal flap will be fashioned. It can also be produced if the corneal surface is excessively wet.
Poor/acceptable (b): Do not proceed until the keratometry is less than 41 D. This indicates a small corneal flap will be created. There is an increased risk of a free corneal cap; adjust for a larger hinge. Check pressure carefully.
Not acceptable (c): Remeasure, as the applanation lens is not properly seated.

Figure 13-31. *Excellent/acceptable* (a): Meniscus is smaller than the tonometer ring, indicating IOP above 65 mm Hg. Proceed.
Poor/unacceptable (b): Meniscus is larger than the tonometer ring, indicating IOP below 65 mm Hg. Do not proceed. High risk of thin or perforated corneal flap.
Fair/borderline acceptable (c): Meniscus equal in size relative to the tonometer ring, indicating borderline IOP. Confirm the corneal surface is dry and the suction ring is seated well, then retest. There is a higher risk of corneal flap problems, especially thin flap.

Pneumatic Ring Vacuum Pressure

The pneumatic suction ring is placed differently for the right and left eyes with the Chiron Classic Automated Corneal Shaper, but always with the flat edge pointing temporally. Thus the handle is directed toward the surgeon for left eyes and away for right eyes (Figure 13-32). Once the suction ring is perpendicular to the eye and well seated, the microkeratome is then fully engaged into the tract grooves. When the vacuum pressure is activated, the surgical assis-

final maneuver prior to the microkeratome pass to help ensure that an adequate pressure is present for the critical microkeratome pass.

tant should notify the surgeon of the vacuum pressure achieved. It is best to give control of the vacuum pressure to the surgical assistant to prevent the surgeon from accidentally pressing the suction pedal rather than the microkeratome motor pedal, which could be disastrous to the flap. The maximum vacuum pressure produced by each unit is 23 to 28 mm Hg depending on the altitude. Each surgeon should note the precise reading for his or her unit (Figure 13-33), as it is reproducible for each procedure when full occlusion of the suction ring is created intraoperatively. If full occlusion is not achieved or is lost, the vacuum pressure typically reads a lesser value (Figure 13-34). That is, if the maximum vacuum pressure is typically 25 mm Hg and the

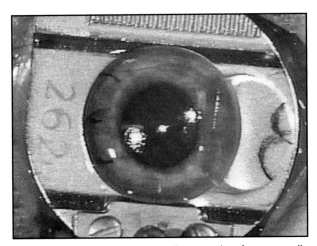

Figure 13-40. Intraoperative photograph of a naturally hydrated stromal bed immediately upon opening the corneal flap. The suction ring can be left in position, but the suction pressure should be turned off. The ring sits nicely within the scleral indentation created to help patient fixation, as can be assessed by the bright fixation reflex. Note the two half circle alignment markings on the corneal flap, which correspond to the two half circles on the uncut temporal corneal.

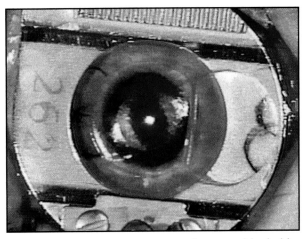

Figure 13-41a. Intraoperative view of a stromal bed ablation pattern during the Chiron Technolas 6.6-mm multi-multizone technique, demonstrating central translucency denoting increased central hydration.

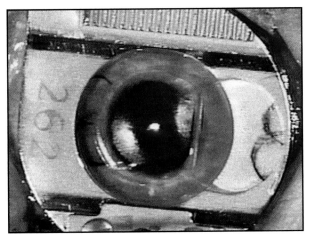

Figure 13-41b. Intraoperative hydration pattern at the conclusion of the procedure demonstrating encroachment on the corneal hinge and diffuse translucency. Peripheral taper of the ablation pattern and increased hydration status of deeper stroma reduce the effective optical zone created.

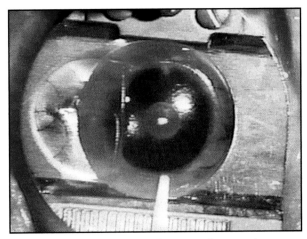

Figure 13-42. Pretreatment technique with air application to prevent central island formation with the Chiron Technolas 6.6-mm seven-zone multi-multizone technique for -10.5 D. Increased incidence of central islands is associated with LASIK due to increased hydration status of the deeper stroma, unless nomogram compensation or technique modifications are made. The amount of pretreatment depends on beam profile, optical zone size, and nomogram. Scanning excimer lasers do not require pretreatment.

13-40 to 13-42). The mid-stroma is more hydrated, which results in an increased incidence of undercorrections and, with broad beam excimer lasers, central islands. The LASIK technique and ablation profile must reflect this fact.

If there is no software adjustment, the pretreatment technique should be used on the inner stroma to remove stromal tissue within the central 3 mm prior to the full refractive correction in order to avoid central islands with broad beam lasers. The central undercorrection is produced because of the naturally increased hydration of the central stroma (Lin 1994) and the acoustic shockwaves (Machat 1992) produced by each pulse, which drive stromal fluid centrally. Other central island theories include the Vortex plume theory (Klyce 1992), which states that plume debris blocks laser pulses centrally, and the Shielding theory (Neuhann 1997), which depicts the plume debris as shielding the central cornea from full correction.

With the Chiron Technolas 116 excimer laser, we performed a pretreatment step followed by a multizone ablation pattern for the spectacle refractive error divided the refractive error into several equal steps with a depth of approximately 40 microns each. We noted that the optical zone size achieved was still smaller than that treated due to the flap masking the peripheral blend zones in light of the increased

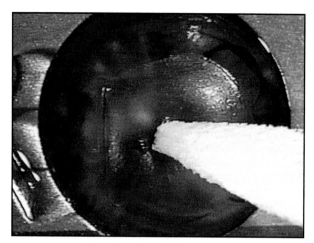

Figure 13-43. Intraoperative photograph demonstrating use of a dry, nonfraying surgical spear to control the intraoperative hydration status of the stromal bed. The nomogram can be adjusted to completely avoid the use of a spear.

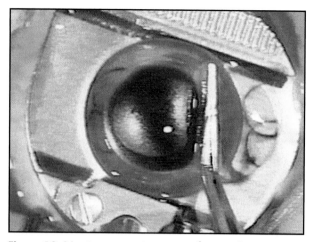

Figure 13-44a. Intraoperative series of views demonstrating closure of the corneal flap following ablation.

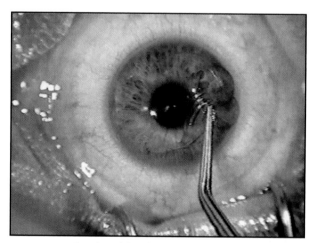

Figure 13-44b. Closed fine forceps or a fine spatula can be inserted along the entire hinge length and used to reflect the corneal flap in one smooth motion.

hydration encountered. The use of air or wiping with a surgical spear or spatula to control the increased hydration status of the inner stroma was also needed (Figure 13-43). A Merocel surgical sponge or other nonfraying spear is specifically recommended. Surgical spears, however, may leave debris on the stromal bed and within the interface and may produce variable dehydration effects upon the stroma. With the VISX Star, a pretreatment program was built into the software program, and a vertex distance corrected ablation was targeted. The VISX Star LASIK algorithm required the targeted correction to be reduced by about 15% compared to our PRK algorithm. For the Summit Omnimed or Apex without international software, a pretreatment utilizing patient training A was performed using the formula of approximately 3 to 4 pulses per diopter of refractive correction programmed followed by the full refractive correction. With the Nidek EC 5000, the scanning slit delivery system avoided the need for any pretreatment as central islands are not observed, but a 30% reduction in the targeted ablation was needed to avoid overcorrections with this unit. Currently with the Chiron Technolas 217, the flying spot scanning delivery system with eye tracking capabilities also negates any need for pretreatment and allows for more flexibility in treatment profiling. With a typical optical zone of 6 mm devoid of central island effects and an ablation blend typically of 9.2 mm, qualitative vision is consistently better during both day and night. The stroma and corneal flap remain more physiologically hydrated throughout the procedure utilizing this scanning method. The flying spot scanning lasers offer the most consistent and programmable method of LASIK that is currently available and is able to effectively treat not only myopia, but hyperopic and mixed astigmatism.

CLOSING THE FLAP

Fine closed tiers or a cyclodialysis spatula of some variety should be inserted nasally the full length of the hinge. The flap should be replaced in one smooth, even motion in an effort to minimize irregular astigmatism (Figures 13-44a through 13-44d). Avoidance of irregular astigmatism is the greatest challenge in lamellar surgery.

In cases in which a good, but somewhat thin, corneal flap is created or in which excessive drying of the corneal flap has occurred, it is best to first place a few drops of BSS on the flap for approximately 10 seconds to allow for hydration and even some swelling of the corneal flap. This technique will thicken the corneal flap and allow for easier manipulation and placement. Corneal tissue swells in relationship to time—not the amount of fluid—so excessive irrigation is not required. Furthermore, if fluid has accumu-

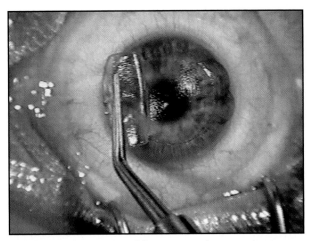

Figure 13-44c. Use closed forceps or a fine spatula to insert along the entire hinge length and reflect the corneal flap.

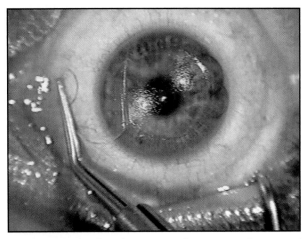

Figure 13-44d. Filtered BSS is used to irrigate the corneal flap and hinge prior to repositioning of the corneal flap.

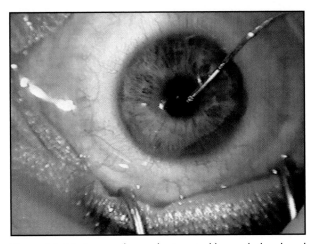

Figure 13-45. A cannula can be inserted beneath the closed flap, if desired, to irrigate out debris and epithelium within the interface.

lated in the medial canthus, the corneal flap may become edematous during the ablation; therefore, it should be dried.

Most surgeons remove the pneumatic suction ring immediately following the lamellar incision to simplify flap closure and realignment. As stated, patients do not require a fixation device if the stroma is left relatively moist during the ablation. Self-fixation is compromised with excessive drying of the stromal bed during the ablation. Replacement of the cap can even be performed with the suction ring still in position and has the dual advantage of maintaining fixation and preventing contamination of the interface. For the left eye, the suction ring may be twisted clockwise to allow room for the maneuver with the right hand.

INTERFACE IRRIGATION

The key element to irrigating the interface is to irrigate with the flap closed, creating a one-way valve system to prevent debris within the fornices from washing back (Figure

13-45). The interface can also be irrigated beneath the flap, and the excess fluid can be simultaneously aspirated utilizing an aspirating speculum as described in the Kritzinger-Updegraff method. Irrigation of the interface provides a cleaner interface devoid of debris that may potentially reduce the incidence of epithelial ingrowths by clearing any trapped epithelial cells. With the stromal bed and cap moist, alignment is easier, as the cap literally floats into position and irregular astigmatism may be reduced. This LASIK step has become a standard part of the procedure over the last 3 years and has not only improved the final flap alignment but ensured a pristine interface. The primary disadvantage of interface irrigation is that flap adhesion is prolonged. In general, a wet spear is passed away from the hinge to literally smooth the corneal flap into position and squeegee the excess fluid from the interface. A dry surgical spear can also be used along the flap edge to promote a more rapid seal.

FLAP ALIGNMENT

Once the flap is replaced and the interface irrigated, the correct position of the flap is confirmed through two primary methods. First, the alignment markings are examined to ensure that the ends are approximated; and second, ensure an even and well-approximated gutter exists between the cap edge and peripheral cornea (Figure 13-46). If correct placement is not achieved, the cap can easily be refloated with additional interface irrigation. With a small hinge, alignment may be difficult to achieve, as the flap is more mobile and multiple attempts may sometimes be required. Once the flap is closed and properly aligned, a wet surgical spear may be used quite effectively to smooth the flap and maintain the health of the epithelium. The surgical spear is moistened with BSS and always passed temporally, starting at the nasal hinge each time. With the superior hinged flap of the Hansatome, the wet spear is passed inferiorly away from the hinge. Minor misalignments are often corrected

Figure 13-46. Clinical photograph of a LASIK-treated eye in the immediate postoperative period, demonstrating excellent flap apposition as indicated by a smooth corneal flap edge and the appearance of a fine symmetrical peripheral gutter.

Figure 13-47. Clinical photograph of a retroilluminated corneal flap during the immediate postoperative period to assess for corneal striae. Retroillumination is the best technique to detect fine corneal striae secondary to flap misalignment, which may be associated with irregular astigmatism.

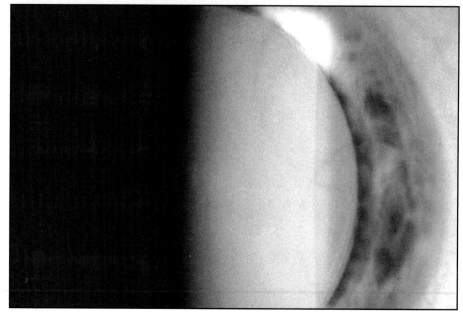

with this technique; however, flap rotations cannot be corrected, as flap striae will be produced and irregular astigmatism increased. Therefore, flap rotations should be treated by refloating the flap into the correct position. If striae are evident postoperatively, the cap is always misaligned and typically rotated several degrees and must be realigned as soon as possible, as striae become quite difficult to eliminate within days (Figure 13-47).

There are two important concepts to grasp with respect to corneal flap realignment:

First, the corneal flap is elastic in nature and has a tendency to shrink away from the stromal bed margins. For proper realignment and to avoid epithelial ingrowth, the flap edges must approximate the bed margins. A wet surgical spear can be quite effective in helping stretch the corneal

flap into position. Any excessive drying of the corneal flap, such as when compressed air is used, or in a highly myopic patient who is treated with a prolonged ablation time will result in flap shrinkage and require rehydration. The elastic nature of the corneal flap is fundamental in the formation of corneal striae.

Second, the radius of curvature of the stromal bed is altered during ablation, especially for very high degrees of myopia and hyperopia correction. In myopia, the stromal bed is flattened, creating a shorter radius of curvature and increasing the amount of corneal flap relative to the stromal bed. That is, horizontal corneal striae with the classic Corneal Shaper head and vertical striae with the Hansatome will be far more prevalent in high myopes. It is important to smooth the flap vertically with the classic Corneal Shaper and horizontally with the Hansatome when treating high myopia to ensure that any striae formed are outside the visual axis. A wet surgical spear is effective, however a partially expanded but squeezed spear will provide greater friction over the flap surface where a gap is evident and one is attempting to approximate the gutter. In the case of hyperopia, especially consecutive hyperopia following PRK or LASIK, the radius of curvature of the stromal bed is steepened, creating a corneal flap that is somewhat smaller than the bed. In the case of severe hyperopia or when correcting even mild overcorrections following myopic LASIK, it is not unusual to have a symmetrically wide peripheral gutter that may possibly invite epithelial ingrowth.

ENHANCING FLAP ADHESION

Most surgeons wait 2 to 5 minutes for adhesion of the flap. Some who utilize less interface irrigation find less than 1 minute adequate to create a secure seal. One technique to enhance re-adhesion is to use a dry surgical spear and lightly dab the gutter to draw fluid out of the interface. Similarly, the interface fluid can be expressed with a cannula, spatula, or wet spear. Compressed air at 1 to 2 liters per minute can also be used to dry the flap and flap edge to enhance adhesion time, but is not recommended since striae may be produced and the epithelium becomes more friable. The central cap epithelium is maintained moist with the wet surgical spears passed temporally over the flap. The small amount of fluid within the interface must literally be pumped out by the negative internal pressure created by the endothelial cell pump; therefore, all techniques are designed to aid this action. If the corneal flap gutter is asymmetric or greater than .5 mm, a wet, squeezed spear, the blunt side of fine tiers, or a similar tool to stretch or iron the flap edges away from the cap center to approximate the peripheral gutter is effective. The flap surface must be relatively dry for the tiers to work. If too much force is used, the entire flap will move.

TESTING FLAP ADHESION

There are multiple methods of assuring adequate cap adhesion. The primary method is known as the Slade striae test and involves depressing the peripheral cornea with fine tiers or forceps and observing for striae transmission onto the cap itself. If the epithelium is too moist, it will be impossible to determine if corneal striae are evident on the cap. The second essential test is known as the lid or "blink" test and involves re-examination of the integrity of flap adhesion after allowing the patient to blink several times. If there is any movement of the edges of the flap, the eyelid speculum must be reinserted and the flap edges smoothed with a wet or squeeze-dried surgical spear. A viscous lubricating agent should be avoided intraoperatively, as this will inhibit and delay flap adhesion.

It is important to carefully insert and remove the eyelid speculum to avoid engaging the flap edge. If the flap edges are retracted significantly by more than 1 mm and fail to smooth out with the wet spear, a dry technique can be used. The epithelial surface is allowed to dry somewhat, then the side of fine tiers are used to iron the edges out toward the peripheral gutter. If the irregularity or retraction is significant, the flap should be refloated. Occasionally, the striae test is positive but the blink test results in movement of the flap edge. In general, waiting 30 seconds after the striae test is adequate for removal of the speculum. Currently, we prefer to keep the epithelium moist by wiping a wet spear across the flap repeatedly during flap re-adhesion, then removing the speculum after 1 to 2 minutes without performing a striae test. Some surgeons, including ourselves, advocate having the patient wait 15 to 30 minutes following surgery with their eyes closed for at least the first 5 minutes and rechecking flap position at the slit lamp prior to discharging them.

REMOVING THE EYELID SPECULUM

The final step of LASIK is to remove the eyelid speculum. Although this would initially appear to be a simple step, beginning LASIK surgeons often cause flap displacement or striae at this time by allowing the speculum to touch the flap. The patient is instructed to keep both eyes open and look straight up at the laser fixation light. The speculum is then elevated away from the globe so that the blades of the speculum are well away from the corneal surface. The speculum arms are then retracted by turning the speculum screw with the surgeon's other hand, and the speculum is manipulated out of the palpebral fissure by disengaging the upper then the lower lid as the patient is directed to look down then up.

IMMEDIATE POSTOPERATIVE MEDICATIONS

Postoperative lubrication aids not only in epithelial health but also reduces the friction over the flap caused by blinking. We personally instill TobraDex, Ciloxan, and Voltaren into the eye immediately postoperatively and ask the patient to keep his or her eyes closed for 5 minutes. The eyelids can be taped closed for minutes or hours to prevent blinking, however, we have rarely found this to be necessary. Some surgeons place an eye shield over the eye at this time, but we advocate only sunglasses while awake and reserve the eye shield for sleeping.

The entire LASIK procedure is typically less than 10 minutes in duration and can take as little as 3 to 5 minutes, including flap adhesion, once proficiency is achieved. Consistency of technique is more important than speed to maintain a similar hydration status of the stroma intraoperatively. Each step must be executed properly to ensure a safe outcome.

CHAPTER 14

Personal LASIK Technique

Stephen G. Slade, MD
John F. Doane, MD

My laser in situ keratomileusis (LASIK) technique has developed as an ongoing modification of the original technique I learned when I began doing lamellar refractive surgery with myopic keratomileusis (MKM) after studying with Lee Nordan, MD in 1983. Nordan was one of the first surgeons to perform MKM in the United States, having learned the technique directly from Barraquer. Many aspects of my technique, such as not wearing gloves and avoiding handling the cornea as much as possible, are based on this classical teaching. The general approach is one of minimalism and extreme discipline and concentration. There are many differences in my current technique and my technique when I started. I leave out several steps, such as marking the cornea and checking pressure, that I would not leave out if I were doing my first 200 or 300 cases.

> The general approach is one of minimalism and extreme discipline and concentration. I leave out several steps, such as marking the cornea and checking pressure, that I would not leave out if I were doing my first 200 or 300 cases.

PATIENT SELECTION

Candidates for LASIK procedures should have a stable refraction and healthy corneas. Relative contraindications for LASIK should include patients with keratoconus, autoimmune disease, or patients with poor epithelium. Patients should undergo an "engaged" informed consent with their surgeon and be fully informed of the risks of the procedure. They must understand that irreversible complications do happen and can result in blindness.

PREOPERATIVE PREPARATION

In most cases, a patient's preoperative preparation includes an oral sedative such as Valium (5 to 10 mg) prior to the procedure. Immediately before prepping, one drop of a topical anesthetic (Proparacaine) should be instilled and then one more drop before the keratectomy. No preoperative miotic is used.

SURGICAL LOGISTICS

The proper laser room environment is critical for optimal laser performance. The laser is set up per the manufacturer's recommendations (Figures 14-1 and 14-2). The temperature should be maintained between 18° to 24°C, and the humidity should be kept at a stable level and below 50%. In addition, several air filtration units should be used continuously in the laser room to keep the atmosphere surgically clean and to achieve standard laser ablation rates.

Laser beam calibration is achieved by fluence testing. In the case of the Chiron Technolas laser, appropriate fluence

> The temperature should be maintained between 18° to 24°C, and the humidity should be kept at a stable level and below 50%.

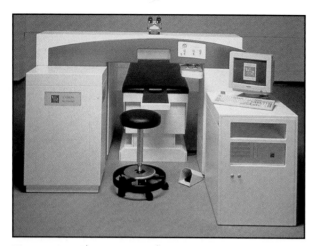

Figure 14-1. Chiron excimer laser set-up.

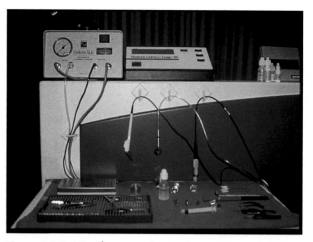

Figure 14-2. Microkeratome instrument set-up.

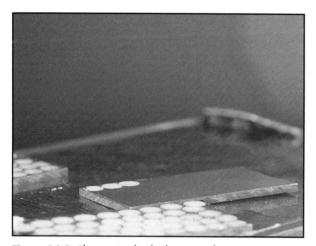

Figure 14-3. Fluence is checked on test plates.

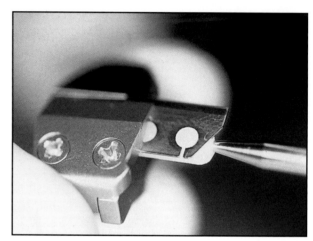

Figure 14-4. Assemble the Hansatome.

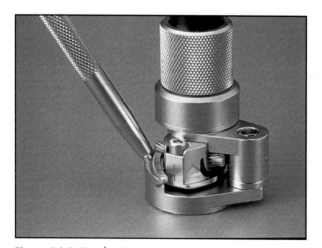

Figure 14-5. Test the Hansatome.

is defined as 65 ± 2 pulses to make a predetermined ablation pattern on fluence plates supplied by the manufacturer. The surgeon is able to test beam alignment and homogeneity, as well as the fluence, with these fluence plates (Figure 14-3).

The microkeratome is assembled and tested prior to use

(Figure 14-4 and 14-5). A trial pass of the keratome through the suction ring is recommended. The vacuum pump must also be tested.

The surgical set-up is minimal and laid out on a sterile drape: one Merocel sponge, a curved forceps, and a syringe full of balanced salt solution (BSS) with an ASICO LASIK cannula (Figure 14-6). There are no other instruments.

SURGICAL TECHNIQUE

The surgical field is prepared by irrigating the conjunctival fornices with a sterile solution to clear the eye of any particulate debris. The peri-ocular skin is prepared in typical fashion for ocular surgery. The field is draped with an aperture drape (3M 1020) making certain to include the cilia and lid margins in the adhesive backing of the drape so that they will not be in the path of the keratome on the passage over the suction ring (Figure 14-7). I use an ASICO locking lid speculum on 98% of the cases and an ASICO wire nonlocking speculum on rare exceptions (Figure 14-8). Either locking or nonlocking speculums can be used as long as they maximize exposure to enable clear passage of the microkeratome.

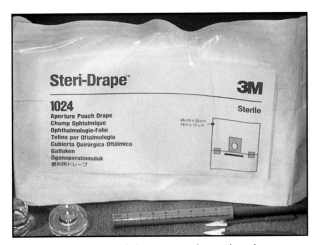

Figure 14-6. A surgical drape is used to isolate the eye.

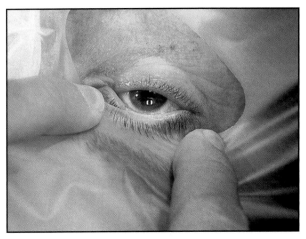

Figure 14-7. The upper and lower lid and lashes are isolated from the surgical field.

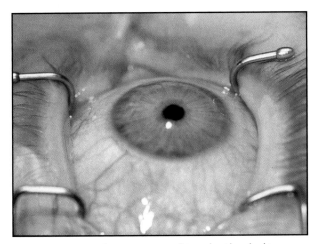

Figure 14-8. Good exposure is achieved with a locking eyelid speculum.

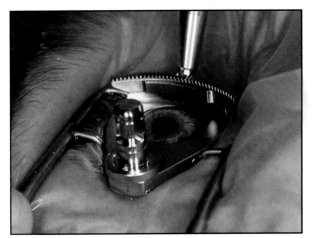

Figure 14-9. The suction ring is applied.

Prior to placing the LASIK suction ring, the patient's head should be positioned so the chin and forehead are in the same frontal plane. The iris must be perpendicular to the beam. The cornea should be centered between the lids for maximum exposure. Just prior to placement of the suction ring, BSS is irrigated over the surface of the cornea and suction ring. The LASIK suction ring of the Hansatome is slightly decentered superiorly by 1 mm depending on the size and appearance of the cornea (Figure 14-9). The vacuum pump is activated. The keratome is placed into the suction ring and advanced by depressing the pedal, the keratome is reversed and the vacuum is stopped (Figure 14-10).

At this point, the surgeon can proceed to ablate the stromal bed. The patients' head alignment is checked so the chin and forehead are in the same frontal plane. The corneal flap is reflected superiorly with the curved forceps (Figure 14-11). The laser focus is achieved over the pupillary center. The computer screen is checked to make certain all of the appropriate data is entered. The ablation is then completed. When the larger zones of ablation or astigmatism are being

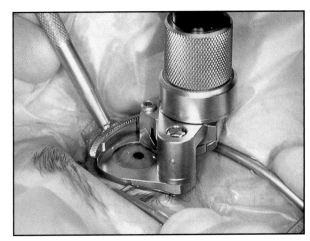

Figure 14-10. The Hansatome is advanced.

Prior to placing the LASIK suction ring, the patient's head should be positioned so the chin and forehead are in the same frontal plane.

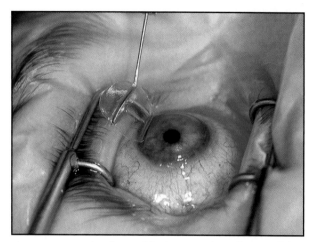

Figure 14-11. The flap is lifted superiorly with curved forceps.

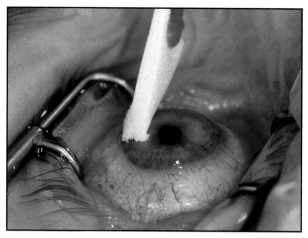

Figure 14-12. The excimer ablation is carried out while protecting the flap.

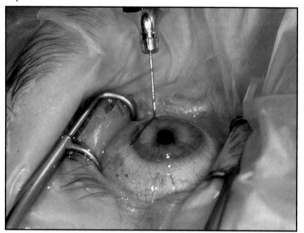

Figure 14-13. The flap is replaced with a cannula, starting superiorly under the flap.

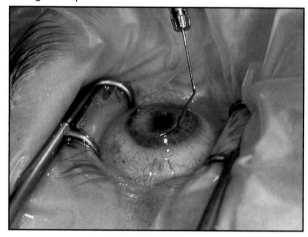

Figure 14-14. The flap is replaced with a cannula moved inferiorly.

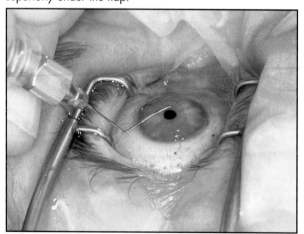

Figure 14-15. The flap interface is irrigated.

When the larger zones of ablation or astigmatism are being completed, the surgeon must protect the flap and hinge from ablation by holding an instrument over this area if necessary.

completed, the surgeon must protect the flap and hinge from ablation by holding an instrument over this area if necessary (Figure 14-12).

When the ablation is complete, the flap is positioned back onto the stromal bed using the cannula (Figure 14-13 and 14-14). The cannula is placed underneath the flap and irrigation is completed to clear any remaining debris from the interface (Figure 14-15). The Merocel sponge is moistened and squeezed dry and then used to squeegee the flap in the direction of the hinge (Figure 14-16). The flap is inspected to assure that there are no wrinkles and for proper position by making certain an equal gutter/keratectomy edge distance is present throughout the circumference (Figure 14-17). Depressing the peripheral cornea with closed blunt-tipped forceps completes a striae test (Figure 14-18). When striae pass well into the flap 360°, appropriate apposition has been achieved. During this phase it is recommended to keep a micro-drop of BSS over the central corneal epithelium to maintain its integrity. There is no specific waiting time with this technique.

The case is completed by carefully removing the specu-

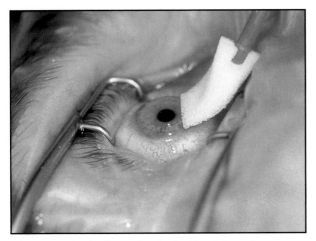

Figure 14-16. The flap is brushed with a Merocel sponge.

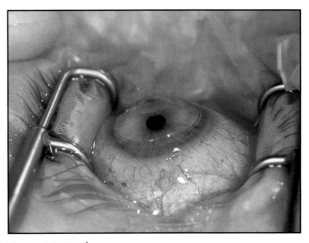

Figure 14-17. The gutter test.

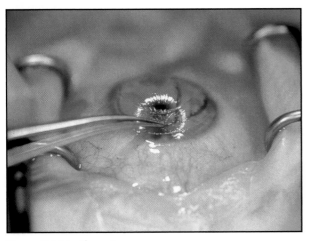

Figure 14-18. The striae test.

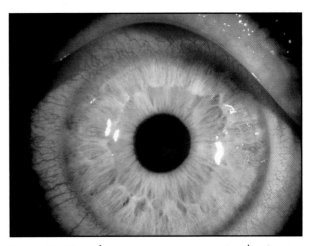

Figure 14-19. A clear cornea on postoperative day 1.

lum and drape. The eye is re-examined to make certain the flap is in proper position. Immediately postoperatively, several drops of an antibiotic agent (Ofloxacin) are instilled. The eye is not taped or shielded, rather the patient is instructed to wear a shield at night. On the first postoperative examination, the cornea should be remarkably clear (Figure 14-19). Flap apposition should be checked and no stromal edema should be present. The patient should be placed on topical prophylactic antibiotics four times per day for 4 days and seen again in approximately 1 month. Topical steroids are optional.

There are a few principles that are most important in

> The surgeon does not have to be fast but must be efficient during at least two phases (when the suction pump is engaged and the flap is off). The surgeon must manage fluids properly: cutting a wet cornea, maintaining an even hydration state during the ablation, and keeping the gutter dry during the post-ablation phase. The surgeon must key in on the first postoperative visit appearance to detect any potential complications and manage them aggressively.

this technique. The surgeon does not have to be fast but must be efficient during at least two phases (when the suction pump is engaged and the flap is off). The surgeon must manage fluids properly: cutting a wet cornea, maintaining an even hydration state during the ablation, and keeping the gutter dry during the post-ablation phase. The surgeon must key in on the first postoperative visit appearance to detect any potential complications and manage them aggressively.

CONCLUSION

LASIK can become an important part of any refractive surgical practice, but the surgeon must fully appreciate the risks as well as the benefits and be intimately familiar with standard and emergency procedures related to corneal surgery. The surgical staff must be thoroughly trained and familiar with every detail of the surgical facility, equipment, and instrumentation. This procedure, while very effective, can challenge even the most confident surgeons.

Strict adherence to the surgical protocol will help prevent significant complications and yield excellent, predictable results. As in any surgical procedure, the surgeon must be prepared for any eventuality.

T A B L E 15-3.
PRE-SURGERY CHECKLIST

Preparation and Assembly of the Chiron Microkeratome (ACS)

- Inspect the head in the open position and make sure that the blade holder moves freely inside its groove and is placed correctly with the groove for the eccentric placed posteriorly.

- Check external and internal gears for absolute smoothness without friction.

- Check the blade edge carefully under high magnification with the microscope.

- Insert the blade on the blade holder using the magnet.

- Check that the blade is inserted correctly and seated firmly on the blade holder.

- Close the head using the knurled collar smooth side towards the head.

- Insert the thickness plate until a click is heard, and then while holding it firmly with two fingers, firmly tighten the screw.

- Apply the stop mechanism and position it, as well as adjust the calibration screw correctly (first generation microkeratomes)— modern ones have a fixed stop mechanism).

- Inspect the movement of the blade and gear system for smoothness with the motor test tool.

- Once again ensure that the calibration of the stop has been set correctly.

- Simulate the movement by allowing the head of the microkeratome to advance for a few millimeters along the suction ring (the motor not yet attached).

- Activate the motor and listen to its hum; it must be constant, uniform, with the same intensity.

- Attach the head to the microkeratome motor/handle, taking care not to over-tighten, particularly if there is resistance.

- Engage the head of the microkeratome in the suction ring track and allow it to move forward and backward. Watch for smoothness of the movement and try not to allow the stop to engage as this will cause unnecessary wear and tear on the motor ("dry-run").

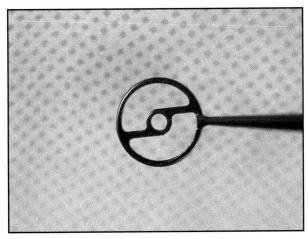

Figure 15-10. Ruiz central-paracentral corneal marker (with pararadial segment).

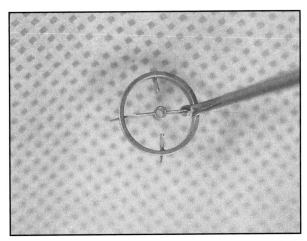

Figure 15-11. Central-paracentral corneal marker (radial).

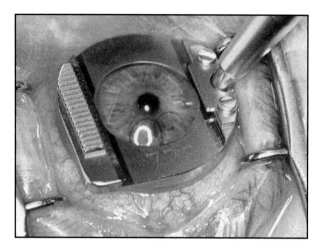

Figure 15-12. Positioning of the nonadjustable suction ring (LASIK).

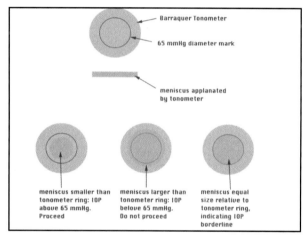

Figure 15-14. Barraquer's intraoperative tonometry (reticle).

It is incumbent upon the surgeon to ensure that the microkeratome has been assembled correctly and is functioning perfectly.

tioning perfectly. The proper positioning and plate checking is mandatory to allow for proper thickness resection as well as to prevent entrance into the anterior chamber. The stop mechanism must also be checked to make sure that it is both present and properly calibrated.

The suction ring, particularly the newer suction ring designed for LASIK, is then placed on the sclera and either centered directly around the outer mark of the Ruiz marker or decentered slightly nasally or superiorly, depending on the type of hinge desired (Figure 15-12). With the normal nasal hinge, the handle of the suction ring is placed superiorly for right eye LASIK and inferiorly for left eye LASIK. A helpful hint is that the serial number on the suction ring should always be temporal.

When the surgeon feels that the suction ring has been symmetrically and perfectly placed, the eye is then stabi-

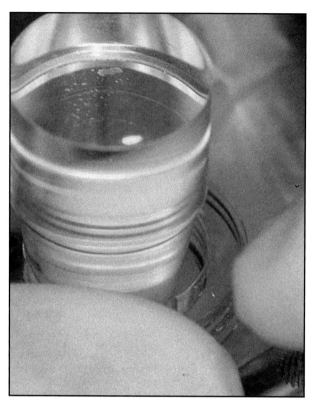

Figure 15-13. Intraoperative tonometry.

If a keratectomy is performed under the conditions of inadequate pressure, a thin flap will result.

lized by placing the index finger on the protruding corneal surface. The suction is engaged by pushing the appropriate pedal and then releasing it. Stabilization of the eye with the surgeon's index finger prevents the occasional drift of the eye once suction is engaged. The surgeon then waits a few seconds until sufficient suction is achieved, which is normally indicated by firmness of the globe as well as dilation of the pupil. The patient usually remarks that he or she can no longer see. All of these are helpful hints that good suction is achieved; however, checking the intraocular pressure (IOP) using the Barraquer tonometer is mandatory (Figure 15-13). This should be done when both the corneal surface and the tonometer are dry, otherwise a falsely low IOP reading may occur.

The applanation area of the cornea should be well within the circular mire inscribed on the inferior surface of the tonometer (Figure 15-14). If the applanation is just at or slightly exceeds the margin of the mire, then inadequate suction is present, and the keratectomy should not be performed. If a keratectomy is performed under the conditions of inadequate pressure, a thin flap will result.

Many surgeons use the 7.2 mm applanation disc, which is engaged in the dovetail of the suction ring track and then depressed to ensure that the diameter of the resection will be 7.2 mm or larger. With the LASIK suction ring, if adequate

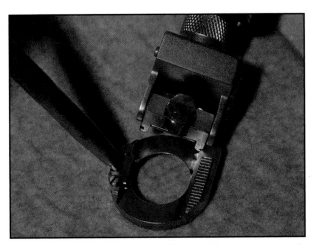

Figure 15-15. Training to insert the microkeratome correctly in the suction ring. The microkeratome is tilted and brought close first to the guide situated alongside the toothed runner.

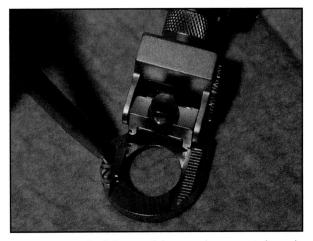

Figure 15-16. The left part of the microkeratome is brought close to the suction ring.

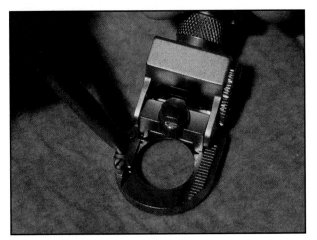

Figure 15-17. Both the right and left parts of the microkeratome rest on the suction ring.

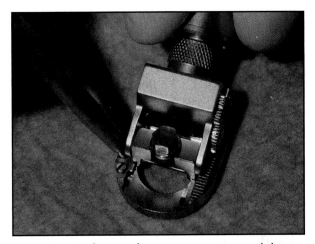

Figure 15-18. The microkeratome progresses until the two lateral wings come correctly into contact with the ring guides.

IOP has been checked using the Barraquer tonometer, this applanation step may be considered optional, as a large flap will always be created.

INADEQUATE SUCTION

If good exposure of the globe is not obtained for adequate suction, the lid speculum can be changed. Replacement of the locking lid speculum with the Barraquer wire lid speculum allows the suction ring to override the Barraquer speculum and depress it, thus proptosing the globe. Alternately, in some cases, the use of no lid speculum may facilitate suction.

When good suction still cannot be obtained, even after manipulation of the lid speculum, consideration may be given to use a retrobulbar injection of BSS or anesthetic. This is fraught with the potential complication of penetration of the globe or optic nerve as well as inducement of conjunctival chemosis, which may prevent adequate suction. Alternatively, the surgery can be rescheduled and

LASIK can be attempted again after the swelling of the globe and conjunctiva has resolved.

THE MICROKERATOME CUT

The surface of the cornea is moistened with BSS, taking care not to allow the BSS to coat the gear mechanism. The wet corneal surface facilitates the progression of the microkeratome over the epithelium; however, excess liquid may hit the laser lens and disturb the laser emission as well as damage the microkeratome motor. The microkeratome is then inserted into the dove-tail track on the gear side first, then depressed with the index finger over the hexagonal plate screw to depress the microkeratome head into the opposite track. The microkeratome head is moved to its starting position where the gears are engaged (Figures 15-15 to 15-27).

At this point, the operative field should be inspected to make sure that nothing will potentially block the progression of the microkeratome, such as the speculum, drape,

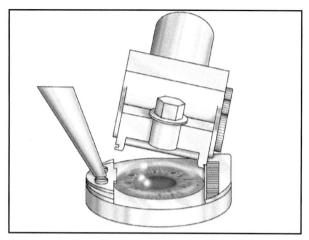

Figure 15-19. Engage dovetail gear side first.

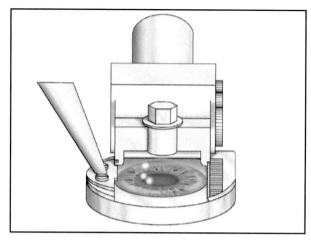

Figure 15-20. Flatten the head into the track.

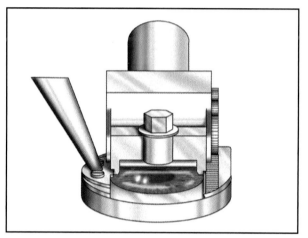

Figure 15-21. Move forward to engage both sides and first gear ("wobble test").

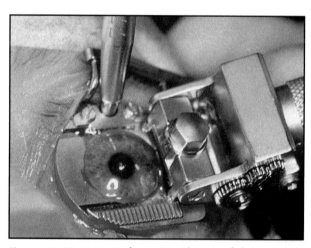

Figure 15-22. Cutting phase: introduction of the microkeratome in the suction ring.

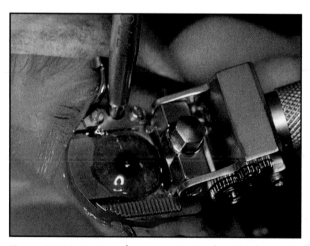

Figure 15-23. Cutting phase: positioning the microkeratome flat on the track.

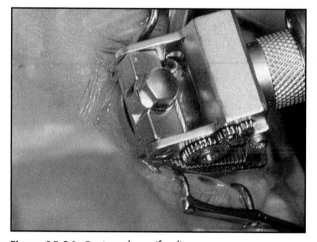

Figure 15-24. Cutting phase (final).

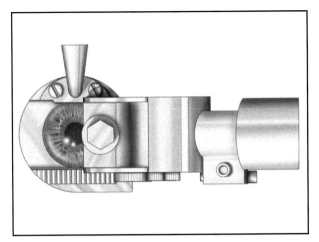

Figure 15-25. Microkeratome in the track, gears engaged.

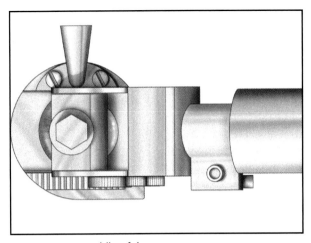

Figure 15-26. Middle of the pass.

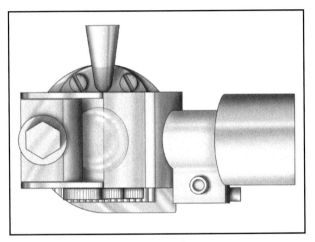

Figure 15-27. Pass complete, stop hits.

lashes, conjunctiva, eyelid skin, etc. The surgeon should be comfortable using arm supports, if desired, and the power cord and suction tubing should be free of traction. The pedals should be properly positioned so that either the surgeon or his or her assistant can activate them easily and safely.

Once again, looking through the operating microscope of the laser, the plate positioning is verified. While supporting the microkeratome handle in a neutral position or supporting only the power cord of the microkeratome in a neutral position, the forward motion of the microkeratome is activated by depressing the appropriate pedal. When the stop is complete, the reverse pedal is activated to retract the microkeratome. The microkeratome is then removed from the suction ring, and the suction pump is switched off.

This is the ideal time to determine whether a free cap

> The wet corneal surface facilitates the progression of the microkeratome over the epithelium; however, excess liquid may hit the laser lens and disturb the laser emission as well as damage the microkeratome motor.

has been created. Although this is a very infrequent occurrence, the free cap is normally in the head of the microkeratome and can either be left there until replacement or transferred to the antidesiccation jar to await replacement. When the suction is off and the suction ring is still in place, a free cap that is not in the microkeratome head can be easily found on the cornea or suction ring and placed in the antidesiccation jar.

> Although this is a very infrequent occurrence, the free cap is normally in the head of the microkeratome.

IN SITU EXCIMER LASER ABLATION

In the normal case with a hinge, the suction ring and microkeratome are passed off to the assistant. If the laser has been properly programmed and is ready for ablation, the corneal flap is flipped over nasally or superiorly onto the perilimbal conjunctival surface using a blunt spatula or the open jaws of a tying forceps without traumatizing the flap by grasping the tissue (Figures 15-28 to 15-30). I have found that a circular rim of an instrument wipe that is placed over the circumferential sclera approximately 1 mm peripheral to the limbus is the ideal surface to lay the flap, as it keeps the flap away from the tear film and prevents tear film debris from getting into the interface (Figures 15-31 and 15-32).

Some surgeons prefer to keep the suction ring in place with the suction turned off and fold the flap back onto the suction ring. We have not found this to be useful for several reasons: one of the surgeon's hands will always be occupied by holding the ring, the ring will frequently not stabilize the globe, especially if the patient is anxious and blinking, and finally, the flap may dry and adhere to the suction ring, creating a situation in which the hinge may tear if the cap is not rehydrated when the suction ring is removed.

It is important to be as atraumatic as possible to the epithelium of the flap and the peripheral cornea, as any

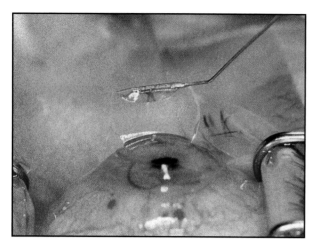

Figure 15-28. Elevating the corneal flap.

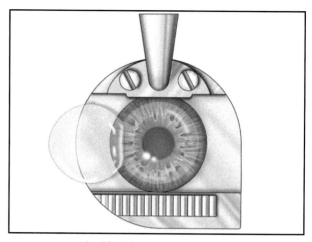

Figure 15-29. The lifted flap is placed nasally on the suction ring (kept in place with no suction).

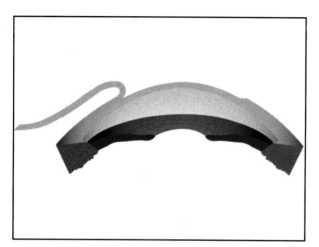

Figure 15-30. The flap is lifted and placed nasally (diagram with lateral view).

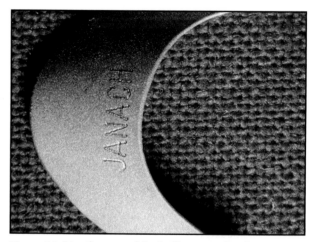

Figure 15-31. Close-up of the half-moon collar that prevents the flap from laying on the conjunctiva (Janach).

irregularities or corneal abrasions induce a foreign body sensation with subsequent lacrimation and eyelid squeezing, which will jeopardize good adhesion of the flap to its underlying bed.

The exposed corneal surface is now ready for ablation with the excimer laser. Any wet spots in the bed should be patted with a Merocel sponge to allow even hydration of the bed. Usually ablation should commence approximately 30 seconds following the lifting of the flap to allow consistent hydration of the stroma so that it is neither overhydrated nor overly dry, which could affect the ultimate refractive outcome. The patient is instructed to refixate on the fixation light in the laser, and the excimer ablation is begun (Figures 15-33 to 15-35).

> Corneal abrasions induce a foreign body sensation with subsequent lacrimation and eyelid squeezing, which will jeopardize good adhesion of the flap to its underlying bed.

During the ablation, particularly with astigmatic, and hyperopic ablations requiring large optic zones, the surgeon must protect the internal portion of the hinge to prevent it from being accidentally ablated. The following techniques are useful to protect the hinge during ablation:

- The flap should be fully retracted using a spatula, and the gutter of the hinge should be dried of any retained fluid. It is important, however, not to overstretch the flap, which can cause a crease to develop.
- Closed McPherson forceps along the internal corneal edge of the flap should allow slight flap retraction as well as shield it from accidental ablation.
- Shield the hinge with a spatula specifically designed for this purpose (Figures 15-36 to 15-38).
- A damp Merocel sponge may also be used to shield the margin of the hinge as well as facilitate retraction; however, it does not allow as stable and complete coverage as the previous techniques.

During the photoablation, the patient is constantly coaxed to maintain fixation on the fixation light. Some

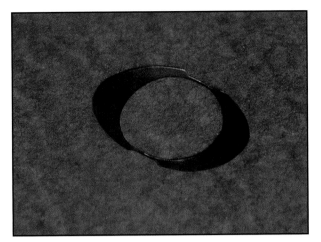

Figure 15-32. Double half-moon collar.

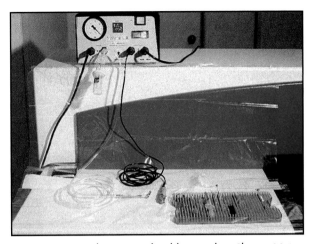

Figure 15-33. The surgical table on the Chiron Vision Keracor 117.

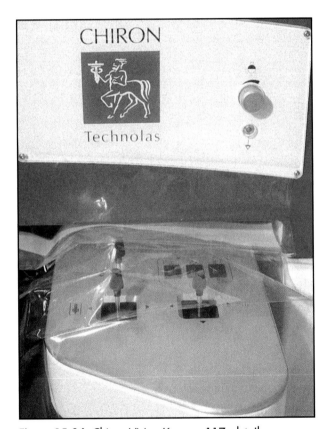

Figure 15-34. Chiron Vision Keracor 117: detail.

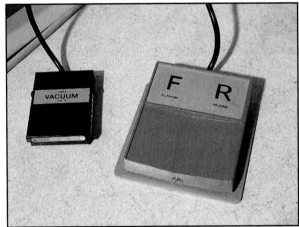

Figure 15-35. The two foot switches of the Chiron microkeratome.

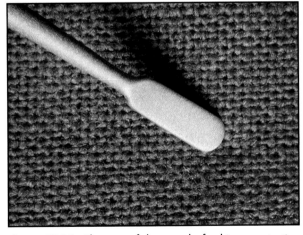

Figure 15-36. Close-up of the spatula for hinge protection during ablation.

lasers provide an active eye tracking mechanism, which assists in maintaining good centration of the ablation. The coaxial illumination of the laser microscope should be minimal and only the least amount of oblique illumination used to allow the surgeon to ensure that the patient is maintaining good fixation without creating excessive glare for the patient, who is striving to see the fixation target.

The surgeon should follow the protocol that applies to the specific laser he or she is using. If obvious fluid is building up in the center of the ablation, the ablation should be

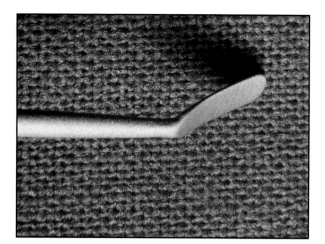

Figure 15-37. Lateral view of the above spatula.

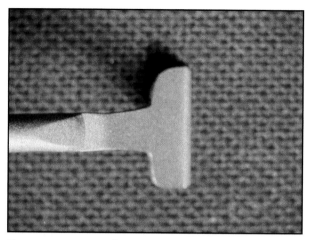

Figure 15-38. ASICO hinge retracting and protecting spatula.

suspended and the fluid removed with a Merocel sponge. Alternately, the fluid may be wiped away with a spatula. With some lasers that use a multizone ablation approach, it is recommended that the fluid be wiped with a spatula between each of the zonal ablations. In the case of astigmatic ablation, in which the ablation extends peripherally, the surgeon must be aware of the axis of ablation and protect the hinge when the ablation extends in that direction. There is also a tendency, as previously mentioned, for fluid to pool at the base of the hinge. This fluid should also be removed, especially if the ablation is approaching this area.

Once the ablation has been completed, a drop or two of BSS may be placed on the stromal side of the flap, especially if the ablation has been prolonged and the flap may have dried. Also, moistening the flap if the suction ring has been left in place prevents adhesion of the flap to the suction ring. Once the flap has been slightly moistened, the spatula or closed Kelman-McPherson forceps are placed underneath the hinge, and the flap is gently flipped back into place on its stromal bed.

REPLACING THE FLAP

If the ablation has been brief and the flap has maintained good hydration and form, it may be allowed to remain in place without further manipulation. In the vast majority of cases, however, it is preferable to irrigate the interface once the flap has been replaced using BSS with either a 25- or 27-gauge BSS irrigation cannula or one of the newer cannulas designed specifically for interface irrigation. The purpose of the irrigation is twofold: 1.) to remove interface debris; and 2.) to allow a smooth layer of BSS, which facilitates the flap "floating" back into its original position.

The cannula or spatula is then used to stroke the flap from the hinge temporally (or inferiorly with the Buratto superior hinge technique), and then the flap is gently "painted" into place using a slightly moist Merocel sponge. The painting motion is continued until the flap is both aligned

> The purpose of the irrigation is twofold: 1.) to remove interface debris; and 2.) to allow a smooth layer of BSS, which facilitates the flap "floating" back into its original position.

and distended properly, and the gutter starts to appear. The gutter should appear symmetrical around the margin of the keratectomy. The painting motion is continued until the flap is slightly dry and a matte finish is seen through the surgical microscope, which allows the surgeon to ensure that perfect realignment and adherence of the flap is being achieved (Figures 15-39 and 15-40).

A drop of BSS is then placed on the corneal dome to maintain hydration of the epithelium without allowing the drop to disperse into the gutter, which would potentially reduce flap adherence. If the gutter is moistened, this should be gently removed with a Merocel sponge.

The flap is then allowed to dry naturally for approximately 2 to 5 minutes, maintaining a drop of BSS on the corneal dome, while allowing the periphery of the flap and the gutter to remain dry. The length of this waiting time is dependent upon the surgeon's experience and comfort level that the flap is well-adhered. After the time has passed, a blunt instrument, such as a dry Merocel sponge, an olive-tipped spatula, or closed .12 forceps, is used to depress the corneal periphery near the limbus, inducing striae formation, which can be seen radiating into the flap (Slade's striae test). The patient should be advised that this pressure will occur, as unexpected pressure will alarm the patient, causing him or her to blink and dislodge an otherwise perfect flap.

> If there is any doubt in the surgeon's mind that the flap is not perfectly aligned or that striae can be seen, the flap should be refloated and the procedure repeated as previously described.

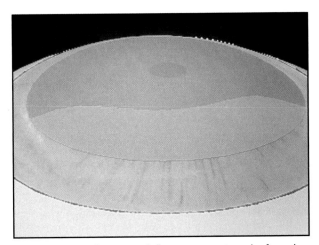

Figure 15-39. The corneal flap is repositioned after photoablation.

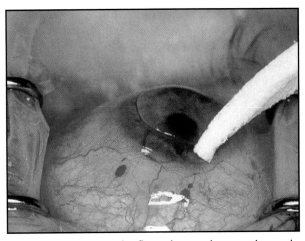

Figure 15-40. Drying the flap edges in the sutureless techniques in the foreground, the circular epithelial marking is useful for correct repositioning (the operation was a free cap).

The margins of the flap should be aligned perfectly with the margins of the keratectomy and no striae or folds should be apparent. If there is any doubt in the surgeon's mind that the flap is not perfectly aligned or that striae can be seen, the flap should be refloated and the procedure repeated as previously described.

The speculum may then be removed. It is imperative that the speculum be removed very gently, and the assistance of the technician is helpful, as the patient has a natural tendency to blink during speculum removal. One must also take care to avoid touching the cornea and dislodging the flap. Likewise, the assistant should maintain lid retraction while the drape is being removed to prevent the sharp margins of the drape from touching the cornea, causing either a corneal abrasion or flap displacement.

The patient is then allowed to blink normally, and this is observed through the operating microscope (blink test). The flap should appear well-adhered and remain in perfect position. A few drops of a broad spectrum antibiotic are instilled and, once again, the patient is allowed to blink with the surgeon observing that the flap is well-adhered without any sign of movement or decentration.

POSTOPERATIVE CARE

The patient is brought to a waiting area where he or she receives postoperative instructions. At this time, we like to examine the patient at the slit lamp to once again reassure ourselves that the flap is in perfect position with good adherence and that there is no unexpected debris in the interface. If there is an unacceptable amount of debris in the interface, the patient is taken back to the laser suite and the flap is once again lifted, cleaned, and refloated.

With topical anesthesia, the patient is allowed to leave the office with a pair of sunglasses and a plastic shield to be placed over the eye while he or she is sleeping. Alternately,

the patient may be discharged with the plastic shield in place, instructed to begin the postoperative drops and strictly advised not to rub the eye.

In the case of peribulbar or retrobulbar anesthesia, horizontal and vertical Steri-Strips are applied to maintain lid closure. A pressure bandage should be avoided, as this will cause undue posterior pressure, which may dislodge the flap once the patient regains ocular motility.

ADDITIONAL CONSIDERATIONS

When an astigmatic ablation is planned, the axis of the steep meridian should be marked preoperatively with the patient at the slit lamp. Normally, the 12 o'clock and 6 o'clock vertical axes are marked. Once the patient is reclining in the laser chair, the Mendez ring is used to again mark the axis of astigmatic correction. This prevents inaccurate axis marking due to cyclotorsion of the eye, frequently seen in anxious patients. Once again, consideration needs to be given to hinge protection with these astigmatic ablations, especially in with-the-rule situations in which the ablation is horizontal.

In cases of LASIK retreatment of previous incisional surgery, consideration should be given to making a thicker flap with a 200-micron plate, taking particular care not to separate the previous keratectomy when handling of the flap.

In cases of hyperopic ablation, the hinge must also be carefully protected. This is a situation in which the superior hinge, created with the Buratto down-up technique, comes in handy.

> In cases of LASIK retreatment of previous incisional surgery, consideration should be given to making a thicker flap with a 200-micron plate.

SUMMARY

With the widespread use of LASIK, we have now seen a major paradigm shift in keratomileusis surgery from the carving of the refractive correction on the cap away from the eye, to the refractive ablation in situ directly on the eye. Thus, a previous extraocular technique has now become an ocular technique.

The use of the excimer laser now allows the refractive surgeon to correct the refractive error much more precisely than previously obtained with cryolathe or other mechanical or microkeratome techniques. With the excimer laser, we are able to obtain homogeneous, uniform lenticular ablations that are well-centered over the pupil and are also smooth and tapered so that they facilitate the spontaneous reattachment of the flap.

The continued evolution of microkeratome technology with automated movement to create a smoother, more regular resection, as well as the new Chiron Hansatome that creates a large corneal flap with a superior hinge, has allowed the surgeon to obtain the best anatomical and visual results with minimal complications and induced irregular astigmatism.

In conclusion, LASIK provides the surgical refraction correction that patients desire. It allows for a virtually instantaneous improvement of uncorrected vision with minimal discomfort, which leads to greater patient satisfaction.

ATLAS OF SURGICAL TECHNIQUE

CASE 1

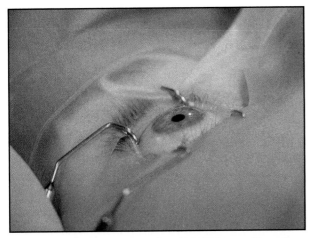

Figure A-1. The Buratto speculum (ASICO) is positioned.

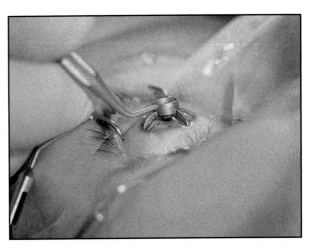

Figure A-2. Epithelial marking using the Buratto radial marker.

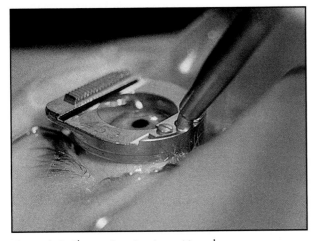

Figure A-3. The suction ring is positioned.

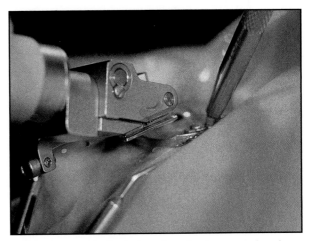

Figure A-4. Final check that the microkeratome has been assembled correctly prior to use.

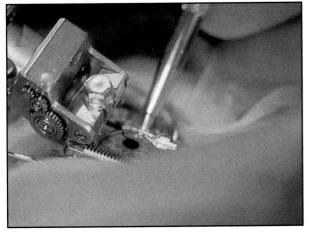

Figure A-5. The microkeratome is positioned on the toothed track of the ring.

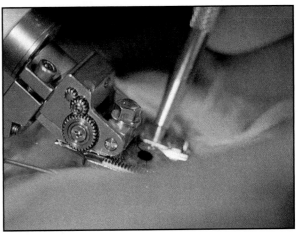

Figure A-6. Initiation of the microkeratome's forward movement.

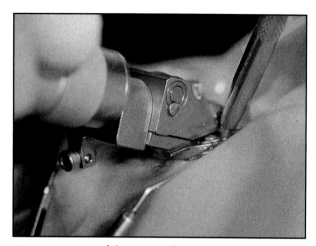

Figure A-7. Start of the cutting phase (posterior view).

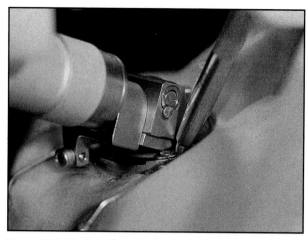

Figure A-8. Cutting phase (side posterior view).

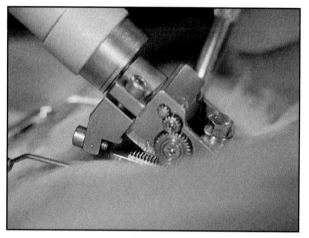

Figure A-9. Final cutting phase: return of the microkeratome.

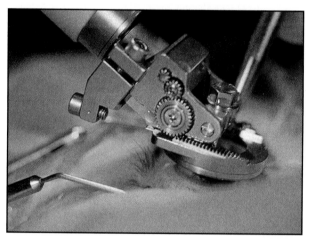

Figure A-10. The ring and microkeratome are removed from the cutting surface.

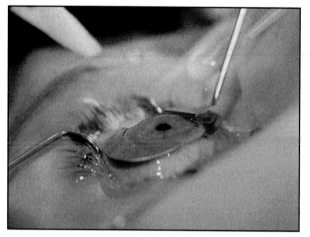

Figure A-11. The half-moon is positioned on the conjunctival surface.

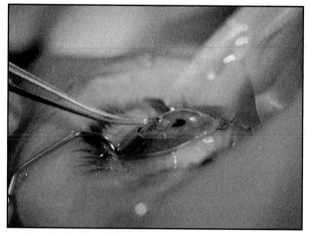

Figure A-12. The flap is raised with the Buratto forceps (ASICO).

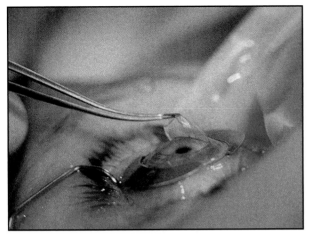

Figure A-13. The flap is raised.

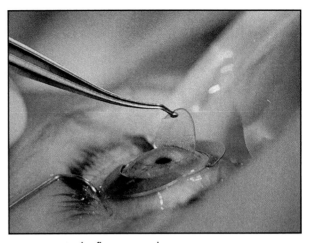

Figure A-14. The flap is raised.

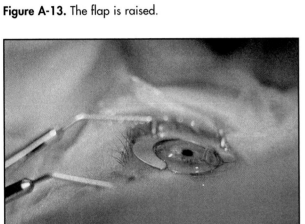

Figure A-15. The flap is placed on the half-moon support.

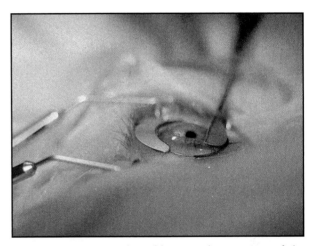

Figure A-16. In situ photoablation with protection of the hinge base using the Buratto spatula (ASICO).

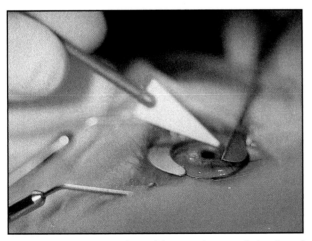

Figure A-17. In situ photoablation: drying of the liquid meniscus at the base of the hinge between ablation pulses.

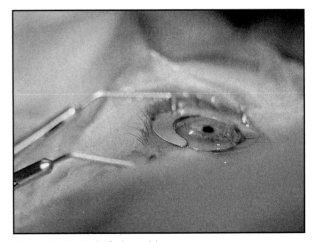

Figure A-18. End of photoablation.

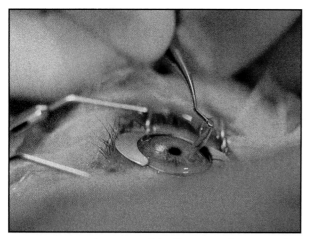

Figure A-19. Replacement of the flap using the Buratto forceps (ASICO).

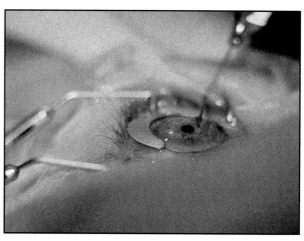

Figure A-20. Irrigation of the interface using a three-hole cannula (ASICO).

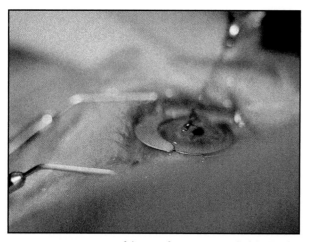

Figure A-21. Irrigation of the interface using a 3-hole cannula.

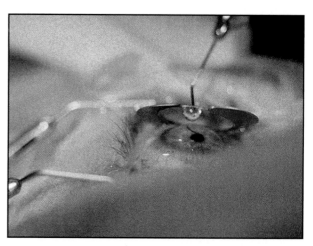

Figure A-22. Irrigation of the interface using a 3-hole cannula.

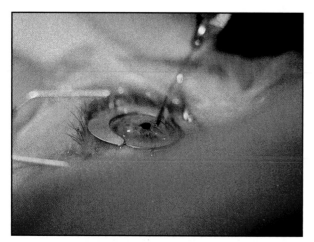

Figure A-23. Maintain a moist corneal dome.

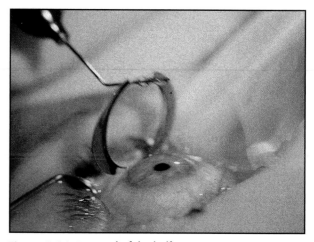

Figure A-24. Removal of the half-moon support ring.

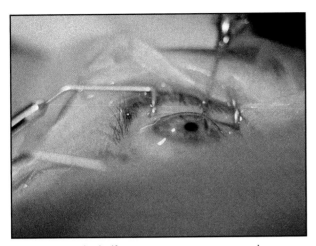

Figure A-25. The half-moon support ring removed.

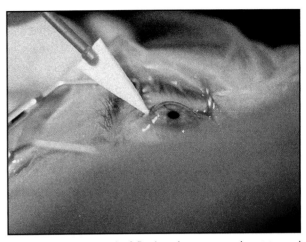

Figure A-26. Removal of fluid in the gutter with a Merocel sponge.

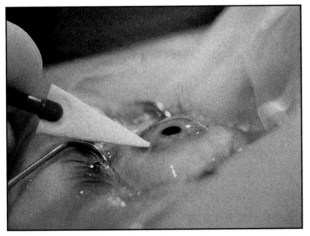

Figure A-27. Checking the adhesion (Slade striae test) by drying with a Merocel sponge.

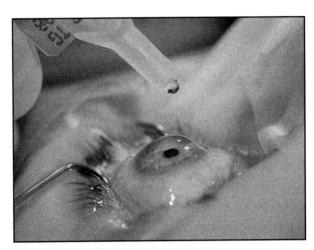

Figure A-28. Medication.

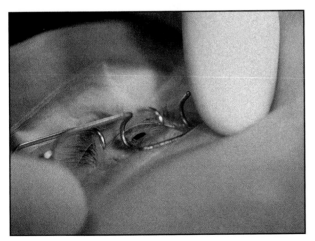

Figure A-29. The speculum is removed.

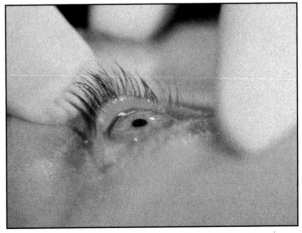

Figure A-30. The eye is examined and the adhesion is checked using the adhesion test.

Case 2

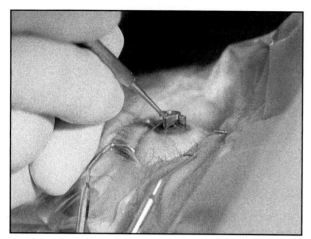

Figure A-31. Epithelial marking with the Buratto marker (ASICO).

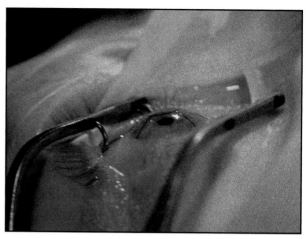

Figure A-32. The speculum is positioned and the eye is centered under the laser.

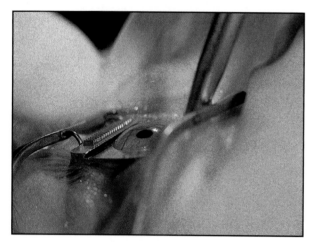

Figure A-33. The suction ring is positioned.

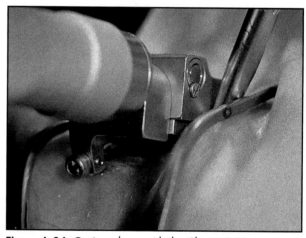

Figure A-34. Cutting phase with the Chiron ACS.

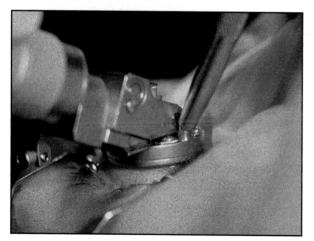

Figure A-35. Cutting phase with the Chiron ACS.

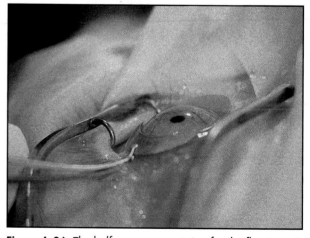

Figure A-36. The half-moon support ring for the flap is positioned.

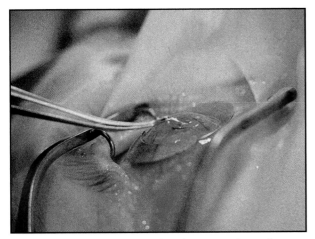

Figure A-37. The flap is raised and positioned nasally.

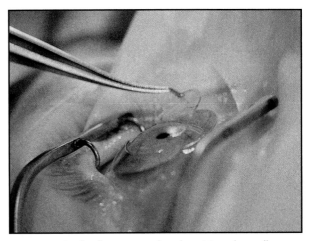

Figure A-38. The flap is raised and positioned nasally.

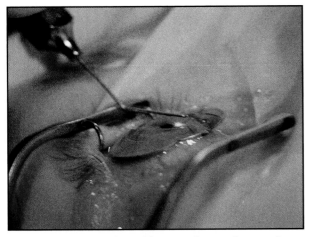

Figure A-39. In situ photoablation with smoothing and protection of the hinge base.

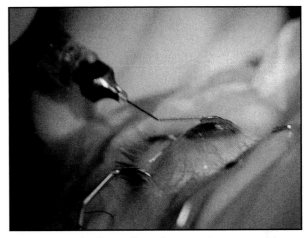

Figure A-40. The flap is flipped over and repositioned in its original position.

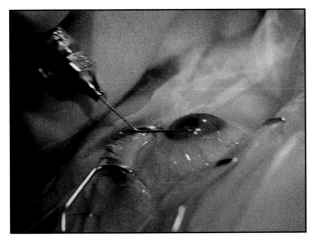

Figure A-41. Irrigation of the treated surfaces.

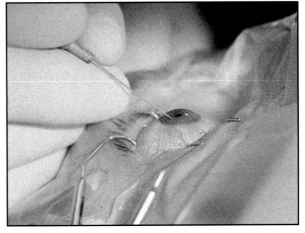

Figure A-42. Spatula used to smooth and distend the flap.

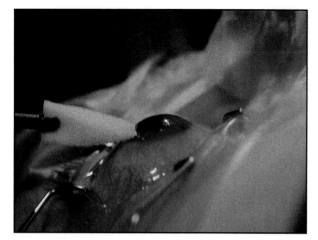

Figure A-43. Dehydration of the gutter.

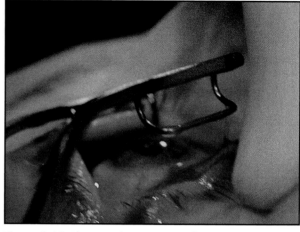

Figure A-44. The speculum is removed.

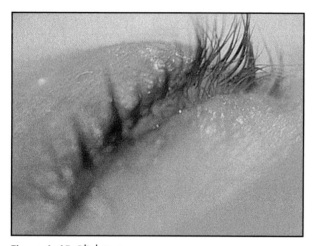

Figure A-45. Blink test.

CASE 3

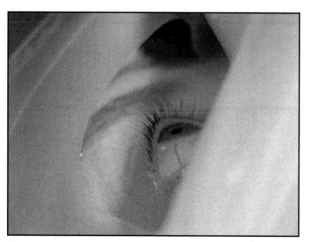

Figure A-46. The patient is positioned under the microscope's laser and draping is begun.

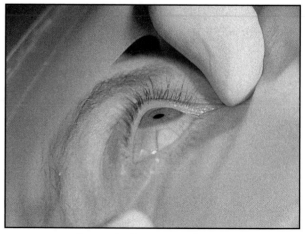

Figure A-47. The sterile drape is applied and excludes the inferior eyelashes from the operating field.

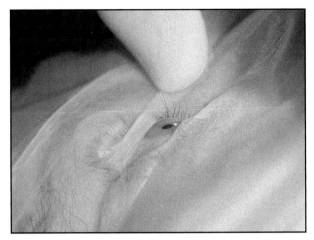

Figure A-48. The sterile drape is applied and excludes the superior eyelashes from the operating field.

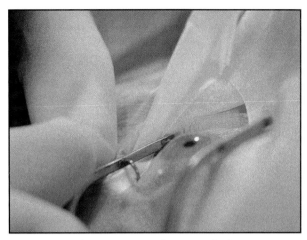

Figure A-49. The Buratto speculum is applied.

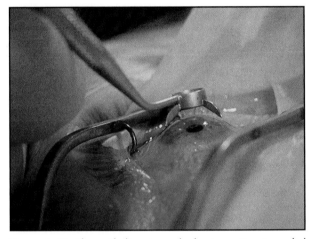

Figure A-50. The epithelium is marked using a Buratto radial marker.

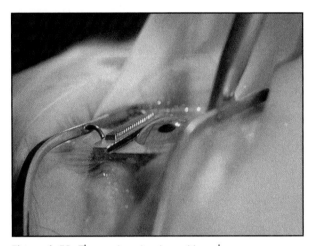

Figure A-51. The suction ring is positioned.

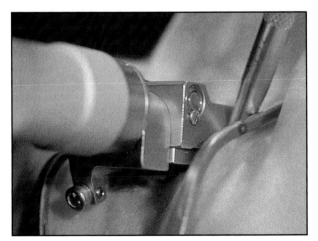

Figure A-52. Cutting phase with the Chiron ACS.

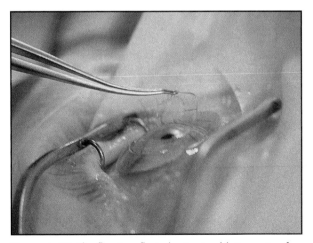

Figure A-53. The flap is reflected prior to ablation using forceps (ASICO).

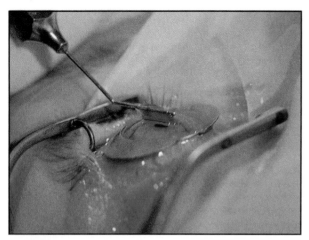

Figure A-54. The flap is flipped over and placed laterally using a needle cannula, then photoablation is performed.

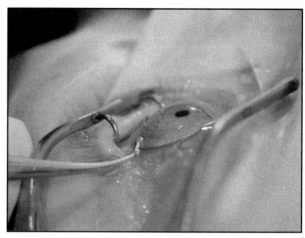

Figure A-55. The half-moon ring (ASICO) used to support the flap is removed.

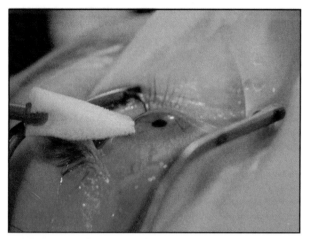

Figure A-56. Dehydration of the cut edges and striae test for adhesion.

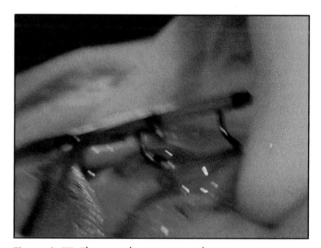

Figure A-57. The speculum is removed.

Personal LASIK Technique

Michiel S. Kritzinger, MD
Stephen A. Updegraff, MD

The most common sight-threatening complication following lamellar corneal surgery is irregular astigmatism.[1,2] Although earlier studies attributed this problem to the suturing required for myopic keratomileusis, irregular astigmatism can still be a major complication of laser in situ keratomileusis (LASIK), or automated lamellar keratoplasty (ALK), in which no sutures are used,[3] especially when compared to surface ablation techniques. When a corneal flap or cap is returned to the stromal bed, micro-irregularities can exist resulting from folds on the epithelial surface. Another complication of lamellar surgery, which, with time can be sight-threatening, is the presence of debris such as meibomian secretions or epithelial nests within the interface. We have designed instrumentation and developed techniques that incorporate low flow irrigation with repositioning of the corneal flap or cap, which we call low flow tectonic keratoplasty. The goal is to minimize irregular astigmatism and reduce or eliminate debris in the interface.

> The goal is to minimize irregular astigmatism and reduce or eliminate debris in the interface.

The original Ruiz marker was designed primarily to prevent the surgeon from inverting a free corneal flap by having a single pararadial mark temporally. Some alignment of the corneal cap was obtained by making sure that this pararadial mark was symmetrically aligned across the gutter. We developed a marking system that utilizes seven radials and one pararadial. The radial marks ensure proper orientation of the entire cap/flap. Each of the blades on this marker is very short so as to minimize the amount of ink

that is placed on the corneal surface. The surface area of ink is actually less on this marker than on the original Ruiz marker. This reduces the incidence of visually significant epitheliopathy from the ink marks, which can lead to disappointing visual acuities in the immediate postoperative period. The broad cross hair marks on the peripheral cornea, outside the bed, are used to maintain laser ablation centration by aligning with the reticule of the laser microscope. When the cornea is marked, the frontal plane of the patient's head should be 90° to the point of fixation. Centering the marker over the corneal light reflex of a normally light constricting pupil will ultimately accurately center the laser ablation. The suction ring is centered over the concentric circular mark of the Kritzinger-Updegraff (KU) marker. After the keratectomy is performed, the flap is folded back nasally. The peripheral markings of the KU marker are still visible. Thus, these are used as a visual cue to line up the cross hair of the reticule, which corresponds to the exact fixation prior to the keratectomy. It is very important not to chase the patient's eye by moving the bed. Rather, move the patient's head gently to achieve centration if the eyes have drifted. Improper alignment of the patient's head does not mean the bed has moved but rather the patient's head has moved and thus must be oriented back to the position you had initially worked so hard to achieve.

The technique for repositioning a lamellar flap or cap is based on the dilution principle and plate tectonics. A steady flow of fluid is more effective in removing debris than short bursts of smaller volumes of fluid from a syringe or bulb delivery. We use BSS from an intravenous set-up. The flow is adjusted so that it is constant and does not "jet" the cap/flap, but rather "floats" the flap with fluid steadily exiting from under the entire edge of the flap. The KU irrigation cannula creates fluid flow patterns that aid in the removal of interface debris. The surgeon uses a two-handed technique by irrigating with one hand and aspirating with the other. A 19-gauge cannula is used for aspiration. The patient is fixating so that the apex of the globe is in line with the microscope. This will allow the fluid to flow from underneath the cap or flap peripherally and out past the limbus into the fornices. The fornices are aspirated first. This removes debris and meibomian secretions that have flowed downhill. After approximately 15 to 20 seconds of central irrigation, the irrigating cannula can be moved toward the hinge and gently swept back and forth from the hinge, then held centrally again. This allows any epithelium entrapped by the blade at the hinge to be freed and irrigated out. Once the fornices are cleared of fluid and debris, the aspiration cannula can be moved towards the gutter, and with a low flow irrigation, the cap can be nudged with a KU manipulator so that the radial marks are exactly aligned. This is like plate tectonics, in which the earth's crust constantly moves on a bed that is more fluid. However, this is a controlled repositioning so that as the flap floats into position, the peripheral marks are realigned. Once this is achieved, the gutter should be aspirated for 270°, while there is steady irrigation. This again removes debris that could have become lodged at the edge of the keratectomy. Aspiration of the gutter is continued as the irrigating cannula is gently withdrawn, taking note of the approximation of the radial and pararadial marks. We use a curved KU flap manipulator to smooth the flap from the center to the periphery in making sure the radial and pararadial marks are realigned. If alignment is not achieved, the irrigating cannula is once again reintroduced and the aspiration is performed in the gutter. The cap is then allowed to be adjusted on a bed of fluid.

To date, we have not experienced any dislocation of caps/flaps postoperatively. We discourage the use of air blown on the corneal surface and believe it can cause cracks in Bowman's membrane, as well as push debris accumulated in the gutter back under the flap. Aspiration or Merocel sponges that wick fluid from the gutter in an outward motion from under the flap work well to ensure cap adherence. A drop of balanced salt solution (BSS) is placed on the central cornea during these maneuvers to prevent epitheliopathy. We always utilize the Slade striae test to confirm adherence, and then we remove the speculum. Once again, adherence and alignment of the flap is reconfirmed with the "blink test" prior to placing clear shields over the patient's eyes.

We have demonstrated, in a prospective study, the usefulness and safety of low flow tectonic keratoplasty.[4] We do notice an early hyperopic shift because the irrigating fluid creates stromal edema at the edge of the keratectomy, thus effectively creating more central flattening. This resolves in 2 to 3 days.

Another major advantage of this technique is that it allows the surgeon to safely and predictably retreat patients by lifting the corneal flap. Many experienced LASIK surgeons create another keratectomy when retreating patients, due to the risk of introducing debris and irregular astigmatism when lifting a flap. These risks are higher when lifting a corneal flap because the overlying epithelium at the edge of the keratectomy tears and does not have a sharp edge as with the primary keratectomy. Utilizing the marking and irrigating techniques, the corneal flap can be realigned and the torn edges tend to "float" into position. We have developed the KU corneal flap elevator that creates a sharper edge and aids in lifting flaps that are more than 3 months postoperatively. We do not recommend lifting flaps that are older than 12 months. This application is particularly useful in treating penetrating keratoplasty corneas, in which we have demonstrated that waiting 4 weeks after the primary keratectomy to perform the ablation significantly reduces retreatment for these patients.[5]

KEY POINTS OF THE KRITZINGER LASIK TECHNIQUE

PATIENT POSITIONING FOR LASIK

1. Ensure the patient's head and body lie in a straight line.
2. The chin must be horizontal and level.
3. Check that the green HeNe beam is in the center of the reticle of the operating microscope.
4. Switch on the red HeNe beam and superimpose it on the green light.
5. Check that the red laser beam is absolutely centered on the two superimposed red/green HeNe beams.
6. Position the two lights on the center of the pupil using the joystick.
7. Increase the illumination intensity—the pupil constricts, enabling better centration.
8. Decrease illumination after alignment of the head and eye.
9. Observe the bright red reflex from the retina.
10. Properly position the patient.
11. Refrain from using the joystick in the XY axis once the above steps are completed since the patient is now perfectly aligned.

Should the HeNe lights become decentered, adjust the patient's head; do not use the XY joystick to make any adjustments since this will decenter the ablation. Only use the focus joystick to keep the beams superimposed.

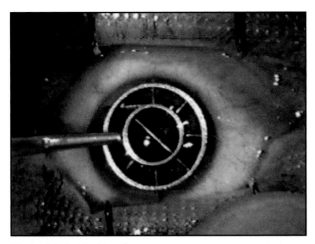

Figure 16-1. Marking the cornea.

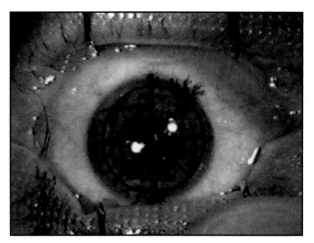

Figure 16-2. Corneal markings.

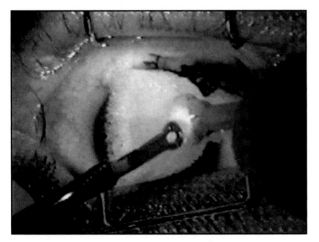

Figure 16-3. Remove excess gentian violet.

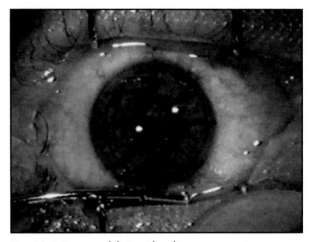

Fig. 16-4. Remove debris with saline.

STEPS OF THE LASIK PROCEDURE

1. Preoperative topical anesthetic: Instill no more than one-half hour before surgery because the drops can damage the epithelium. Do not use more than 5 drops instilled 5 to 10 minutes apart. The first drop is any routine anesthetic eye drop followed by .5% Marcaine four times, 5 to 10 minutes apart. Also put 5 cc of .5% Marcaine in a 250 ml BSS bottle connected to the irrigation needle for eye and surgical interface cleaning. This also improves postoperative discomfort and pain.

2. Clean and drape the patient, cover the head and forehead, and leave the lower face exposed to monitor the head and chin position, especially when performing the laser surgery.

3. Use 3M or Johnson and Johnson Transpore to cover the eyelashes—a gauze swab with transpore on the side of the eye to prevent fluid from running into the patient's ear, causing irritation and head movement during treatment.

4. Insert a wire Barraquer speculum. With difficult patients, use a Lieberman wire blade screw speculum.

5. Mark the cornea with gentian violet ink using the KU marker (Figures 16-1 and 16-2).

6. Remove excess ink with saline from the 250 ml BSS bottle and KU irrigation and aspiration needle system (Figure 16-3).

7. Clean and dry the cornea and fornices well with a damp microsponge to prevent mucus and water from coming onto the surgical interface (Figures 16-4 and 16-5).

8. Test the vacuum on your thumb. The minimal reading should be no less than 22 pounds per square inch (psi).

9. Run the microkeratome across the track to ensure smooth transition forward and backward.

10. Apply the suction ring to the cornea, check the vacuum reading, and feel corneal pressure with your finger. Ideal pressure is 22 psi. If the suction is low, cut the suction tube shorter. This will increase the psi to 22.

11. Engage an 8.5 applanation lens. Check the meniscus because it will indicate the size and sometimes the thickness of the flap that will be cut (Figure 16-6).

12. Remove the applanation lens, and wet the cornea and

> If the suction is low, cut the suction tube shorter. This will increase the psi to 22.

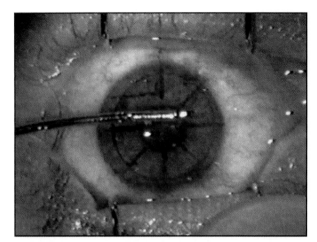

Figure 16-5. Irrigate fluid from the cornea.

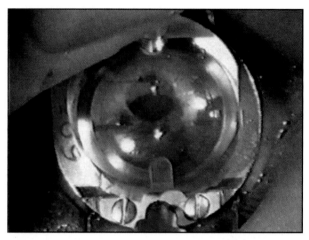

Figure 16-6. Suction ring and applanation lens.

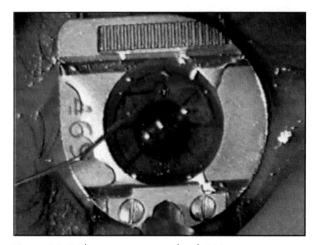

Figure 16-7. The cornea is wetted with BSS.

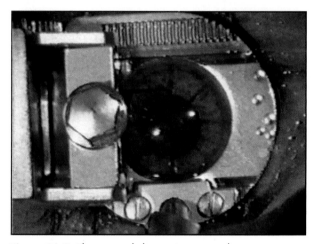

Figure 16-8. The corneal shaper is engaged.

suction ring with BSS solution (Figure 16-7).

13. Engage the corneal shaper (Figure 16-8).

14. Run the device forward and backward by pressing on the foot pedal. Ensure a smooth ongoing cut and do not stop halfway because this causes a jagged cut in the cornea. Support the cord only, do not hold the motor (Figure 16-9).

15. Break suction (via the foot pedal) and remove the suction ring as soon as possible after the cut is made.

16. Never take your eyes off the operating field through the microscope while performing the suction/cutting process! You will miss critical signs of bad suction and end up with defective flaps.

17. Clean and dry the fornices and canthus with a Collibri forceps prior to lifting the flap. This prevents BSS from coming into contact with the surgical bed interface of the corneal stroma (Figures 16-10 through 16-12).

18. First realign the patient with the red/green HeNe lights, then lift the flap. This prevents unnecessarily drying out of the corneal stromal bed.

> Never take your eyes off the operating field through the microscope while performing the suction/cutting process!

19a. Ablate the stroma. Do not wait more than 10 seconds before starting the laser treatment because unnecessary drying of the corneal stromal bed will induce an overcorrection (Figure 16-13).

19b. Protect the flap up to its base nasally with a damp merocel sponge. This will prevent double laser treatment on the nasal aspect of the cornea.

20. Flip the cornea back into position with the KU spatula (Figure 16-14).

21. After replacing the flap, wash the interface and underneath the flap with the KU irrigation and aspiration cannulas. This will create a one way flow of BSS from under the flap to the fornices, thus preventing new foreign material from slipping underneath the flap again (Figure 16-15).

22. Float the flap into position (Figure 16-16).

23. Realign the flap with the original radial markers and express excessive fluid from the flap interface with the KU spatula.

24. Stroke the flap radially and dry the gutter with the KU aspiration cannula, then dry the flap and gutter with a dry

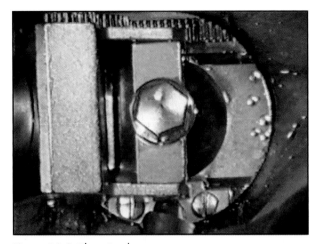

Figure 16-9. The microkeratome cut.

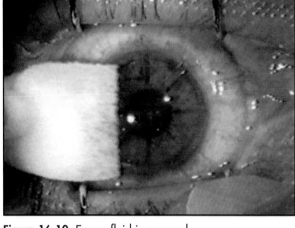

Figure 16-10. Excess fluid is removed.

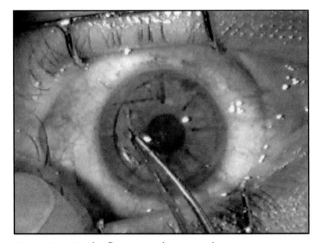

Figure 16-11. The flap is gently grasped.

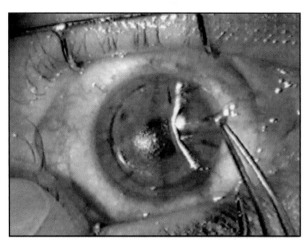

Figure 16-12. The flap is pulled back naturally.

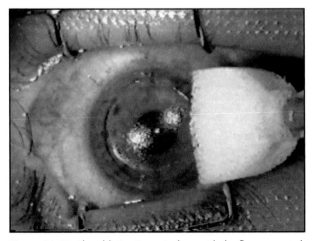

Figure 16-13. The ablation is carried out with the flap protected.

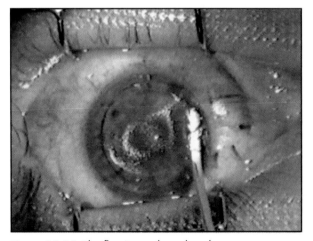

Figure 16-14. The flap is gently replaced.

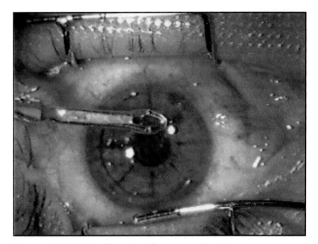

Figure 16-15. The flap interface is washed.

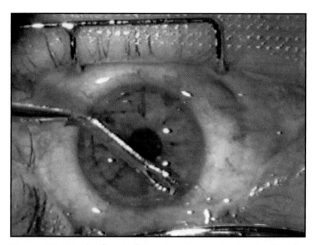

Figure 16-16. The flap is floated and smoothed to realign the corneal markers.

microsponge (Figure 16-17).

25. Test the flap adherence with striae reflection.

26. Instill Ofloxacin drops, patch the eye with an eye shield, and keep it closed behind the shield until the following morning.

GENERAL USEFUL HINTS FOR LASIK SURGERY

THE MACHINE

1. Always assemble the head of the microkeratome and insert the blade yourself. Never leave it for the nursing staff to do.

2. The suction tubing of the suction ring can be cut shorter to increase the suction power of the machine. You can do this if you've got too low psi (ideally 22 psi).

3. Always do the "pre-flight" check yourself. Make sure the microkeratome and suction ring, especially the handle of the ring, is cleaned perfectly. Make sure the opening in the handle is open because after some use it can clog up and have an effect on the suction power of the machine.

4. If the motor feels rough while running, do not use it.

> Always wash the excessive gentian violet off because it can cause an epithelialitis.

MARKING THE CORNEA

1. Always wash the excessive gentian violet off because it can cause an epithelialitis as well as an inflammatory response in the interface of the cornea after surgery.

2. Before lifting the flap, always dry the cornea and fornices with a damp microsponge to prevent foreign material and water from entering the surgical interface.

CUTTING THE FLAP

1. The better the suction, the bigger and thicker the flap.

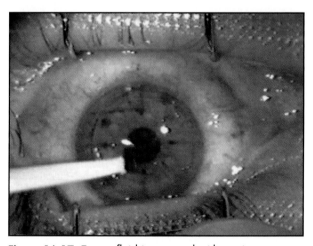

Figure 16-17. Excess fluid is removed with a microsponge.

> If you suspect pseudosuction, turn the handle and suction ring while the suction is on.

Beware of pseudosuction.

2. If you suspect pseudosuction, turn the handle and suction ring while the suction is on to get rid of the conjunctival plug creating it.

3. Tilt the suction ring slightly to the side of the handle to help increase pressure at the port of the suction ring. If there are problems with the application of the suction ring, push slightly down on the wire speculum to open up the eyelids and position the eye more anteriorly.

THE FLAP

1. If you see that you have cut a defective flap, do not lift it. Leave it in place, dry it, and cut a new flap 3 months later.

2. If you are not happy with the flap you have cut, do not laser the stroma. Rather, repeat LASIK in 2 to 3 months (by cutting a new flap).

3. If the flap is too thin, there are islands of Bowman's

> If you see that you have cut a defective flap, do not lift it. Leave it in place, dry it, and cut a new flap 3 months later.

membrane, or there is a doughnut effect, you have experienced pseudosuction or the patient has broken the suction by squeezing the eyelids while you were cutting the flap.

4. With fresh flap folds, you must immediately take the patient back to the theatre, lift the flap, and hydrate it to get rid of the folds. Then stroke the flap to unfold the folds. If the folds are older than approximately 6 months, you will be unable to remove them all. If they are causing visual distortions or problems, do a transepithelial photorefractive keratectomy or phototherapeutic keratectomy on the flap by removing it and leaving the stroma to re-epithelialize.

5. If you are ever doing enhancement surgery on patients from other doctors and scarring or haze is on the flap, there were likely problems with the flap. It was either too thin or had an epithelial flap. Cut a new flap rather than lifting the old flap. A bad flap almost always equals a bad operation.

> A bad flap almost always equals a bad operation.

SURGICAL INTERFACE

1. Whenever you see foreign bodies, especially if they are near the visual axis, wash them out as soon as possible, as they will never disappear. They cause a greyish foreign body reaction in the stroma and flap, interfere with vision, and induce glare and halos.

2. If you see epithelial cell nests, wash and scrape them out immediately because they will cause corneal melting.

3. Foreign bodies in the interface can be:

- Red blood cells. They disappear by themselves so it is not necessary to wash them out.

- White blood cells. Wash them out immediately.
- Chemical substances like gentian violet. Wash them out because they induce stromal haze and keratitis.
- Conjunctival mucus. Wash it out.
- Pieces of lint. Wash them out because they can give a greyish foreign body reaction.
- Meibomian secretions. Wash them out.
- Cut eyelashes. Wash them out.
- Beauty spots, eyeliner, mascara, and eye shadow. Wash these out.
- Metal dust from blades and microkeratomes. Try to them wash out, however this is not always easy to do.
- If infection occurs postoperatively at the edge of the flap, always remember the infection is *coming from the outside*; thus, do not lift the flap, as it will spread the infection.
- As a general rule, do not lift the flap or try to rinse the interface while there is an *active* infection present.

REFERENCES

1. Updegraff SA, Ruiz LA, Slade SG. Corneal topography in lamellar refractive surgery. In: Sanders DR, Koch DD, eds. *Corneal Topography*. Thorofare, NJ: SLACK Incorporated; 1994.

2. Nordan LT, Fallor MK, Myopia keratomileusis: 74 corrected non-amblyopic cases with 1-year follow-up. *J Refract Corneal Surg.* 1986;2:124-128.

3. Arenas-Archila E, Sanchez-Thorin JC, Naranjo-Uribe JP, Hernandez-Lorano. Myopic keratomileusis in situ: a preliminary report. *J Cataract Refract Surg.* 1987;17:424;435.

4. Updegraff SA, Kritzinger MS. A prospective evaluation of flow tectonic lamellar keratoplasty: A new technique for LASIK and ALK. Presented at the International Society of Refractive Surgery; October 1995; Atlanta, Ga.

5. Updegraff SA, Kritzinger MS, Slade SG. Therapeutic lamellar surgery: ALK homoplastic grafting and LASIK. Presented at the International Society of Refractive Surgery; July 1995; Minneapolis, Minn.

TABLE 17-1. COMPARISON OF DRY AND WET TECHNIQUES	
Dry technique	Wet technique
Advantages:	
Faster visual rehabilitation (hours)	Lower incidence of flap fold or wrinkles
Lower incidence of epithelial islands or debris	
Disadvantages:	
Higher incidence of flap folds or wrinkles	Slower visual rehabilitation due to edema (24 to 72 hours)
Higher incidence of epithelial islands or debris	

The assistant goes through the patient's data once and double-checks with the technician to ensure that the proper attempted correction is given. Once the centration of the laser aiming beams is confirmed, the surgeon activates the laser with the foot pedal and ablation is given. When ablation is complete, the surgeon switches the suction off and removes the mask from the eye.

If the ablated surface appears to be irregular, it is possible to make it smooth in the following manner: a wet Merocel is passed over the ablated surface. Then, a 9-μm PlanoScan phototherapeutic keratectomy (PTK) ablation is usually sufficient to make the surface regular.

REPOSITIONING THE FLAP

Repositioning the flap can be performed using two techniques (Table 17-1):
1. The dry technique: A small suction tube with moderate suction or the Pallikaris LASIK suction tube is moved over the area of the bed to remove epithelial cells or debris that could be left in the interface. No direct irrigation of the corneal bed or stromal surface of the flap is performed. One or two drops of BSS solution are placed at the area of the hinge. The flap is then replaced into the stromal bed. The corneal surface is thoroughly irrigated with BSS using an irrigation-aspiration cannula so that debris and excessive epithelial cells are removed (Figure 17-5).
2. The wet technique: The ablated bed and stromal surface of the flap are irrigated thoroughly (flushed) with BSS using an irrigation-aspiration cannula. A wet Merocel sponge is used to remove excessive moisture, and this manipulation is repeated several times until all the potential cells and debris are totally removed. The effectiveness of the Merocel movement can be aided by pressing on the surface of the sponge with an air cannula as it is moved across the stromal bed (Figure 17-6). This technique is repeated twice, once

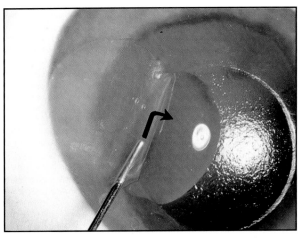

Figure 17-5. The dry technique: one or two drops of BSS are placed on the corneal bed at the hinge of the flap. An air cannula is inserted beneath the epithelial surface of the flap. The cannula is moved slowly temporally (arrow), parallel to the corneal surface, and the fluid on the bed allows the flap to settle gently in its primary position.

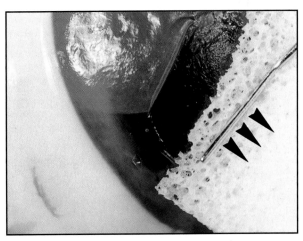

Figure 17-6. The wet technique: a wet Merocel microsponge is used to remove excessive moisture, and this manipulation is repeated several times until cells and debris are totally removed from the surface of the globe. The Merocel movement can be aided by pressing it with an air cannula (arrows).

nasally and once temporally, starting from the base of the flap. The flap is then repositioned using an air cannula as described in the dry technique.

Two Merocel sponges are used to gently manipulate the cornea so that the marks on the flap are properly aligned with the corresponding marks on the peripheral corneal ring.

When the flap is repositioned in the correct orientation, the surface of the cornea is dried using air through an aquarium air pump or with exposure to room air for 5 minutes. Dehydration of the corneal surface allows the flap to adhere onto the bed. Adequate adherence of the flap is detected by

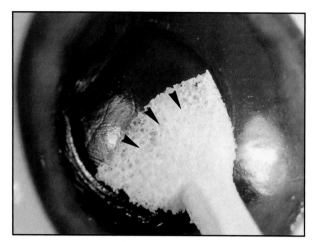

Figure 17-7. A Merocel sponge just wet in its periphery is used to lightly press the center of the cornea for a few seconds.

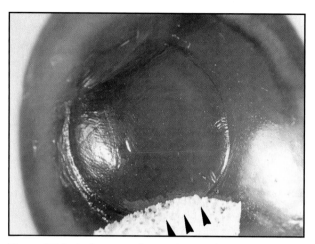

Figure 17-8. A dry spear (arrows) is used to remove excessive moisture from the borders of the aligned flap, aiding its seal to the bed.

depressing the peripheral cornea with the tip of a cellulose sponge. The formation of radiating lines that extend to the flap (striae sign) indicates that the flap is adhered to the bed.

A Merocel sponge that is wet at the end is used to lightly press the center of the cornea for a few seconds (Figures 17-7 and 17-8). Following that, a light "massage" is applied to the cornea with the wet sponge and one drop of diclofenac sodium (a combined antibiotic-steroid solution [Tobradex] and 1% cyclopentolate). A bandage soft contact lens is applied only in cases in which there is an epithelial defect. Eye patching is rarely necessary and sutures are reserved for the rare case of a free cap that will not adhere to the stromal bed with normal dehydration techniques.

> A bandage soft contact lens is applied only in cases in which there is an epithelial defect.

POSTOPERATIVE LASIK CARE

At the end of the procedure, the patient is given oral and written instructions regarding early postoperative care and is helped to the recovery room. The most important instruction is not to rub the operated eye. Thirty to 60 minutes

later, the surgeon re-evaluates the flap under the operating microscope or at a slit lamp to ensure that the flap has not displaced.

If the flap is irregularly positioned, it should be lifted back and repositioned, however, this will increase the risk for epithelial cell accumulation at the stromal-flap interface. The patient is re-examined on the following day to ensure complete healing from the surgical trauma.

SUGGESTED READING

1. Automated Corneal Shaper. Operator's manual. Rev 1.4. Chiron Vision Corporation, March 1994.
2. Pallikaris IG, Papatzanaki ME, Siganos DS, Tsilimbaris MK. A corneal flap technique for laser in situ keratomileusis. *Arch Ophthalmol.* 1991;109(12):1699-1702.
3. Pallikaris IG, Papatzanaki ME, Siganos DS, Tsilimbaris MK. Tecnica de colajo corneal para la queratomileusis in situ mediante laser. Estudios en humanos. *Arch Ophthalmol* (Spanish ed). 1992;3(3):127-130.
4. Pallikaris IG, Siganos DS. Excimer laser in situ keratomileusis and photorefractive keratectomy for correction of high myopia. *J Refract Corneal Surg.* 1994;10(5):498-510.
5. Pallikaris IG, Siganos DS. Laser in situ keratomileusis to treat myopia: early experience. *J Cataract Refract Surg.* 1997;23(1):39-49.

Personal LASIK Technique

Stephen F. Brint, MD, FACS

My laser in situ keratomileusis (LASIK) technique has evolved with the procedure—through the work and collaboration of dedicated surgeons from all over the world. I have used the VISX Star, Summit Apex Plus, and the Chiron Technolas 117 excimer lasers to perform LASIK. My early experience with the Steinway microkeratome for myopic keratomileusis (MKM) procedures, through its evolution and subsequent manufacture and distribution by Chiron Vision, led me to continue using the ACS (Automated Corneal Shaper) microkeratome as I began performing LASIK. Although it is does not approach the cost of an excimer laser, the microkeratome is not only expensive but also the most important tool in LASIK. It enables us to create a corneal flap and thus preserve the outer layers of the cornea.

The Chiron ACS consists of three major parts: the shaper head, the motor, and the suction ring with its handle. The importance of proper assembly and maintenance of the ACS cannot be over-emphasized; the ACS must be disassembled and cleaned after every procedure.

The insertion of the thickness plate is one of the most important steps during assembly. The thickness plate determines the thickness of the flap. We normally recommend using a 160-µm plate, although the 180-µm plate is routinely used when the cornea thickness allows, which I feel leads to smoother, more manageable flaps. Why is a thickness of 160 to 180 µm used? In general, the thinner the flap, the less stable it is and the easier it will wrinkle and form striae, which leads to irregular astigmatism and loss of vision. In contrast, the thicker the flap, the more stable it is. However, less tissue is available for ablation in high myopia with a thicker flap. Considering this, a thickness of 160 µm is probably the best compromise in higher amounts of myopia. In a very thin cornea, a thickness of 130 µm may alternatively be used, but thicker or thinner flaps should be avoided.

With regard to possible complications, the thickness plate is the single most important part of the ACS. Should the surgeon forget to insert it or should the thickness plate be improperly seated, the eye will be penetrated during the cut. This results in iris damage, damage to the lens, and possible vitreous loss. Amazingly, these complications have actually occurred in a small number of cases. It should be our foremost duty to prevent a complication as fatal and as easy to avoid. The only way to do this every time with utmost security is by using a checklist. The newer microkeratomes, such as the Hansatome, have fixed plates to avoid this problem. Only a standardized procedure that involves the routine use of a checklist will guarantee maximum results. We use several checklists that summarize all key items and contain the absolute minimal requirements to successfully complete the LASIK. These include materials set-up, ACS assembly and testing, patient preparation, and a final surgeon's checklist. ACS assembly and performing the laser testing is completed by our assistants, but the surgeon is responsible for performing a final test immediately prior to LASIK. I designed a very simple checklist that is attached to my laser within easy view of both my assistant and myself. My standard procedure is to review the settings of the laser and the performance of the fluence, cassette, and Axicon alignment tests. Prior to patient entry into the laser suite, I carefully go through this final checklist. The best way to avoid complications is to use a standardized proce-

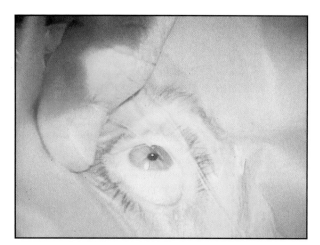

Figure 18-1. A 3M 1020 open drape is used to retract the eyelashes and eyelids.

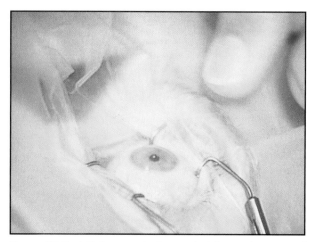

Figure 18-2. A Lieberman locking-style lid speculum is used for maximum exposure.

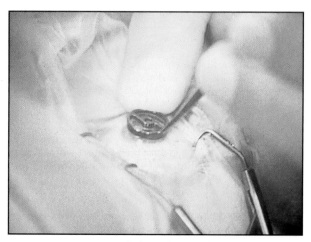

Figure 18-3. A pararadial mark is applied to the cornea, taking care to use a minimum amount of gentian violet.

dure that involves checklists. With the Summit Apex Plus, the morning "start-up" consists of He Ne alignment, beam homogeneity (fluence), laser disc alignment, and Axicon lens alignment. We also cut a polymethylmethacrylate (PMMA) disc.

Careful patient preparation cannot be over-emphasized. During preparation for LASIK in the preoperative area, the patient receives instruction and information regarding the procedure. The eye(s) are irrigated to remove tear film debris, initial topical anesthesia is applied (Proparacaine), and the operative eye is marked with a color-coded sticker. Patients wear surgical caps and booties, and a blanket is provided in the preoperative area and laser suite (the required ambient temperature makes the area uncomfortably cold for most patients).

I isolate the lashes very carefully using a modified 3M 1020 drape (Figure 18-1). A locking Lieberman style lid speculum, which gives maximum exposure and slightly proptoses the globe, is then inserted and slowly opened (Figure 18-2). The disadvantage is the discomfort to the patients, especially in small lid apertures and deep-set eyes. In any case, the speculum must be strong enough to withstand forced closure of the lids. Otherwise, the patient might forcefully close his eyes during the cut, which would dislodge the suction ring and keratome, resulting in the dissection of an irregular cap.

The position of the patient's head is rechecked and adjusted once the patient has been prepared for the procedure. The head must be in a horizontal plane to avoid decentration of the ablation, which can occur when the head is tilted.

To insure proper flap repositioning, it is mandatory to mark the cornea prior to the cut. Both radial and pararadial marks are used (Figure 18-3). The pararadial marks are important in case a free cap is dissected, as they will insure that the flap is replaced properly, with the stromal side down. Marking or not marking can mean the difference

between a minor nuisance (free cap, replaced properly as marked) and a major complication (free cap, replaced epithelial side down and lost during the first night) (Figure 18-4). The suction ring is now placed on the eye with slight nasal decentration to allow for a more nasal placement of the hinge, therefore out of the way of the ablation. Except in the cases of average keratometry of less than 41.5, which result in a smaller flap and hinge and need to be well-centered (Figure 18-5). Anticipating the possibility of later retreatment with recutting a new flap, slight nasal decentration is recommended for the initial procedure; this insures a fresh beginning when the suction ring is later placed centrally for the enhancement cut.

Adequate suction is verified using an applanation tonometer on a dry cornea to check the pressure. The applanated area must be smaller than the reference circle engraved in the tonometer (Figure 18-6). After tonometry indicates that the intraocular pressure is high enough and after careful irrigation with balanced salt solution (BSS) (Figure 18-7), the microkeratome is inserted into the suction

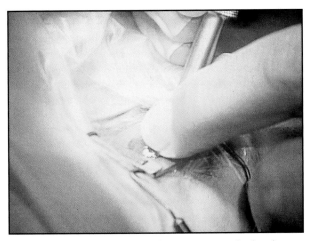

Figure 18-4. The suction ring of the ACS is applied to the eye and decentered slightly nasally.

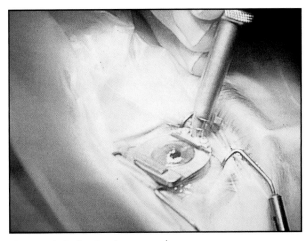

Figure 18-5. Suction is engaged.

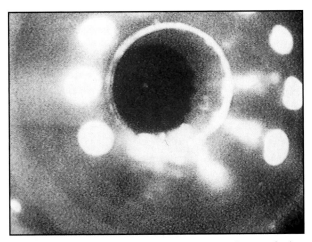

Figure 18-6. The Barraquer tonometer is used to verify that the applanated area is well within the circular mire on the lucite tip of the Barraquer tonometer.

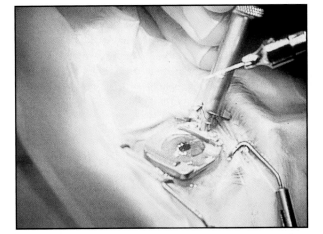

Figure 18-7. BSS drops are instilled on the cornea, avoiding the track of the suction ring.

ring (Figure 18-8). Prior to making the cut, verification that the prospective path of the ACS across the eye is unobstructed is mandatory (Figure 18-9).

In summary, there are three essential steps that guarantee a perfect cut:
- tonometry to verify sufficient pressure
- a moist cornea (not wet)
- the path of the ACS must be unobstructed

These essential steps are again verified using our checklist.

Once the cut is completed, I carefully remove the suction ring, turn down the direct illumination, and immediately loosen the lid speculum for patient comfort. I use blunt, smooth, open tying forceps to lift the flap and lay it smoothly to the nasal side (Figure 18-10). During a 30-second period to permit consistent corneal hydration, I will focus and center the red fixation beam over the central pupil. During the ablation, I constantly monitor centration and focus. The flap hinge is protected from inadvertent ablation using a

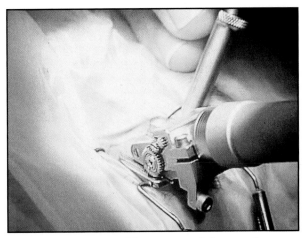

Figure 18-8. After careful inspection of the microkeratome head, ensuring that the appropriate footplate is present, well-positioned, and the stop is on, the gears are engaged in the track and the microkeratome forward foot pedal is engaged.

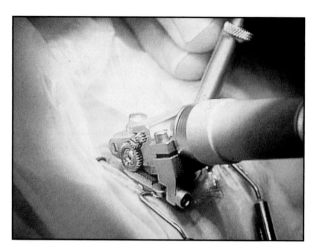

Figure 18-9. The microkeratome's forward motion is stopped by the action of the stopper.

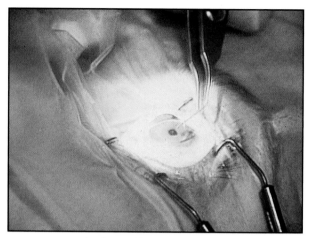

Figure 18-10. The flap is lifted and rotated nasally using the open blades of a tying forceps, taking care not to actually grasp the flap.

blunt metal instrument (I use a Tooke knife); do not use a Merocel sponge, as it will be penetrated by the laser energy. A Merocel sponge is used to remove any visible fluid that frequently collects at the hinge of the flap.

The 3.0 software presently being used with the Summit Apex Plus in the CRS study allows single-zone treatment (surgeon adjusted from 1 to 6.5 mm) from 1 to 9.9 diopters (D) of myopic ablation (Figure 18-11). We generally use a 6 mm zone up to 7 D at the corneal plane per US Food and Drug Administration approval for this amount of myopia. From 7 to 15 D (the software actually allows 22 D) of myopia I use the aspheric program, which creates a 5 mm ablation that smoothly blends out to 6.5 mm, removing less tissue in these higher myopes. Central island prevention treatment is integrated into all ablations and is generally set to deliver an additional 10% of the total anticipated ablation pulses to the central 2.5 mm treatment area (Figure 18-12).

Toric correction is provided by the toric laser disc (Figures 18-13 through 18-19), which is placed and aligned to the minus cylinder axis in the Emphasis cassette. The laser displays the appropriate disc to select after the desired refractive correction is entered. Laser discs are supplied in a consignment similar to intraocular lenses. Up to 5 D of astigmatism may be corrected simultaneously with the myopia creating a very smooth ablation surface of 5 x 6.5 mm size (soon to be enlarged to 6 x 6.5 mm) (Figure 18-20 and 18-21).

Likewise, hyperopia to 6 D (L disc) (Figures 18-22 through 18-24) and compound hyperopic astigmatism (P disc) can be corrected with a 6.5 mm ablation zone. Blending out to 9.5 mm with the Axicon lens (Figures 18-25 through 18-27) creates predictable and stable hyperopic treatment. As the Chiron ASC microkeratome generally creates an 8.5 mm flap (depending on the steepness of the cornea), the new Hansatome, which creates a larger flap, is preferred for these larger hyperopic ablations.

Once the ablation is over, I place a drop of BSS on the bed, then sweep the flap temporally with closed tying forceps

(Figure 18-28). I follow with irrigation of the interface with the Slade cannula (ASICO)—the primary purpose of which is to allow the flap to float back to its original position as well as to remove any potential debris (Figure 18-29). The flap is then painted into place with a moistened Merocel sponge (Figure 18-30), and position is checked primarily by making sure the gutter is symmetrical all the way around, as well as by verifying the alignment of the corneal marks. Once the flap is perfectly centered, a 2 to 3 minute drying period allows the flap to adhere while the central epithelium is kept moist with repeated drops of BSS. After flap adhesion is verified, the lid speculum is carefully removed (Figure 18-31). The patient is then asked to blink while looking up and down, which again verifies flap adhesion. Ciloxan and Voltaren eye drops are instilled prior to the patient sitting up and leaving the laser suite.

After surgery, patients are escorted into an exam lane for slit lamp check followed by postoperative instructions; Tobradex eye drops and nonpreserved artificial tears are instilled and written instructions are reviewed. At the slit lamp, I verify proper adhesion, centration, and smoothness of the flap. Patients are instructed to use an eye shield (in the postoperative pack) during the night for 4 days. In addition, Tobradex (qid for 4 days) is prescribed; no medication other than artificial tears is used thereafter. We check the patients the first day after surgery and return them to the care of their co-managing doctor for the 1-week (5 to 10 days after surgery) postoperative exam. Other routine exams are scheduled after 4 to 8 weeks, 4 to 6 months, 12 to 14 months, and 24 to 26 months.

Frequent evaluation of our clinical results is facilitated by an up-to-date outcomes database. Uncorrected visual acuity is the main criteria used to assess the effectiveness of a refractive procedure. This data is collected and entered into our outcomes program for every postoperative visit. Current statistics of this type allow us to not only make informed decisions about nomogram adjustments, but also give our patients a very real picture of the success of the LASIK procedure (Figures 18-32 through 18-43).

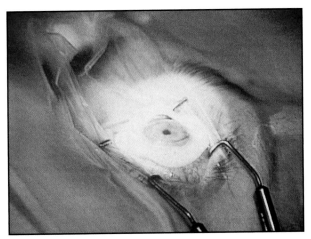

Figure 18-11. The laser ablation takes place with the He Ne beams diverging and centered at the 3 and 9 o'clock positions.

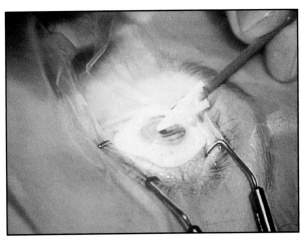

Figure 18-12. During long myopic ablations, the bed may be dried periodically to avoid central island formation.

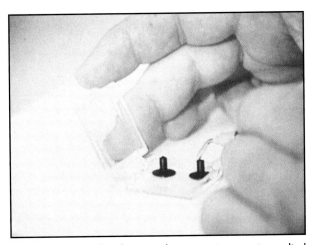

Figure 18-13. A dust-free, single-use suction cup is applied to the pneumatic forceps for transferring the laser disc to the Emphasis cassette.

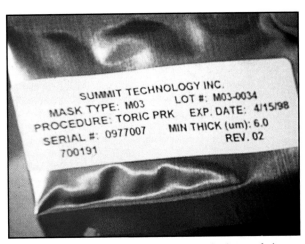

Figure 18-14. A toric laser disc is supplied in a foil type wrapper.

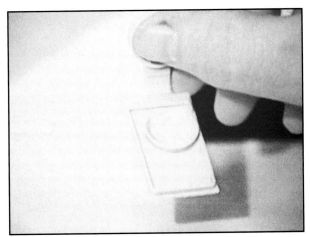

Figure 18-15. The laser disc is removed from the foil wrapper and stored in a contact lens case.

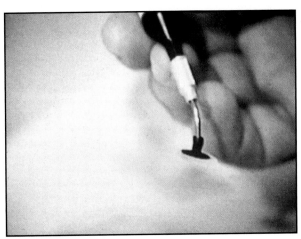

Figure 18-16. The disc is grasped by the suction cup from the contact lens case.

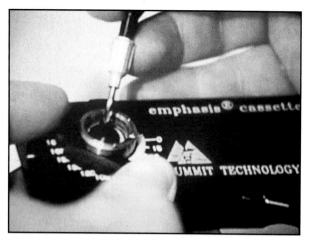

Figure 18-17. The disc is firmly seated in the Emphasis cassette and locked into place.

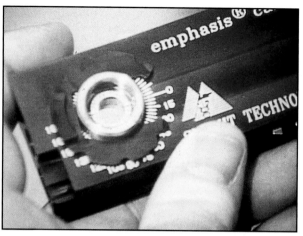

Figure 18-18. The toric disc is aligned with the minus cylinder axis, taking care to avoid error of parallax.

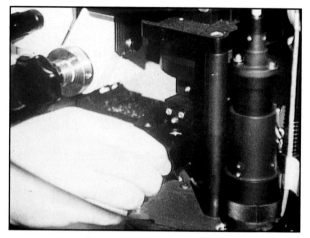

Figure 18-19. The Emphasis cassette is inverted and inserted into its slot and locked into place in the laser down tube.

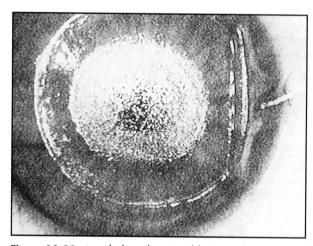

Figure 18-20. A with-the-rule toric ablation is demonstrated with the minus cylinder axis along the 180° meridian.

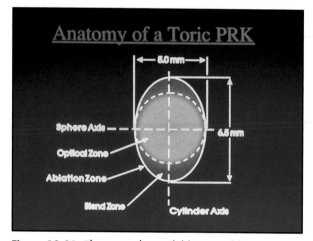

Figure 18-21. The currently available toric ablation pattern of 5 x 6.5 mm, soon to be enlarged to 6 x 6.5 mm.

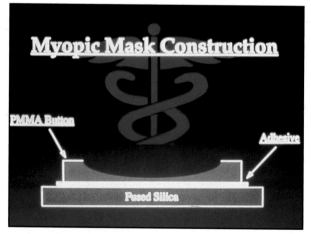

Figure 18-22. The PMMA laser disc, mounted on a silica plate, is typical of the myopic and toric disc.

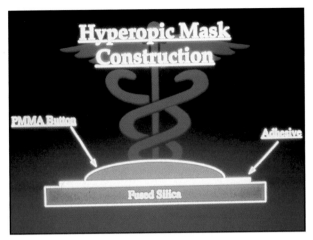

Figure 18-23. Hyperopic disc construction.

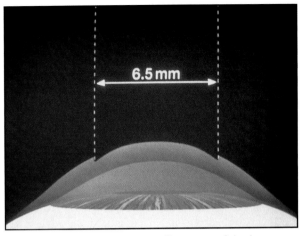

Figure 18-24. A diagrammatic illustration of the hyperopic correction obtainable using the L-mask.

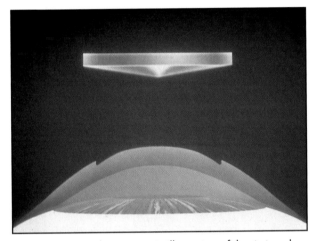

Figure 18-25. A diagrammatic illustration of the Axicon lens in place, which diverges the laser light.

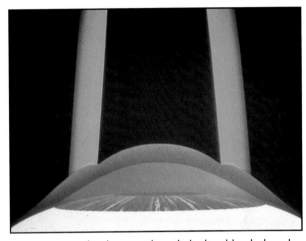

Figure 18-26. The divergent laser light then blends the edge off of the hyperopic ablation, extending the transition zone out to 9.5 mm.

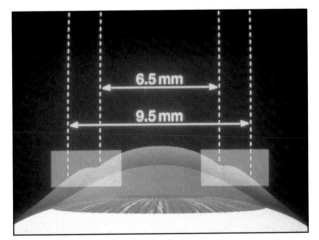

Figure 18-27. The 6.5 mm hyperopic ablation blended out to 9.5 mm, with the aid of the Axicon lens.

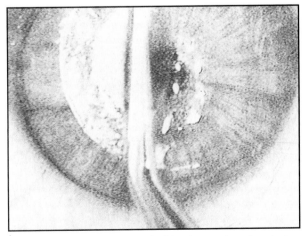

Figure 18-28. The flap is stroked back into place by placing closed tying forceps underneath the hinge and flipping the flap back into place.

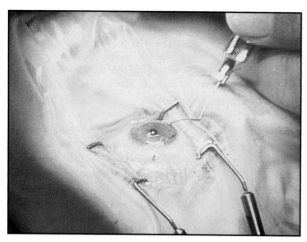

Figure 18-29. The Slade irrigating cannula is used to irrigate the interface, removing any potential debris and creating a lake of fluid, which allows the flap to float back into perfect position.

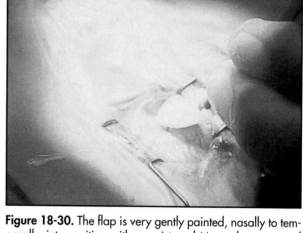

Figure 18-30. The flap is very gently painted, nasally to temporally, into position with a moistened Merocel sponge and then allowed to dry in place for 3 minutes.

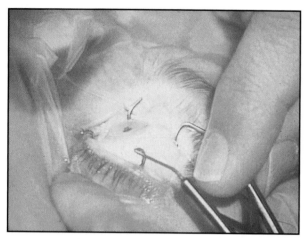

Figure 18-31. The lid speculum is carefully removed with the aid of an assistant to prevent dislodging the flap while removing it and the drape.

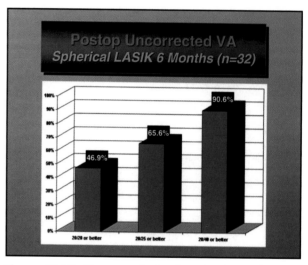

Figure 18-32. Uncorrected visual acuity 6 months post-spherical LASIK.

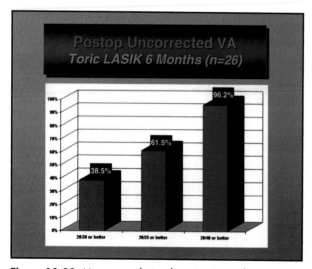

Figure 18-33. Uncorrected visual acuity 6 months post-toric LASIK.

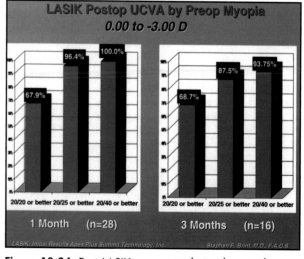

Figure 18-34. Post-LASIK uncorrected visual acuity by pre-operative myopia of 0 to -3 D.

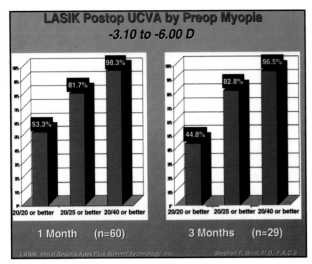

Figure 18-35. Post-LASIK uncorrected visual acuity by preoperative myopia of -3.1 to -6 D.

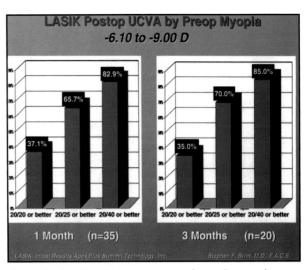

Figure 18-36. Post-LASIK uncorrected visual acuity by preoperative myopia of -6.1 to -9 D.

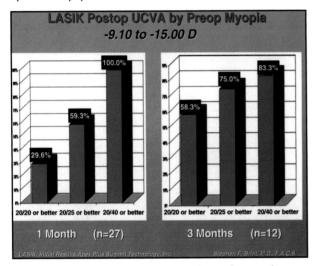

Figure 18-37. Post-LASIK uncorrected visual acuity by preoperative myopia of -9.1 to -15 D.

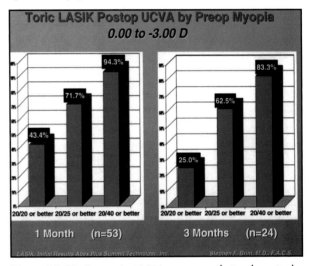

Figure 18-38. Post-toric LASIK uncorrected visual acuity by preoperative myopia of 0 to -3 D.

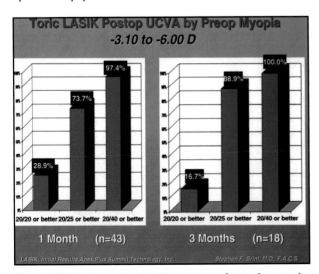

Figure 18-39. Post-toric LASIK uncorrected visual acuity by preoperative myopia of -3.1 to -6 D.

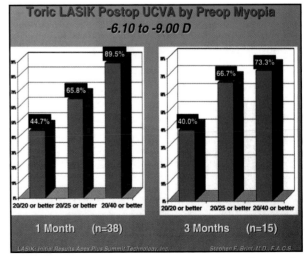

Figure 18-40. Post-toric LASIK uncorrected visual acuity by preoperative myopia of -6.1 to -9 D.

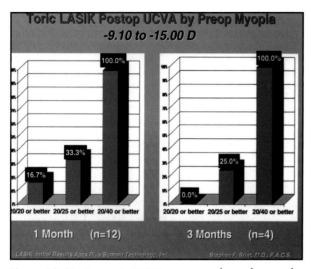

Figure 18-41. Post-toric LASIK uncorrected visual acuity by preoperative myopia of -9.1 to -15 D.

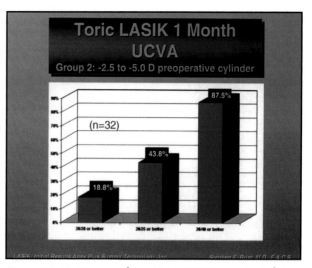

Figure 18-42. One month post-toric LASIK uncorrected visual acuity.

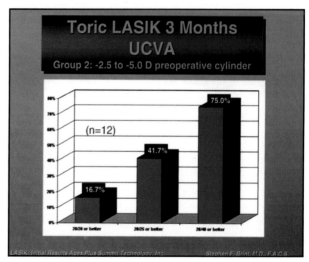

Figure 18-43. Three months post-toric LASIK uncorrected visual acuity.

CHAPTER 19

Personal LASIK Technique

Roberto Zaldivar, MD

PREOPERATIVE PATIENT PREPARATION

The preparation for laser in situ keratomileusis (LASIK) begins when the patient enters our surgical center. The atmosphere is designed to be attractive, relaxing, and professional. The staff is carefully selected to ensure that each patient receives a consistent impression of confidence and compassion. By emphasizing our concern for the comfort of each individual patient, we have found that little preoperative sedation is required. Of course, some patients will still be excessively anxious and can be treated with preoperative alprazolan.

The patient is prepared with a hair net prior to entering the laser room. The eyelids are carefully cleaned and the eye is washed with a commercial iodine eye scrub. A gauze pad is placed over the temporal aspect of the peri-orbital region in order to absorb any fluid drainage from the eye during LASIK (Figure 19-1). The eye is anesthetized with topical .5% proparicaine immediately before LASIK to minimize the epithelial toxicity. The fornices are washed with balanced salt solution (BSS) to ensure that the conjunctival surface is free of debris (Figure 19-2).

Once the patient has been brought into the laser room, constant reassurance is provided during the entire procedure. Surgical gloves are generally not worn during LASIK.

PLACING THE EYELID SPECULUM

Micropore surgical tape is placed over the lashes of the lower lid. This serves the dual purpose of removing eye-lashes from the operative field and protecting the lower lid from potential injury caused by the rotation of the Hansatome. A locking wire lid speculum is then carefully inserted under both the eyelids, ensuring that the corneal surface is not traumatized (Figure 19-3).

CORNEAL MARKS

The corneal alignment markings are then placed with the Zaldivar corneal marker (Figure 19-4). This step is performed with the minimal amount of gentian violet in order to avoid epithelial toxicity.

MICROKERATOME CUT

The suction ring of the Chiron Hansatome is then placed over the corneal surface with downward pressure on the handle of the suction ring as well as digital pressure on the lateral aspect of the ring itself. The aperture of the ring should sit symmetrically on the cornea or displaced slightly superiorly to account for the superior hinge (Figure 19-5). The suction is then applied and pupillary dilation and digital pressure confirm the elevated intraocular pressure. The cornea is then moistened with 3 to 4 drops of BSS (Figure 19-6). The head and motor of the Hansatome are then inserted onto the suction ring (Figures 19-7 and 19-8). The Hansatome is fully advanced and then reversed (Figure 19-9). When the head has been fully reversed to the original position, both the microkeratome head and suction are removed from the eye. The flap is reflected superiorly with

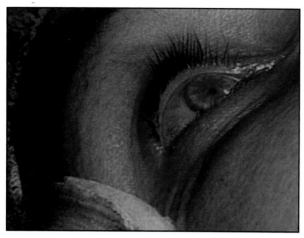

Figure 19-1. A gauze pad is placed over the temporal aspect of the peri-orbital region to absorb any fluid drainage from the eye during LASIK.

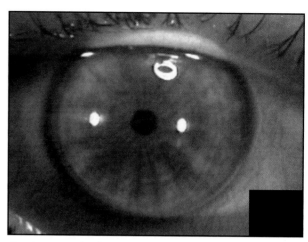

Figure 19-2. The fornices are washed with BSS solution to ensure that the conjunctival surface is free of debris.

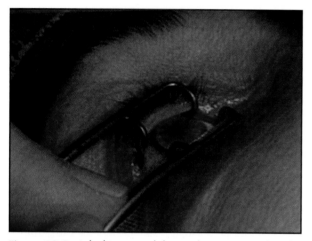

Figure 19-3. A locking wire lid speculum is inserted under both eyelids.

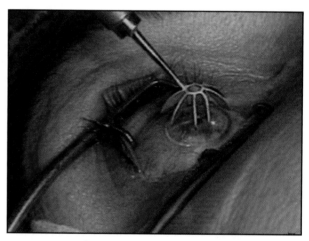

Figure 19-4. The corneal alignment markings are then placed with the Zaldivar corneal marker (ASICO).

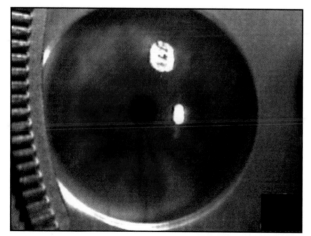

Figure 19-5. The aperture of the Hansatome suction ring is displaced slightly superiorly to account for the superior hinge.

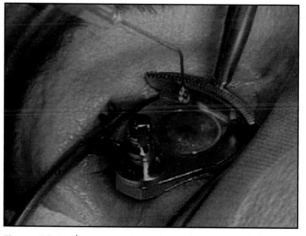

Figure 19-6. The cornea is moistened with 3 to 4 drops of BSS.

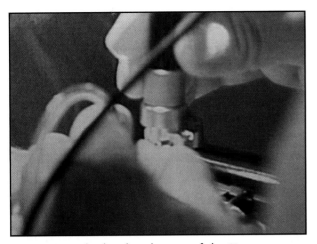

Figure 19-7. The head and motor of the Hansatome are inserted onto the suction ring.

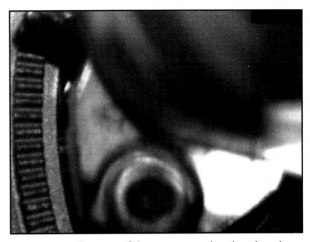

Figure 19-8. The gear of the Hansatome head is placed into the track of the suction ring.

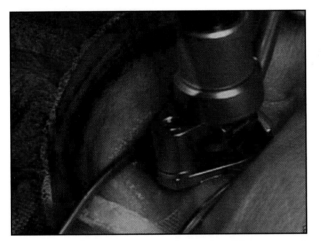

Figure 19-9. The Hansatome is advanced and then reversed.

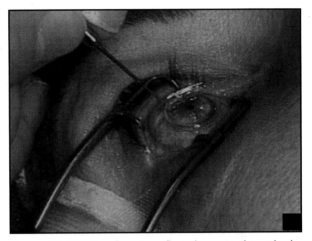

Figure 19-10. The flap is reflected superiorly with the Zaldivar flap spatula (ASICO).

the Zaldivar flap spatula (ASICO), with careful attention given to minimizing the distribution of the any BSS solution on the corneal surface (Figures 19-10 and 19-11). Stromal hydration is carefully controlled with gentle strokes with the tip of a Merocel sponge to ensure that the stromal bed has uniform hydration (Figure 19-12).

EXCIMER LASER ABLATION

The Nidek EC 5000 excimer laser is my choice for at the Instituto Zaldivar for the correction of myopia and myopic astigmatism, and the Chiron 117c laser is used for hyperopia and hyperopic astigmatism. The other locations of our network use the Nidek EC 5000 for both myopia and hyperopia, as well as for astigmatism. A small fan has been installed on the side of my Nidek laser, which is activated at the time of the ablation. While this small amount of increased air circulation has not increased the refractive effect of the ablation, it does help dissipate the odor of the ablated cornea that the patients can find so disturbing.

The focusing beams are aligned on the corneal surface (Figure 19-13). During the excimer ablation, the microscope lights are reduced to facilitate fixation. The superior flap hinge is protected with a dry Merocel sponge in my right hand (Figure 19-14). My left hand is gently placed under the patient's chin. This provides excellent control of the patient's head position as well as providing reassurance during the ablation. The stromal surface is monitored through the procedure, and the stromal bed is wiped with the dry tip of the same sponge if there are any areas of excessive stromal hydration.

FLAP REPLACEMENT

When the ablation is complete, several drop of BSS are placed on the stromal surface of the corneal flap and the flap is reflected back into position. The flap interface is irrigated for only 2 to 3 seconds (Figure 19-15). Excessive irrigation is avoided, as this will increase the time for flap adhesion. Since the stromal bed has been wiped with the Merocel

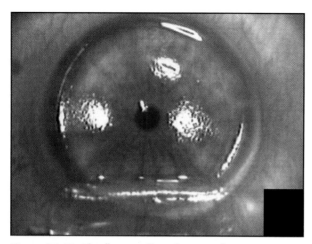

Figure 19-11. The flap is reflected superiorly.

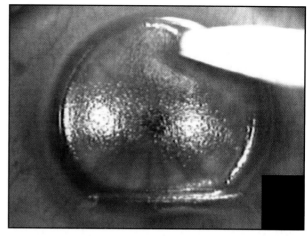

Figure 19-12. The stromal hydration is carefully controlled with gentle strokes from the tip of a Merocel sponge.

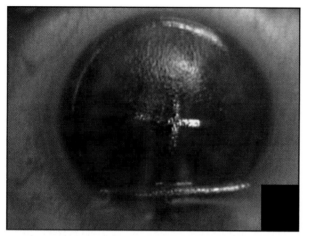

Figure 19-13. The focusing beams of the Nidek EC 5000 excimer laser are aligned on the corneal surface.

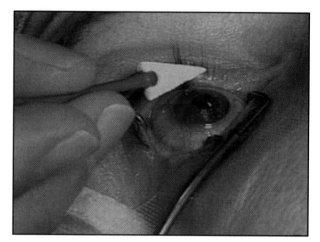

Figure 19-14. The superior flap hinge is protected with a dry Merocel sponge.

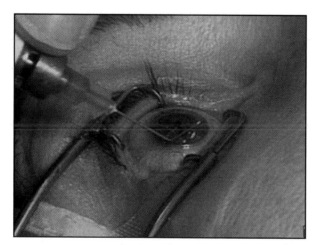

Figure 19-15. The flap interface is irrigated for 2 to 3 seconds.

sponge during the excimer ablation, little interface debris will be present in the interface.

The flap is massaged from the center of the flap to the mid-periphery with the Zaldivar flap spatula for about 30 seconds (Figures 19-16 and 19-17). If there are any concerns about the flap alignment, it is refloated and then massaged and stroked again. I have found that this technique has significantly reduced the incidence of postoperative flap striae. A dry Merocel sponge is then placed along the peripheral cornea to remove any residual surface fluid (Figure 19-18).

Air is then gently applied along the flap edge for 3 to 5 seconds (Figure 19-19). The air is applied at only 1 liter per minute through a large bore plastic tube to avoid excessive pressure. Application of the air allows rapid adhesion of the corneal flap and therefore reduces the waiting time necessary after flap replacement. Excessive air should be avoided, as it can cause the flap to shrink. With minimal interface irrigation, massage of the corneal flap, and the application of air to the corneal surface, I have found that adequate flap adhesion usually occurs within 1 minute.

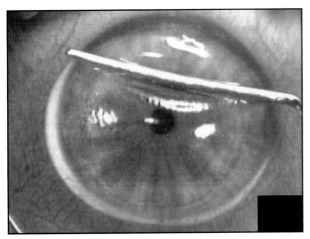

Figure 19-16. The flap is massaged from the center of the flap to the mid-periphery with the Zaldivar flap spatula for approximately 30 seconds.

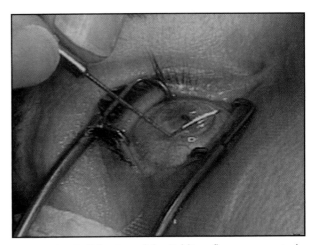

Figure 19-17. Side view of the Zaldivar flap massage technique.

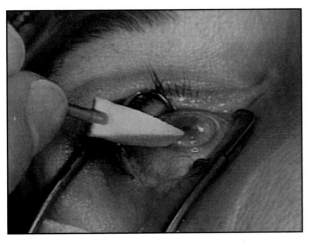

Figure 19-18. A dry Merocel sponge is used to remove peripheral corneal fluid.

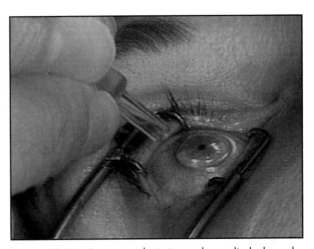

Figure 19-19. Compressed air is gently applied along the flap edge for 3 to 5 seconds.

POSTOPERATIVE CARE

Topical medications are then placed on the cornea, which include .3% tobramycin and Voltaren as well as an ocular lubricant (Figures 19-20 and 19-21). Immediately after LASIK, the cornea is clear, the patient is comfortable, and vision is quite good (Figure 19-22). The eyelid speculum is carefully removed to avoid disturbing the flap (Figure 19-23). The patient is reassured that the procedure was successful and is given postoperative instructions (Figure 19-24). The flap is checked 30 minutes following LASIK and the following day to ensure stable flap alignment. Routine follow-up is arranged through the patient's referring doctor.

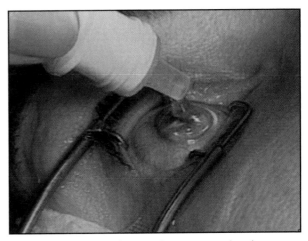

Figure 19-20. Topical .3% tobramycin and Voltaren are placed on the cornea.

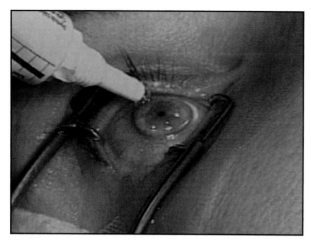

Figure 19-21. An ocular lubricant is placed on the cornea.

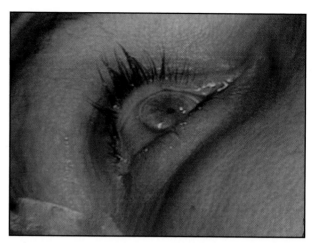

Figure 19-22. Immediately after LASIK, the cornea is clear, the patient is comfortable, and vision is good.

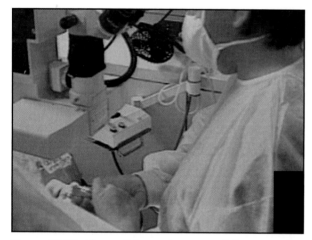

Figure 19-23. The eyelid speculum is carefully removed to avoid disturbing the flap.

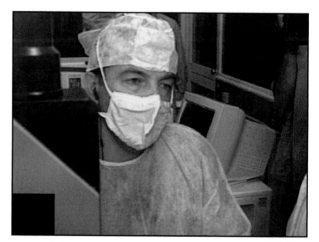

Figure 19-24. The patient is reassured that the procedure was successful and given postoperative instructions.

SECTION FIVE
LASIK Enhancements

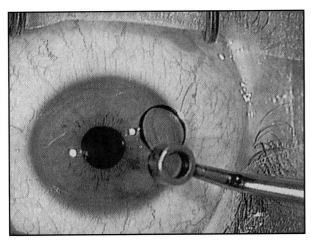

Figure 20-4. Lifting the corneal flap: the marking circles are placed to assist in flap alignment at the end of the procedure.

There are two main methods of performing an enhancement following LASIK: lifting the original flap or recutting another flap.

SURGICAL TECHNIQUES

There are two main methods of performing an enhancement following LASIK: lifting the original flap or recutting another flap. During the first 6 months following the original LASIK procedure, we recommend that patients have the flap lifted and the ablation performed in the original plane. The flap is quite easy to lift up to 6 months postoperatively. While we have lifted flaps up to 14 months following LASIK, this technique becomes progressively more difficult after the 6-month period. Although patients can experience 24 hours of discomfort following this procedure due to the epithelial defects that often occur along the edge of the flap, this technique is much safer because it has none of the risks associated with another pass of the microkeratome.

After 6 postoperative months, we recommend that the flap be recut. This technique offers the advantage of a comfortable eye postoperatively without epithelial defects and a rapid rehabilitation of vision, usually by the next postoperative day. However, recutting the flap is associated with all the risks of the original lamellar procedure, which include corneal perforation, flap configuration problems, free flaps, and lost flaps. There are also added risks associated with recutting a cornea that has already had a lamellar cut and is centrally flattened because of the original LASIK stromal ablation, including a higher risk of a centrally thin or perforated flap and the potential to generate a free corneal wedge of tissue where the two flaps intersect if the original flap has not adequately healed.

LIFTING THE ORIGINAL FLAP

In preparing the eye, the surgeon should avoid liberal use of topical anesthetic as is commonly done for PRK because topical anesthetics are toxic to the corneal epithelium, which is preserved with LASIK. Irrigation of the fornices with balanced salt solution (BSS) removes debris from the tear film. Preoperative antibiotics and Voltaren are instilled routinely, and 2 to 3 mg of lorazepam are given sublingually 10 to 15 minutes prior to the procedure.

The patient is taken to the slit lamp biomicroscope, and the edge of the flap is marked with a sharp instrument such as the Fine forceps, the Suarez, or the Machat spreader. This initial step, which was developed at TLC, is essential because it allows simple, rapid reopening of the flap with minimal epithelial trauma and maximal postoperative comfort. It is not necessary to create an epithelial defect, which can cause the patient discomfort following the procedure, but only to indent the epithelium sufficiently to allow detection of the mark under the excimer laser operating microscope. If the flap edge is not marked at the slit lamp biomicroscope, it may be impossible to discern the flap edge under the surgical microscope because of the lack of the tangential illumination.

The patient is then aligned underneath the surgical microscope and the eye is thoroughly anesthetized in the fornices prior to the insertion of the eyelid speculum. As with the original LASIK procedure, it is useful to use a drape or tape the eyelashes underneath the eyelid speculum to ensure that they do not interfere with the flap. The Probst tape tucker provides a convenient and painless method of tucking the eyelid tape or surgical drape into the conjunctival fornices so that the eyelashes are completely separated from the operative area. The adjustable titanium Lieberman eyelid speculum offers excellent exposure and the locking mechanism ensures that patient eyelid squeezing is minimized.

The cornea is then marked temporally with one or two 3.75 mm optical zone markers that have been covered with gentian violet (Figure 20-4). In the primary LASIK procedure, two optical zone markers of different sizes (3.25 mm and 3.75 mm) for four-point alignment are used so that the flap can be correctly oriented using the disparate circle sizes should the unusual complication of a free flap occur. When performing an enhancement procedure by lifting the flap with an intact hinge, the risk of a free flap is minimal, so two different sized optical zone markers are not necessary. These corneal marks are placed in a straddling position over the flap edge so that both the flap and the peripheral cornea are marked. It is helpful to place one of the markers over the indented epithelial mark as well, as this will further facilitate finding the lamellar plane of the original LASIK incision. The correct repositioning of the flap following the enhancement procedure is indicated by the proper realignment of these corneal marks.

A spreader is then inserted at the interface indicated by the demarcated flap edge (Figures 20-5 and 20-6). The marking allows precise placement of the spreader and therefore minimizes unnecessary trauma to the surrounding tis-

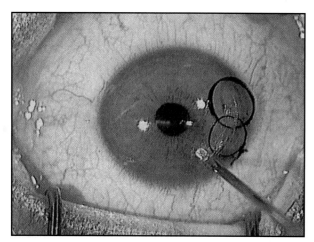

Figure 20-5. Lifting the corneal flap: the Machat spreader is inserted under the corneal flap and the temporal edge of the flap is gently opened.

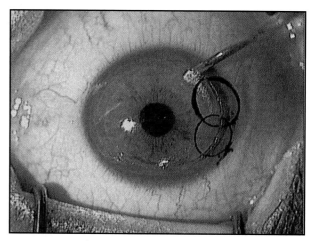

Figure 20-6. Lifting the corneal flap: the Machat spreader has been moved circumferentially in order to open the temporal aspect of the flap.

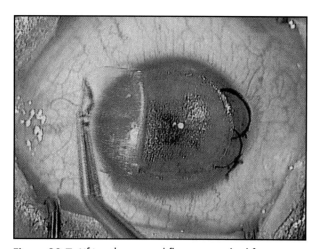

Figure 20-7. Lifting the corneal flap: nontoothed forceps are used to reflect the flap nasally.

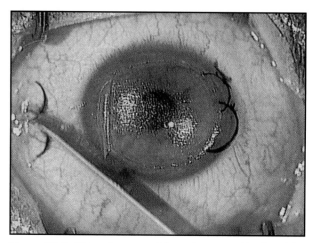

Figure 20-8. Lifting the corneal flap: the stromal bed and the undersurface of the corneal flap are gently scraped to remove debris or epithelium.

sue. A gentle down and inward pressure is usually sufficient to place the spreader within the lamellar plane of the LASIK flap. This step can also be performed at the slit lamp, creating a one to two o'clock pocket to insert the spreader. The spreader is passed along the healed cut edge peripherally. Typically, the flap adhesion is along the cut edge of Bowman's layer for approximately .5 to 1 mm. The spreader should be moved and oriented so that the lamellar dissection is only along the flap edge. The tendency to further insert the spreader beneath the flap should be avoided because this may insert epithelial cells underneath the flap and contribute to postoperative epithelial ingrowth. Once the flap edge has been sufficiently dissected, the flap is gently grasped with nontoothed forceps, and with slow and steady nasal traction it can be reflected back onto the conjunctiva (Figure 20-7). During this step, it is important not to reposition or regrasp the flap, as this can result in epithelial displacement.

Once the peripheral healed edge along Bowman's layer has been opened, the strength of the stromal adhesion is extremely variable. While the most consistent factor associated with strong stromal adhesion is increased postoperative time, patients with aggressive wound healing characteristics and patients with flap problems, such as stromal melt or haze, may also have increased stromal adherence. Epithelial ingrowth within the interface tends to prevent adhesion of the flap to the stromal bed, allowing the flap to be lifted more easily in this region. If a strong adhesion is encountered, a blunt instrument such as the cyclodialysis spatula found on the other end of the Machat spreader is inserted beneath the flap and a gentle lamellar dissection is performed. Some surgeons have advocated using filtered BSS to dissect the interface, however this will alter the stromal hydration and, therefore, can affect the efficacy of the enhancement excimer ablation.

Once the flap has been reflected back, the interface is

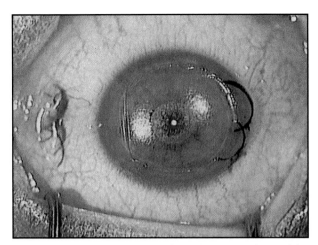

Figure 20-9. Lifting the corneal flap: the excimer laser ablation is performed centered on the center of the pupil. The pretreatment protocol has been performed using the Chiron Technolas Keracor 116 excimer laser at 3 mm.

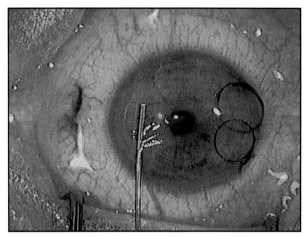

Figure 20-10. Lifting the corneal flap: after the flap has been replaced, a cannula is placed beneath the flap and it is "refloated" into its original position as indicated by the realignment of the corneal markings.

inspected with high magnification for any evidence of epithelium or debris that has been introduced underneath the flap. Any epithelium that is hanging over the peripheral edge of interface bed, present on the stromal interface, or present on the reflected flap surface, must be removed by gently scraping those affected areas with a sharp surgical blade that is regularly inspected and cleaned of the epithelial debris that accumulates on its surface (Figure 20-8). If this process is carefully and meticulously performed, the risk of epithelial ingrowth is similar or less than the risk of epithelial ingrowth associated with recutting the corneal flap, and the complications associated with recutting are avoided.

The ablation is then performed according to the preoperative calculations (Figure 20-9). Since the patient has free movement of the eye during the enhancement procedure, constant verbal encouragement must be given to patients to fixate on the fixation light and to resist squeezing their eyes, which can cause Bell's phenomenon to occur. The pneumatic suction ring without the actual application of suction can be used to stabilize the eyes of patients unable to maintain their eye position or patients with nystagmus. The central corneal stroma can be dried with filtered air, a surgical spear, or wiped with a spatula in order to avoid central accumulations of fluid and central island formation. Scanning excimer laser systems such as the Chiron Technolas 217 or broad beam excimer laser systems equipped with a pretreatment nomogram as developed by Machat, such as the VISX Star, do not require central island compensation techniques.

Following the ablation, the reflected flap and stromal bed along the hinge are hydrated with several drops of BSS. An instrument such as the blunt forceps or a cyclodialysis spatula is inserted underneath the nasal hinge of the reflected flap and the flap is gently replaced by one smooth motion temporally (Figure 20-10). The interface is then thoroughly irrigated with filtered BSS injected through a flat cannula

such as a hydrodissection needle or a flattened blunt-tipped 25-gauge cannula that has been inserted along the lamellar plane underneath the flap. The irrigation can be used for up to 10 seconds to remove debris, fibers, and small air bubbles that are often noted on close inspection of the flap interface. Excessive fluid irrigation should be avoided, as it can result in the corneal flap swelling, poor flap adhesion, and incorrect flap alignment. After the interface irrigation, the cannula is gently withdrawn to allow the flap to "float" into its correct position. Wet surgical spears are then lightly wiped from nasal to temporal flap positions to remove the remaining interface fluid. Generally, perfect flap alignment is observed at this point; however, if the corneal markings indicate misalignment, the flap should be refloated and wiped again so positioning can be reassessed.

The patient is instructed to maintain fixation on the fixation light for the next few minutes to allow for adequate adhesion to form between the flap and the stromal bed. Filtered compressed air can be used to promote flap adhesion, however this should be used conservatively, as it often results in flap shrinkage along the flap edge. Surgeons should resist the temptation to poke and prod the flap and the flap edge during this waiting period, as this invariably results in a disturbance in the flap alignment and does not speed the process of flap adhesion. If little BSS was used, the flap will generally seal in 1 minute; however, when excessive amounts of BSS irrigation are used, flap adhesion can take as long as 5 minutes. The majority of flaps will form an adequate adhesion in 2 to 3 minutes.

The final check of the corneal flap involves the assess-

Proper flap alignment is confirmed not only by the realignment of the circular corneal markings, but also by the edge gape test, the Probst air surface test, and the retroillumination test.

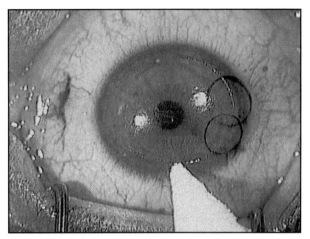

Figure 20-11. Lifting the corneal flap: the *gutter test* involves examining the small gap between the peripheral flap and the cornea. Asymmetry found on the gutter test indicates that the flap may not be accurately placed. The *Slade striae test* is performed by gently pressing on the corneal edge peripheral to the flap to ensure that the striae are transmitted through to the flap, indicating good flap adherence.

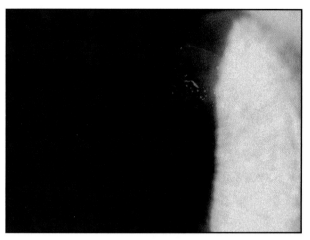

Figure 20-12. Machat epithelial ingrowth grade 1. The thin, almost transparent line of epithelial ingrowth is visible near the flap edge.

ment of two factors: the flap alignment and the flap adhesion. Proper flap alignment is confirmed not only by the realignment of the circular corneal markings, but also by the edge gape test, the Probst air surface test, and the retroillumination test. The edge gape test involves a quick circumferential check of the flap edge to ensure that excessive gape is not present in one location, indicating that the flap may be displaced in the opposite direction (Figure 20-11). The Probst air surface test involves gently blowing filtered air over the center of the flap until the surface partially dries. Any ripples or lines identified when the microscope illumination light reflects off the dried corneal surface may indicate that corneal striae and/or flap misalignment are present. It is important not use an excessive amount of air because this can cause flap dehydration and shrinkage. The retroillumination test also allows the identification of subtle flap striae by projecting the fixation beam directing through the center of the pupil with the surgical microscope illumination light turned off. If any problems are identified with the corneal flap it should be refloated.

Tests of the flap adherence include the striae test and the blink test. The Slade striae test involves gently pressing along the cut corneal edge peripheral to the flap with blunt forceps to ensure that the striae are transmitted through to the flap, indicating that it is well-adhered to the stromal bed. The side of blunt forceps can then be wiped peripherally along the flap edge to confirm the flap adherence, smooth the flap edges, or realign the flap edges. The blink test is performed after the lid speculum has been carefully

> Tests of the flap adherence include the striae test and the blink test.

removed from the eye with great care so that the arms of the speculum do not touch the flap edges. The patient is asked to blink several times, the eyelids are opened, and the flap edges are examined once again. Occasionally, a slight displacement of the superior edge of the flap with a few associated striae will be noted. If the flap is displaced, it must be refloated, and if the flap is not demonstrating adequate adherence, it must be left to stabilize with the eyelid speculum in place for 1 or 2 more minutes and then retested. If flap striae are present only in the superior position, they can be eliminated by instructing the patient to look down, smoothing the striae with the side of the blunt forceps or a Merocel sponge, and then waiting another minute for re-adhesion.

Epithelial ingrowth occurs following the original LASIK or the retreatment procedure in approximately 2% of cases. Epithelial ingrowth that is greater than 2 mm, progressive, or associated with flap melting should be removed. The flap is lifted and replaced in the same manner described for performing a LASIK enhancement procedure. Once the flap is lifted, the flap and the stromal bed are scraped with a sharp instrument until the epithelium is completely removed. Machat has devised the following grading system for epithelial ingrowth.

Grade 1: Thin ingrowth, 1 to 2 cells thick, limited to within 2 mm of the flap edge, transparent, difficult to detect, well-delineated white line along the advancing edge, no associated flap changes, nonprogressive. No retreatment required (Figure 20-12).

Grade 2: Thicker ingrowth, discreet cells evident within the nest, at least 2 mm from the flap edge, individual cells are translucent, easily seen on a slit lamp, no demarcation line along the nest, corneal flap edge rolled or gray, no flap

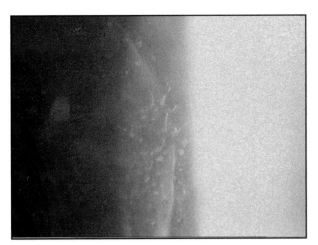

Figure 20-13. Machat epithelial ingrowth grade 2. Discreet areas of epithelial ingrowth are visible associated with the rolled and gray flap edge.

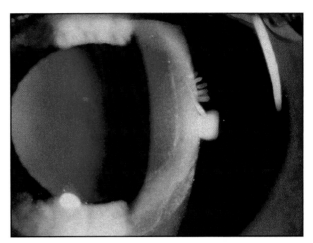

Figure 20-14. Machat epithelial ingrowth grade 3. Pronounced epithelial ingrowth with thick, opaque areas of epithelial cells extending beyond 2 mm from the flap edge. The corneal flap melt is associated with confluent haze along the exposed stromal bed.

edge melting or erosion, usually progressive. Requires non-urgent treatment within 2 to 3 weeks (Figure 20-13).

Grade 3: Pronounced ingrowth, several cells thick, greater than 2 mm from the flap edge, ingrowth areas are opaque, obvious on a slit lamp, white geographic areas of necrotic epithelial cells with no demarcation line, corneal flap margins rolled with thickened whitish-gray appearance. Progression results in large areas of flap melting from collagenase release from the necrotic epithelium. Confluent haze develops peripheral to the flap edge as the flap pulls away leaving the exposed stromal bed in contact with the surface epithelium. Urgent treatment is required with close follow-up, as recurrences are more common due to the altered flap edges (Figure 20-14).

RECUTTING A LASIK FLAP

Six months after the original LASIK procedure, the corneal flap becomes very adherent, making the process of lifting the flap more difficult and time-consuming, which invariably results in more epithelial defects and some degree of flap distortion. For these reasons, we recommend recutting the flap after this postoperative period. Many high-volume LASIK surgeons routinely recut a new flap for retreatment at 3 months or earlier, however the risks and benefits of this technique must be considered. At TLC, we use the Chiron Vision Automatic Corneal Shaper (ACS) microkeratome for our LASIK procedures.

The advantages of performing a second microkeratome pass are that the basic dynamics of the original LASIK procedure are unchanged, the nomogram for the excimer ablation is still applicable, and excessive

The advantages of performing a second microkeratome pass are that the basic dynamics of the original LASIK procedure are unchanged, the nomogram for the excimer ablation is still applicable, and excessive flap and flap edge manipulation are avoided, so postoperative pain and discomfort are minimized.

flap and flap edge manipulation are avoided, so postoperative pain and discomfort are minimized. Additionally, because there is less displacement of the epithelial cells around the rim of the flap, theoretically the incidence of epithelial ingrowth would be expected to be less than after the original flap is manually relifted. However, this has not been found to be clinically significant since we began scraping and cleaning the undersurface of the flap and the stromal bed during LASIK enhancements performed by lifting the flap.

The disadvantages of performing the second microkeratome pass are three-fold. The eye is once again subjected to the risks of the previous microkeratome pass, which include ocular perforation, thin flaps, short flaps, free flaps, or an irregular flap. Additionally, the corneal contour has now been altered so that the central cornea is significantly flattened, often to less than 40 D as measured by computerized videokeratography. While clinically this does not seem to cause a problem with flap creation because the peripheral edge of the cornea where the microkeratome engages is still the original steepness, this does increase the risk of free, perforated, and thin flaps. Finally, performing a second microkeratome pass requires that an additional lamellar cut be made in the cornea. Most surgeons will perform the second lamellar cut at the same depth as the original cut, however, this can result in a loose lamellar wedge of stromal tissue if the postoperative period has been too short, and adequate healing of the original lamellar cut has not occurred. We prefer to wait at least 6 months, with a minimum of 3 months before the second lamellar cut to ensure that a firm bond has occurred

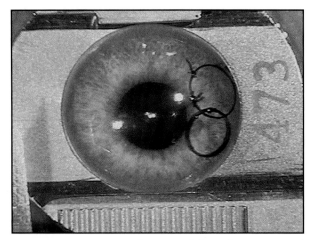

Figure 20-15. Recutting the corneal flap: the two corneal markings are made with different sized optical zones to assist with the corneal flap alignment in the event of a free flap. The pneumatic suction ring has been placed on the globe and has been decentered nasally about .5 to 1 mm in order to compensate for the hinge of the flap during the excimer ablation.

> We generally perform the second microkeratome pass at 200 μm to compensate for the flatter cornea and to minimize the risk of creating a free wedge of cornea.

between the original flap and the stromal bed, and we generally perform the second microkeratome pass at 200 μm to compensate for the flatter cornea and to minimize the risk of creating a free wedge of cornea.

The technique used to perform the second microkeratome pass is identical to the original LASIK procedure. The microkeratome is religiously and systematically checked prior to each procedure using the "look, listen, and feel" tests. The microkeratome is examined under the microscope to ensure that the blade quality is excellent, the stopper is in place, the plate number is correct and fully inserted, and the blade oscillation is consistent. The microkeratome is run through the pneumatic suction ring to ensure smooth passage. A change in the pitch of the microkeratome motor as it advances and reverses can provide clues about improperly assembled equipment or a weak motor. The head of the microkeratome and the plate screw are felt to ensure that they are firmly attached.

After the eye has been appropriately prepared and anesthetized and the lid speculum has been placed as previously described, the cornea is peripherally marked using the Machat marking technique with two optical zone markers of different sizes so that a free flap could be appropriately replaced and reoriented if necessary. The pneumatic suction ring is placed on the eye and displaced .5 to 1 mm nasally on the cornea to displace the hinge of the corneal flap more medially—away from the area of ablation (Figure 20-15). The suction ring can

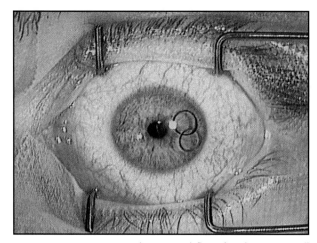

Figure 20-16. Recutting the corneal flap: for deep or small orbits, downward pressure on the eyelid speculum will proptose the eye and increase exposure, allowing suction to be successfully achieved with the pneumatic suction ring.

also be displaced slightly inferiorly to avoid cutting through excessive superior corneal neovascularization.

The authors utilize the following technique for small orbits and deep-set eyes when it is often difficult to get adequate suction; this technique can be used successfully for all eyes (Figure 20-16). Downward pressure on the eyelid speculum will cause the eye to proptose, increase the tautness of the conjunctiva, and cause the palpebral opening to increase slightly, allowing placement of the pneumatic suction ring with firm downward pressure for 1 to 2 seconds to create a firm seal before the suction is activated. The suction is then applied and the level verified by the meter on the base unit to ensure adequate suction has been achieved.

Once suction is achieved, the pneumatic suction ring is lightly supported; downward pressure on the suction ring can result in prolapsing conjunctiva and elevation of the eyelid speculum above the plane of the microkeratome, which makes smooth passage of the microkeratome extremely difficult. The suction ring should not be torqued because this may result in a loss of suction. The IOP is then checked with the Barraquer applanation tonometer to confirm a level greater than 65 mm Hg.

The experienced LASIK surgeon does not need to check the size of the LASIK flap when using the fixed LASIK suction ring, as the size of the flap can be predicted by the preoperative curvature and diameter. The corneal surface is wetted with several drops of BSS in order to ensure smooth passage of the microkeratome and minimize epithelial defects. The dovetail of the microkeratome is then gently rotated into the track of the pneumatic suction ring and advanced (Figure 20-17). If the microkeratome gears do not engage, the foot pedal is depressed briefly, first to engage the gears of the microkeratome into the track of the pneumatic suction ring, and next to perform the second microkeratome cut. Once the microkeratome has been fully

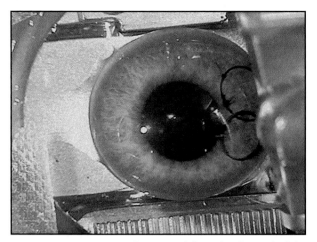

Figure 20-17. Recutting the corneal flap: the dovetail of the microkeratome is gently inserted into the track of the pneumatic suction ring by tilting the microkeratome.

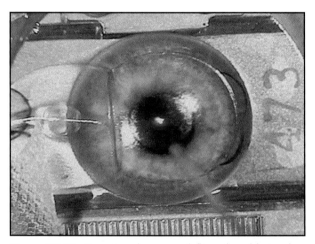

Figure 20-19. Recutting the corneal flap: the ablation has been performed with the Chiron Technolas Keracor 116 excimer laser with the multizone ablation protocol to 5 mm.

advanced nasally, it is fully reversed and gently removed from the track of the pneumatic suction ring.

The suction ring may be left in place to stabilize the eye, however, the suction itself is released so the period of high pressure in the eye with its associated retardation of the ocular perfusion is minimized. The corneal flap is then reflected nasally onto the edge of the pneumatic suction ring and the excimer ablation is performed (Figures 20-18 and 20-19). When the ablation process is completed, the stromal bed, as well as the reflected corneal flap, is wetted generously to ensure that there is no adhesion of the epithelial surface of the corneal flap to the suction ring. The flap is then gently replaced in the same manner described previously, and the suction ring is removed from the eye after the patient has been instructed to maintain his or her eye in the primary position. The flap is floated and then the alignment and positioning are checked in the same manner as previously described (Figures 20-20 and 20-21).

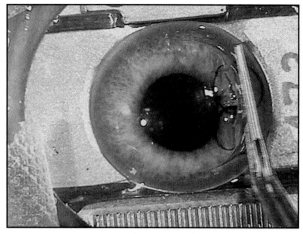

Figure 20-18. Recutting the corneal flap: closed blunt forceps are used to reflect the cut flap nasally with one smooth movement across the flap.

If the microkeratome cut is thin, perforated, asymmetrical, or short, some surgeons advocate performing PRK 1 week after with a transepithelial approach; however, this approach can yield postoperative corneal haze and irregular astigmatism. The best management of an intraoperative flap complication is to close the flap and realign the flap edges as closely as possible, and then recut a new flap with a 180 µm or a 200 µm depth plate 3 months later.

POSTOPERATIVE CARE

The postoperative regimen is identical for the two lamellar procedures. Two days of rest are recommended. At TLC, our postoperative protocol following LASIK involves the use of fluorometholone .1% and ofloxacin .3% four times a day for 4 days. Patients are instructed to avoid rubbing or squeezing the eyes, particularly during the first postoperative day and extending through the first postoperative week. By 24 to 48 hours postoperatively, the visual recovery is usually complete and the flap and cornea are clear.

If epithelial defects are bothersome, a contact lens with a topical nonsteroidal anti-inflammatory drop such as Voltaren, and a corticosteroid-antibiotic combination drop such as Tobradex for the first 24 to 48 hours will provide increased postoperative comfort.

RESULTS OF LASIK ENHANCEMENTS

The results of LASIK enhancements performed at TLC were retrospectively reviewed for a total of 209 cases with follow-up ranging from 1 to 12 months. The average preoperative spherical equivalent (SE) refractive error was -1.95 ± .78 D SE (range: -4.5 to -.38 D SE). Follow-up data were not available for each interval in some cases. The total number of cases recorded for follow-up was 159 cases at 1 month, 122 cases at 3 months, 51 cases at 6 months, and 9 cases at 1 year.

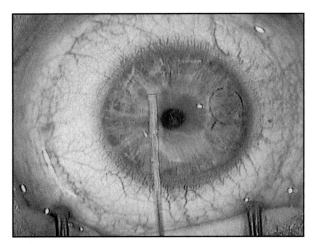

Figure 20-20. Recutting the corneal flap: the flap is refloated by inserting the cannula underneath the flap and slowly injecting BSS.

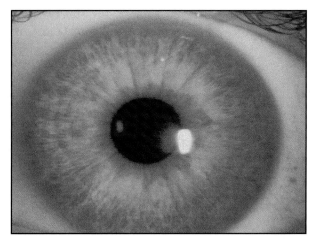

Figure 20-21. Recutting the corneal flap: the first day post-LASIK enhancement by recutting the flap. The corneal surface is smooth, the flap is barely visible, and the cornea is clear.

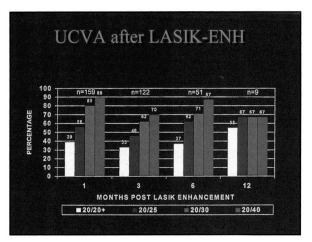

Figure 20-22. Uncorrected visual acuity after LASIK-ENH.

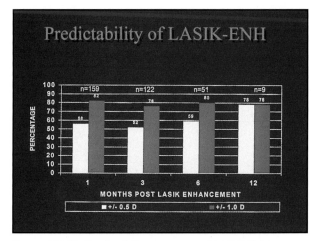

Figure 20-23. Predictability outcomes of LASIK-ENH.

This retrospective review of the data found that many post-LASIK enhancement patients do not return for follow-up. Those that do return have generally not achieved 20/20 UCVA and therefore are seeking further treatment. Therefore, there is a negative bias in the data because the most successful patients are not represented.

The efficacy of the procedure was evaluated by determining the percentage of eyes that achieved each level of acuity (Figure 20-22). At 3 months follow-up, 31.1% of eyes achieved at least 20/20 visual acuity, and 71.3% of eyes achieved at least 20/40. At 6 months follow-up, 37.3% of eyes achieved at least 20/20 visual acuity, and 88.2% of eyes achieved at least 20/40. At 12 months follow-up, 44.4% of eyes achieved at least 20/20 visual acuity, and 66.7% of eyes (six of nine eyes) achieved at least 20/40. Because these results are for enhancement procedures alone, they add to the postoperative LASIK eyes that achieved 20/40 or better UCVA from the primary procedure. Because many highly myopic eyes have a reduced BCVA

prior to surgery, these UCVA results tend to underestimate the success of the procedure. We have adjusted our excimer ablation nomograms so that now virtually all patients achieve at least 20/30 UCVA.

The predictability of the enhancement procedure was also evaluated (Figure 20-23). At 3 months follow-up, 51.6% of eyes were within ± .5 D of emmetropia, and 76.2% were within ± 1 D of emmetropia. At 6 months follow-up, 58.8% of eyes were within ± .5 D of emmetropia, and 86.3% were within ± 1 D of emmetropia. At 12 months follow-up, 77.8% of eyes were within ± .5 D of emmetropia, and 77.8% were within ± 1 D of emmetropia (Figure 20-24). The scattergram of the attempted and achieved refractive results illustrates that only one eye was significantly overcorrected and the majority of the eyes outside ± 1 D of emmetropia were undercorrected.

The average SE refractive error was found to be -.33 ± .84 D at 1 month, -.63 ± .92 D at 3 months, -.69 ± 1.1 D at 6 months, and -.67 ± .9 D at 12 months. Analysis of variance

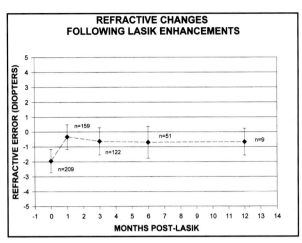

Figure 20-24. The scattergram demonstrates the predictability of LASIK enhancements at 6 months follow-up of 51 eyes. Only one eye was significantly overcorrected, while the remaining eyes not within 1 D of emmetropia were undercorrected.

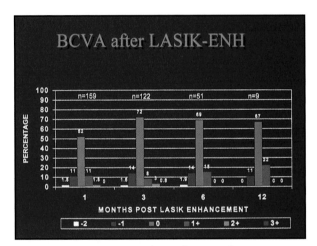

Figure 20-26. Best-corrected visual acuity after LASIK-ENH.

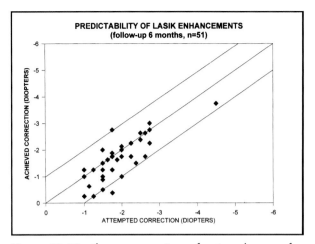

Figure 20-25. The postoperative refractive change after LASIK enhancements for the 1, 3, 6, and 12-month follow-up data. While there was a significant myopic regression in the myopia between the first and third postoperative month, after this point refractive stability was achieved with no significant change in the average SE refractive error.

1.9% lost two lines, and no patient had a greater visual loss, while a gain of one Snellen line was achieved in 15% of eyes. At 12 months post-LASIK, 11% of eyes lost one line of Snellen acuity, while a gain of one Snellen line was achieved in 22% of eyes, with no eyes gaining or losing greater amounts of BCVA. These results indicate that LASIK is a relatively safe procedure with few eyes experiencing a significant loss in BCVA.

COMPLICATIONS

Epithelial ingrowth that required removal occurred in two eyes, and flap striae was treated in one eye. Both these complications were treated without a loss in BCVA or a significant change in the refractive outcome.

One eye lost two lines of BCVA at the 1 month follow-up visit because of moderate haze that had developed at the flap interface. Further follow-up will determine if this haze will resolve, however our past experience has shown that haze generally fades with time, even post-LASIK. Haze is very uncommonly observed post-LASIK, occurring in approximately one in 1000 cases.

A patient returned on the fourth postoperative day with discomfort. While the epithelium was approximately 50% healed into the center of the cornea, a close examination found that the corneal flap had dislodged and was attached by a thin hinge to the nasal cornea. Because the dislodged flap was in poor condition and was felt to be extremely thin, it was removed and the epithelial defect was allowed to continue to close. Eight months following this procedure, a refraction of -4.5 + 2 x 180 gave a BCVA of 20/20. Surface PTK/PRK excimer ablation was then performed using the VISX Star excimer laser. The PTK mode was used to ablate through 55 µm of epithelium to ensure a smooth stromal

indicated a significant difference in the refractive change over time; however, further analysis with the Tukey-Kramer Multiple Comparisons Test indicated that only the refractive change from the 1 to the 3 months was significant (Figure 20-25). There was not significant change in the average SE refractive error from 3 to 6 or 12 months. Therefore, while significant regression was initially noted following the enhancement procedure, stability of the refractive result was achieved approximately 3 months following the enhancement procedure.

The safety of the LASIK enhancement procedure was reviewed for a change in the postoperative BCVA (Figure 20-26). At 3 months post-LASIK, 14% of eyes lost one line of Snellen acuity, and 1.6% lost two lines. No patient had a greater visual loss. Conversely, a gain of one Snellen line was achieved in 8% of eyes, two Snellen lines in 3% of eyes, and three Snellen lines in .8% of eyes. At 6 months post-LASIK, 14% of eyes lost one line of Snellen acuity, surface, and then the residual refractive error and astigmatism were treated by PRK. One month following this procedure, the UCVA had improved to 20/25.

This study found that no eyes lost more than two lines of BCVA, and between 1.6% to 1.9% of eyes lost two lines of BCVA after the LASIK enhancement procedure. The FDA phase III PRK excimer laser trials found 1% of eyes treated with the VISX laser and 3% of eyes treated with the Summit laser lost a similar amount of BCVA.[16,17] Lindstrom noted that for PRK to be considered approvable by the FDA, less than or equal to 5% of eyes could lose two lines of Snellen acuity, and less than or equal to .2% of eyes could lose five lines of Snellen acuity (serious adverse reaction).[18] Therefore, the loss in BCVA found in this study of LASIK enhancements is comparable to the results of the FDA PRK trials, and significantly less than what would be considered approvable by the FDA.

The majority of the eyes in this study had no change in their BCVA or gained BCVA. Since spectacle-corrected myopes experience a magnification effect that can effectively increase their preoperative BCVA, and high myopes can experience a number of other postoperative ocular problems unrelated to refractive surgery, the UCVA and BCVA results following LASIK must be considered as a situation unique to high myopes. Despite these considerations, more than 98% of our eyes at 6 months follow-up were within one line of their preoperative BCVA.

> More than 98% of our eyes at 6 months follow-up were within one line of their preoperative BCVA.

CONCLUSIONS

Initial undercorrections and regression result in a significant number of post-LASIK eyes with residual myopia. This refractive error is effectively treated with a LASIK enhancement procedure that can achieve excellent visual acuity and good stability. The uncommon complications of corneal flap striae, epithelial ingrowth, and even dislodged/lost flaps can be effectively managed without compromising the BCVA. LASIK enhancements allow the refractive surgeon to further improve the results of the original LASIK procedure in an efficacious, safe, and predictable manner.

REFERENCES

1. Pallikaris IG, Siganos DS. Excimer laser in situ keratomileusis and photorefractive keratectomy for the correction of high myopia. *Journal of Refractive Surgery.* 1994;10:498-510.
2. Knorz MC, Liermann A, Seiberth V, et al. Laser in situ keratomileusis to correct myopia of -6.00 to -29.00 diopters. *Journal of Refractive Surgery.* 1996;12:575-684.
3. Brint SF, Ostrick M, Fisher C, et al. Six-month results of the multicenter phase I study of excimer laser myopic keratomileusis. *J Cataract Refract Surg.* 1994;20:610-615.
4. Kremer FB, Dufek M. Excimer laser in situ keratomileusis. *Journal of Refractive Surgery.* 1995;11(suppl)S244-S247.
5. Sher NA, Hardten DR, Fundingsland, et al. 193 nm excimer laser photorefractive keratectomy of high myopia. *Ophthalmology.* 1994;101:1575-1582.
6. Krueger RR, Talamo JH, McDonald MB, et al. Clinical analysis of excimer laser photorefractive keratectomy using a multiple zone technique for severe myopia. *Am J Ophthalmol.* 1995;119:263-274.
7. Rajendran B. Janakiraman P. Multizone photorefractive keratectomy for myopia of 8 to 23 diopters. *Journal of Refractive Surgery.* 1995;11(suppl):S298-S301.
8. Pop M, Aras M. Multizone/multipass photorefractive keratectomy: six month results. *J Cataract Refract Surg.* 1995;21: 633-643.
9. Sher N, Frantz JM, Talley A, et al. Topical diclofenac in the treatment of ocular pain after excimer laser photorefractive keratectomy. *J Refract Corneal Surg.* 1993;9:425-436
10. Fagerholm P, Nystrom-Hamberg H, Tengroth B, Epstein D. Effect of postoperative steroids on the refractive outcome of photorefractive keratectomy for myopia with the Summit excimer laser. *J Cataract Refract Surg.* 1994;20(suppl):212-215.
11. Fitzsimmons TD, Fagerholm P, Tengroth B. Steroid treatment of myopic regression: acute refractive and topographic changes in excimer photorefractive keratectomy patients. *Cornea.* 1003;12(4):358-361.
12. Talley AR, Hardten DR, Sher NA, et al. Results one year after using the 193 nm excimer laser for photorefractive keratectomy in mild to moderate myopia. *Am J Ophthalmol.* 1994;118(3):304-311.
13. Maguen E, Salz JJ, Nesburn AB, et al. Results of excimer laser photorefractive keratectomy for the correction of myopia. *Ophthalmology.* 1994;101:1548-1557.
14. Maguen E, Machat JJ. Complications of photorefractive keratectomy, primarily with the VISX excimer laser. In: Salz JJ (ed). *Corneal Laser Surgery.* St. Louis: Mosby; 1995.
15. Epstein D, Fagerholm P, Hamberg-Nystrom H, Tengroth B. Twenty-four-month follow-up of excimer laser photorefractive keratectomy for myopia. Refractive and visual results. *Ophthalmology.* 1994;101:1558-1564.
16. Brancato R, Tavola A, Carones F, et al. Excimer laser photorefractive keratectomy for myopia: results in 1165 eyes. *J Refract Corneal Surg.* 1993;9:95-104.
17. Garty DS, Muir MGK, Marshall J. Photorefractive keratectomy with an Argon fluoride excimer laser: a clinical study. *J Refract Corneal Surg.* 1991;7.420-435.
18. Garty DS, Muir MGK, Marshall J. Photorefractive laser keratectomy. 18 month follow-up. *Ophthalmology.* 1992;99:1209-1219.

SECTION SIX
Postoperative Care

Postoperative LASIK Management

Jeffery J. Machat, MD

The postoperative needs of laser in situ keratomileusis (LASIK) patients can vary considerably. Most LASIK patients require minimal follow-up care and improve over time, even when minor flap irregularities exist. In fact, patients often need to be encouraged to return for all their follow-up visits, as the postoperative course is typically very smooth and uneventful. However, flap complications such as visually significant flap striae or flap melts can require multiple corrective surgeries and often involve frequent follow-up monitoring and repeated counseling. Postoperative medications and examination schedules vary considerably between surgeons, with the common element being that most patients will do well with very little intervention (Figures 21-1 and 21-2).

GENERAL CONCEPTS FOR POSTOPERATIVE LASIK CARE

POSTOPERATIVE MEDICATIONS

At TLC The Laser Center, we currently use Tobradex (tobramycin .3%-dexamethasone .1%, Alcon) four times a day for 4 days and intensive lubrication for 7 days. Patients also receive Ciloxan (ciprofloxacin .3%, Alcon), two doses preoperatively and postoperatively to reduce the bacterial load of the conjunctiva and within the fornices. In general, topical steroids are not routinely required after the first 4 postoperative days, and their need within the postoperative regimen at any stage remains unclear. Short-term topical steroids will reduce inflammation and improve eye comfort.

Nonsteroidal anti-inflammatory agents (NSAIDs) are used immediately after LASIK in the postoperative recovery room in order to reduce the immediate postoperative burning and irritation and improve eye comfort. Frequent lubrication is also strongly recommended.

Although most patients exhibit good refractive stability by 1 month, a subset of patients, particularly higher myopes, may regress an additional 1 to 3 D over the proceeding 3 months. Broad beam profiles appear to regress somewhat more. While it has been proposed that a 4-week tapering regimen of topical steroids may have a role, we have used this in a number of cases and the effect has been inconsistent. Our current practice for regression or undercorrection following LASIK is retreatment. Overall, the intrastromal ablation of LASIK has far less tendency for regression than the surface ablation of PRK because less wound healing occurs in the deeper stroma, however exaggerated wound healing with up to 3 D of regression is evident in some highly myopic patients.

FOLLOW-UP EXAMINATION SCHEDULE

LASIK patients are typically examined on day 1 to specifically examine the flap, then at 1 week and 1 month to measure the visual and refractive performance of the eye. The eyes are then re-examined at 3, 6, and 12 months to check refractive stability. The first day visit is the most important, as it represents the first opportunity to assess the corneal flap position and alignment. It is far easier and safer to intervene with corneal flap displacement or alignment problems at this early stage (Figures 21-3 and 21-4). At the 1-week visit, temporary glasses or disposable contact lens-

Figure 21-1. Clinical photograph of a LASIK-treated left eye in the early postoperative period demonstrating preserved corneal clarity with minimal conjunctival injection. The patient was treated for -6 D sphere with 20/20 -2 vision recorded from the first postoperative day.

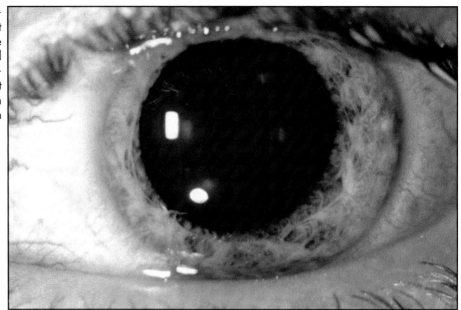

Figure 21-2. Clinical appearance of the left eye treated with LASIK in the early postoperative period demonstrating a clear cornea and minimal inflammation.

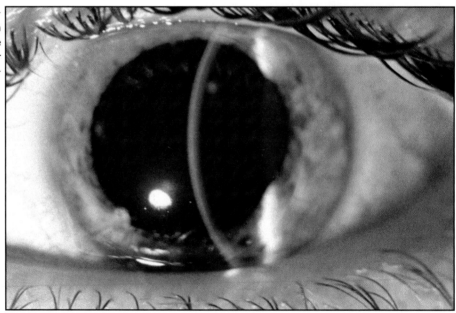

es may be fitted; and at the 3-month visit, enhancement is planned and performed. Enhancement of lower myopes may be performed as early as 1 month because refractive stabilization is far more rapid and the corneal flap can be easily lifted.

REFITTING WITH CONTACT LENSES

Patients requiring enhancement surgery due to undercorrection or myopic regression may be fitted with temporary glasses or contact lenses. It is important to wait at least 1 week prior to fitting a patient with contacts to ensure that the flap is secure. Disposable contacts are preferable, as the prescription may be quickly updated at little expense and have the least effect on the recovering cornea. Rigid gas

permeable lenses should not be used, as they will alter corneal topography pending retreatment. Early visual rehabilitation of patients is essential for improving overall patient satisfaction, as even 1 D of undercorrection following treatment of a -10 D myope will result in blurred vision. Although the postoperative undercorrected vision greatly exceeds the uncorrected visual acuity (UCVA) preoperatively, it will not compare to the best-corrected vision preoperatively. A stronger disposable contact lens prescription is commonly required postoperatively, as there may be excessive central clearance. The fit is on the midperipheral cornea and tends to be similar to the preoperative fit or steeper. Disposable contact lenses are well tolerated, and lubrication should be encouraged.

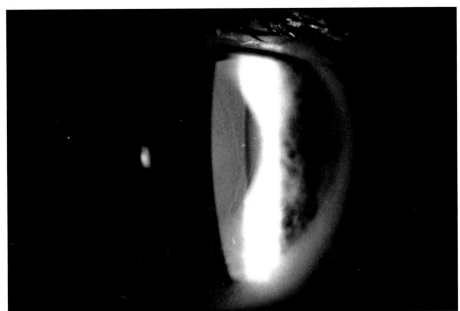

Figure 21-3. Clinical detection of fine corneal flap striae during slit lamp biomicroscope examination with optical section during the early postoperative period. Uncorrected vision was 20/60 with best-corrected vision reduced by one line with qualitative blur.

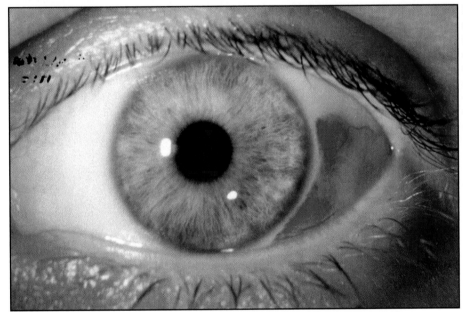

Figure 21-4. Clinical appearance of a LASIK-treated eye on the first postoperative day demonstrating a common pattern of excellent corneal clarity associated with a subconjunctival hemorrhage. Reduced suction ring manipulation and suction time diminish both inflammation and incidence of subconjunctival hemorrhages. The patient was treated for -7.75 D with mild astigmatism, reading 20/30 on the first-day examination.

IMMEDIATE POSTOPERATIVE CARE

EYE SHIELD USE

During the immediate postoperative period, care must be taken to avoid displacement of the flap. Patients are instructed to absolutely avoid rubbing their eyes or squeezing their eyelids forcefully for the first week. Patients are instructed to keep their eyes protected nightly for the first 4 nights.

Protective sunglasses are provided for the patients and placed over the eyes immediately after the postoperative flap check. Sunglasses should initially be worn during the day to reduce light sensitivity and ensure that the patient does not touch his or her eyes. At night, the patient is instructed to use the eye shield over the operative eye(s). The eye shield should be clear, as patients often have good functional vision although still quite blurry; one patient described this accurately as "Vaseline vision," reducing qualitative vision while quantitative vision is dramatically improved. The eye shield should be used nightly and when taking a nap. This is a conservative regimen; some surgeons do not utilize an eye shield whatsoever and have not observed corneal flap displacement. Other extremely cautious surgeons insist that their patients wear an eye shield

It is important to recognize that the eye should never be pressure patched even with an epithelial defect, as eye movement may dislodge the flap.

for 48 hours as well as nightly for 1 week. Each surgeon will select a regimen based upon his or her personal comfort level and clinical experience.

It is important to recognize that the eye should never be pressure patched even with an epithelial defect, as eye movement may dislodge the flap. A light pressure patch, or more preferably, taping the eyelid shut is useful in the case of a free corneal cap. Although ointment is avoided preoperatively because of the possibility of it becoming entrapped within the interface, it is acceptable to utilize ointment postoperatively once the epithelium is intact.

Lastly, some surgeons strongly advocate the insertion of a bandage contact lens immediately postoperatively for 1 to 12 hours.[1] The bandage contact lens provides improved initial comfort and is believed by some to help prevent flap displacement. The authors, however, do not recommend the use of a therapeutic contact lens for routine cases, and only utilize bandage lenses when a significant epithelial defect occurs. In fact, bandage contacts have been associated with not only infections but occasionally with flap displacement, as the lens can become lodged in the lower fornix and catch the inferior flap edge. Removal of these contact lenses may also be traumatic but can usually be simplified by instilling copious topical anesthetic and Genteal to ensure that the eye is numb and the lens is floating off the flap surface. Alternatively, while having the patient look up, fine forceps can be used at the slit lamp to grab the inferior edge of the contact and pull it gently away from the eye.

CLINICAL FINDINGS

Some patients describe a burning or irritation in their eyes during the first 1 or 2 hours postoperatively. During this time, patients are feeling the cut edge of the flap, which has yet to re-epithelialize, and there is also an increase in prostaglandin release. This sensation can be reduced considerably by placing two drops of Voltaren preoperatively and at 5 minutes postoperatively. Lubrication (Genteal) every half-hour the first day and every hour the second day, also helps—especially in high myopes. Using this Voltaren and lubrication regimen will reduce a patient's discomfort. Additionally, increasing the topical steroid regimen for 1 to 2 days in cases of severe postoperative pain both post-photorefractive keratectomy (PRK) and post-LASIK may help improve the comfort level. Any patient seen the next morning in extreme discomfort likely has displaced his or her corneal flap unless a large epithelial defect occurred but was not protected with a bandage contact lens.

In a small scale experiment, I've used a dilute proparacaine solution made by taking a 2.5 ml bottle of tears supplement and adding 10 to 20 drops of proparacaine. I instructed the patients to use this during the first couple of hours to provide temporary relief. I also explicitly warned the patient not to use more than one drop every half-hour and to discard the bottle at the end of the evening. I am very concerned about doing this routinely, however.

Vision immediately postoperatively is usually quite blurry and improves rapidly over the first 12 to 24 hours. However, the occasional patient will sit up immediately after surgery and be overwhelmed at the dramatic subjective and objective improvement in his or her UCVA (see Figure 21-4). The quality of the immediate postoperative vision is related to the quantity of the myopic correction and the quality of the corneal flap epithelium. In order to maximize the postoperative comfort and uncorrected vision, the surgeon must make every effort to preserve the integrity of the corneal epithelium throughout the LASIK procedure. The most effective means of promoting a rapid visual recovery include:

1. minimizing topical anesthetic use
2. limiting flap manipulation
3. maintaining the hydration of the epithelium during the ablation, which can be simply accomplished by laying the flap on the moist conjunctival surface
4. lubricating the flap frequently with a wet surgical spear while flap re-adhesion occurs.

Conjunctival injection and edema that is evident at the conclusion of the case disappears rapidly, leaving only the occasional subconjunctival hemorrhage on the first postoperative day. The corneal cap alignment markings are barely visible within minutes to hours (Figure 21-5). The line of the cut epithelium along the flap edge is visible immediately after LASIK but becomes virtually impossible to discern on the first postoperative day.

The corneal flap may be a little edematous, appearing somewhat gray and thickened. Edema can be caused by prolonged interface irrigation or can occur when large epithelial defects are present on the surface of the flap. Fortunately, flap edema clears within 12 to 24 hours in most cases. A traumatic, excessively long, or complex procedure will also leave the flap more edematous. An edematous corneal flap will be less adherent to the stromal bed and may become displaced more easily; therefore, close follow-up is required until the flap edema resolves. Increasing topical steroid use may help reduce corneal flap edema more rapidly. These patients often have a much higher risk of a grade 2 or 3 epithelial ingrowth with flap melting and should be watched closely for this. The patient should also be treated aggressively if ingrowth does occur. Increasing topical steroids and lubrication with virtually daily follow-up is the recommended treatment for LASIK flap edema. I personally avoid hypertonic solutions in these cases. Occasionally, a bandage contact lens is very helpful. While a contact lens

> An edematous corneal flap will be less adherent to the stromal bed and may become displaced more easily; therefore, close follow-up is required until the flap edema resolves.

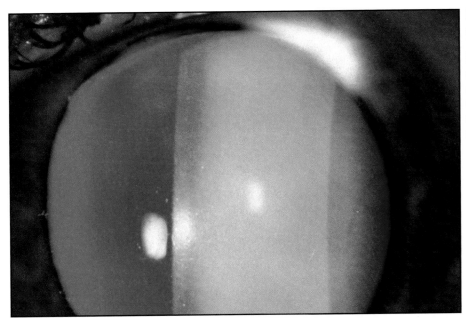

Figure 21-5. Clinical appearance of -13 D LASIK treated eye 10 to 15 minutes postoperatively demonstrating rapid clearing of alignment markings, rapid clearing of residual corneal flap edema, intact epithelium, and absence of corneal striae on retroillumination.

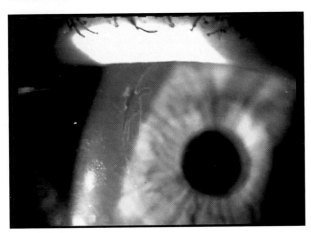

Figure 21-6. Small epithelial defects are often present in older patients in the superior region of the flap.

The incidence of epithelial ingrowth will be higher in these patients so follow-up should be adjusted to monitor more closely for this complication, typically weekly examinations for the first month are recommended.

may guard against flap displacement, it may also promote further flap edema and induce flap striae in some cases.

Corneal epithelial defects should be evaluated in the immediate postoperative period. Small epithelial defects are often present in older patients or contact lens wearers in the superior region of the flap (Figure 21-6), but may occur anywhere along the flap edge (Figure 21-7). Small defects less than 2 mm in size that are not causing discomfort are best monitored and treated with the standard postoperative drops with lubrication. These small defects usually heal within 24 to 48 hours. The incidence of epithelial ingrowth will be higher in these patients so follow-up should be adjusted to monitor more closely for this complication, typically weekly examinations for the first month are recommended. Larger epithelial defects are best covered with a contact lens and monitored daily until the defect heals completely. Topical NSAIDs can be used in these cases to improve the patient's discomfort. Without these interven-

tions, these patients can have significant postoperative discomfort, which can cause excessive lacrimation and eyelid squeezing with the potential for flap displacement.

The cut edge of the flap is visible as a thin peripheral line on the first postoperative day. If a second cut has been made in the case of LASIK enhancements 6 months after the primary procedure, two lines are visible on the peripheral cornea (Figure 21-8). These lines represent the first cut at 160 or 180 microns and the second cut at 200 microns. Rarely, some bleeding may be visible from cut peripheral corneal vessels immediately after LASIK or on the first postoperative day (Figure 21-9). This will invariably resolve without treatment. A faint interface haze is occasionally visible on the first postoperative day (Figure 21-10), which usually fades by the first postoperative week. Very occasionally, an air bubble will be visible under the flap immediately after LASIK or on the first postoperative day (Figure 21-11). This does not require corrective surgery, as it will absorb on its own within a few days.

MEDICATIONS

At the conclusion of the procedure (Figures 21-12 through 21-13), Ciloxan and Tobradex drops are instilled. One or two drops of Voltaren are also given immediately following LASIK to enhance postoperative comfort; however, no additional topical NSAID is required unless an epithelial defect is present. Topical steroids are helpful in reducing postoperative inflammation, and we will routinely

Figure 21-7. Clinical appearance of LASIK treated eye immediately postoperatively demonstrating a small epithelial defect along the flap edge. Epithelial disruption is most common along the flap margin and increases the incidence of epithelial ingrowths.

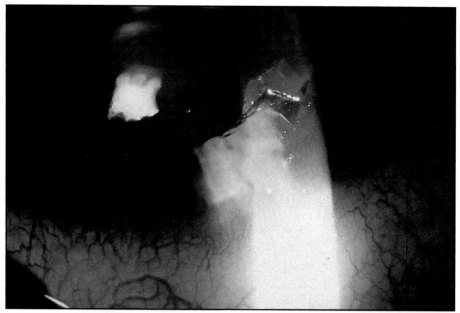

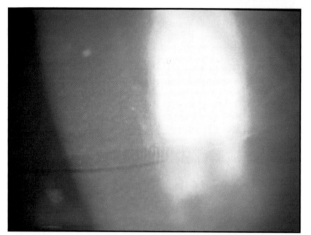

Figure 21-8. If a second cut has been made in the case of LASIK enhancements 6 months after the primary procedure, two lines are visible on the peripheral cornea.

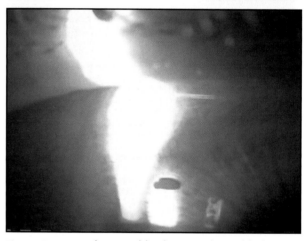

Figure 21-9. Rarely, some bleeding may be visible from cut peripheral corneal vessels immediately after LASIK.

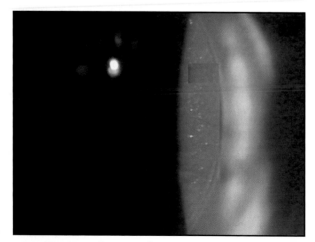

Figure 21-10. A faint interface haze is occasionally visible on the first postoperative day.

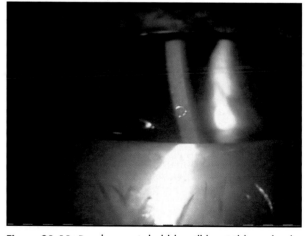

Figure 21-11. Rarely, an air bubble will be visible under the flap immediately after LASIK.

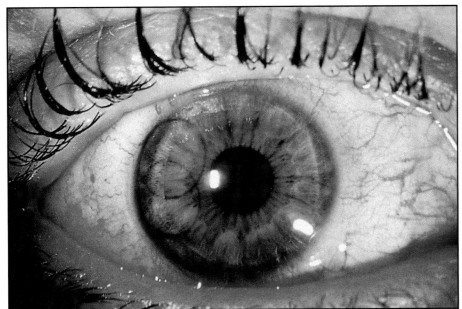

Figure 21-12. Clinical appearance of a LASIK-treated eye during the immediate postoperative period with visible alignment markings.

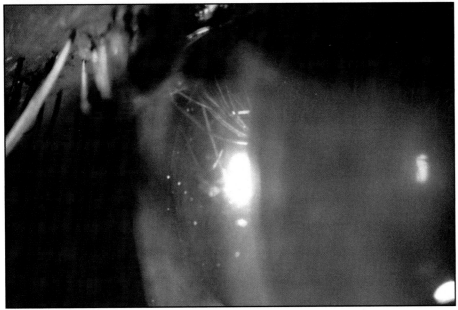

Figure 21-13. Clinical appearance of a LASIK-treated eye during the immediate postoperative period demonstrating intact epithelium with well-positioned corneal flap and clear corneal interface. Corneal flap status with respect to epithelial defects, edema, displacement, and interface opacities are assessed 15 to 60 minutes postoperatively prior to discharging the patient.

place the patient on an antibiotic-steroid regimen, Tobradex qid for 4 days.

In evaluating the role of NSAIDs with LASIK, we performed a double blind randomized study and determined that the instillation of two drops of Voltaren (diclofenac sodium .5%, CIBA Vision Ophthalmics) 5 minutes preoperatively and 5 minutes postoperatively improved the comfort of our patients dramatically during the immediate postoperative period. In the clinical study, 204 eyes of 109 patients were treated with LASIK and the need for Voltaren perioperatively was assessed. Patients were randomly divided into two groups, one group consisting of 54 patients who received Voltaren and another group of 55 patients who did not. All patients had an uneventful primary LASIK procedure. Two experienced optometrists questioned the patients

30 minutes following their procedure and the following morning. Both optometrists and the surgeon were blinded as to which patients had received Voltaren. Patients were questioned about symptoms of pain, irritation, and burning. While all patients in both groups were comfortable by the next morning, 3 patients (5 eyes) who received Voltaren and 41 patients (77 eyes) in the non-Voltaren-treated group complained of moderate or greater discomfort symptoms at 30 minutes post-LASIK. In both groups, most symptoms dissipated by 2 hours, although some patients in the non-Voltaren-treated group had persistent burning for as long as 6 hours. As stated, all patients were equally comfortable the following morning when examined for their day 1 postoperative visit, however the overall patient experience was more positive for those patients that received Voltaren, with

100% stating that the procedure was easier than expected compared to 86% in the non-Voltaren-treated group. Since most refractive surgery patients are derived from word-of-mouth advertising from past patients, the use of Voltaren peri-operatively has become an integral part of our LASIK regimen. We do not generally use topical NSAIDs after the first postoperative day, as associations have been made with the use of continued or excessive use of topical NSAIDs and subepithelial infiltrates and LASIK flap melts.

The role of lubrication postoperatively has also not been fully appreciated to date. Maintaining a well hydrated epithelial surface speeds visual recovery and helps prevent epithelial breakdown. Dry eye symptoms are often intensified by all refractive procedures, including LASIK; therefore, we recommend the liberal use of lubricating agents and that punctal plugs be considered both preoperatively and postoperatively in symptomatic dry eye patients. Genteal has been the mainstay of our dry eye therapy, as it comes in a 15 ml bottle, but the sodium perborate preservative becomes inactivated upon enzymatic breakdown by the tear film. Our success with preservative-free single dose units or minums has been quite variable as patients do not find them as convenient, reducing compliance.

EARLY POSTOPERATIVE CARE

The most important element of the first-day examination is to rule out flap displacement or misalignment. Typically, flap displacement occurs during the first 24 to 48 hours, particularly within the first few hours, and rarely without trauma thereafter. Significant flap displacement occurs in approximately 1 in 1000 patients in our experience. If the flap is displaced, simply keep the flap well hydrated with hourly preservative-free lubricating drops and both eyes closed until it can be replaced. The eyelid can be taped shut to protect the flap, however pressure patching in any form should be avoided, as this will promote the development of flap striae. It is said that if the flap is significantly displaced, it can be discerned from the doorway of the exam room, as the patient will be in severe discomfort, which is quite unlike other first postoperative day LASIK patients.

Any flap misalignment that could affect the postoperative result in any way should be corrected within the first few postoperative days. Flap displacements should be corrected as soon as possible. The longer the flap is allowed to remain misaligned, the more difficult it will be to correct the flap striae. Flap striae are relatively easy to smooth out with proper techniques utilized during the first postoperative day or so and then become progressively more difficult to remove.

The UCVA should be checked prior to any examination. Although the quantitative visual acuity may be impressive on the first postoperative day, it should be recognized that the qualitative vision is often still poor. The vision will also fluctuate greatly over the first few days. Typically, patients will read 20/100 or better, with most in the 20/40 to 20/60 range, and a number of patients will be 20/30 or better. It is not surprising to have mild to moderate myopes 20/20 the first day. The preoperative refractive error has a direct correlation with not only the final outcome, but also the speed of visual acuity recovery quantitatively and qualitatively. Patients with less than 9 D of myopia do exceedingly well, with near perfect results reported for moderate myopes. Above -10 D, the results are more variable with many of these patients requiring more than one procedure.

Preoperative cylinder also greatly affects immediate postoperative visual recovery, as treatment of cylindrical corrections is less predictable. It is important to counsel patients preoperatively with respect to the anticipated quantitative and qualitative vision expected.

It must be recognized that patients never complain if they see better than expected, but they will always be disappointed if the vision falls short of their expectations. In general, severe myopes have the same expectations as mild myopes, even with appropriate preoperative counseling. It is also somewhat surprising that despite a preoperative refraction of > -9 D, high myopes will often inquire about enhancement procedures for less than 1 D of residual myopia and less than 1 D of astigmatism. Patients also have tremendous difficulty remembering the level of their uncorrected preoperative vision. While measurement of the uncorrected preoperative vision has no real clinical significance for the myopic LASIK procedure, this value can be useful postoperatively to demonstrate to patients just how much the uncorrected vision has improved. There is definitely a psychology to assessing the visual acuity results of patients on the first postoperative day, as one must not only be very encouraging but enthusiastic. The 20/200 line should first be displayed and then gradually descend the chart to enable the patient to recognize his or her improvement. If one begins with the 20/20 line it will be disappointing, even to those capable of reading it since the qualitative vision is not 100% as yet.

A baseline refraction can usually be measured on the first postoperative day, although best-corrected vision is often still reduced by one to three lines. Lower myopes retain and regain their best-corrected vision faster. Manifest refraction is typically within 1 D for moderate to severe myopes, and within 2 D of emmetropia for severe myopes. Severe myopes often have manifest refractive errors disproportionately high relative to their UCVA. That is, they may have an UCVA of 20/40 but have a noncycloplegic refraction of -2 D rather than the expected -1 D. This is due to multiple factors—from accommodative spasm, which can even occur in older presbyopes, to central island formation—but is usually due to the multifocal nature of the postoperative cornea. The topographical change induced by the intrastromal ablation creates this multifocal cornea.

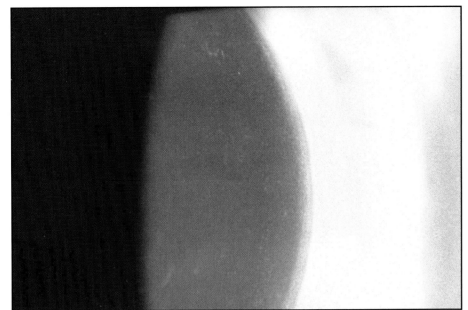

Figure 21-14. High magnification clinical appearance of a corneal flap during the immediate postoperative phase demonstrating an almost imperceptible flap edge. Corneal flap edges are notably smooth and flat, with an evenly symmetrical peripheral gutter indicating excellent flap apposition.

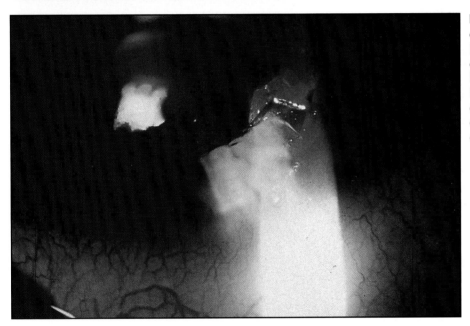

Figure 21-15. Clinical appearance of a LASIK-treated eye immediately postoperatively demonstrating a small epithelial defect along the flap edge. Epithelial disruption is most common along the flap margin and increases the incidence of epithelial ingrowths.

Corneal examination reveals an almost imperceptible flap edge (Figure 21-14), as the peripheral gutter has been filled in by epithelium. There is often slight stippling or superficial punctate keratitis in the area of the alignment markings because gentian violet dye is toxic to the corneal epithelium. There may also be small epithelial defects apparent (Figure 21-15), typically along the flap edge but also centrally if excessive drying of the flap surface occurred intraoperatively (Figure 21-16). Stromal edema of the cap may persist for 24 to 48 hours, but rarely longer, and is an uncommon finding with good technique (Figure 21-17). Persistent edema not related to epithelial breakdown is not normal and may indicate infection, flap nonadhesion with epithelial ingrowth, nonspecific diffuse inflammatory interface keratitis (previously known as Sands of the Sahara) and must be carefully assessed.

Interface clarity is dependent upon technique and the amount of debris within the patient's tear film. Interface irrigation after the replacement of the corneal flap has virtually eliminated the earlier problems with interface debris. Small amounts of debris and lint fibers may be observed (Figure 21-18), however, these are clinically insignificant both visually and physiologically, as the stroma is quite inert and an inflammatory reaction will rarely ensue (Figures 21-19a and 21-19b). In general, interface debris bothers the doctor more than the patient. Removal of foreign particles is only performed if clinically significant and should be done early or at the time of enhancement (Figure

Figure 21-16. Postoperative clinical appearance of irregular epithelium following LASIK with focal areas of keratitis related to intraoperative drying of surface epithelium, gentian violet marking dye, and topical peri-operative medications (topical anesthetic and aminoglycoside antibiotics). The interface is clear with the exception of minimal fine particle dusting. The corneal flap clarity was restored with preservative-free lubrication.

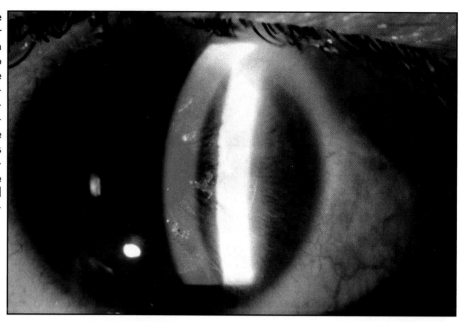

Figure 21-17. Clinical appearance of the left eye following LASIK for -8 D demonstrating minimal eyelid edema with 20/25 unaided vision at day 1.

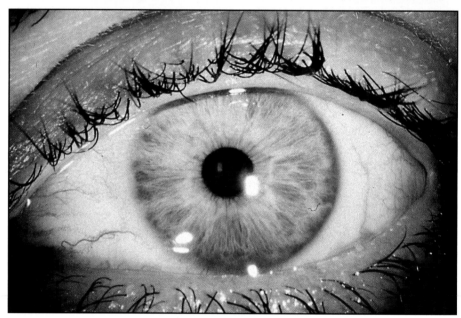

21-20). The most clinically significant indication for immediate removal of a lint fiber is partial extension of the fiber from the wound margin, enabling it to act as a wick for infection. Some surgeons however, routinely examine the interface at the slit lamp upon completion of the case and will irrigate any visible debris; however, the risk of displacement, flap edema, infection, and even epithelial breakdown and ingrowth from further manipulation may be increased.

CLINICAL FINDINGS AFTER 3 TO 4 WEEKS

The UCVA has typically reached the maximal level expected, and the eye has usually regained its best-corrected visual acuity (BCVA) level, although very severe myopes greater than -12 D may require months. The eye requires approximately 1 month to begin stabilizing, with subjective complaints of glare and ghosting beginning to dissipate (Figures 21-21 through 21-22). The qualitative vision has improved to the preoperative level at this time in the overwhelming majority of patients.

The refractive error can be measured and determined quite accurately. Some patients who achieved better than 20/25 vision initially with near plano refractive errors may have regressed by 1 D or more. The healing pattern and stabilization occurs about three to four times faster than with PRK. Consideration of repeat surgery for enhancement of the refractive and visual result is performed after 4 to 12 weeks and can be planned at this visit, with retesting performed the day of the procedure, ideally after 3 months for high myopes (Figure 21-23).

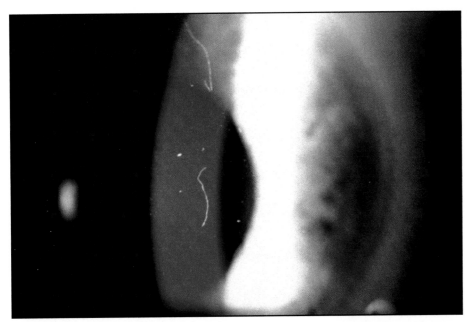

Figure 21-18. Clinical appearance of lint fibers with interface postoperatively. Interface opacities are of limited clinical significance, as the patient is subjectively unaware of them and inflammatory reactions to foreign matter are very infrequent.

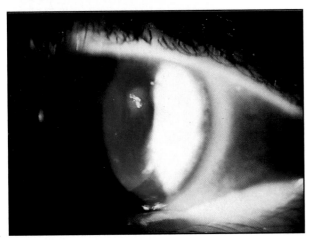

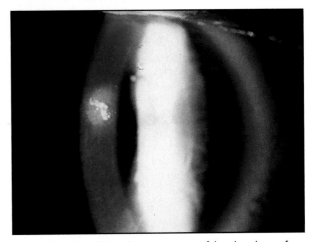

Figure 21-19a. Clinical appearance of a localized interface inflammatory reaction surrounding foreign matter under low magnification. Lint fibers are one of the most commonly encountered and frustrating interface opacities. The patient was closely monitored but not treated, as there was no associated patient symptoms, no clinical progression, and discernible visual sequelae.

Figure 21-19b. Clinical appearance of localized interface inflammatory reaction surrounding foreign matter under medium magnification.

Corneal examination reveals a clear interface, although a small amount of interface debris may be present. The flap edges are well-healed and a faint white ring along the cap edge may become apparent. The white ring represents scarring along the cut surface of Bowman's layer and is about .5 mm in diameter (Figure 21-24). In a small number of patients, epithelium is observed to be invading the interface along one edge or circumferentially. Epithelial ingrowth that is active at this stage must be managed surgically by lifting and cleaning the interface and flap undersurface. Epithelial ingrowth should be treated if it is greater than 2 mm, the visual axis is threatened, vision is affected, it is associated with flap edge erosion or other changes in flap

integrity, vacuolated cells, or geographic plaques of white necrotic cells are visible (see Chapter 34).

Corneal topography demonstrates central flattening, although the optical zone size often appears smaller than attempted (Figures 21-25a and 21-25b). There are two explanations for this:
1. The hydrated stroma makes the peripheral blend zone less effective.
2. The corneal flap may somewhat mask the ablation pattern.

LASIK appears to be quite unlike ALK in this regard, as the ALK flap aids the small 4.2 mm (typically) refractive resection in creating a 5.5 mm effective optical zone. With

Figure 21-20. Peripheral interface opacity consisting of lint fibers in this clinical example. It is important to keep all gauze and eye pads that can produce lint away from the operative field and surgical instruments.

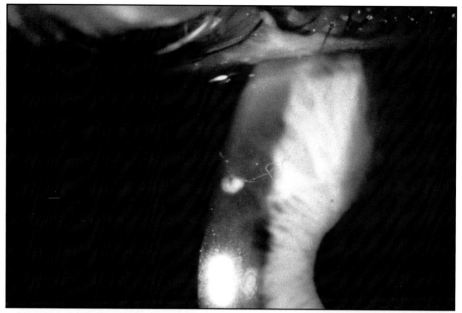

Figure 21-21. Clinical appearance of a LASIK treated left eye 2 months postoperatively demonstrating clear corneal interface. Unaided vision was 20/30 on the first postoperative day, following -7.25 D spherical correction, with gradual improvement to 20/20 by 1 month and slight regression back to 20/30, but with improved qualitative vision.

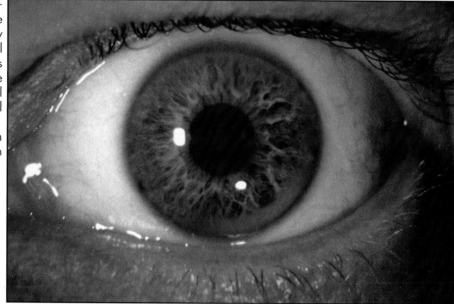

RK, the effective optical zone is far greater than the surgical optical zone. With PRK, however, the surgical optical zone and effective optical zone are equivalent; and with LASIK, the effective optical zone appears to be smaller than the surgical optical zone. Transition zone blending with LASIK may actually act to diminish the effective optical zone observed on topography since it blends a 5 mm zone out to 6 mm or 6.5 mm, accounting for symptoms of night glare with LASIK (Figures 21-26 and 21-27). The ablation transition zone used with the Chiron 217 scanning excimer laser extends the true of optical zone from 6 mm out to 8 or 9 mm for LASIK, which dramatically improves the quality of night vision.

Corneal videokeratography (Figures 21-28a through 21-28c) after LASIK may demonstrate a number of patterns, such as central circular or elliptical flattening (Figure 21-29), decentration (Figures 21-30a through 21-32), nasal steepening (Figures 21-33a through 21-34b), and central island formation. Decentration of the ablation is not related to centration of the flap. If the ablation is performed with a dilated pupil or with an active suction, the ablation may be decentered superotemporally due to the shift in pupil alignment. That is, the center of the pupil appears to be more superior and more temporal than is actually the case. Similarly, some surgeons utilize pilocarpine 1% to constrict the pupil, but this may result in a superonasal shift. A non-pharmacologically manipulated pupil provides the most ideal circumstance for achieving good centration. Additionally, centration toward the visual axis and not the pupillary center may be preferable in some cases in which a

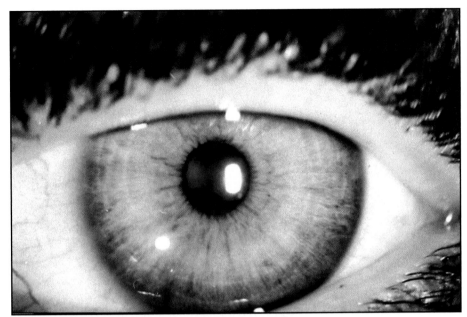

Figure 21-22. Clinical appearance of a LASIK-treated left eye 3 months postoperatively demonstrating a clear cornea. Unaided vision was 20/40 on the first postoperative day following -4.25 -2.5 x 10 toric ablation, with gradual improvement to 20/25 by 1 week and no regression of effect observed.

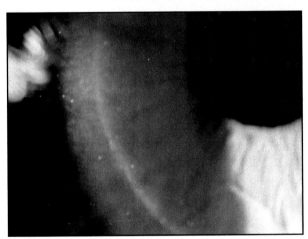

Figure 21-24. Clinical appearance of a LASIK-treated eye 12 months postoperatively demonstrating .5 mm white peripheral scarring along the corneal flap edge. No clinical significance noted.

large angle kappa exists, as is the case for RK. Other causes of abnormal topography include the development of induced cylinder from a large broad hinge. Fluid accumulation along the hinge or a short flap may also result in inadequate treatment nasally, resulting in a nasal step. Typically, a nasal step does not produce any clinical symptoms, although some patients describe peripheral visual distortions.

Central island formation can occur in both the clinically dramatic and clinically subtle varieties. Patients with significant central islands often have reduced best-corrected vision, induced myopia and cylinder, and complaints of visual distortions. Unlike the post-PRK central islands, the post-LASIK islands appear to be more stable and less likely to resolve with time (Figure 19-35), which is likely related to the absence of epithelial remodeling and an inert stro-

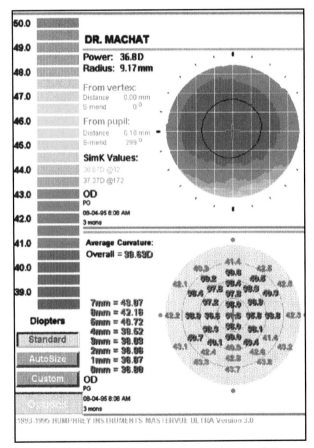

Figure 21-23. Postoperative videokeratography following LASIK for -9 D with multizone technique. Postoperative refraction -1 D at 3 months. No right glare.

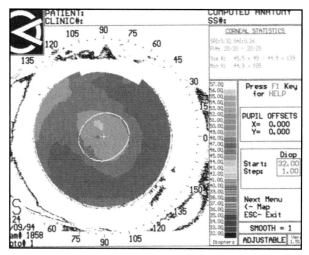

Figure 21-25a. Preoperative videokeratography prior to LASIK for -13.5 D.

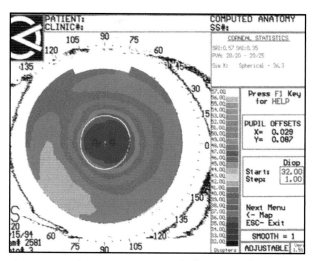

Figure 21-25b. Postoperative videokeratography demonstrating central flattening following multizone LASIK. The effective optical zone is smaller than anticipated due to a corneal flap masking effect of peripheral taper. Postoperative uncorrected vision was 20/60, preoperative best-corrected vision was 20/25.

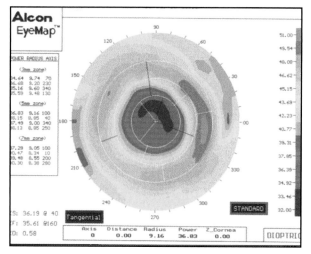

Figure 21-26. Videokeratography post-LASIK demonstrating a small effective optical zone despite a 6.6-mm attempted optical zone.

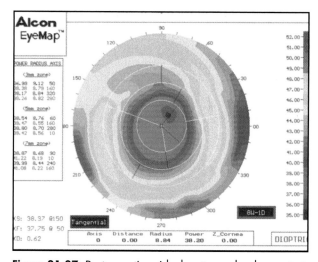

Figure 21-27. Postoperative videokeratography demonstrating a small effective optical zone post-LASIK for high myopia.

mal bed. Patients should be monitored monthly until the refraction and topography indicate stability, then treatment of the central island is arranged with careful attention to the location, height, and size of the island. Treatment can usually be performed by 4 to 6 weeks, but very large islands can be considered for treatment as early as 1 week. It should be noted, however, that virtually all LASIK patients, minutes after their procedure, will demonstrate central islands on videokeratography, and treatment before 1 month carries additional risk.

Night glare is not an uncommon complaint after refractive surgery, however most improve over time. Since any residual myopic refractive error or even hyperopic refrac-

tive error will exacerbate a patient's night glare. One alternative is to treat the residual myopia with a 6 mm optical zone, or preferably larger, if adequate tissue remains—this often dramatically reduces night glare. Alternatively, patients with residual error can be provided with night driving glasses that have anti-reflective coating and prescription that is overminused by -.5 D to -1 D.

IOP measurements are underestimated after refractive surgery. Refractive surgery flattens the cornea, which distorts the IOP calculations with the Goldmann tonometer as well as with noncontact tonometry readings. In general, they underestimate the true IOP; this is directly proportional to the amount of myopia treated. For example, a patient

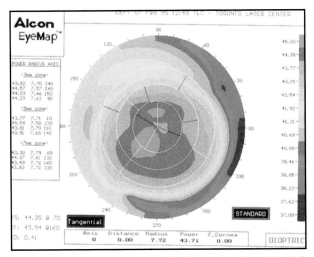

Figure 21-28a. Preoperative videokeratography of the left eye with refraction of -9.5 + 1 x 80.

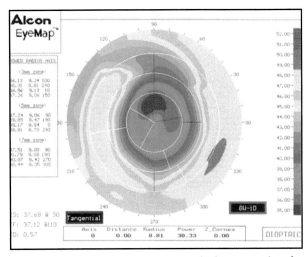

Figure 21-28b. Postoperative LASIK videokeratography of a well-centered ablation. Postoperative refraction was -.75 + 1 x 17 at 1 month.

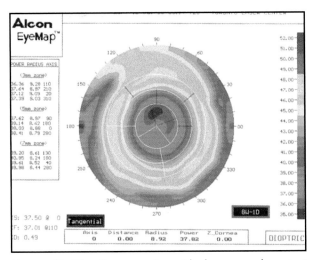

Figure 21-28c. Postoperative videokeratography at 4 months with myopic regression to -2.5 + 1 x 10. Note the smaller optical zone.

> IOP measurements are underestimated after refractive surgery.

treated for -3 D of myopia likely has his or her IOP underestimated by 2 mm Hg. A patient treated for -6 D will likely have his or her IOP underestimated by 4 mm Hg. Neither the refractive procedure performed nor the presence of haze following PRK makes a difference. Factors resulting in underestimated IOP include the degree of refractive error treated and thinness of the cornea postoperatively. All patients with a family history of glaucoma should be treated with LASIK, rather than PRK, as they have a higher incidence of steroid response. All patients who have pigment dispersion syndrome should be warned that their pressures could be falsely low. Their doctors should be notified as well.

The only interface opacity that is of any significance is

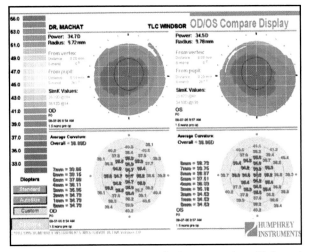

Figure 21-29. Postoperative videokeratography of bilateral primary elliptical LASIK for extreme myopia and astigmatism. OD: -10.5 + 1.5 x 100; OS: -11.75 + 2.5 x80. Postoperative refraction: OD: -1 + .5 x 96; OS: -1.5 sphere. Uncorrected visual acuity: OD: 20/30; OS: 20/80. The patient desired repeat LASIK OS and decided against monovision despite his presbyopic age group.

epithelium. Virtually every other material from lint to blood to make-up, or metallic debris from microkeratome blades, has not been found to be a problem. Occasionally, one will notice an inflammatory reaction around a foreign body. However, this is usually very self-limited. While the interface debris is not attractive to look at for the surgeon or co-managing doctor, all should rest assured that it is absolutely inert and will not affect the vision now or decades from now.

CLINICAL FINDINGS AFTER 3 MONTHS

The UCVA and BCVA has stabilized in virtually all patients. A number of extremely high myopes and compli-

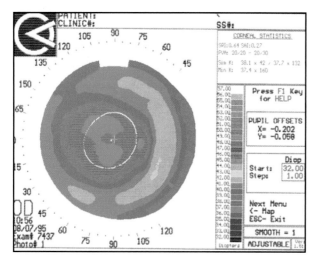

Figure 21-30a. Right eye with mid temporal decentration following bilateral LASIK for -8 D OU. Right eye had 20/30 UCVA with -.5 D refractive error. The patient was asymptomatic OU. The nasal step is evident on videokeratography OU.

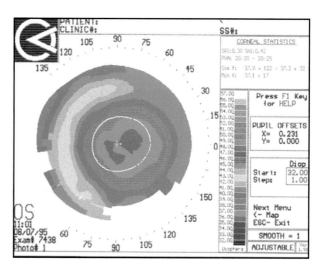

Figure 21-30b. Left eye with mild temporal decentration following bilateral LASIK for -8 D OU. Left eye plane with 20/20 UCVA. The patient was asymptomatic OU. The nasal step is evident on videokeratography OU.

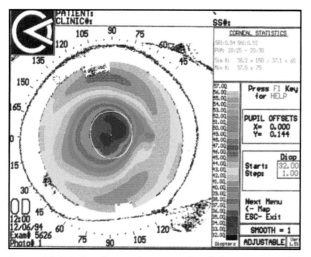

Figure 21-31. Small optical zone evident following LASIK for extreme myopia. Minimal decentration.

> The only interface opacity that is of any significance is epithelium.

cated patients may continue to demonstrate improvement over an entire year, as with all forms of lamellar surgery. Qualitative vision and night visual disturbances dramatically improve over the first 3 months, but continue to improve over 6 months or longer.

The refractive error is measured with cycloplegia to accurately quantify the residual refractive error when enhancement is considered. Myopic regression of severe myopes usually ceases after 3 months, and enhancements are performed between 3 and 6 months. Mild myopes who demonstrate stability earlier may be enhanced after 6 weeks. Corneal examination may reveal interface haze in a very small number of patients centrally and in a greater number

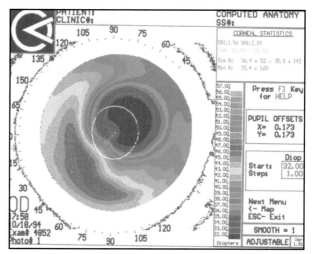

Figure 21-32. Clinically significant decentration following LASIK for high myopia with greater than 2 mm decentration. Etiology was related to performing LASIK with a dilated pupil. Elevated SRI indicated irregular astigmatism. Preoperative refractive error of -15 D, decentration resulted in gross undercorrection with induced cylinder. Correction involves reablation centrally with residual error beneath the corneal flap. There are no concerns with blending zones as with PRK.

of patients peripherally. There is definite haze formation in a select number of high myopes who undergo LASIK and have a propensity toward aggressive wound healing. Interface fibrosis makes lifting the flap extremely difficult for reablation. Interface debris remains unchanged from prior examinations, but occasionally appears to disappear. The white ring that demarcates the flap edge may increase in intensity over the first 3 months but is not readily apparent in many patients (Figures 19-36 and 19-37). In higher myopes, fine microstriae may be visible when the flap is

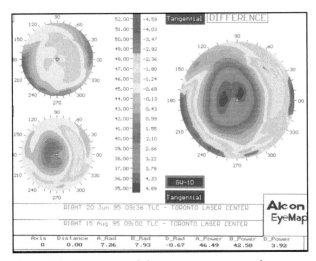

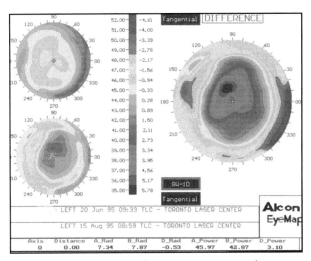

Figure 21-33a. A nasal hinge creates a nasal step on videokeratography (right eye map). Although the difference map demonstrates central flattening, postoperative videokeratography, subset B map, demonstrates a nasal area of steepening secondary to the LASIK hinge.

Figure 21-33b. A nasal hinge creates a nasal step on videokeratography (left eye map). Although the difference map demonstrates central flattening, postoperative videokeratography, subset B map, demonstrates a nasal area of steepening secondary to the LASIK hinge.

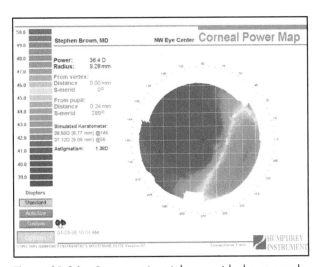

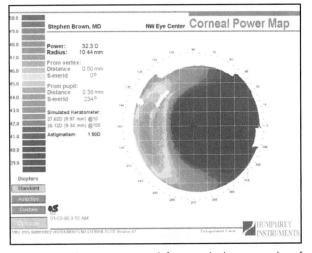

Figure 21-34a. Postoperative right eye videokeratography of a highly myopic patient with large nasal steps evident OU. The patient was well-centered OU, but a large nasal hinge gives the appearance of temporal decentration. Preoperative refraction: OD: -13 -3 x 90. Postoperative refraction: OD: -1 -3 x 95. No loss of BCVA was observed.

Figure 21-34b. Postoperative left eye videokeratography of a highly myopic patient with large nasal steps evident OU. Preoperative refraction: OS: -16 -3 x 100. Postoperative refraction: OS: -3.75 -1.75 x 105. No loss of BCVA was observed.

transilluminated through a dilated pupil. These occur because the flap is replaced onto the ablated stromal bed with a shorter radius of curvature. Corneal topography typically demonstrates little change from the 1-month examination, although slight regression may be identified.

LASIK RETREATMENTS

The need for and timing of retreatment of myopic LASIK cases is usually dependent on the degree of preoperative refractive error. The greater the refractive error, the

longer the recommended delay in scheduling retreatment, and the higher the enhancement rate. For example, in a patient requiring retreatment who was treated for -3 D, treatment can be performed as early as 4 to 6 weeks. The flap can be lifted easily at this time and enhanced. However, if the patient was severely myopic (greater than -9 D), at least 3 months should pass before enhancement is scheduled to allow for refractive stability.

There are two basic techniques in performing a LASIK enhancement: repeating the primary LASIK technique and cutting a new flap or lifting the original corneal flap and re-

Figure 21-35. Small 2 D central island following LASIK for -8 D.

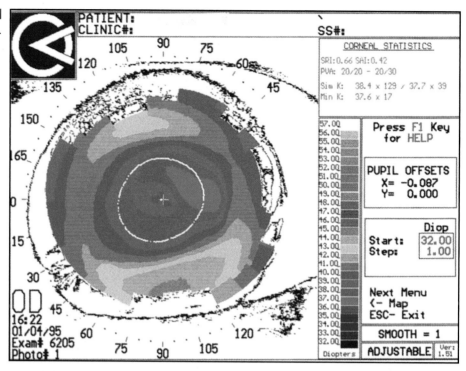

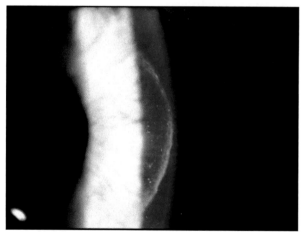

Figure 21-36. Clinical appearance of a LASIK-treated eye 9 months postoperatively, demonstrating white peripheral scarring along the corneal flap edge. Width and presence of peripheral scarring may be related to the size of the peripheral gutter at the conclusion of the procedure.

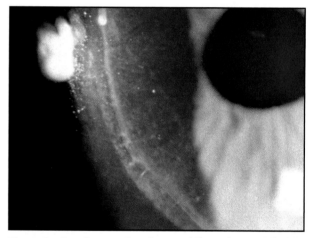

Figure 21-37. The peripheral corneal flap edge may thicken and retract over 3 to 6 months. This may be in association with epithelial ingrowth, or not. It must be observe closely, especially if epithelial ingrowth is evident.

ablating. The main factor in selecting which technique to use is how much time has elapsed since the initial flap was created. Lifting the flap is easier to perform earlier in the postoperative course. The second, and clinically more relevant issue, is whether the primary flap was of good quality. If not, a new flap should always be cut. Therefore, it is important to always document the quality of the corneal flap at the time of the primary procedure. Lifting the corneal flap allows for a safe and predictable means of enhancing LASIK patients, although this is less comfortable than cutting a new flap.

While RK enhancement of LASIK rather than repeat

Degree of preoperative myopia	Earliest time to enhance
< -3 D	4 to 6 weeks
-3.1 D to -6 D	6 to 8 weeks
-6.1 D to -9 D	8 to 12 weeks
> -9 D	> 12 weeks

LASIK is a viable but not preferred option, PRK over LASIK is associated with a very high incidence of corneal haze and should be avoided.

With the proper technique, lifting the flap even at 3 to 4

months is not difficult. As one approaches 6 months, it becomes increasingly difficult. Although in some cases there is no problem in lifting the flap well past 1 year, other cases exhibit extreme difficulty even at 4 to 6 months. The more peripheral and central haze that is noted in the flap interface, the more interface fibrosis that is present and the greater the difficulty encountered when attempting to lift the flap.

The first step in lifting the corneal flap is demarcating the flap edge for 1 clock hour at the slit lamp utilizing a Suarez or Machat spreader. It should be recognized that the peripheral .5 mm margin of the corneal flap is the area of greatest adherence along which the cut edge of Bowman's layer has healed. By depressing the spreader posteriorly and nasally at the flap edge, the flap interface can be identified and dissected open. The spreader is then passed along the margins of the original flap once the patient is positioned under the laser and the flap peeled back. The epithelium is somewhat disrupted along the margins, which accounts for the several hours of discomfort experienced by these patients postoperatively. Any epithelium noted along the undersurface of the flap or along the peripheral stromal bed should be debrided to avoid epithelial ingrowth. Ablation of the residual refractive error can then be performed on the stromal bed.

As one becomes more comfortable with LASIK, the more likely it is that greater consideration will be given to cutting a new flap for LASIK enhancement. It is faster and more comfortable, but clearly involves more risk. With proper technique, the risk of cutting a new flap can be reduced. When it is necessary to cut a new flap, the longer a surgeon waits beyond the 3-month mark, the better. I do not recommend cutting a new flap before 3 months because a free wedge of stromal tissue may be produced, which may result in induced cylinder. (I know this from experience and prefer to wait 4 months.)

One essential ingredient in safely cutting a new flap is ensuring good residual thickness to the cornea to allow for the creation a thicker new corneal flap. When cutting the new flap, I use a 200-micron plate when possible and center the eye rather than decenter it nasally. Therefore, my recut begins before the initial point of where the original cut started. This recut will go beneath the previous flap and works extremely well.

In cases that have healed poorly, such as those with a peripheral stromal melt or scarring following an old resolved epithelial ingrowth, lifting the flap may encourage a recurrence of the ingrowth. Therefore, it is best in these cases to recut a new corneal flap unless an area of active epithelial ingrowth is still evident. Even well after 6 months, if an area of epithelial ingrowth is still evident and not scarred, lifting the corneal flap may be the preferred technique for retreatment so that the epithelial cells may be cleaned from the interface.

The final issue surrounds the correction to be targeted.

> As one becomes more comfortable with LASIK, the more likely it is that greater consideration will be given to cutting a new flap for LASIK enhancement.

The amount of ablation required is often less than the refraction measured. The unaided visual acuity level should be considered when programming the target correction. That is, it is not uncommon to have a patient see 20/40 unaided but refract to -2 D, more than would otherwise be expected for this level of uncorrected vision. A target correction of -1 D represents a more reasonable treatment plan for a patient capable of seeing 20/40 uncorrected and should be programmed accordingly. Central island formation and other topographical abnormalities will greatly exaggerate this discrepancy between uncorrected vision and level of myopia measured. Therefore, planning an enhancement should involve a review of the postoperative map and a difference map in cases of topographical abnormalities.

LASIK Retreatment Conclusions

The three most important surgical technique points are:
1. In general, LASIK retreatment should be performed by lifting the flap between 1 and 6 months or by cutting a new flap after a minimum of 4 months.
2. For lifting the corneal flap, the key element is preoperatively demarcating the flap edge at the slit lamp.
3. For cutting a new corneal flap, the key element is using a thicker depth plate when possible and centering the suction ring on the eye so as to begin the new flap temporal to the original flap.

> For cutting a new corneal flap, the key element is using a thicker depth plate when possible and centering the suction ring on the eye so as to begin the new flap temporal to the original flap.

LATE POSTOPERATIVE CARE

Examination of patients at 6 and 12 months is important primarily to ensure that stability of cycloplegic refraction has been maintained. These are also the most essential visits to monitor return of BCVA and subjective reduction of night glare. If irregular astigmatism and night glare persist beyond 6 months, they may very well be permanent. The clinical appearance of the flap is typically unchanged over the first year beyond the 3-month examination (Figures 19-38 and 19-39). Enhancement procedures can also be performed at this time; however, a new flap must be recut since the strong adherence peripherally and even centrally will be fully formed, making lifting the original flap more complex and difficult.

A central cornea iron line can be identified in some

Figure 21-38. Clinical appearance of a LASIK-treated eye 14 months postoperatively demonstrating a naturally clear cornea with no change in refractive stability from 6 weeks following -7 D correction. The patient achieved -.75 D refractive endpoint with 20/30 visual acuity.

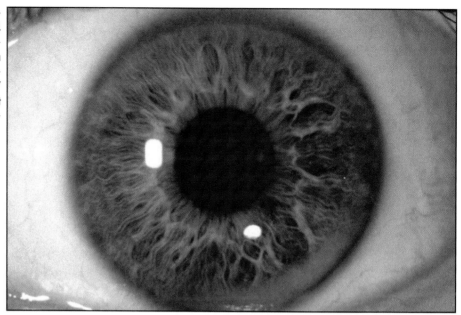

Figure 21-39. Postoperative videokeratography PRK for -7 D with a pretreatment multizone technique. UCVA was 20/20 with +.75 D refraction in a 27-year-old patient 1 year postoperatively.

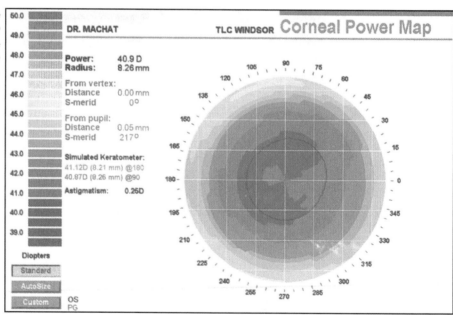

patients after LASIK (Figure 19-40). It is more common in patients with larger myopic corrections. While dry eye is a relatively common complaint after refractive surgery, LASIK does not seem to be associated with this problem to the same degree as PRK. Patients may complain of a foreign body sensation and slightly diminished vision at their LASIK follow-up. Corneal examination may demonstrate inferior corneal superficial punctate keratitis (Figure 19-41). Frequent lubrication with nonpreserved ocular lubri-

cants are very effective in improving the symptoms and temporary or permanent punctal plugs should be considered in these cases.

REFERENCE

1. Montes M, Chayet AS, Castellanos A, Robledo N. Use of bandage contact lenses after laser in situ keratomileusis. *Journal of Refractive Surgery.* 1997;13(suppl):S430-431.

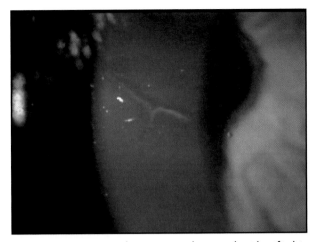

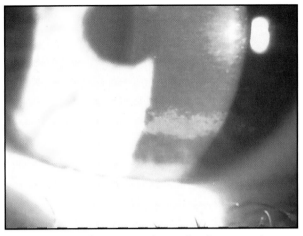

Figure 21-40. A central cornea iron line can be identified in some patients after LASIK.

Figure 21-41. Inferior corneal superficial punctate keratitis after LASIK.

Co-managing the LASIK Patient

Dennis W. Kennedy, OD

PREOPERATIVE LASIK PATIENT EVALUATION

INTRODUCTION

You may have heard the expression "laser vision correction can literally improve quality of life." Having been involved in this incredible "new" technology for more than 5 years, I can honestly say I have witnessed this time and time again. I cannot begin to describe the personal satisfaction I have experienced since I began caring for patients following this treatment option. My involvement with laser vision correction has revitalized my entire approach to primary eyecare. I now feel qualified to effectively offer my patients a complete understanding of all refractive options, including contact lenses, spectacles, and refractive surgery.

Our patients come to us for the best possible advice regarding their vision. I feel it is our obligation to have a comprehensive understanding of all refractive options and provide this information to them. Ultimately, it is the patient's choice—not ours—as to which refractive option may best suit him or her, but the patient needs as much information as possible to make an informed decision.

REFERRAL SOURCE = INCREASED PATIENT BASE

Referrals are the greatest measurement of "success." I have co-managed more than 500 laser vision correction procedures to date. Of the 500+ procedures I have managed through my practice, close to 70% of these patients came to

me by referral. These patients do not "come alone." They bring their entire family with them. They also refer their friends and neighbors. Why? They have found a new specialist. Their "new doctor" is currently practicing the latest technology.

Why are these patients not seeking advice and guidance from their own doctor? It is obvious that, as a profession, we are not discussing laser vision correction as an option. Patients indicate that they perceive their doctor as unwilling to offer this option, for whatever reason, or that they lack knowledge about this new technology.

DELEGATE AUTHORITY TO CREATE PATIENT AWARENESS

I have taught my chairside assistants to recognize potential candidates for laser surgery and contact lenses as they take the patient's case history. Once these patients have been identified, they are asked this simple question, "Would you care to have the doctor discuss the various new technologies with contact lenses or laser surgery as an alternative to glasses to correct your vision?"

When patients respond affirmatively, I become committed to discussing these options with them. As involved as I am with refractive surgery, I found myself not offering all options to every patient, especially if I felt I was going to fall behind in my schedule. Too often as conservative clinicians we pre-determine who would or would not be interested in other options. Since delegating the responsibility of asking patients if they are interested in discussing other options, I have been pleasantly surprised by how many patients were waiting for me to discuss these alternatives with them.

PATIENT EDUCATION

Properly educating patients can be time consuming. Without assistance, you cannot possibly devote enough time during your busy schedule to accomplish this task.

THE LASER VISION COORDINATOR

Recognizing the need for help with patient education, I came upon the idea of the "laser vision coordinator." My practice coordinator, who had undergone photorefractive keratectomy (PRK) in 1993, was and still is an enthusiastic advocate of this technology. She was the perfect choice. Having had the procedure herself, she could relate to potential candidates better than anyone else in my practice.

Together we felt a structured protocol was necessary to move patients through the process of learning about all methods of refractive surgery. My laser vision coordinator developed an organizational flow chart so that each step involved in educating the patient about his or her options is systematically covered in detail (Figure 22-1). This process has proven to be well-organized, effective, and time efficient.

DOCTOR AND LASER VISION COORDINATOR SHARING PATIENT EDUCATION

Once the patient indicates the desire to discuss laser vision correction as an option, I bring my laser vision coordinator into the examination room before I begin discussing it. I want my coordinator to understand what level my discussion with the patient has reached. This makes for a smooth transition as I transfer the educational responsibility to the coordinator. The total time I may spend discussing this option with the patient is less than 3 to 4 minutes. This allows me time to continue seeing other patients without interrupting my schedule.

TYPICAL PATIENT QUESTIONS

Is Laser Vision Correction Safe and Effective?

Patients often ask me about the safety and effectiveness of laser vision correction. I generally respond by stating the following, "I have been in private practice for over 25 years and have established a very successful practice. My approach to patient care has always been conservative. At this stage of my career I do not need to refer patients for a procedure that will burden my day with managing complications resulting from this treatment option. I can honestly

> I can honestly say that the best part of my day is when my laser patients come in for their follow-up appointments.

say that the best part of my day is when my laser patients come in for their follow-up appointments. These patients are truly the most enthusiastic patients I have ever had the pleasure to care for."

PATIENT COUNSELING

The process of determining a suitable candidate for LASIK is the same as it would be for any refractive surgery procedure. The key to a successful outcome is through a comprehensive education of the patient with emphasis on risks, benefits, and limitations. If the patient and the co-managing doctor have a complete understanding of these risks, benefits, and limitations, as well as a true understanding of the patient's expectations, the chances of success are greatly enhanced. The more information the patient receives prior to his or her surgery date, the more likely the chances of having a satisfactory outcome. I can assure the reader it is far easier to deal with clinical complications than it is to deal with the emotional side of unfulfilled expectations.

> I can assure the reader it is far easier to deal with clinical complications than it is to deal with the emotional side of unfulfilled expectations.

> If the patient and the co-managing doctor have a complete understanding of these risks, benefits, and limitations, as well as a true understanding of the patient's expectations, the chances of success are greatly enhanced.

SHARED RESPONSIBILITY FOR PATIENT PREPARATION

The co-managing doctor is not alone in preparing the patient for surgery. The center director and the center's staff are your adjunct personal for use in patient preparation and consultation. They will become your greatest allies with this endeavor. There are certain areas of responsibility that the primary doctor and the center director are responsible for.

ROLE OF THE CO-MANAGING DOCTOR

The preoperative role of the co-managing doctor generally covers the basics, whereas the details are covered by the center:

1. Determine patient eligibility.
   - Refractive status
   - Ocular and general health
2. Inform and educate the patient of the risks, benefits, and limitations of laser vision correction.

Note: Your involvement with this process can be at whatever level you feel comfortable with. It is not necessarily the role of the co-managing doctor to go into great detail about risks, benefits, and limitations of the surgery. Your

Patient name _____

Beginning date_____

REFRACTIVE SURGERY FLOW SHEET

Date

_____ In office consultation with co-managing Dr. and patient   _____
_____ In office consultation with surgical coordinator and patient   _____

_____ Dispense patient packet
      TLC brochure / fee outline / video / business card   _____

_____ Follow up phone call with patient / one wk. after apt.   _____

_____ Dispense: Informed Consent / True and False /   _____
      "Fill in the blank" consent to surgery risks

_____ Patient returned signed informed consents   _____

_____ Schedule surgery date at TLC   _____

_____ Faxed referral form to TLC   _____

_____ Schedule post op visits in our office   _____

_____ Charge and collect co-management fee   _____

DATE OF SURGERY _____ TYPE OF SURGERY _____

_____ *Day of surgery / progress call* - Comments:_____
       _____
       _____

_____ Patient wishes to hold on surgery at this time. Keep on Mailing / Phone recall list.
       Date: _____
_____Inform patient of next monthly seminar.   Date of seminar _____

{each item is to be initialed after completion }

Figure 22-1. The refractive surgery flow sheet.

TABLE 22-1.
LASIK

Indicated	Caution	Contraindicated
High myopia	Endothelial dystrophies (cell count >1500)	Endothelial dystrophies (cell count <1500)
High astigmatism	Flat corneas	Monocular patients
Keloid formers	Small orbits	Herpes zoster Ophthalmicus
Long RGP CL history	ABM dystrophy (mild)	ABM dystrophy (moderate to severe)
Forme fruste keratoconus (Normal corneal thickness age >35 years old)	Post-RK surgery	Abnormal eyelid closure
Medication intolerance or noncompliance	Post-PKP	Active collagen vascular disorder
Steroid responder	Vitreal syneresis	Systemic vasculitis
Rapid visual recovery desired		Keratoconus
		Thin corneas

center director and staff are highly trained in this field and will provide your patients with extensive knowledge regarding laser vision correction.

3. During the educational process, the doctor must completely understand the patient's expectations. Managing the "complication" of unsatisfied expectations can be the most challenging aspect of laser vision correction.

ROLE OF THE CENTER DIRECTOR

The role of the center director is to:

1. Continue the educational process of the patient through the surgical informed consent that covers in detail the risks, benefits, and limitations of the procedure.
2. Restate and examine the patient's expectations.
3. Provide additional testing to determine patient candidacy when necessary.
4. Consult with the co-managing doctor when needed.
5. Consult with the patient.
6. Coordinate the surgical date and post-surgical follow-up appointments.
7. Address financial considerations.
8. Address postoperative patient management issues that require consultation.
9. Be available on a 24-hour basis for any and all help that the co-managing doctor feels is necessary.

REFRACTIVE ERROR CONSIDERATIONS

- Myopia range -1 to -15 D (corneal thickness is a limiting factor)
- Astigmatism (with myopia) -.5 to -8 D
- Hyperopia range +.75 to +6 D (spherical equivalent)
- Astigmatism (with hyperopia) +.5 to + 4 D

Hyperopia refractive error examples: +4 +2 x 180, the spherical equivalent is just +5, but the procedure is limited to +6 in any one meridian.

1. +2 +4 x 180 = candidate
2. +3 +4 x 180 = noncandidate for "full" correction (7 D in vertical meridian)

BCVA is no less than 20/40 in the weakest eye. Anything less than 20/40 is considered clinically monocular and is not a candidate under any circumstances. The exception would be a patient who has BCVA below 20/40 in both eyes. The surgical approach would be a monocular procedure. If the postoperative BCVA is equal to or better than the preoperative values, then the other eye can be operated on.

GENERAL AND OCULAR HEALTH CONDITIONS

As with any surgical procedure, there needs to be a complete understanding of the patient's general and ocular health. There are, however, far fewer health contraindications to LASIK than PRK due to the reduced wound-healing nature of LASIK. Many systemic health conditions that are absolute contraindications with PRK, such as autoimmune diseases, immunosuppressed or immunocompromised patients, or any systemic illnesses that affect wound healing, become relative contraindications with LASIK. The absolute ocular contraindications for PRK are essentially the same for LASIK. These include clinical keratoconus, monocular patients (either actual or functional), severe dry eye, exposure keratopathy, and herpes zoster ophthalmicus. To summarize, it is always safe to avoid any patient with active general or ocular disease until such a condition has resolved or become stable (Table 22-1).

PREPARING THE LASIK CANDIDATE

Preparing the LASIK candidate is essentially the same as it would be for PRK. As I described previously, the patient should have a complete understanding of all the risks and limitations of the procedure as well as a complete

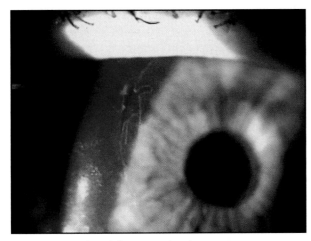

Figure 22-2. Edge defect immediately postoperative.

risks and limitations of the procedure as well as a complete understanding of the postoperative course of events.

CONTACT LENS REMOVAL PRIOR TO SURGERY

The timing of contact lens removal is not and should not be clear-cut and concise. The cornea must recover fully from any mechanical compromise caused by the lenses themselves. The minimum time contact lenses should be removed preoperatively with soft lenses is 48 hours, 4 to 6 weeks with rigid gas-permeable lenses, and 6 or more weeks with polymethylmethacrylate lenses. The actual time contact lenses should be removed is when the cornea has re-established its "natural" contour. This may involve several weeks or even months of monitoring with serial topography or keratometry and manifest and cycloplegic refractions.

POSTOPERATIVE CARE OF THE LASIK PATIENT

The postoperative care of the LASIK patient requires less chair time than with PRK, but by no means is patient management routine. The clinician must have a complete understanding of all clinical findings so that a satisfactory outcome can be obtained. The following postoperative LASIK guide was developed to help the co-managing doctor have a better understanding of expected results from day 1 through 1 year. This guide was created from my personal experience of observing several thousand PRK and LASIK patients during the past 4 years. There are many different approaches to the medical management of any surgical procedure. This guide is just one such approach.

My hope is that the following guide to LASIK co-management provides clinicians with enough information to enthusiastically accept this exciting new challenge. As I have indicated earlier, co-managing the laser vision correction patient is profitable, but the emotional rewards are beyond description. You will never be involved with patient care that fulfills you in so many different ways than with

this treatment option.

"If your patients are going from your office to mine, it isn't that I'm better, just that I'm willing to talk about their options."

LASIK POSTOPERATIVE CARE SURVIVAL GUIDE

DAY 1 POSTOPERATIVE LASIK VISIT:
DETERMINE FLAP POSITION

Purpose of visit
1. Evaluate flap position and integrity.
2. Establish completion of epithelial migration from the flap edge to the adjacent tissue, thus creating a complete intact "envelope" of epithelium across the gutter/seam created by the microkeratome.
3. Establish presence/absence of infection.
4. Evaluate uncorrected visual acuity (UCVA).
5. Evaluate refractive error and best-corrected visual acuity (BCVA).
6. Consultation of expected symptoms and visual quality/abilities.

Test
1. UCVA
2. Biomicroscopy
3. Manifest refraction
4. BCVA
5. Do not evaluate intraocular pressure (IOP) at this visit (do not disturb the flap).

Expectations
1. UCVA: expect 20/30 to 20/50. Range: 20/15 to 20/100.
2. Biomicroscopy: The gutter/seam created by the microkeratome should have complete epithelial closure at the 24-hour postoperative visit but typically heals within 6 hours. It is important to document any residual epithelial defect, as any persistent defect is a potential site for epithelial ingrowth (Figure 22-2). You cannot diagnose epithelial ingrowth at day 1, just the potential for ingrowth. Epithelial ingrowth will be discussed at the One Week Visit section of this chapter.

> You cannot diagnose epithelial ingrowth at day 1, just the potential for ingrowth.

a. The flap adherence mechanism: Three of the four mechanisms that hold the flap down are in place at 1 day. They are:
  1. The stroma is composed of glycoprotein and has the consistency of Velcro. This enables the flap stroma to mesh with the stroma within the bed. This occurs within seconds.

2. The endothelial pump pulls the flap down. This occurs within minutes.

3. The intact epithelial envelope that was created when the epithelium, from the surface of the flap, migrated to the adjacent corneal surface epithelium. This occurs within 6 to 12 hours.

4. The cut edge of Bowman's layer forms a thin scar along the incision seam. This occurs within 6 to 12 weeks.

b. <u>Debris under the flap:</u> The interface should be clear and free of debris; however, should any debris be noted, do not attempt to remove it. Do not "play with the flap."

Scattered debris at the interface level is common, and because it is inert, it will not create complications or affect the final result. Debris at the interface bothers the doctor, not the patient.

Occasionally, a fiber or piece of lint extends out from beneath the flap. The patient should be referred back to the center for removal because it can act as a wick for infection.

c. <u>Flap edema:</u> The flap may be edematous but should resolve within the next 24 to 48 hours. This may result in temporarily reduced BCVA.

d. <u>Flap striae:</u> Striae will be discussed in detail in the One Week Postoperative Visit section; however, since striae can occur during the surgical procedure and up to 1-week postoperatively, it needs to be discussed here as well.

> Clinically significant striae are striae that, in your opinion, interfere with BCVA.

Etiology of Striae

Striae occurs from three main causes:
1. The patient squeezing or rubbing the lids.
2. Poor flap placement (this is more common with flat corneas that have narrower hinges).
3. High myopia with excessive flattening of the stromal bed.

Location of Striae

Striae within the flap may be noted at the day 1 visit, and if it is clinically significant,* the patient should be referred back to the center as soon as possible. Striae can be located near the seam/gutter or centrally.

- Seam/gutter: If the striae are at the seam and create an excessive gap, the patient should be referred to the clinic.
- Centrally: If the striae are near or within the central pupillary area, the patient should be referred to the clinic.

Both of these conditions need immediate attention.

Clinically significant striae are striae which, in your opinion, interfere with BCVA. This usually involves striae that extend across the visual axis. If there is any doubt about their significance, it is advised you reevaluate this condition at the 1-week visit.

Treatment of Striae

Striae can be treated several months postoperatively but are far easier to treat within the first 1 to 2 weeks. After this period, they become significantly more difficult to remove or "iron out" (Machat technique). The Machat Technique involves lifting the flap, refloating it, then stretching the flap edge to the seam/gutter. If you detect striae with no loss of BCVA, just document and observe it. There is no need to "fix" a condition that is not clinically significant.

e. <u>Decemets folds (striae):</u> Mild striae or folds may be located at the level of decemets membrane that is related to corneal edema. This should not be confused with flap striae. This phenomenon is rare and generally noted in patients over 40 years of age. It usually resolves without the need for surgical intervention.

4. Manifest refraction: There are many factors that affect the immediate or 1-day postoperative refractive results. Do not become alarmed with BCVA that is less than optimal at day one. Patients can be either significantly hyperopic or myopic at day one, then emmetropic at week one. If in your opinion the eye is "white and quiet" (excluding subconjunctival hemorrhages) and the flap is intact and in proper position, the patient should be reassured and instructed to return in 1 week. It is at the 1-week visit that the manifest refraction can best be analyzed.

Hyperopic Shift (Immediately Postoperatively)

It is important that the patient be made aware of normal postoperative "hyperopic shift." Reading glasses may be dispensed for temporary use during this normal healing phase. This is especially true in patients over 40 years old who expect to return to work the next day. It is suggested you keep several drug store half eyes on hand to loan out. Instruct the patient that he or she will become less and less dependent on these glasses during the healing phase. This obviously depends on the individual refractive status of each patient.

5. Symptoms: Typically, the LASIK patient is asymptomatic at the 1-day visit. Exceptions to this include a foreign body sensation as a result of a persistent epithelial defect at the gutter/seam. This is especially prevalent in patients who have poor epithelial adherence (ie, anterior basement membrane dystrophy [ABMD]). ABMD is associated more with long-term contact lens wearers and patients over 50 years old.

> The LASIK patient, just as with the PRK patient, must be seen daily until full re-epithelialization has occurred.

Use of a Bandage Contact Lens with LASIK

With ABMD there may be an epithelial defect on the face of the flap. This condition may require the insertion of a bandage contact lens immediately following surgery. If this is the case, you must evaluate the epithelium and remove the bandage contact lens when full re-epithelialization has occurred. As with PRK, during re-epithelialization, a copious amount of lubrication is recommended.

Removal of the Bandage Contact Lens with LASIK

Great care must be followed when removing the bandage contact lens so as not to disturb the flap.

Liberally lubricate the eye with Genteal or a similar lubricant until the lens separates from the cornea. The lens must literally float on the corneal surface before attempting to remove it. When you achieve complete lens/cornea separation, gently drag the lens inferiorly and remove it from the sclera, thus avoiding the flap entirely.

6. Dry eye: Although this subject could fall under the general topic of symptoms, I feel it deserves special note.

Many patients pursue PRK/LASIK as a treatment option because they can no longer wear their contact lenses due to dry eyes. I can assure you the symptoms of dry eyes do not improve following surgery, in fact this symptom may become more significant immediately postoperatively.

The afferent pathway from the cornea to the lachrymal gland is interrupted as a result of the surgery and may take several months before it re-establishes communication to the gland. This applies to reflex tearing only but ultimately has an effect on overall dry eye symptoms.

Dry eye management with the use of unpreserved tear substitute PRN should be encouraged. Punctual occlusion should be considered depending on the severity of symptoms. Punctual occlusion is very effective but underutilized.

7. Glare: Virtually every refractive surgery patient experiences glare at day 1. This condition gradually resolves itself during the first 3 to 6 months. Patient reassurance is recommended.

8. Medications: Use Tobradex qid for the first 4 days unless there is a persistent epithelial defect. Patients are instructed to lubricate with Genteal or another tear supplement every hour or PRN. They are sent home with Ativan, or a similar product, to help with sleep for the first night only.

If, in your opinion, there is any potential for infection, such as a persistent epithelial defect, you may extend the antibiotic treatment for as long as necessary. Any persistent defect that lasts longer that 3 days should be reported to the center.

CLINICAL PEARLS

Quantitative versus qualitative vision needs to be discussed at this time. The patient is generally very excited about his or her "new" vision, but he or she may also note that there is a "Vaseline-like" appearance to everything. Tell the patient that immediately postoperatively the quality of vision is less than perfect. This is due to the fact that the laser, while reshaping the cornea, disturbs the natural corneal cell alignment. It generally takes 1 to 4 weeks for nature to realign the corneal cells, thus allowing vision to sharpen. This process takes place very slowly. There is a slight improvement in the quality of vision that occurs each day. Advise the patient that we achieve quantity of vision at day 1, but quality of vision takes time. Patience needs to be stressed at this time.

Undercorrection: If there is a significant undercorrection, I will introduce the possibility of enhancement, but I also indicate that it may be too early to be sure. I add that we will re-evaluate this possibility the following week. Continue to reassure.

Overcorrection: If there is a significant overcorrection, suggest temporary reading glasses and indicate that during this healing period a certain amount of regression will take place. Also, irregularity early on produces hyperopia. This induced hyperopia is generally associated with reduced BCVA and will improve with time. It is important not to alarm the patient of an overcorrection possibility until you are certain this is the case.

Note: Do not use the words "undercorrected or overcorrected," as they can be interpreted as a surgical mistake. It is very important that the clinician and the patient understand that the target correction was correct and it is not an undercorrection or an overcorrection in the true sense of the word, rather an under or over-response related to each individual patient. Explain that it is the initial goal to be slightly farsighted at this point and with time there will be a gradual reduction in the farsightedness as the patient heals. It should be stressed that each patient has a different healing response to surgery; some respond more and others respond less. Time and patience is the best medicine.

It is important for the clinician to understand that we can virtually enhance any refractive outcome. Therefore we should never show concern but rather confidence that the final result should be satisfactory.

> Advise the patient that although we achieve quantity of vision at day 1, quality of vision takes time.

> Do not use the words, "undercorrected or overcorrected," as they can be interpreted as a surgical mistake.

WEEK 1 POSTOPERATIVE LASIK VISIT:
ESTABLISH FUNCTIONAL VISION WITH THE USE OF DISPOSABLE CONTACT LENSES IF NECESSARY
Purpose of visit

1. Determine UCVA
2. Ensure flap position and corneal integrity
3. Evaluate manifest refraction and BCVA
4. Evaluate IOP
5. Discuss expected visual rehabilitation

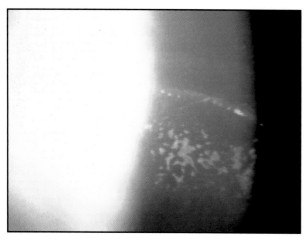

Figure 22-3a. Early epithelial ingrowth (nests) 1 week postoperatively: appears like oil droplets.

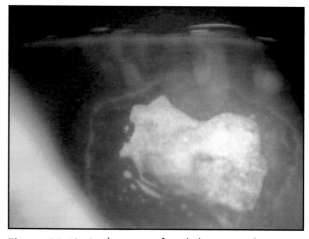

Figure 22-3b. Implantation of epithelium 2 weeks postoperatively.

Tests

1. UCVA
2. Biomicroscopy
3. Manifest refraction
4. Applanation tonometry

Expectations

1. UCVA: Expect 20/15 to 20/40, with a range between 20/15 to 20/80 depending on the preoperative refractive error.

2. Biomicroscopy: The gutter/seam should be barely visible at this time.

   a. Interface material: This can be debris (unimportant—inert) or epithelial cells (important—can lead to ingrowth).

   b. Epithelial ingrowth: It is at this 1-week visit that epithelial ingrowth can first be detected. Epithelial ingrowth occurs in 2 to 2.5% of the cases. Progressive ingrowth that is clinically significant and affects flap integrity occurs in less than .5% of the cases, the other 2% are nonprogressive and stable. Although this condition is rare, we must be able to properly recognize and manage it.

The great majority of ingrowth (98%) occurs because the flap epithelium, which should migrate across the gutter/seam, migrate around and then under the flap and into the interface. The exact etiology of this is uncertain. This ingrowth develops from the gutter/seam peripherally and first appears like oil droplets (Figure 22-3a). These oil droplets are, in fact, epithelial nests. They can be found anywhere along the edge of the flap, but most often they are observed at the superior and inferior temporal aspect of the flap. These epithelial nests can also be found wherever there was a persistent edge defect of the flap.

The other 2% are islands of implanted epithelial cells. These occur during the procedure as the blade "drags" epithelial cells into the interface (Figure 22-3b).

If you detect epithelial nests at this visit you must care-

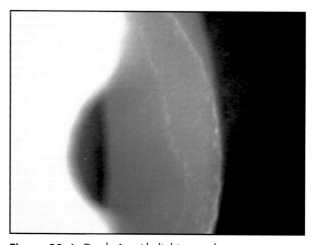

Figure 22-4. Grade 1 epithelial ingrowth.

fully observe this condition, as it can become an aggressive complication. If you are unsure of the existence of ingrowth, it is advised that the patient be asked to return in 7 days. Ingrowth that is carefully observed and properly treated does not and should not complicate the final visual result. However, ingrowth that is not identified and properly managed can become a clinically significant complication. Clinically significant ingrowth is typically treated at 1 month. Treatment involves lifting the flap and scraping the cells from the undersurface of the flap and the surface of the bed. This is the only treatment for ingrowth.

Ingrowth can be classified into three categories according to the Machat Epithelial Ingrowth Grading System:

- Grade 1: This is, by far, the most common variety. Thin ingrowth, usually one to two cells thick, nonprogressive, limited to within 2 mm of the flap edge, transparent, and often difficult to detect. It often has a well-delineated faint white line along the advancing epithelial edge and no associated flap edge changes. No treatment is required, but is usually observed during routine retreatment for refractive error (Figure 22-4).

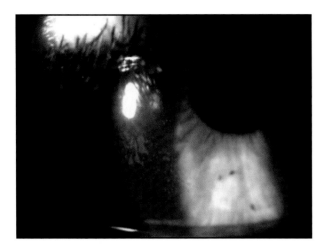

Figure 22-5. Grade 2+ epithelial ingrowth.

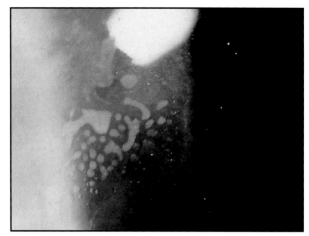

Figure 22-6. Grade 3 epithelial ingrowth.

- Grade 2: Thicker ingrowth; discreet individual cells evident within the nest; usually cells appear vacuolated and translucent, easily detected at the slit lamp, usually at least 2 mm extension, corneal flap edge is usually somewhat thickened, may be rolled or gray, slight melting or erosion of the flap edge may be evident; no demarcation line along the edge of the epithelial nest; typically means it will progress. Requires nonurgent treatment within 2 to 3 weeks. It is easily remedied (Figure 22-5).
- Grade 3: Very pronounced and thickened ingrowth several cells deep: white geographic areas of necrotic epithelial cells, corneal flap margins classically rolled with thickened whitish-gray appearance clinically and eroded. Progression can result in large areas of flap melting due to epithelium sandwiching stroma and the release of collagenase from necrotic epithelium. Confluent haze develops peripheral to the flap edge as the flap pulls away, leaving the exposed stromal bed in contact with surface epithelium. Urgent treatment is required, schedule as soon as possible. Ideally it is advised to treat ingrowth before it progresses to this stage. Grade 3 is difficult to treat because abnormal flap edges invite recurrence of epithelial ingrowth and re-initiates cycle (Figure 22-6).

3. Manifest refraction: The manifest refraction at the 1-week period generally gives us enough information to predict the final refractive outcome.

It is suggested that you fog the patient 3 D while explaining that "I am going to blur the eye chart then slowly change the lenses to improve your vision."

For this reason, you will note the expected values listed below may seem a little high. In reality, they are more representative of the actual refractive result. Too often we tend to overminus the refractive surgery patient. This leads to inaccurate counseling regarding enhancements.

CLINICAL PEARLS

Do not examine the postoperative patient in dim illumination, as it causes pupillary dilation. This dilation can cause pupil/treatment zone interaction and reduce visual acuity as much as two to three lines on the Snellen chart.

Overminus stimulates accommodation and pupillary constriction. This draws the pupil away from the edge of the ablation zone and increases visual acuity. For this reason it is not uncommon to see the laser vision correction patient accept more minus power than is consistent with unaided visual acuity.

This phenomena gradually becomes less significant during the first 3 postoperative months.

The main factor that affects the manifest refraction at this visit is the preoperative prescription. Expectations:
- a. Preoperative = -1 to -6, expect +.5 D Sph to +1 D Sph
- b. Preoperative = -6.25 to -10, expect +1 D Sph to +1.75 D Sph
- c. Preoperative = -10.25 and above, expect +1.5 D Sph to +2.5 D Sph

Thus the refraction can range from +.50 to +2.5 over "target" and still may not require an enhancement when fully stabilized.

If the refraction is:
- > +2.5 = possible overcorrection
- < +1 = possible undercorrection

Stabilization of Refractive Error

Generally, all patients will become stable with their refractive results between 1 and 3 months. For this reason, enhancements should not be considered before the 1-month period and then only when complete stabilization has occurred.

Regression

Most regression occurs between 2 to 4 weeks postoperatively depending on the preoperative prescription.

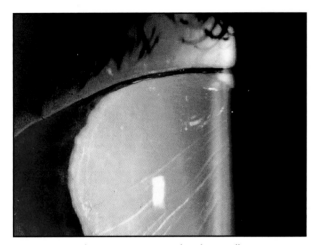

Figure 22-7. Flap striae as viewed with retroillumination.

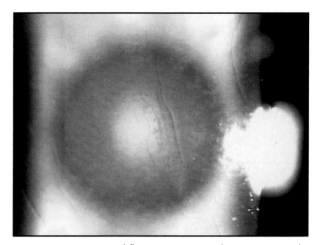

Figure 22-8. Untreated flap striae 13 months postoperatively.

Generally, we will see approximately 90% of the desired result during this time period.

Disposable Contact Lenses

If you detect patient anxiety as a result of significant residual refractive error, then it is suggested you re-establish BCVA with contacts or glasses as soon as possible. Daily wear disposable contact lenses can and should be fit at the 1-week period (assuming intact epithelium).

Average enhancement time frame by refractive error:
- < 3 D = 4 to 6 weeks
- 3 to 6 D = 6 to 8 weeks
- 6 to 9 D = 8 to 12 weeks
- > 9 D = 12 weeks or more

Very important:

4. BCVA: Expected BCVA could be equal to or better than the preoperative BCVA at this visit. Do not become alarmed if there is a loss of BCVA. The majority of times, this apparent loss of BCVA will resolve without further medical intervention. As stated before, each patient reacts to surgery in a different way and heals at a different pace. We have to be able to distinguish between clinical issues that require retreatment and those conditions that will resolve with time.

The main etiology of decreased BCVA at the 1-week postoperative visit is irregular astigmatism. Irregular astigmatism can be located within the flap (epithelium, Bowman's, anterior one-third of the stroma) or the bed (the stromal surface that received the laser beam).

  a. Flap: If the irregular astigmatism is located within the flap it can be either epithelial, stromal, or striae that can involve both the epithelium and the stroma.

- Epithelial: Significant superficial punctate keratitis due to insufficient tear production can cause irregular astigmatism and should be treated with either copious amounts of tear substitute or punctal occlusion.
- Stromal: Stromal edema often resolves on its own. Hyperosmotics can be utilized and are effective.

  3. Striae: This is by far the most significant cause of irregular astigmatism. Striae needs to be confirmed

> **Striae is not a self-limiting condition. If it is clinically significant, it must be retreated at the clinic.**

and, if necessary, evaluated for possible retreatment. Striae is not a self-limiting condition. If it is clinically significant, it must be retreated at the clinic.

Striae can be detected at any time postoperatively, but as we indicated earlier, the sooner you establish clinically significant striae, the easier it is to remedy. It is clinically significant if the striae crosses the visual axis. This generally occurs when the flap is torqued away from the gutter/seam by more than 1 mm. This obviously reduces BCVA and is generally associated with irregular astigmatism and hyperopia.

Subtle striations may not be detected until the 1-week postoperative visit and can best be detected with retroillumination through a dilated examination (Figure 22-7). With the application of fluorescein stain, striae can be highlighted by pooling along the folds. The more apparent the pooling, the more significant the folds.

Significant striae can only be treated by lifting the original flap and smoothing or "ironing" them out. Some surgeons have suggested sutures to reduce striae, but this should not be necessary if detected early and treated appropriately. Striations that are not properly recognized and subsequently treated can result in permanent loss of BCVA. This could necessitate the removal of the flap to reduce the distortion created by the folds (Figure 22-8).

  b. Bed: Irregular astigmatism that is located on the surface of the bed is the result of an abnormal or a decentered ablation pattern.

- Abnormal ablation patterns can be the result of poor laser beam homogeneity, unequal stromal hydration and poor patient fixation. If the irregularity is subtle, it may not create subjective symptoms. However, if the irregularity is severe, it can reduce BCVA. One of the more common forms of this abnormality is central islands.

Central islands: This can only be observed with

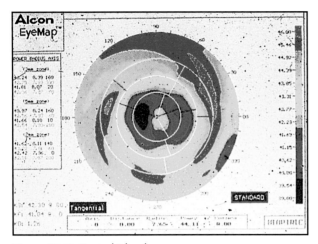

Figure 22-9. Central Island.

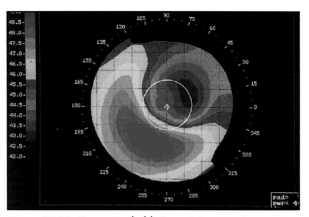

Figure 22-10. Decentered ablation >1.5 mm.

corneal topography (Figure 22-9). There are several theories as to the etiology of the formation of central islands. One of the more popular theories is the Acoustic Shock Wave Theory: Broad beam lasers push stromal fluid peripherally, then as the fluid returns, it forms a pool of moisture centrally blocking the laser beam from ablating tissue. Subjective symptoms may include: monocular diplopia and/or ghosting of images.

Unlike central islands with PRK that generally resolve with time due to epithelial remodeling, central islands with LASIK may need to be retreated with the excimer laser. The original flap is lifted and a few pulses in a 3-mm area are utilized to literally flatten the island. There is no urgency to this complication other than relieving the patient's symptoms. Typically, treatment is indicated between 1 to 3 months. Treatment can take place sooner if the symptoms are very severe, however treatment is rarely performed earlier than 1 month postoperatively.

Decentered ablation: Management of this condition can be challenging for both the co-managing doctor as well as the surgeon. Decentered ablations greater than 1.5 mm (Figure 22-10) and central islands manifest similar subjective symptoms. These symptoms include glare, monocular diplopia, and blur. A differential diagnosis can only be confirmed by corneal topography.

Treatment of this condition requires exceptional surgical skill. Current laser technology in the United States limits the surgeon's ability to treat irregular corneal surfaces such as decentered ablation patterns. The laser systems that have been approved by the US Food and Drug Administration are not capable of customized ablation patterns. Whatever surface irregularity is present before the laser beam is applied will be "mimicked" after the ablation.

Advanced laser technology is available. It is called Topo-Link or topography-assisted laser ablation (see Chapter 40). It couples the corneal topographer with the excimer laser. With this new technology, the laser beam can be directed by computer to the portion of the cornea that requires ablation and avoids that portion of the cornea that

does not require ablation, thus leaving the corneal surface uniform.

It is important to understand that the FDA-approved laser systems are excellent and can effectively treat the majority of refractive disorders.

5. Resumption of normal activities are indicated at the 1-week visit:

- Resume exercise, including swimming
- Resume sports (use common sense with contact sports)
- Resume wearing make-up
- Resume all normal activities

CLINICAL PEARLS

Rule of Thumb

Lower myopes (less than -6 D):

- heal less
- regress less
- stabilize quicker
- less glare
- less dry eye symptoms
- quality of vision returns faster
- can retreat sooner

Higher myopes (greater than -6 D):

- heal more
- regress more
- more glare
- more dry eye symptoms
- stabilize slower
- quality of vision returns slower
- takes longer to stabilize, thus there is a longer time before retreatment

If all clinical findings are within the normal range, the next postoperative visit should be in 3 weeks. This will be considered the 1-month postoperative evaluation.

Shorten the recall visit if there are any concerns at the 1-week visit, such as potential striae complications or epithelial ingrowth. In these cases, the patient should be

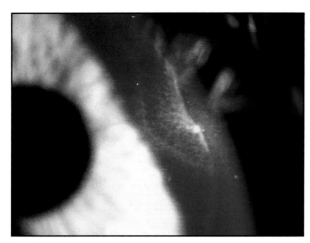

Figure 22-11. Grade 2 epithelial ingrowth with a slight edge roll that appears stable as no advancing nest is evident, less than 2 mm.

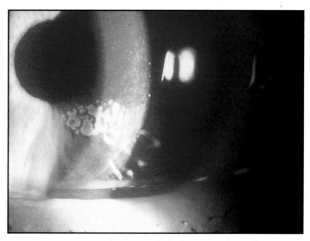

Figure 22-12. Grade 3 epithelial ingrowth with a geographic pattern.

seen in 1 week for further evaluation, do not wait 3 weeks.

The next scheduled visit is at 1 month.

ONE-MONTH POSTOPERATIVE LASIK VISIT:
DETERMINE IF AN ENHANCEMENT IS NECESSARY
Purpose of visit
1. Recheck flap position and corneal integrity
2. Measure UCVA
3. Determine manifest refraction and BCVA
4. Evaluate IOP
5. Plan enhancement possibility

Test
1. UCVA
2. Biomicroscopy
3. Corneal topography/keratometry
4. Manifest refraction
5. Applanation tonometry

Expectations
1. UCVA: 20/15 to 20/40, or in the case of monovision target near visual acuity.
2. Biomicroscopy: The cornea should be clear and the flap edge may be undetectable at this visit. However, there may be a slight edge roll of < 1 mm, scarring at the edge of the seam of < 1 mm, and/or a grade 1 ingrowth, but these conditions are considered nonprogressive and therefore need only be documented and observed (Figure 22-11).

Any epithelial ingrowth that exceeds 2 mm (Figure 22-12) needs to be evaluated by the center for possible treatment. Ingrowth that is less than 1.5 mm may not advance

> We must always remember that although it is rare, untreated epithelial ingrowth can lead to stromal melt. If this melt occurs within the pupillary margin, this can result in permanent loss of corneal tissue resulting in glare symptoms with possible loss of BCVA.

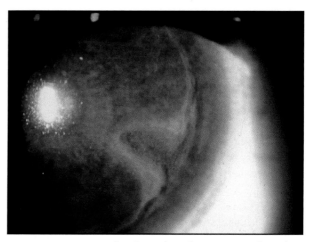

Figure 22-13. Stromal melt resulting from untreated grade 3 epithelial ingrowth.

and therefore may not need to be treated. If there is any question about ingrowth, it is always safe to have the center evaluate the patient and make a judgment as to the degree of the condition. We must always remember that although it is rare, untreated epithelial ingrowth can lead to stromal melt (Figure 22-13). If this melt occurs within the pupillary margin, it can result in permanent loss of corneal tissue and the need for surgical removal of the flap with possible loss of BCVA. Generally, if there is no evidence of ingrowth at 1 month you will not see it develop.

3. Corneal topography/keratometry: With corneal topography there should be a well-centered ablation pattern. As described in the 1-week visit, any decentration of the ablation should be < 1.5 mm. If there is decentration > 1.5 mm, it could result in a variety of symptoms including glare, monocular diplopia, and blur. At this time, an incomplete circular ablation pattern (Figure 22-14a) is not unusual and is generally due to incomplete healing. This will typically take 2 to 3 months to resolve and is not associated with loss of BCVA (Figure 22-14b). With keratometry, the mires

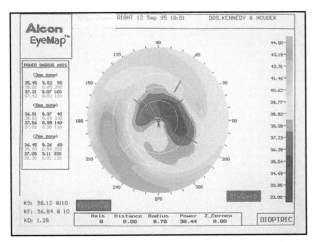

Figure 22-14a. Incomplete circular ablation pattern due to incomplete healing 3 weeks post-LASIK.

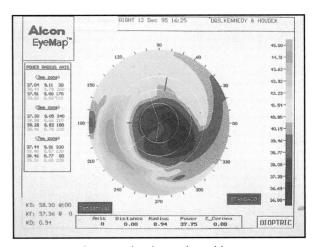

Figure 22-14b. Completed circular ablation pattern 4 months post-LASIK.

should be relatively sharp with the possibility of slight micro-irregularity.

4. Manifest refraction: The results at this postoperative time period depend on the patient's preoperative refraction and age.

    <u>a. Myopia between -.75 D to -6 D sph</u>

    All ages: The refraction should be within .25 D to .5 D of target

    <u>b. Myopia between -6.12 D to -15 D sph</u>

    Age 18 to 39: Refraction should be within .5 D to .75 D of target

    Age 40 to 65: Refraction should be within .25 D to .5 D of target

The greater the myopia and the younger the patient, the more regression you can expect. Conversely, the lower the myopia and older the patient, the less regression you will observe.

5. Applanation tonometry: It is generally accepted that applanation tonometry is the standard of care when evaluating IOP. The noncontact tonometer may be used to determine IOPs post-PRK/LASIK, but we have found that the results are not as consistent as with applanation measurements.

Recent studies have demonstrated that patients who have undergone PRK or LASIK surgery consistently demonstrate IOPs 3 to 4 mm Hg lower than their preoperative measurements.

Goldmann applanation is based on a normal corneal thickness of 550 μm and a normal curvature cornea. With laser refractive surgery we may reduce corneal thickness by as much as 50 to 150 μm and flatten the cornea by several diopters.

Since the cornea is thinner following laser surgery, there is less corneal resistance and we obtain lower pressure readings. It is important to understand that the actual IOP is unchanged. Our measurements have a lower value as a result of less corneal resistance and altered curvature, not as

a result of lower intraocular fluid volume.

Example: Preoperative IOPs of 18 mm Hg by Goldmann applanation may read 15 mm Hg postoperatively with a patient treated for -5 D. Because the cornea has been thinned at the point of applanation (centrally), we are obtaining lower than normal readings.

6. Consultation: If the patient's results are within all expected parameters both visually and physically, continued reassurance is recommended. Schedule a return visit in 2 months.

If there are any structural issues, such as possible epithelial ingrowth or clinically significant striae, the patient should be reassured that although he or she may not be healing exactly as expected, vision will improve with time or can be corrected. If there are any questions regarding these issues, the patient should be returned to the center.

Refractive issues: Too often we make assessments regarding the residual refractive error at this visit. Although it is true that with low to moderate myopia the refractive results can be stable at 4 to 6 weeks, it is not unusual with higher degrees of myopia and hyperopia to take an additional 4 to 6 weeks to stabilize. Caution: do not preempt your discussion regarding enhancements until complete stabilization has occurred.

Enhancements of low to moderate myopia: If complete stabilization has been established, retreatment can be performed anytime after 6 weeks. Retreatment at this time is performed by lifting the original flap and re-ablating the stromal bed. After 6 months, a new corneal flap must be cut.

The next scheduled visit is at 3 months.

THREE-MONTH POSTOPERATIVE LASIK VISIT:
FINAL DETERMINATION FOR ENHANCEMENT
Purpose of visit

1. Measure UCVA
2. Recheck flap and corneal integrity
3. Determine manifest refraction and BCVA

4. Evaluate IOP

5. Discuss potential enhancement of residual refractive error

Test

1. UCVA

2. Biomicroscopy

3. Corneal topography/keratometry

4. Cycloplegic refraction

5. Applanation tonometry

Expectations

1. UCVA: At this visit there should be stabilization of refractive error. We should be at or near our target.

2. Biomicroscopy: The flap should be intact without clinically significant striae, and a thin white scar along the seam (Bowman's layer) should be visible (Figure 22-15). There may be a slight roll anywhere along the edge of the seam as well as a grade 1 epithelial ingrowth. These are all normal observations at this visit.

3. Corneal topography/keratometry: A well-centered ablation pattern should be present as well as sharp keratometry mires.

4. Cycloplegic refraction: It is suggested that a cycloplegic refraction be performed at this visit. It is easy to overminus the patient in an attempt to obtain BCVA. This often leads to over-referrals for enhancements.

Enhancement Qualifications

The patient becomes a candidate for enhancement if:

- the refractive error is =/> .75 from the target
- visual acuity is 20/40 or less
- residual astigmatism =/> 1 D
- stabilization of refractive error has been established

5. Applanation tonometry: Tonometry results should be consistent with the readings from the 1-month visit.

6. Consultation: Careful consideration regarding enhancements should be made. Many patients are not unhappy with their vision regardless of the result. As concerned practitioners, we tend to place our expectations on the patient and often convince them that an enhancement is necessary. My clinical experience has shown that most patients do not want to undergo further surgical procedures.

> As concerned practitioners, we tend to place our expectations on the patient and often convince them that an enhancement is necessary. My clinical experience has shown that most patients do not want to undergo further surgical procedures.

CLINICAL PEARLS

Patients whose corneal pachymetry readings were initially borderline, as with high myopia, should be enhanced between the 3- and 6-month visit. This is so we can lift the original flap and not have to make a new cut. Be aware that

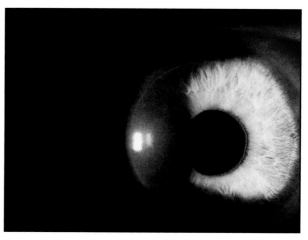

Figure 22-15. Classic faint white line along the seam (Bowman's scar) 3 months post-LASIK.

some patients, especially those with high preoperative prescriptions may not have adequate tissue for enhancement, respective of timing.

It should be our responsibility to advise rather than recommend. Whatever the refractive result, it is important we stress patience. Time and/or enhancement procedures generally resolve most complications.

The next scheduled visit is at 6 months postoperatively.

SIX-MONTH POSTOPERATIVE LASIK VISIT: DETERMINE STABILITY

Purpose of visit

1. Evaluate UCVA

2. Evaluate corneal integrity

3. Evaluate cycloplegic refraction and BCVA

4. Evaluate IOP

Test

1. UCVA

2. Biomicroscopy

3. Corneal topography/keratometry

4. Cycloplegic refraction

5. Applanation tonometry

Expectations

1. UCVA: At this visit there should be stabilization of refractive error. We should be at or near our target. Enhancement qualifications are the same as described at the 3-month visit.

2. Biomicroscopy: The flap should be intact without clinically significant striae, and a thin white scar along the seam (Bowman's layer) should be visible.

3. Corneal topography/keratometry: A well-centered ablation pattern should be present as well as sharp keratometry mires.

4. Cycloplegic refraction: It is suggested that a cycloplegic refraction be performed at this visit. It is easy to over minus the patient in an attempt to obtain BCVA. This often leads to over-referrals for enhancements.

5. Applanation tonometry: Tonometry results should be

consistent with the readings from the 1- and 3-month visit.

6. Consultation: Generally, the refractive status is stable at this visit. With the absence of any clinical issues, the patient is instructed to return in 6 months and yearly thereafter. It is important to stress the importance of annual examinations to assure good ocular health. It is critical that the patient understand that his or her eyes are still "myopic" and thus subject to all inherent risks of myopia.

7. The next scheduled visit is 1 year postoperatively. The patient is again reminded that yearly comprehensive examinations are necessary not only to confirm stability of their surgical outcome but also to assure good ocular health is maintained.

SECTION SEVEN
LASIK Results and Evaluation

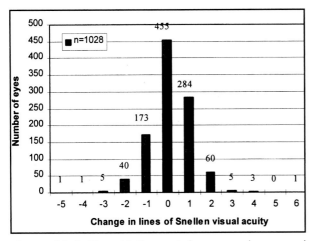

Figure 23-8. (Summit) Change in best spectacle-corrected visual acuity at the last postoperative visit (n = 1028).

Of the 25 intraoperative flap complications, there were 10 free flaps, eight incomplete flaps, four flap buttonholes, one thin flap, one thick flap, and one bilaminar flap.

23-3. Two of these 15 eyes subsequently underwent uncomplicated LASIK several months later. Only two of these 25 eyes with intraoperative flap complications lost two or more lines of BSCVA, both due to flap buttonholes. BSCVA changed from 20/15 to 20/25 and from 20/20 to 20/40 in these two eyes.

Postoperative complications consisted of eight partially dislocated and four totally dislocated flaps. In each case, the flaps were repositioned within 1 to 2 days after surgery with no loss of BSCVA greater than one line. Twenty eyes developed epithelial ingrowth that was significant enough to warrant flap revision and removal of epithelium from the stromal bed. One patient developed bilateral keratitis of the flap interface 24 hours after surgery, but microbial cultures were negative. It was hypothesized that the inflammation was a response to materials that may have been introduced into the cornea at the time of surgery. The keratitis resolved in both eyes and unaided visual acuity was 20/25 and 20/20. Two eyes developed significant flap folds that were not recognized at the 24-hour postoperative visit. Only one of the 40 eyes with postoperative complications lost two or more lines of BSCVA from 20/20 to 20/40. This occurred in one of the eyes with postoperative flap folds.

Postoperative complications consisted of eight partially dislocated and four totally dislocated flaps.

Epithelial ingrowth was significant enough to warrant surgical removal in 20 (1.4%) eyes. However, in the majority of eyes, epithelial ingrowth either resolved spontaneously or remained at a clinically insignificant level. None of the eyes with epithelial ingrowth requiring flap revision lost two or more lines of BSCVA.

TABLE 23-1.
SUMMIT INTRAOPERATIVE FLAP COMPLICATIONS

Type	Number	Ablates	> 2 lines of lost BCVA
Free	10	4	
Normal	5	2	
Small	5	2	
Incomplete	8	2	
Hole	4	2	2
Thin	1	1	
Thick	1	1	
Split/bilaminar	1		
Totals	25	10	2 (1 ablated)[*]

[*]*Lines lost: 2 (20/16 to 20/25) and 2 (20/20 to 20/40)*

TABLE 23-2.
SUMMIT POSTOPERATIVE COMPLICATIONS

Type	Number	> 2 lines of loss of BSCVA
Slippage, partial	8	0
Slippage, total	4	0
Epithelial ingrowth	20	0
Keratitis, culture negative	2	0
Flap folds	2	1[*]
Totals	36	1

[*]*Lines Lost: 2 (20/20 to 20/40)*

THE NIDEK INVESTIGATION

The mean preoperative spherical equivalent refraction of this consecutive series of 119 eyes was -5.25 D (range: -1 D to -14.25 D). Mean preoperative cylinder was 1.1 D (range: 0 D to 4 D). At the time of analysis, data was available for 119 eyes at the 3-month postoperative visit. Twenty-five eyes received spherical laser ablation and 94 eyes received toric ablation.

The change in spherical equivalent refraction 3 months after LASIK is shown as a function of attempted correction in Figure 23-9. Sixty-three percent (75 of 119) of eyes were within ± .5 D of intended correction, and 81.5% (97 of 119) were within ± 1 D.

Figure 23-10 shows UCVA 3 months after LASIK after exclusion of 12 eyes that were intentionally undercorrected for monovision. 85% of eyes (91 of 108) achieved UCVA of 20/40 or better, and 44.9% of eyes (48 of 108) saw 20/20 or better.

For spherical ablation (n = 25), the mean vector-induced astigmatism was .06 D (.3 D SD) with no significant axis orientation. Toric ablation (n = 94) reduced the preoperative cylinder magnitude by 94.9 %. The mean axis error (±SD)

TABLE 23-3.
SUMMIT BSCVA FOR 15 INTRAOPERATIVE FLAP COMPLICATIONS AND NO LASER ABLATION

Case	Preop BSCVA	Final BSCVA	Change in BSCVA (lines)	Intraoperative flap complication
1*	20/20	20/16	+1	Free flap
2	20/20	20/20	0	Free flap
3	20/20	20/16	+1	Free flap
4	20/16	20/20	-1	Free flap
5	20/20	20/20	0	Free flap
6	20/25	20/30	-1	Free flap
7*	20/20	20/20	0	Incomplete flap
8	20/20	20/20	0	Incomplete flap
9	20/20	20/20	0	Incomplete flap
10	20/20	20/20	0	Incomplete flap
11	20/16	20/16	0	Incomplete flap
12	20/30	20/25	+1	Incomplete flap
13	20/20	20/20	0	Buttonhole in flap
14	20/16	20/25	-2	Buttonhole in flap
15	20/20	20/20	0	Split/bilaminar flap

Subsequently had uncomplicated LASIK

was 4.5 (±25) for cylindrical ablations below 1 D, -.8 (±10.8) for cylindrical ablations of 1 D to 2 D, and .9 (±5.2) for cylindrical ablations above 2 D.

The change in BSCVA 3 months after LASIK is shown in Figure 23-11. Thirty-seven eyes gained one or more lines of BSCVA; 12 eyes lost one or more lines of BSCVA; and 70 eyes showed no change in BSCVA. One eye (.8%) lost two or more lines of BSCVA, changing from 20/15 preoperatively to 20/25 postoperatively.

There were 10 complications: three were intraoperative and seven (2.4%) were postoperative (Table 23-4). All three of the intraoperative flap complications were free flaps; laser ablation proceeded uneventfully and the flaps were repositioned. None of these three eyes lost lines of BSCVA as a result of flap complications.

None of the eyes with postoperative complications lost two or more lines of BSCVA. Postoperative complications included one partially dislocated and one totally dislocated flap. In both cases, the flaps were repositioned on the first postoperative day with no loss of BSCVA. Three eyes developed epithelial ingrowth that was significant enough to warrant flap revision and removal of epithelium from the stromal bed. There were no cases of keratitis in this investigation. Two eyes developed significant flap striae that required flap repositioning. Neither of the eyes with flap striae lost BCVA.

> None of the eyes with postoperative complications lost two or more lines of BSCVA.

DISCUSSION

The Emory Summit and Nidek investigations are in agreement with previous reports of safety and efficacy of LASIK for the correction of myopia,[1-4,6-8,11-21] This chapter reports the results of 1028 consecutive eyes undergoing LASIK for myopia with a Summit excimer laser and 119 consecutive eyes undergoing LASIK with a Nidek laser at the Emory Vision Correction Center. The patients in these two investigations had myopia ranging from -1 to -21.5 D.

Eyes from the Summit investigation received spherical laser ablations, and astigmatism was corrected with Arc-T at the time of LASIK or as an enhancement procedure. In contrast, eyes from the Nidek investigation received either spherical or toric laser ablation depending on the presence of astigmatism. A comparison of LASIK outcomes of Summit and Nidek eyes is therefore limited by the different techniques that were employed in the two investigations to treat astigmatism. Follow-up in the Nidek group was 3 months, and none of the eyes received enhancement procedures; follow-up in the Summit group averaged 9.5 months and enhancement data were included. Three months after primary LASIK, 63% of Nidek-treated eyes achieved a postoperative spherical equivalent that was within .5 D of intended outcome compared to 58% of Summit-treated eyes after 9.5 months including enhancement data (p = .35).

Comparison of outcomes for two different excimer lasers can be potentially misleading, as one can erroneously compare the relative accuracy of the laser algorithms that the two systems currently use instead of a true comparison. Figures 23-12a and 23-12b show average refractive out-

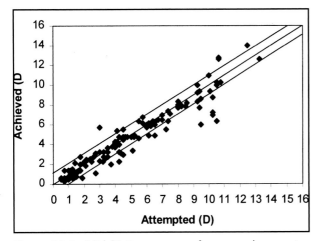

Figure 23-9. (Nidek) Scattergram of attempted correction versus achieved change in spherical equivalent at 3 months postoperatively (n = 119).

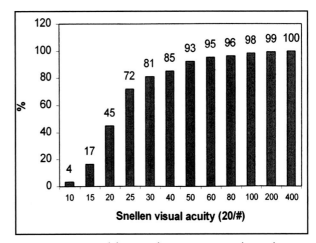

Figure 23-10. (Nidek) Cumulative uncorrected visual acuity data at the last postoperative visit, excluding 12 monovision eyes (n = 107).

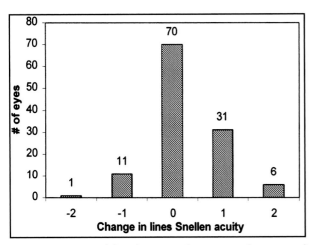

Figure 23-11. (Nidek) Change in best spectacle-corrected visual acuity at 3 months after LASIK (n = 119).

T A B L E 23-4.
NIDEK POSTOPERATIVE COMPLICATIONS

Type	Number	> 2 line loss of BSCVA
Slippage,		
partial	1	0
total	1	0
Epithelial ingrowth	3	0
Flap striae	2	0
Total	**7**	**0**

come with respect to time for two theoretical laser systems. In Figure 23-12a, laser "A" achieves an outcome that is consistently closer to emmetropia than laser "B" at all postoperative time intervals. The fact that the error bars are identical in magnitude for "A" and "B" indicates, however, that there is no true difference between the two laser systems. Improvement of the laser nomogram for "B" will eliminate the difference in outcome that was observed. In Figure 23-12b, laser "A" still achieves an outcome consistently closer to emmetropia than "B." However, the variability of refractive outcome is much less for laser "B" as evidenced by the smaller error bars. In this situation, there is a true difference between lasers in that laser "B" will achieve a better average refractive outcome than laser "A" after modification of the laser "B" nomogram. In addition to laser "B" having less variability in outcome (smaller error bars), we would expect the percentage of eyes achieving a postoperative refraction within .5 D of intended outcome to be higher for laser "B." Therefore, true differences in the potential out-

come of the two laser systems can be inferred from a comparison of the standard deviation of average refractive outcome or by a comparison of the percentage of eyes within .5 D of intended outcome. Comparison of UCVA data is misleading and is confounded by patient age, preoperative BCVA worse than 20/20, and the current accuracy of laser nomograms for the two systems.

The vector analysis of toric Nidek ablations revealed that 94.5% of the preoperative cylinder was corrected by laser ablation. The average axis error was small, and the standard deviation of mean axis error was lower for the larger cylindrical ablations. We hypothesize that the 5.2° standard deviation for cylindrical ablations over 2 D is a reasonable estimate of alignment error. It is likely that the larger standard deviation that was observed for the lower cylindrical ablations was confounded by measurement error in determination of cylinder axis (during refraction) together with small random changes in cylinder as a result of the corneal flap being created and reflected back into position.

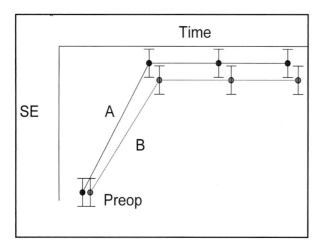

Figure 23-12a. Theoretical comparison of two excimer laser systems (A and B) showing mean refractive outcome (y) with respect to time (x). Laser A achieves an average postoperative spherical equivalent refraction that is closer to emmetropia than laser B for all postoperative intervals. The magnitude of the error bars are identical for A and B, indicating that there is no intrinsic difference between A and B. Modification of the nomogram for laser B would eliminate the difference in mean refractive outcome between A and B.

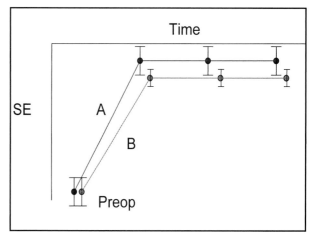

Figure 23-12b. As with Figure 23-12a, laser A again achieves an average postoperative spherical equivalent refraction that is closer to emmetropia than B at all postoperative intervals. However, in this example, the error bars are smaller for laser B, indicating that B is potentially more accurate than laser A. Modification of the laser nomogram for laser B would achieve a more accurate average refractive outcome than would be possible for laser A, allowing a larger percentage of eyes to achieve a spherical equivalent refraction within .5 D of intended outcome.

The intent to treat analysis of procedure safety for the Summit investigation included all cases performed during the "surgical learning curve" for surgeons who did not have previous microkeratome experience. The Summit LASIK safety data therefore provides a realistic indication of procedure safety for surgeons who perform the procedure with no previous lamellar surgery experience.

In our investigations, the percentage of eyes losing two or more lines of BSCVA was 4.6% for Summit and .8% for Nidek. The difference can be explained in part by differences in the incidence of intraoperative flap complications. The three Nidek flap complications were all free flaps, which did not prevent the surgeon from proceeding with laser ablation, with no loss of BSCVA. In contrast, there were buttonhole flaps in the Summit study that were associated with loss of BCVA. One other possible explanation for the difference in loss of BSCVA is a difference in the occurrence of irregular astigmatism or videokeratographic pattern in the two groups; however, videokeratographic and gas-permeable contact lens over-refraction data for the two groups has not been analyzed.

> The percentage of eyes losing two or more lines of BSCVA was 4.6% for Summit and .8% for Nidek.

The Summit investigation documented a learning curve whereby the intraoperative complication rate for inexperienced lamellar surgeons decreased from 9% (2 of 22) in the first quarter of the study to 2.7% (4 of 148) in the fourth quarter (data not shown).[10] Our data is in agreement with that of Gimbel, who also demonstrated the existence of a learning curve for LASIK (Incidence and management of intra/peri-operative complications in 1000 consecutive LASIK cases. Gimbel HV. Annual Meeting of the American Academy of Ophthalmology, October 1997, San Francisco).

Perhaps the most important issue in interpretation of LASIK outcomes is examination of the data in relation to the safety and efficacy data of alternative procedures such as PRK. This allows an assessment of the range of myopia that can reasonably be treated with each procedure. The upper limit of myopia for LASIK is governed by the increased incidence of optical side effects that would occur as one decreased the multizone ablation diameters to minimize ablation depth. The upper limit of myopia for PRK is limited by the increased likelihood for corneal scarring when higher dioptric corrections are performed.[22-30] The lower limit of myopia at which LASIK would be considered can be determined by the loss of BSCVA in relation to that for PRK. A previous report of LASIK performed at Emory Vision Correction Center stratified the outcome with respect to preoperative myopia.[31] This allowed comparison of safety and efficacy data with McCarty's large PRK study.[32] Patients with less than 5 D of preoperative myopia had a 1.1% incidence of loss of 2 or more lines of BSCVA following LASIK and increased to 7.3% for patients with 10 D or more of preoperative myopia. In McCarty's series, 4% of eyes lost two or more lines of BSCVA for myopia below 5 D; this increased to 8% for myopia between 5 and 10 D and to 22% for myopic PRK above 10 D. While it is undesirable for any patient to lose BSCVA, fewer patients undergoing LASIK lost two lines or more of BSCVA than did patients undergoing PRK in McCarty's study in each category of myopia studied. Comparison of efficacy showed that LASIK and PRK were equivalent for myopia below 5 D, and LASIK was superior for myopia above 5 D. The actual lower limit of myopia for LASIK should be a personal decision for each surgeon and patient and is dependent on the particular surgeon's LASIK intraoperative complication rate.

> Fewer patients undergoing LASIK lost two lines or more of BSCVA than did patients undergoing PRK.

LASIK can correct larger amounts of myopia than PRK because LASIK avoids breach of Bowman's layer, except at the margin of the corneal flap that is created with the microkeratome. Additional advantages of LASIK over PRK include a more rapid recovery of vision, less postoperative discomfort, less need for postoperative management, and the ability to refine or adjust the outcome of the initial surgery more easily. Disadvantages of LASIK compared to PRK include the potential for intraoperative complications caused by the microkeratome, the need for more skill on the part of the surgeon and operating room team, and the additional cost and complexity of the microkeratome required for surgery.

In summary, we have demonstrated the safety and efficacy of LASIK for correction of myopia and myopic astigmatism. LASIK at Emory Vision Correction Center is comparable in safety and efficacy to PRK below 5 D of myopia and superior to PRK above 5 D. The Emory LASIK system is now the preferred method for treating myopia up to -15 D.

REFERENCES

1. Pallikaris IG, Papatzanaki ME, Stathi EZ, Frenschock O, Georgiadis A. Laser in situ keratomileusis. *Lasers Surg Med.* 1990;10(5):463-8.

2. Pallikaris IG, Papatzanaki ME, Siganos DS, Tsilimbaris MK. A corneal flap technique for laser in situ keratomileusis. Human studies. *Arch Ophthalmol.* 1991;109(12):1699-702.

3. Pallikaris IG, Siganos DS. Excimer laser in situ keratomileusis and photorefractive keratectomy for correction of high myopia. *J Refract Corneal Surg.* 1994;10(5):498-510.

4. Brint SF, Ostrick DM, Fisher C, et al. Six-month results of the multicenter phase I study of excimer laser myopic keratomileusis. *J Cataract Refract Surg.* 1994;20(6):610-5.

5. Kremer FB, Dufek M. Excimer laser in situ keratomileusis. *J Refract Surg.* 1995;11:S244-7.

6. Fiander DC, Tayfour F. Excimer laser in situ keratomileusis in 124 myopic eyes. *J Refract Surg.* 1995;11:S234-8.

7. Salah T, Waring GO III, el-Maghraby A, Moadel K, Grimm SB. Excimer laser in-situ keratomileusis (LASIK) under a corneal flap for myopia of 2 to 20 D. *Trans Am Ophthalmol Soc.* 1995;93(163):163-83.

8. Salah T, Waring GO III, el-Maghraby A, Moadel K, Grimm SB. Excimer laser in situ keratomileusis under a corneal flap for myopia of 2 to 20 diopters. *Am J Ophthalmol.* 1996;121(2):143-55. Comments.

9. Carr JD, Nardone R, Stulting RD, Thompson KP, Waring GO III. Risk factors for epithelial ingrowth after LASIK. *Invest Ophthalmol Vis Sci.* 1997;38(4):S232.

10. Stulting RD, Balch K, Carr JD, Walter K, Thompson KP, Waring GO III. Complications of laser in-situ keratomileusis. *Invest Ophthalmol Vis Sci.* 1997;38:S231.

11. Kremer I, Blumenthal M. Myopic keratomileusis in situ combined with VISX 20/20 photorefractive keratectomy. *J Cataract Refract Surg.* 1995;21(5):508-11.

12. Kohlhaas M, Lerche RC, Draeger J, Arnott E, Williams K. Keratomileusis with a lamellar microkeratome and the excimer laser. *Ophthalmologe.* 1995;92(4):499-502.

13. Bas AM, Onnis R. Excimer laser in situ keratomileusis for myopia. *J Refract Surg.* 1995;11:S229-33.

14. Guell JL, Muller A. Laser in situ keratomileusis (LASIK) for myopia from -7 to -18 diopters. *Journal of Refractive Surgery.* 1996;12(2):222-8.

15. Marinho A, Pinto MC, Pinto R, Vaz F, Neves MC. LASIK for high myopia: 1-year experience. *Ophthalmic Surgery and Lasers.* 1996;27:S517-20.

16. Helmy SA, Salah A, Badawy TT, Sidky AN. Photorefractive keratectomy and laser in situ keratomileusis for myopia between 6 and 10 diopters. *Journal of Refractive Surgery.* 1996;12(3):417-21.

17. Gimbel HV, Basti S, Kaye GB, Ferensowicz M. Experience during the learning curve of laser in situ keratomileusis. *J Cataract Refract Surg.* 1996;22(5):542-50. Comments.

18. Knorz MC, Liermann A, Seiberth V, Steiner H, Wiesinger B. Laser in situ keratomileusis to correct myopia of -6 to -29 diopters. *Journal of Refractive Surgery.* 1996;12(5):575-84.

19. Kim HM, Jung HR. Laser assisted in situ keratomileusis for high myopia. *Ophthalmic Surgery and Lasers.* 1996;:S508-11.

20. Condon PI, Mulhern M, Fulcher T, Foley NA, O'Keefe M. Laser intrastromal keratomileusis for high myopia and myopic astigmatism. *Br J Ophthalmol.* 1997;81(3):199-206.

21. Pallikaris IG, Siganos DS. Laser in situ keratomileusis to treat myopia: early experience. *J Cataract Refract Surg.* 1997;23(1):39-49.

22. Talamo JH, Siebert K, Wagoner MD, Yeh E, Telfair W. Multicenter study of photorefractive keratectomy for myopia of 6 to 8 diopters. VISX moderate myopia study group. *Journal of Refractive Surgery.* 1995;11(4):238-47.

23. Siganos DS, Pallikaris IG, Margaritis VN. Photorefractive keratectomy with a transition zone for myopia from -7 to -14 diopters. *Journal of Refractive Surgery.* 1996;12(2):S261-3.

24. Rajendran B, Janakiraman P. Multizone photorefractive keratectomy for myopia of 8 to 23 diopters. *Journal of Refractive Surgery.* 1995;11:S298-301.

25. Zato MA, Matilla A, Gomez T, Jimenez V. Multizone versus monozone in the treatment of high and moderate myopia with an excimer laser. *Ophthalmic Surgery and Lasers.* 1996;27:S466-S470.

26. Chan WK, Heng WJ, Tseng P, Balakrishnan V, Chan TK, Low CH. Photorefractive keratectomy for myopia of 6 to 12 diopters. *Journal of Refractive Surgery.* 1995;11:S286-S292.

27. Kremer I, Gabbay U, Blumenthal M. One-year follow-up results of photorefractive keratectomy for low, moderate, and high primary astigmatism. *Ophthalmology*. 1996;103(5):741-8.

28. Rogers CM, Lawless MA, Cohen PR. Photorefractive keratectomy for myopia of more than -10 diopters. *J Refract Corneal Surg*. 1994;10(2):S171-S173.

29. Sher NA, Hardten DR, Fundingsland B, et al. 193-nm excimer photorefractive keratectomy in high myopia. *Ophthalmology*. 1994;101(9):1575-82.

30. Moller-Pedersen T, Vogel M, Li HF, Petroll WM, Cavanagh HD, Jester JV. Late onset corneal haze after photorefractive keratectomy for moderate and high myopia. *Ophthalmology*. 1997;104(3):369-73.

31. Carr JD, Stulting RD, Thompson KP, Waring GO III. Laser in-situ keratomileusis. In: Abbot RL, Hwang DG, eds. *Ophthalmology Clinics of North America*. WB Saunders Co: Philadelphia, Pa; 1997:533-542.

32. McCarty CA, Aldred GF, Taylor HR, et al. Comparison of results of excimer laser correction of all degrees of myopia at 12 months postoperatively. *Am J Ophthalmol*. 1996;121:372-383.

CHAPTER 24

The CRS LASIK Study

Guy M. Kezirian, MD, FACS
J. Charles Casebeer, MD

INTRODUCTION

Refractive surgeons in the United States were faced with an unexpected dilemma in late 1995 and early 1996 when the US Food and Drug Administration (FDA) approved the Summit Apex and VISX Star lasers for use in photorefractive keratectomy (PRK).

Aware of international reports about the benefits of laser in situ keratomileusis (LASIK) and the risks of PRK, many surgeons preferred to use the lasers to perform LASIK rather than PRK. However, so-called "off-label" use of approved devices presented liability risks, and of more immediate concern, it was uncertain whether the treatment algorithms for PRK would work for treatments performed beneath a surface layer.

In response, the CRS LASIK study was launched as a collaborative effort to study the use of FDA-approved lasers in LASIK. The project began in April 1996 with the original goal of evaluating the safety and efficacy of the lasers in LASIK and developing a modification of the PRK nomogram to perform LASIK ablations.

It met with immediate success. Within 2 months, more than 50 surgeons were enrolled, and by November the number of participants had increased to more than 100. It has grown since then to more than 230 surgeon participants. Originally, the study set out to evaluate the two lasers in

> The CRS LASIK study was launched with the original goal of evaluating the safety and efficacy of the lasers in LASIK.

their FDA-approved range of treatments. Now, the study administers several protocols to study treatments beyond the approved range, including high myopia, astigmatism, and hyperopia.

This article describes the administrative and clinical features of the project and includes a report of the approved range of study results.

METHODS

ADMINISTRATIVE ORGANIZATION

The study was originally designed as an independent off-label study, but within a few months of its organization, it was required to submit an application for an Investigational Device Exemption (IDE) investigation under FDA supervision. This requirement added a significant administrative burden to the project but also provided the opportunity to study LASIK treatments beyond the approved range of the lasers.

Four groups participate in the study's administration, and each plays a specific and vital role. CRS Clinical Research, Inc is the administrating sponsor of the study. CRS is a non-profit clinical research company located in Scottsdale, Ariz, and incorporated in California. Participants in CRS include J. Charles Casebeer, MD as chairman; Stephen Slade, MD, of Houston Texas; Luis Ruiz, MD, of Bogota, Colombia; Marguerite McDonald, MD, of New Orleans, La; Richard Lindstrom, MD, of Minneapolis, Minn; and George Waring, MD, of Atlanta, Ga.

The International Society of Refractive Surgery (ISRS) acts as the participating peer group affiliated with the study. The president-elect of ISRS, Jeffery Robin, MD, of Cleveland, Ohio, became involved early in the project and suggested that involving the ISRS would bring added credibility to the grassroots effort. The role of the affiliated peer group is to provide an institutional presence and forum for communication. Meetings of investigators are often held in conjunction with meetings of the ISRS, and the ISRS has offered its *Journal of Refractive Surgery* as an avenue for publication of study reports.

Data.Site, Inc (formerly RSS) of Kansas City, Mo, was contracted to provide online databasing services for the project. The involvement of Data.Site provides the study with state-of-the-art online communications, permitting online data entry and custom generated reports. In addition, the service includes online discussion forums for investigators to share information among themselves using an electronic bulletin board.

To coordinate communication between these groups and to facilitate interaction with investigators, CRS USA, Inc retained the services of SurgiVision Consultants, Inc, a refractive surgery consulting firm located in Paradise Valley, Ariz. SurgiVision Consultants, Inc is run by Guy M. Kezirian, MD, FACS.

The current medical monitors of the study include J. Charles Casebeer, MD; Dan Durrie, MD; Stephen Slade, MD; Dick Lindstrom, MD; and Jeff Robin, MD. Rounding out the administrative group is George Waring, MD, who provides consulting services to the study, and a growing group of advisors who offer assistance in their field of expertise. Currently, the advisory group consists of Jack Holladay, MD (optics), Casimir Swinger, MD (keratomes), Steve Brint, MD (Summit Laser), Ron Krueger (contrast sensitivity), and Lanny Hale (imaging).

FUNDING

To maintain independence from industry, the study is funded solely by the participating surgeons. As a collegiate effort, any qualified ophthalmologist interested in participating is invited to join provided they meet the published requirements and comply with study procedures.

Self-funding has many benefits. Dissociating funding from the commercial interests of the device opens the study to a broad range of considerations that might otherwise be unaffordable. For example, one of the main thrusts of the study has been to provide each surgeon with a treatment nomogram developed from his or her individual outcomes. This has been expensive, and has limited significance to the device per se, but it has immediate utility to the investigators. Furthermore, independent funding ensures that negative outcomes can be communicated among investigators (and to the

profession) without concern for proprietarial consequences.

The drawbacks of self-funding are obvious. Enrollment fees prohibit some surgeons from participating. They add to the expense of performing the procedures in a field that is already at risk from high costs. The limitations of surgeon funding restrict the rate at which the study can grow. Nevertheless, self-funding allows the project to maintain independence and is seen as essential to the project's goal of independent validation of the procedure.

FDA CONSIDERATIONS: IDE VERSUS PRIDE

As previously mentioned, the restructuring of the project as an IDE under FDA supervision was imposed on the study, but it was not undertaken by choice. In turn, however, the FDA has allowed the protocols to be modified as new information is obtained. For example, treatment algorithms can be modified according to outcomes as treatment nomograms become more established. This distinction of the project from the usual IDE format, with the ability to modify protocols to consider new information, has been termed a PRIDE, or practical reality IDE.

The following aspects distinguish a PRIDE from a typical IDE. They are:
1. As a physician-sponsored project, it may not necessarily lead to a pre-marketing application (PMA) for the commercialization or relabeling of the lasers.
2. Outcomes may be communicated to the investigators as they occur rather than be held in confidence.
3. Protocols may be modified as information is learned about the device and the procedure.

The PRIDE structure has enabled the CRS LASIK study to develop at a more rapid pace than would otherwise be possible. It has prevented countless complications from being repeated once they are identified since the protocols have been revised to avoid them. The PRIDE model works. It works for physicians, who can rapidly refine their outcomes; it works for patients, who receive state-of-the-art care as it develops; and it works for the FDA, which can avoid being cast in the role of denying public access to current treatments.

PROTOCOLS

Three protocols are currently being administered in the CRS LASIK study in progress to evaluate three ranges of treatment.

Outcomes for each of the protocols are reported online using Data.Site software. Safety and efficacy criteria consider visual, refractive, and healing outcomes. Adverse events and complications are tracked according to specific definitions. Surgeons have ongoing access to their results through data downloads using interactive software that generates customized reports.

Approved Range IDE

The approved range IDE protocol evaluates the Summit Apex and VISX Star lasers in their FDA-approved range of treatment. For the Apex, this includes spherical myopia treatments of 1.5 diopters (D) to 7 D at the corneal plane. For the Star, this includes spherical myopia treatments from 1 D to 6 D, astigmatic treatments of 1 D to 4 D, and spherocylinder treatments in the same ranges.

The treatment algorithms for the two lasers are significantly different. The VISX laser incorporates a central pretreatment in each procedure to prevent the formation of central islands. The Summit Apex algorithm does not include central island pretreatment, although some surgeons use the patient training mode of the laser to create a similar effect. Treatment diameters in the two lasers are similar, although the contour of the ablations may differ slightly.

Examinations are performed preoperatively at the time of surgery, at 1 day, and at 3 months following surgery.

The FDA has limited the approved range IDE to 103 surgeons and 6180 eyes. Eyes operated beyond those limits are not sent to the FDA but are evaluated locally in the study database.

High Myopia and Astigmatism

The IDE expansion to high myopia and astigmatism evaluates the Summit Apex Plus and VISX Star lasers for myopia treatments beyond the approved ranges up to 14 D of myopia and astigmatic treatments up to 5 D (VISX) or 6 D (Summit). VISX Star lasers are capable of performing treatments in this range with only software modifications. Summit surgeons, however, are required to upgrade their lasers from Apex to Apex Plus.

The Summit Apex Plus laser differs from the Apex in several respects: The beam is collimated, which improves homogeneity. Central island pretreatment is incorporated into the program, and cylinder corrections are made possible through use of an ablatable laser disc. Apex Plus surgeons can select from three treatment modalities: a single zone PRK treatment, a multizone aspheric treatment that includes a peripheral blend zone, and a toric program to treat astigmatism using the ablatable disc. The PRK and aspheric multizone treatments allow surgeon selection of the treatment diameter. For the CRS LASIK study, the diameters are standardized.

The FDA has allowed 20 of each type of laser (40 total) and 4000 eyes (8000 total) in this protocol. This protocol began in May 1997 and is expected to conclude by the end of 1999. Patients are observed for 6 months following surgery.

Hyperopia

In September 1997 approval was received by CRS for a protocol to evaluate spherical hyperopia treatments with the Summit Apex Plus and VISX Star lasers. The approval allows the same 40 lasers to be used that are enrolled in the high myopia and astigmatism study, and permits a total of 4000 eyes to be operated.

This study is seen as a forerunner to other studies, therefore it was designed as a first-level evaluation of hyperopic treatments. For example, only primary procedures are allowed and only for emmetropic targets (monovision targets are excluded). Patients with prior history of strabismus or amblyopia are excluded, and the minimum age for patient enrollment is 35. The purpose of the rigid design was to prevent confounding variables from confusing the results. Study of other subgroups—such as monovision treatments, treatments after other refractive procedures, and treatment of hyperopic astigmatism—will follow.

For this study, the Summit Apex Plus lasers require only a software modification, but the VISX Star lasers require the installation of new hardware. Based on the outcomes of other studies, it was decided to avoid the large diameter treatments that are used in PRK designed to avoid regression and to use 6 to 6.5 mm ablations instead. Smaller diameter ablations in LASIK have not been found to undergo the same regression that is encountered in hyperopic PRK and may provide better optical results. This decision has prevented the need for large-flap microkeratomes, which are new, still under development, and not widely available.

The first subjects were enrolled in the CRS LASIK study protocol for hyperopia in November 1997. Patients are followed for 1 year after surgery, and the procedures performed under the study are expected to be completed within 2 years.

REPORT DESCRIPTION

Results presented here were operated under the general study group. These eyes are not specifically the eyes in the IDE study. Eyes meeting the following criteria are included:
1. Operated prior to May 1, 1997.
2. Preoperative best spectacle-corrected visual acuity (BSCVA) 20/20 or better.
3. Preoperative manifest cylinder amount of 1 D or less.
4. No cylinder treatments performed.
5. Treatment within the approved range for spherical corrections for each laser (Summit Apex: -1.5 to -7 D, VISX Star: -1 to -6 D).
6. Reports were entered for preoperative, surgical, 1-day postoperative, and 3-month postoperative visits.

RESULTS

INVESTIGATORS

The investigators contributing data in the CRS LASIK study IDE for LASIK in the approved range of the laser are listed in on Page 296. Additional investigators are currently being added. This list includes those investigators who contributed data included in this report.

CRS LASIK Study Investigators

Deepinder Dhaliwal	Pittsburgh, Pa
Dan Durrie	Kansas City, Mo
Bruce Gene	Wichita, Kan
Lanny Hale	Scottsdale, Ariz &
	Hales Corners, Minn
Sarah Hays	Birmingham, Ala
Thierry Hufnagel	Garden City, NY
David Johnson	Zephyrhills, Fla
David Kaye	Fresno, Calif
Keith Liang	Sacramento, Calif
Jose Matos	San Juan, PR
Charles Moore	Houston, Tex
G. Peyton Neatrour	Virginia Beach, Va
David O'Brien	Vero Beach, Fla
Singh Pannu	Ft. Lauderdale, Fla
Mark Phelan	Abilene, Tex
Jeffrey Robin	Beachwood, Ohio
Anthony Sakowski	Richmond, Va
Miguell Santiago	San Juan, PR
Robin Smit	Fresno, Calif
Karl Stonecipher	Greensboro, NC
Vance Thompson	Sioux Falls, SD
Morris Tilden	Longmont, Colo
Robert Tobin	St. Joseph, Mo
Stephen Weinstock	Largo, Fla
Jeffrey Whitman	Dallas, Tex
Stephen Wong	Sacramento, Calif
Michael Woodcock	Fayetteville, NC
James Wootton	Mesa, Ariz
Wendy Wootton	Mesa, Ariz

COHORT FEATURES

There were 1079 eyes reported with the Summit Apex and 563 eyes reported with the VISX Star that met the above criteria. The mean age for both lasers was similar: Summit 40 years (standard deviation [SD] 9.7 years) and VISX 39 years (SD 10.1 years). The female to male ratio for Summit was 1.0, and for VISX it was 1.4 (p < .01). There was no apparent reason for the difference in sex distribution for the two lasers.

UNCORRECTED VISUAL RESULTS

Uncorrected visual results are reported at 1 day and 3 months. Uncorrected vision was 20/40 or better in 81% of eyes operated with the Summit Apex and 85% with the VISX Star (Figure 24-1). At 3 months, these rates improved to 88% with the Summit Apex and 89% with the VISX Star

> Uncorrected vision was 20/40 or better in 81% of eyes operated with the Summit Apex and 85% with the VISX Star.

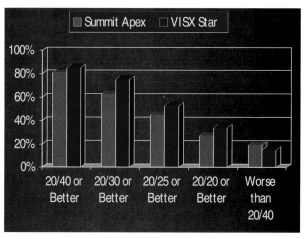

Figure 24-1. Comparison of uncorrected visual acuity results on the first postoperative day for the Summit Apex and VISX Star lasers.

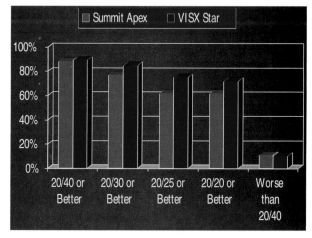

Figure 24-2. Comparison of visual results 3 months after surgery for the Summit Apex and VISX Star lasers.

(Figure 24-2). There was no statistically significant difference between the lasers for either interval.

REFRACTIVE RESULTS

Early on in the study it was recognized that the VISX Star, performing LASIK using the amount of correction provided with the lasers for PRK algorithms, tended to produce overcorrections (hyperopic outcomes). An adjustment was recommended to decrease the treatment amount to avoid widespread overcorrections based on the deviation of results from the programmed amount. The data (Tables 24-1 and 24-2) suggests reducing treatments according to age and treatment amount; however, the protocol allowed sur-

> Early on in the study, it was recognized that the VISX Star, performing LASIK using the amount of correction provided with the lasers for PRK algorithms, tended to produce overcorrections.

TABLE 24-1.
SUMMIT APEX

D	18 to 29	30 to 39	40 to 49	50+
		Age		
-2	3%	-3%	-6%	-7%
-3	5%	2%	6%	3%
-4	2%	-2%	1%	3%
-5	-2%	0%	2%	1%
-6	-4%	-4%	-2%	-0%
-7	-8%	-7%	-6%	-7%

TABLE 24-2.
VISX STAR

D	18 to 29	30 to 39	40 to 49	50+
		Age		
-2	-10%	-12%	-12%	-12%
-3	-7%	-8%	-10%	-10%
-4	-6%	-5%	-10%	-16%
-5	-5%	-11%	-12%	-15%
-6	-4%	-11%	-14%	-15%
-7	-3%	-12%	-17%	-18%

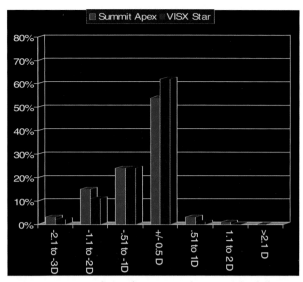

Figure 24-3. Manifest refractive results 3 months following surgery for eyes undergoing spherical corrections.

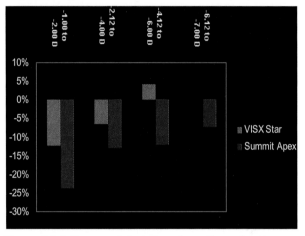

Figure 24-4. Percent of deviation of manifest refractive outcomes measured 3 months following surgery, compared with the programmed correction. Since the algorithms contained in the laser software program were developed for PRK treatments, these results may reveal information about the relationship between PRK and LASIK outcomes after similar treatments.

geons to further modify this formula according to their own experience. The refractive outcomes reported in this chapter include those modifications.

This tendency has not been noted on a systematic basis with the Summit Apex laser, although certain surgeons have noticed a tendency for specific lasers to over- or undercorrect when performing LASIK using a PRK treatment algorithm. Therefore, no recommendation has been made to the group, but surgeons are permitted to incorporate their own adjustments into the treatment amounts.

Given these modifications, it is necessary to consider refractive outcomes in two ways: as absolutes (ie, deviation from plano or targeted amount [nomogram adjusted]) and as a function of the amount of correction programmed into the laser (non-nomogram adjusted).

The absolute or nomogram-adjusted refractive results show that the mean refractive results with the Summit Apex laser were 11% undercorrected from the surgeon's targeted spherical equivalent. For VISX, the mean results were 1% undercorrected from the targeted amount. This difference was statistically significant (p < .001) and suggests that the VISX laser nomogram adjustment achieves a result that is very close to target.

Of course, mean refractive outcomes mean little to individual patients. Figure 24-3 shows the distribution of refractive outcomes at 3 months for each laser. The distribution confirms the tendency of the Summit surgeons to leave patients undercorrected.

Analysis of the refractive outcomes as a function of the programmed amount reveals some interesting trends. Figure 24-3 is a histogram that plots the mean percentage that each laser over- or undercorrected eyes from plano as a function

of the programmed amount. Since the programmed amount is actually the manufacturer's recommended ablation for a PRK treatment, Figure 24-3 may provide information about the relationship between surface (PRK) ablations and LASIK ablations.

Figure 24-4 demonstrates that using PRK treatment amounts for laser programming leads to LASIK undercorrections with both lasers when small refractive errors are treated. When treatment amounts increase, the tendency to undercorrect is reversed, especially with the VISX Star

The CRS LASIK study database (not reported here) shows a tendency for the VISX laser to overcorrect as much as 30% in higher treatments.

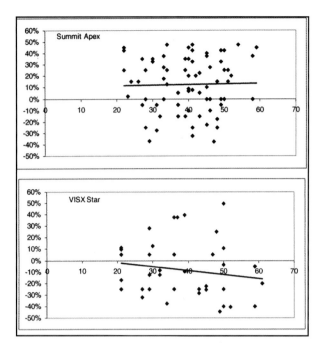

Figure 24-5. Deviation of refractive outcomes from the programmed amount, as a function of age, for eyes undergoing spherical treatments of -4.12 to -6 D of manifest myopia. No clear effect of age on refractive results is apparent, although with the VISX Star laser, the scatter (standard deviation, F test) of outcomes significantly increases ($p < 0.01$) as a function of patient age, as evidenced by the "trumpet" shape of the scatter plot.

laser. Results in the CRS LASIK study database (not reported here) show a tendency for the VISX laser to overcorrect as much as 30% in higher treatments when comparing LASIK outcomes against the programmed amount using the manufacturer's PRK algorithm.

This trend was identified early and has persisted throughout the data collection. It provides the basis for the development of nomograms. However, two potentially confounding factors must be considered before these results are used to develop nomograms, namely age effects and the effect of humidity on refractive outcomes.

The CRS data shows that the effect of age on results is inconsistent (Figure 24-5). To remove the influence of treatment amount on the tendency to over- or undercorrect, as described in the previous paragraph, Figure 24-5 is derived from a small range of refractive corrections using data from treatments in the 4.12 to 6 D range. Data from eyes operated with the Summit Apex laser show no significant effect of age on mean refractive outcomes (Pearson correlation coefficient < .1). The VISX data is more suggestive of an age effect—not for the mean outcomes (Pearson value < .2), but for the predictability of outcomes (ie, scatter of results as

> The CRS data shows that the effect of age on results is inconsistent.

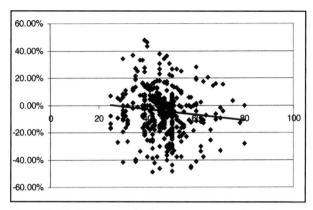

Figure 24-6. Deviation of refractive outcomes from the programmed amount, as a function of the relative humidity in the laser treatment room. The plot shows a trend for undercorrections with higher room humidity. An F test of the data shows a significant increase in scatter with increasing relative humidity ($p < 0.01$).

> The effect of humidity on mean refractive outcomes was not significant.

reflected in the standard deviations of the mean and analyzed using an t test). Possible reasons for these observations are offered in the Discussion section.

Similarly, the effect of humidity on mean refractive outcomes was not significant but became apparent when analyzed for scatter. Figure 24-6 shows a scatter plot of refractive deviations from programmed versus room relative humidity at the time of treatment. This tendency was most apparent when data for similar treatment ranges and ages were used to exclude the effects describe above.

COMPLICATIONS

Best-corrected Visual Acuity

Loss of BSCVA was low in this series as reported 3 months after surgery. Loss of one line or more LogMar

> **Note:** Sampling statistics is a large field that considers many applications, from inspecting items in a production line to predicting outcomes using prior surgical data. Formulae can take many forms, depending on the application at hand, and attempt to define the predictive power of a given sampling method. For the purpose of creating a nomogram, important considerations are the desired confidence interval (typically 1.95 is used), the known or assumed variance of prior results (approximated at .25 D), and the acceptable error of the calculation (typically .25 D). Given these assumptions, at least 20 eyes are needed to calculate each cell of a nomogram.

Loss of two lines or more occurred in less than 1% of VISX eyes and approximately 1% of Summit eyes.

equivalent[1] was encountered in 11% of eyes operated with the Summit Apex laser and 4% of eyes operated with the VISX Star. Loss of two lines or more occurred in less than 1% of VISX eyes and approximately 1% of Summit eyes.

Using LogMar equivalents when calculating loss of BSCVA eliminates the errors that result from algebraic averaging of Snellen equivalents due to the nonlinear progression of Snellen lines. However, it can lead to over-interpretation of results. To avoid over-interpretation, calculations should only be carried out to the appropriate level of significant digits. Since this study did not include reporting of partial lines of acuity, it is not possible to subdivide losses further than whole-line increments. Therefore, in this report, eyes losing .9 lines LogMar equivalent are reported as losing no lines, a report of "one line or more" indicates loss of an entire line or more. This distinction is not often mentioned in the literature but becomes important when considering results from a large series such as this.

Another concern about reports of BSCVA that is often mentioned and that namely limits in the reproducibility of clinical reports of visual acuity may invalidate losses of one line or less as "noise." Figure 24-7 would seem to support this point with near perfect symmetry of the one-line changes on either side of zero.

A survey was sent to each of the surgeons in an effort to evaluate the eventual outcome of the eyes in which one or more lines of BSCVA loss was reported at 3 months. Of the 108 surveys sent, 80% were returned. The operating surgeons reported that they had noticed no abnormalities at the time of surgery in 92% of the eyes that lost one line or more BSCVA. Visual loss was related to decentration of the ablation in only 4% of the eyes. The respondents felt that the cause of visual loss was related to the keratome in 13% of eyes, to the laser in 65% of eyes, and to indeterminate cause in the remainder. Significantly, two-thirds of the eyes that had been subsequently evaluated experienced improvement in BSCVA to preoperative levels; only one third continued to experience visual loss.

Keratome-related complications were reported in the surgical reports of 1.65% of eyes.

Keratome-related Complications

Keratome-related complications were reported in the surgical reports of 1.65% of eyes. These complications, including damage to the stroma, epithelium, small flap, thin flap, as well as epithelial defects. BSCVA loss was not related to reports of keratome-related complications, as there was no statistically significant rate of BSCVA loss in these eyes compared with the overall group. This may be due to the widespread practice of aborting surgery when keratome complications are encountered.

Postoperative Events

Slit lamp abnormalities were noted in 5.8% of eyes. Abnormalities included a broad range of items such as corneal edema (.6%), cornea scar (.1%), epithelial defect (.5%), glare (.2%), discomfort (.5%), interface debris (3.2%), interface epithelium (.6%), and cap thinning (.1%). As can be expected, eyes with slit lamp abnormalities were associated with a significantly increased incidence of lost BSCVA (p < .01).

DISCUSSION

ADMINISTRATIVE RESULTS

By Ophthalmologists for Ophthalmology

The CRS LASIK study is unique in ophthalmology in that it represents a grassroots effort by ophthalmologists to validate new technology and is open to any qualified surgeon on an open enrollment basis.

The entire financial support of the effort is obtained from the participating surgeons who contribute outcomes into a pooled database without any opportunity for direct financial gain. This, in itself, is remarkable and speaks well for the profession's commitment to self-monitoring.

Nevertheless, the success of the study depends on the ability to return benefits to the participants. Benefits include standard-of-care liability protection, surgeon access to technology that is not yet FDA approved, and the ability to improve outcomes through the use of outcomes analysis and grouped databasing.

Regulatory Implications

The project has had regulatory implications for participants and regulators alike. By participating in the regulatory system, the study has made it possible for surgeons to perform and study an off-label procedure without violating federal policies. It has also provided the FDA with an opportunity for detailed "post-approval surveillance" of an approved device. The inability of federal regulators to monitor "real world" application of devices once they are approved has been a long-standing criticism of the regulatory process, and the CRS LASIK study may provide an approach to that problem.

Utilization of Communication Technologies

Without online reporting, the amount of paperwork and added costs for study administration would be unmanageable. The CRS LASIK study has made extensive use of online communications technologies that only recently became available. Data.Site has provided online services and database management. Investigators record and report their results using a computer in their office. The results are transmitted via modem to the central computer and are immediately available for analysis to any authorized participant from anywhere in the world.

Several lessons learned in the process of using this technology are worth mentioning. For example, many surgeons lack any familiarity whatsoever with information technology. This came as a surprise to the study administrators. Many surgeons, despite their great sophistication in other areas, entered the study without ever having turned on a computer. This presented a significant barrier to their participation. Even worse, some were unwilling to learn and were able to participate only after they designated an employee to perform all computer-related tasks. However, since data analysis is done onscreen using computer software, failure to learn to use the study software has usually meant failure to fully benefit from study participation.

Second, early on in the study it became clear that ophthalmologists needed to be involved with the design of the reporting software and could not designate programming duties to non-ophthalmic-trained programmers. Form design, report design, and software architecture all depend on close matching of the software with clinical procedures. What programmers saw as a logical grouping of information often made no sense in the exam room. Once this became apparent, it was necessary to redesign several forms and reports that were technically correct but difficult to use in the clinic. Ophthalmologists had to learn to program, and the programmers had to learn about ophthalmology. It was a tedious exercise but a necessary one.

Another lesson came from the arena of data entry logistics. Nearly all the surgeons in the study voiced a strong preference to continue using their own clinic forms as they examined patients rather than the study forms. This added a step in the reporting process since it meant they had to transcribe the information from their charts onto the study forms before entering the information into the computer. Their reasons for using their own forms included familiarity, matching of their forms to their own exam flows, and a dislike for the "fill in the blank" format of the study forms. However, this presented many obstacles to data reporting and many opportunities for transcription errors.

It became clear that successful use of the online reporting system would not occur unless the study forms were used as the patient chart. This is necessary because the study often demands information that may or may not be obtained in a routine exam, and unless the forms are used in the exam, this may not be apparent until the patient has left the office. By using the study forms as the patient chart, the flow of the exam can be ordered to facilitate gathering information, such as prompting measurement of pupil diameter before dilation is performed. Finally, using the forms in the clinic eliminates the need to fill out the forms later on. This saves time and money and reduces transcription errors. Further, it allows data entry to be performed by nonophthalmic-trained personnel since the design of the computer entry screen matches the design of the report forms, eliminating the need for data entry people to understand the meaning of the information being entered.

However, it is sometimes not easy to convince study investigators and their staff to discard the forms they are currently using in their clinics in favor of new, unfamiliar, and technical-looking forms. Resistance to change is increased when the study forms do not follow a familiar flow, or even worse, when the study forms are in an intermediate stage of development and are not yet perfected. These considerations present barriers to successful study administration and can be difficult to overcome.

Nevertheless, online reporting has been successful. With time, this method is expected to become the standard for clinical trials, especially multi-center, large enrollment trials such as this one.

CLINICAL RESULTS

The visual and refractive results in this series compare well with those from other LASIK series and from reports of PRK.

Some, but not much, investigator-to-investigator variability was observed in the outcomes. This would imply that LASIK is a procedure that can be learned, and done well, by committed surgeons.

The tendency for the PRK algorithm to result in overcorrections, especially with the VISX laser, is interesting. With both lasers, overcorrections increased with the increasing amounts of preoperative refractive error. This would suggest that the PRK algorithms anticipate increasing amounts of regression with higher corrections, and that it is necessary to adjust the PRK treatment algorithms when using the lasers for LASIK.

Relative Humidity Effects

The tendency of increased relative humidity to result in increased scatter of results, and to some degree decrease the effectiveness of the ablation, confirms the need to control room temperature and humidity to within manufacturer-recommended tolerance limits. The effect of relative humidity on ablation efficacy has been suggested to occur through the following mechanisms:

- decreased evaporation of moisture from the stroma

> The tendency of increased relative humidity to result in increased scatter of results, and to some degree decrease the effectiveness of the ablation, confirms the need to control room temperature and humidity.

throughout the treatment, resulting in a wetter "bed" and decreased laser efficacy

- increased accumulation of moisture on the stromal surface during the treatment, resulting in photoablation of surface moisture instead of stromal tissue
- decreased transmission of the laser beam through moister air, wet optics, and humid laser cavities

Of the three mechanisms, the former seems most likely. Regardless, the results of this study confirm that LASIK predictability falls as relative humidity rises. The results support the recommendation to maintain room temperature between 68° and 72°F with relative humidity less than 50%.

Nomogram Development

The development of nomograms for individual surgeons based on their results has been a major focus of the CRS LASIK study. Initially, it was assumed that a single group nomogram could be developed that would be transferable to any user of the same laser type as long as the procedure was performed according to a common standard.

This did not turn out to be the case. Variations in lasers, laser optics, room conditions, and surgical techniques combine to invalidate the concept of a group nomogram and make it necessary to develop nomograms for each surgeon—the so-called personal nomogram. The development and provision of personal nomograms has been a major goal of the CRS LASIK study.

The creation of a nomogram from actual outcomes, as opposed to predicted, theoretical or extrapolated data, requires thousands of eyes to be valid. Since nomograms take the form of a grid and take into account the entire range of refractions and patient ages, a detailed nomogram may include more than 200 individual cells. Sampling statistics require that the calculations for each cell be based on at least 20 eyes, to be used clinically,[1] so more than 4000 eyes would be required to generate the entire table. The generation of a personal nomogram for an individual surgeon would therefore become a lifetime endeavor.

Electronic databasing and pooled results provide a solution to this problem. However, since the results of each surgeon and each laser may differ, the application of pooled data must be limited to trend analysis. Once the general performance of the laser is calculated using the pooled results and put into the form of a reference nomogram, the variation of individual surgeon's results from the group average can be determined. This difference can then be applied to the group results to yield a personal nomogram. With this approach, personal nomograms can be developed after 20 eyes or more have been entered from an individual surgeon.

This approach leverages the power of pooled databasing to yield a nomogram that would otherwise take years to develop. By basing the nomograms on derived data, which consider known and unknown influences, rather than attempting to predict all the parameters that might effect

outcomes and try to control them, the nomograms utilize time-proven principles that developed from the nomograms used for radial keratotomy. In recognition of the contributions made by Casebeer to the development and clinical acceptance of nomograms, the nomograms developed in the CRS LASIK study have been designated as Casebeer LASIK nomograms.

Casebeer LASIK nomograms are based on certain assumptions: the performance trends of the lasers are similar from center to center, the surgeon's technique is consistent, and the variables that are known to affect outcomes are held constant. These assumptions are carefully explained to the participants, and surgeons are warned that the nomograms are a work in progress. We continue to test and modify these assumptions as data accumulates. Further safety is built into the nomograms by adjusting the target to a myopic result. To date, they have been well accepted and seem to be effective.

DIFFERENCES IN SUMMIT APEX AND VISX STAR LASIK OUTCOMES

Some of the differences between the Summit Apex and VISX Star outcomes have already been mentioned:

- The VISX Star seems to be a "hotter" laser than the Summit Apex. The LASIK nomograms for VISX users contain a greater reduction of the PRK treatment amount than the nomograms for the Summit Apex.
- An effect of patient age on outcomes seems to be more apparent with the VISX Star. Older patients seem to experience a greater amount of correction for a given treatment than younger patients with the VISX Star. This effect has not been as consistent with the Summit Apex.

> The VISX Star seems to be a "hotter" laser than the Summit Apex. The LASIK nomograms for VISX users contain a greater reduction of the PRK treatment amount than the nomograms for the Summit Apex.

- There may be a slightly increased loss of BSCVA with the Summit Apex, although there may be a slightly higher rate of improved BSCVA as well. Given the uncertainties of measuring one line of visual loss, this difference may not be due to the lasers but to the examiners.

We have not been able to determine the cause of these differences.

SUMMARY

The CRS LASIK study has met its original goal of studying the FDA-approved Summit Apex and VISX Star lasers for use in LASIK. Participants have benefited from the liability protection that comes with a collaborative effort. By sharing outcomes in a pooled database they have also been able to accelerate their understanding of the procedure. It has been possible to create nomograms that modify the PRK treatment algorithms for LASIK. Much has been learned about the lasers and the procedure.

The CRS LASIK study has gone beyond the original protocol for low myopia and is currently administering protocols for high myopia, astigmatism, and hyperopia. In the future, we hope to evaluate outcomes with other lasers, using other keratomes, and for other treatment indications such as LASIK after radial keratotomy. The project may also grow to consider other technologies, such as refractive implants, thermokeratoplasty, and corneal implants.

Since the CRS LASIK study is completely funded by its participants, future growth will be determined by each project's utility to the participants. This is under continuous review. There are many practical benefits of the project—for surgeons and their patients. The concept of surgeon-based validation of new procedures, without proprietary motivations, is powerful. The independent effort, undertaken by ophthalmologists for the benefit of ophthalmology, reflects a desire for self-regulation that many find appealing.

With the existing logistical infrastructure in place, the project may continue indefinitely. The online reporting software works. Participating practices have made the transition to using report forms as the clinical chart and have systems in place to enter the information online. Surgeons have ready access to their own (and grouped) data and can use that information to improve future outcomes. Enrollment continues to be open to any qualified ophthalmologist who is interested in participating.

LASIK Results from TLC, The London Laser Center

Louis E. Probst, MD
Omar J. Hakim, MD
Bruce D. Nichols, MD
Marion Baird, BSc

TLC, The London Laser Center could be considered the ideal refractive surgery center for gathering laser in situ keratomileusis (LASIK) data. The demographics of London, the nature of the practice of the co-managing optometrists in Ontario, and the consistency of the surgical technique of the two surgeons at the center (BD Nichols and OJ Hakim) allow for an accurate evaluation of LASIK results for the majority of the center's patients.

London is a city of approximately 400,000 people. The town is generally white collar with the largest proportion of millionaires per capita in Canada. London is the home of the University of Western Ontario. With approximately 25,000 students, it provides a very well-educated, young, student-oriented population. These patients have often researched refractive surgery on the Internet prior to coming to the center. These patients tend to have a cautious, yet enthusiastic, approach to refractive surgery.

While the scope of optometric practice in Ontario is currently evolving, at the present time, optometrists in Ontario do not have a TPA (therapeutic agents) to prescribe medications for eye disease. The co-management of cataract surgery has also been somewhat limited to date. The co-management of refractive surgery has, therefore, provided an opportunity for optometrists to expand their scope of practice. While they do not officially prescribe the medications after LASIK, optometrists are able to indicate to

> The co-management of refractive surgery has, therefore, provided an opportunity for optometrists to expand their scope of practice.

patients when the medications should be adjusted or discontinued based on a postoperative schedule provided by the surgeon. This background has lead to a very conscientious approach for the follow-up of LASIK patients.

Approximately 95% of patients return to their optometrists for regular follow-up care. The optometrists are very consistent about faxing follow-up results to the center and providing an excellent database for LASIK results. Many of the patients who are referred to the center live within a 100-mile radius, which makes access and return visits quite convenient. Because the patients have educated themselves to a large degree about LASIK through reading material and the Internet, they are very reliable with their postoperative follow-up.

TLC, The London Laser Center has a consistent set-up with two surgeons (BD Nichols and OJ Hakim). Both surgeons use exactly the same LASIK technique with the same microkeratome plates and nomogram. The preoperative work-up and postoperative medications are also completely consistent.

> Because the patients have educated themselves to a large degree about LASIK through reading material and the Internet, they are very reliable with their postoperative follow-up.

LASIK TECHNIQUE

The patients have their spectacle refraction and subjective refraction performed at the center, along with their

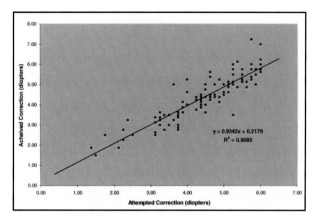

Figure 25-1. Attempted versus achieved correction for myopes plano to -6 D after LASIK treatment (n = 107, SD = .5 D).

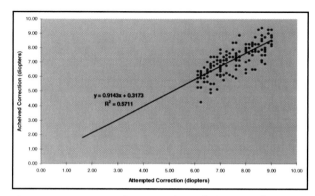

Figure 25-2. Attempted versus achieved correction for severe myopia (6.1 D to -9 D) after LASIK treatment (n = 155, SD = .68).

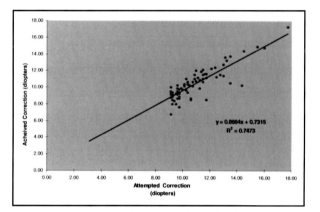

Figure 25-3. Attempted versus achieved refractive results after LASIK for -9.1 D and above (n = 73, SD = .95 D).

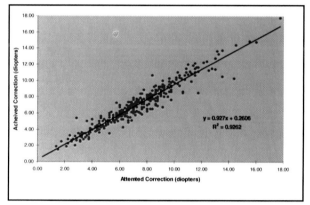

Figure 25-4. Overall attempted versus achieved myopic LASIK correction (n = 335, SD = .73 D).

referral refraction. All patients undergo preoperative screening topography as well as preoperative pachymetry. The patients are counseled on refractive surgery based on the results of these tests. Any patient with a contraindication, including abnormal topography or preoperative ocular abnormalities, is discouraged from having surgery.

The eyelashes are cleaned and the eye is anaesthetized with topical proparicaine. The patient is then taken to the surgical bed and further anesthetic is placed underneath the eyelids. The eyelids are covered with surgical tape. The lid speculum is placed in the eye. The cornea is marked with a peripheral corneal alignment mark. The suction ring is placed in the eye and displaced slightly nasally. The suction is applied and pressure is taken with a Barraquer tonometer to ensure that it is greater than 65 mm Hg. The cornea is then wetted with several drops of balanced salt solution (BSS). The microkeratome is allowed to make a cut across the cornea, and the flap is lifted. The LASIK ablation is carried out according to the standardized nomogram with the Chiron Automated Corneal Shaper and the Chiron Technolas 116 excimer laser. The flap is then replaced and the suction ring removed. Irrigation is performed under-

neath the flap, and the flap is floated back into its correct location. The flap is allowed to sit for 3 minutes to seal into its location.

Generally bilateral procedures are performed, although some unilateral procedures are done in selected cases.

RESULTS

Scattergrams indicate that the results of LASIK procedures are extremely predictable for lower myopia and less predictable for higher ranges of myopia (Figures 25-1 through 25-4). For low myopia of less than 6 diopters (D), more than 81% of eyes were within .5 D of emmetropia, and 96% of eyes were within 1 D of emmetropia. For greater than 9 D of myopia, only 58% of eyes were within .5 D of emmetropia, and 79% of eyes were within 1 D of emmetropia (Figures 25-5 through 25-8).

After one or more LASIK procedures for the overall population, 50% of eyes were 20/20 or better, and 91% of eyes were 20/40 or better. For patients with greater than 9 D of myopia, only 33% of eyes were 20/20 or better and 82% of eyes were 20/40 or better. In the low myopia group, the

LASIK RESULTS FOR TLC CALIFORNIA, BREA

Chang Kim, OD

Robert W. Lingua, MD

Table A and Graph A depict the outcome analysis on 123 consecutive eyes. LASIK was performed on all patients after consultation and informed consent. Inclusion criteria were: target plano, at least 3 months postoperative acuity data, simultaneous sphere and cylinder correction with the VISX Star excimer laser, and no enhancements or previous eye surgery. The range of correction was up to -16.75 sphere and -6.75 cylinder. In more than 700 consecutive LASIK cases, there have been no visually significant keratome complications.

TABLE A.
VISUAL ACUITY OUTCOMES (AT LEAST 3 MONTHS FOLLOW-UP)

Refx range	n = 123	± 20/20	% > 20/20	20/25	% > 20/25	20/30	% > 20/30	20/40	% > 20/40
.5 - 3	50	42	85%	46	92%	49	98%	50	100%
3.1 - 6	46	30	65%	42	91%	44	96%	44	96%
6.1 - 9 +	27	8	33%	16	62%	21	81%	23	86%
ALL	123	80	65%	104	85%	114	93%	117	95%

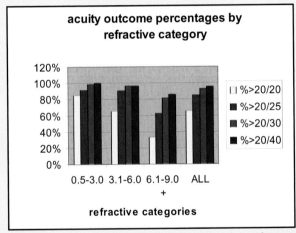

Graph A. Distribution of acuity outcomes within refractive ranges.

In Table C, we examined the change in cylinder amount and axis. The cylinder power was reduced regardless of the accompanying spherical component and to a similar degree among the refractive ranges. The amount of change was fairly stable from the week 1 to the week 4 refraction.

Axis behavior, however, was unpredictable. There was no correlation among the preoperative and week 4 cylinder axes. However, among the week 1 and week 4 data, 75% of resultant axis measurements were within 30°of the week 1 measure, and 57% were within 15°. Thereafter, there was little change, suggesting that the week 4 refraction is acceptable to prescribe.

TABLE B.
ENHANCEMENT RATE PER REFRACTIVE GROUP

		Enhancements	Enhancement %
.5 - 3	144	6	4.10%
3.1 - 6	175	3	1.70%
6.1 - 9	94	3	3.10%
9.1 +	22	4	18%
n = 435			**Average = 6.70%**

TABLE C.
CYLINDER POWER OUTCOME STUDY

Associated sphere n=97

Range	Mean preop cyl	Power	Mean, da 7	Mean, da 30
.5-3	36	-1.45	-.33	-.28
3.1-6	34	-1.64	-.44	-.49
6.1-9 +	27	-1.29	-.55	-.36
ALL	97	-1.46	-.44	-.37

Hyperopic LASIK with the Chiron Technolas Excimer Laser

Maria Clara Arbelaez, MD

INTRODUCTION

Approximately 35% of the total population and more than 50% of the people with refractive errors are hyperopic.[1] As this is a very high percentage of the population, there is significant interest in a method for its surgical correction. Several different approaches have been developed thus far to achieve this aim.

One of the earlier procedures was automated lamellar keratoplasty (ALK), which involved making a deep cut (over 60% of the corneal thickness) across the cornea.[2-4] The intraocular pressure of the anterior chamber would push the attenuated cornea forward, resulting in a "controlled" corneal ectasia that would steepen the central cornea and reduce the hyperopic refraction. The clinical results of this procedure have demonstrated poor visual stability and predictability.

Laser thermokeratoplasty (LTK) utilizing a holmium laser is another approach to the surgical correction of hyperopia.[5,6] The laser beam heats the cornea, thus causing shrinkage of the corneal collagen. The LTK burns are applied in a circular ring of eight spots with a clear zone diameter of 6 to 8 mm. The shrinkage of the peripheral ring of collagen tissue results in an increase in the central corneal curvature, which in turn increases the refractive power of the cornea and reduces hyperopic refraction. LTK has been shown to be effective in the correction of low degrees of hyperopia with minimal astigmatism. Unfortunately, remodeling the collagen fibers over time reverses this change in curvature. Regression following LTK has been consistently identified and therefore has limited the long-term stability of the refractive effect.

Photorefractive keratectomy (PRK) has been shown to be effective for the treatment of low levels of myopia, however haze and regression are more common with higher corrections.[7-12] The treatment of hyperopia with hyperopic PRK (H-PRK) has been shown to be effective for the correction of up to 4 diopters (D) of hyperopia.[13] Regression has been identified as a major postoperative complication, especially above +4 D, due to an overactivation of the re-epithelialization process. The amount of regression seems to be proportional to the spherical equivalent of the hyperopic correction, suggesting that more epithelial thickening occurs with higher curvature change of the cornea. A high incidence of postoperative corneal haze has been reported when H-PRK is performed for greater than +4 D. Of particular concern, there has been a loss of two of more lines of best-corrected visual acuity (BCVA) reported in up to 10% of H-PRK cases.[13]

Laser in situ keratomileusis (LASIK) is the most advanced method available for the correction of myopia. LASIK has been particularly successful for the treatment of high myopes because the intrastromal ablation beneath the corneal flap requires little corneal healing and therefore rarely produces corneal haze, which was a relatively common complication following the correction of high myopia with PRK.[14] LASIK also offers increased convenience for patients with rapid visual rehabilitation and a pain-free post-

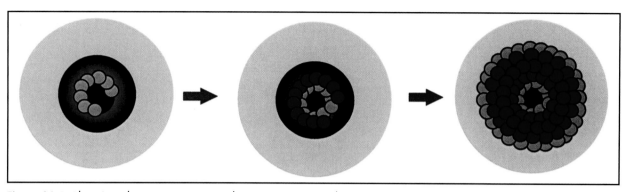

Figure 26-1. PlanoScan hyperopia correction laser scans in a circular pattern over the cornea.

operative course. Myopic LASIK has recently gained increasing popularity over myopic PRK because of these advantages for the correction of high, moderate, and even low myopia.

While there has been several reports of the results of myopic LASIK, little has been reported to date on the correction of hyperopia with hyperopic LASIK (H-LASIK).[15] In contrast to myopic LASIK in which the cornea must be flattened, the central cornea must be steepened in H-LASIK. The regression effect following H-LASIK is minimized as the treatment takes place in the stromal bed. H-LASIK also has the advantage of preserving the Bowman's membrane and allowing for quick visual rehabilitation. Discomfort during the healing process is minimized. The risk of postoperative corneal haze that was relatively common following large correction with H-PRK is almost eliminated with H-LASIK.

> The regression effect following H-LASIK is minimized as the treatment takes place in the stromal bed.

METHODS

The clinical results of H-LASIK performed by one surgeon (MC Arbelaez) were reviewed. The Chiron Technolas Keracor 117c excimer laser with the PlanoScan algorithm with a shot frequency of 25 Hz and the Chiron Automated Corneal Shaper with a flap thickness of 160 microns were utilized in all cases.

The Chiron Technolas PlanoScan hyperopia algorithm scans in a computer-controlled, circular pattern around the central cornea (Figure 26-1). The result is a central steepening effect within a 5 mm optical zone. To achieve a smooth transition out to the uncorrected cornea, the treatment area is extended to 8.5 mm. The PlanoScan hyperopia mode of the Chiron Technolas Keracor 117c laser uses a beam with a 2 mm diameter. The laser spot can be described as a flying spot moving around the treatment surface. Figure 26-2 shows spherical hyperopia treatment with the ablation pattern of spherical hyperopia correction (left side) and the surface of the cornea after ablation (right side).

RESULTS

A total of 91 eyes were treated with H-LASIK. The results were divided into two treatment groups. The low hyperopia group included 70 eyes with a hyperopic preoperative refraction up to +4 D. The mean spherical refraction was +1.78 D (standard deviation [SD] ± 1.11 D). The moderate hyperopia group included 21 eyes with a moderate hyperopic preoperative refraction between +4 and +9 D. The mean spherical refraction was +5.82 D (SD ±1.6) Patient follow-up took place for up to 6 months.

The scattergram of desired versus achieved spherical refractive correction demonstrates the results of 86 eyes with follow-up data at 1 month (Figure 26-3). There are four overcorrected cases (more than 1 D). Only one case is undercorrected by more than 2 D. The predictability was found to be relatively good with 84.9% of the cases (73 out of 86) achieving within 1 D of emmetropia.

After 3 months, the results for 72 eyes were available (Figure 26-4). At this time, one case was overcorrected by more than 1 D, while 70.8% of the cases (51 out of 72) were within 1 D of emmetropia. After 6 months, the results for 36 eyes were available (Figure 26-5). None of the eyes were overcorrected by more than 1 D, two of the eyes were undercorrected by more than 2 D, and 83.3 % of the cases (30 out of 36) were within 1 D of emmetropia. Over the follow-up period, 70.8% to 84.9% of the corrected eyes were within 1 D of emmetropia. A weak regression tendency can be identified when the 1, 3, and 6-month scattergrams are compared.

In order to differentiate the results, we took a closer look at the low hyperopic cases up to +4 D. The cases with a preoperative refraction higher than that were not further

> Over the follow-up period, 70.8% to 84.9% of the corrected eyes were within 1 D of emmetropia.

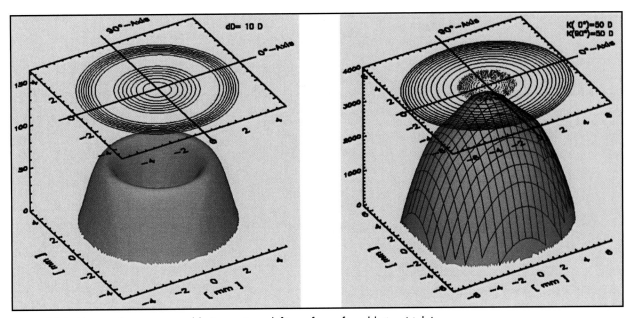

Figure 26-2. Hyperopia treatment: ablation pattern (left); surface after ablation (right).

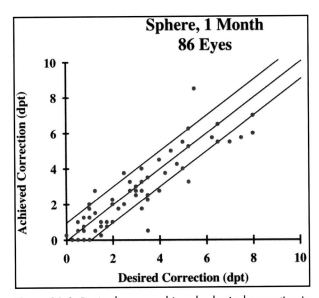

Figure 26-3. Desired versus achieved spherical correction in diopters after 1 month.

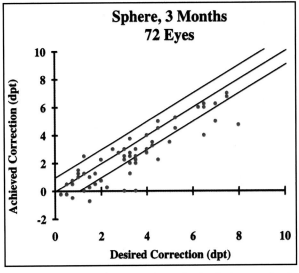

Figure 26-4. Desired versus achieved spherical correction in diopters after 3 months.

analyzed as 21 cases do not give any statistically significant results. Figure 26-6 shows the predictability of the spherical correction. After 1 week, 76% of the spherical refraction parameters had deviation less than 1 D from the expected correction, while 14% were undercorrected by 1 D and 10% were overcorrected by the same amount. One hundred percent of the cases were within ±1 D of emmetropia.

After one month, 71% of cases had deviation less than 1 D from the expected correction, 21% had a deviation over +1 D, and 2% had a deviation of 2 D or more, while 6% had a deviation of at least -1 D. Ninety-eight percent of the cases were within ±1 D of emmetropia.

After 3 months, 59% of the cases had deviation less than

1 D from the expected correction, 27% had a deviation of +1 D, 12% and a deviation of +2 D or more, while 2% had a deviation of -1 D. Eighty-eight percent were within ±1 D of emmetropia. These numbers show a small amount of regression. The percentage rate in the less than ±1 D range of deviation from the expected correction decreased from 76% to 59% after 3 months.

The regression after H-LASIK for the low hyperopes is evaluated in Figure 26-7. The mean preoperative spherical refraction was +1.78 D (SD ±1.11 D). After 3 months, the mean spherical correction was .7 D (SD ±.96 D). After 6 months, the mean spherical correction was .46 D (SD ±.78 D). The low standard deviation values indicate a high level

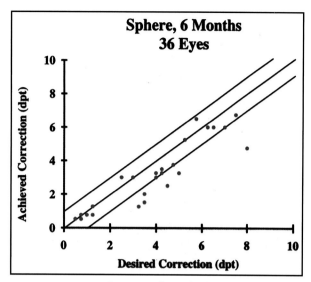

Figure 26-5. Desired versus achieved spherical correction in diopters after 6 months.

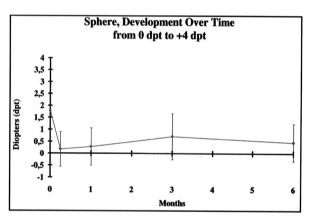

Figure 26-7. Regression of effect over time for low hyperopia.

> Although slight undercorrection and regression does occur after H-LASIK, these results show it is possible to achieve relatively stable outcomes.

of stability during the entire follow-up time. Although slight undercorrection and regression does occur after H-LASIK, these results show it is possible to achieve relatively stable outcomes.

An uncorrected visual acuity (UCVA) (Figure 26-8) of 20/20 in the low hyperopic group was achieved by 29%, 32%, and 37% at the 1-week, 1-month, and 3-month follow-up visits respectively. UCVA of 20/25 in the low hyperopic group was achieved by 40%, 54%, and 56% at the 1-week, 1-month, and 3-month follow-up visits respectively. UCVA of 20/40 in the low hyperopic group was achieved by 67%, 73%, and 80% at the 1-week, 1-month, and 3-month follow-up visits respectively. Over the follow-up period, it was evident that the visual ability increased independent of the level of the UCVA.

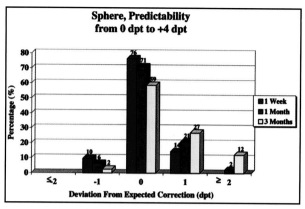

Figure 26-6. Spherical deviation from expected correction (from 0 D to +4 D).

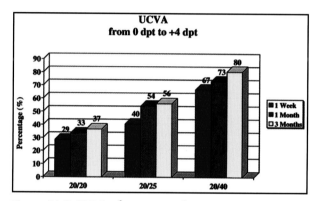

Figure 26-8. UCVA after H-LASIK for 0 D to +4 D.

> There was a relatively high loss of two or more lines of BCVA with values of 12%, 10%, and 10% at the 1-week, 1-month, and 3-month follow-up visits respectively.

Analyzing the BCVA with gained or lost lines in the low hyperopic group, 52% of the operated eyes did not lose or gain any lines after 1 week compared to the preoperative visual acuity (Figure 26-9). After 1 month, 62% of cases, and after 3 months, 76% of cases had no change in BCVA. There was a relatively high loss of two or more lines of BCVA with values of 12%, 10%, and 10% at the 1-week, 1-month, and 3-month follow-up visits respectively.

The relatively high number of patients who lost two or more lines of BCVA may have occurred for several reasons. Hyperopic patients lose the magnifying effect of their glasses after they have a surgical refractive correction. Thus, the images are much smaller postoperatively and not tolerated by all patients in the same way. Another reason is the relatively small optical zone size of 5 mm. This may cause glare and halo effects, which could result in a loss of BCVA. A solution would be a larger optical zone size of 6 mm, which has already been changed by Chiron Vision for the new hyperopia PlanoScan model. The new hyperopia PlanoScan

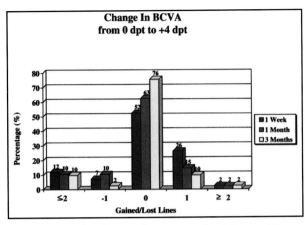

Figure 26-9. Loss of BCVA for H-LASIK for 0 D to +4 D.

The new hyperopia PlanoScan software uses the optical zone size of 6 mm with a transition zone of up to 9 mm.

software uses the optical zone size of 6 mm with a transition zone of up to 9 mm. Preliminary results with the new software show visible improvement. Glare and halo effects appear to be significantly reduced. The safety profile of the new PlanoScan software will need to be further evaluated in terms of the loss of BCVA.

SUMMARY

These results demonstrate that H-LASIK is an effective treatment for hyperopic patients with up to +4 D. For higher hyperopic patients with over +4 D, the procedure is also effective, however greater experience is required in this group. The new PlanoScan algorithm with an optical zone size of 6 mm should improve upon the preliminary results seen with the original PlanoScan algorithm.

REFERENCES

1. Krumpasky G. Epidemiologie der Refraktionsfehler. Jahrbuch der Augenheilkunde. Biermann Verlag; 1995
2. American Academy of Ophthalmology. Automated lamellar keratoplasty, preliminary procedure assessment. *Ophthalmology.* 1996;103(5):852-861.
3. Lyle WA, Jin GJC. Initial results of automated lamellar keratoplasty for correction of myopia: 1-year follow-up. *J Cataract Refract Surg.* 1996;22:31-43.
4. Manche EE, Judge A, Maloney RK. Lamellar keratoplasty for hyperopia. *Journal of Refractive Surgery.* 1996;12:42-49.
5. Cherry PM. Holmium: YAG-Laser to treat astigmatism associated with myopia or hyperopia. *Journal of Refractive Surgery.* 1995;11.
6. Koch DD, Kohnen T, McDonnell PJ, et al. Hyperopic correction by noncontact holmium: YAG laser thermal keratoplasty. Unites States phase IIA clinical study with 1-year follow-up. *Ophthalmology.* 1996;103:1525-1536.
7. Dutt S, Steinert RF, Raizman MB, Puliafito CA. One-year results of excimer laser photorefractive keratectomy for low to moderate myopia. *Arch Ophthalmol.* 1994;112:1427-1436.
8. McDonald MB, Talamo JH. Myopic photorefractive keratectomy: the experience in the United States with the VISX excimer laser. In: Salz JJ, ed. *Corneal Laser Surgery.* St. Louis, Mo: Mosby; 1995.
9. Alamo S, Shimizu K. Excimer laser photorefractive keratectomy for myopia: 2-year follow-up. *Journal of Refractive Surgery.* 1995;11(suppl): S253-S260.
10. Thompson KP, Steinert RF, Daniel J, Stulting D. Photorefractive keratectomy with the Summit excimer laser: The phase III US. results. In: Salz JJ, ed. *Corneal Laser Surgery.* St. Louis, Mo: Mosby; 1995.
11. Krueger RR, Talamo JH, McDonald MB, et al. Clinical analysis of excimer laser photorefractive keratectomy using a multiple zone technique for severe myopia. *Am J Ophthalmol.* 1995;119:263-274.
12. Pop M, Aras M. Multizone/Multipass photorefractive keratectomy: 6-month results. *J Cataract Refract Surg.* 1995;21:633-643.
13. Jackson B, Agapitos PJ, Mintsioulis G, et al. Excimer laser PRK with the VISX Star for low hyperopia. VISX Internet Website Physician Study Data; 1996.
14. Salah T, Waring GO III, Maghraby AE, et al. Excimer laser in situ keratomileusis under a corneal flap for myopia of 2 to 20 diopters. *Am J Ophthalmol.* 1996;121:143-155.
15. Arbelaez M. One-year follow-up of hyperopia (LASIK/PlanoScan). Presented at International Society of Refractive Surgery. 1996 Pre-AAO Conference; Chicago, Ill; October 1996. Abstract.

Hyperopic LASIK with the Summit Apex Plus Laser

Michael A. Lawless, MBBS, FRACO, FRACS, FRCOphth
Gerard I. Sutton, MBBS, FRACO, FRACS

INTRODUCTION

The application of new refractive surgery techniques to hyperopia has historically followed their use in myopia. This is true for keratomileusis, automated lamellar keratectomy, incisional keratotomy, photorefractive keratectomy (PRK), and most recently, laser in situ keratomileusis (LASIK).[1-5] Other technologies, such as holmium thermal keratoplasty and intrastromal implants, have paralleled this evolution but have yet to secure their place in the correction of hyperopic errors.[2,6,7,8]

In contrast to myopia, in which one has to flatten the central cornea, the central cornea must be steepened in order to achieve a refractive correction in hyperopia. The use of PRK for the treatment of hyperopia has had mixed results. Maloney, et al were unsuccessful in correcting hyperopia in rabbits with an erodible polymethylmethacrylate mask and reported paradoxical myopic corrections.[9] Dausch, et al reported moderate success in correcting hyperopia using a scanning process and suction ring mask system.[10] Problems with regression and predictability limited visual outcomes. Koch, et al also had limited success in correcting myopia of up to 3 D with noncontact Holmium YAG laser thermal keratoplasty.[11]

> In contrast to myopia, in which one has to flatten the central cornea, the central cornea must be steepened in order to achieve a refractive correction in hyperopia.

HYPEROPIC PRK

We reported 11 patients in a prospective consecutive study for the treatment of hyperopia with PRK.[12] All eyes had a reduction of hyperopia that was maintained despite some regression. In this study the hyperopic erodible discs used were trial discs. They were designed with the expectation that there would be substantial regression due to wound healing. There was, therefore, an overcorrection factor built into the erodible discs and also into the algorithm for the number of pulses delivered. In this study, after 3 months refraction remained stable with no statistically significant change (p = .67). Within the group overall, however, there were individual variations with the amount of regression being greater in the higher treatment groups. Although refraction was statistically stable by 3 months, keratometry was stable from 6 months (p = .91) and corneal topography was also stable by 6 months (p = .91).

Although no patient lost more than three lines of Snellen acuity at any time, there was a transient drop in best-corrected visual acuity (BCVA) at 1 month due to induced irregular astigmatism. By 9 months, all patients had regained their best spectacle-corrected visual acuity (BSCVA). In the 2 diopter (D) correction group there was a slight loss of contrast sensitivity at higher spatial frequencies, which resolved by 12 months. In the 3 D correction group there was slight loss in higher spatial frequency contrast sensitivity that persisted, and in the 4 D correction group there was a slight reduction of contrast sensitivity at all spatial frequencies, even at 1 year.

HYPEROPIC LASIK WITH THE SUMMIT APEX PLUS LASER

Although we were generally satisfied with hyperopic PRK up to 3 D, the pain, prolonged re-epithelialization with large treatment zones, slow visual recovery, and some loss of contrast sensitivity that persisted meant we were keen to pursue hyperopic LASIK. Hyperopic LASIK can be used to treat naturally occurring hyperopia, to induce monovision in emmetropic patients for the treatment of aphakia, and for hyperopia secondary to overcorrection of myopic errors.

> Although we were generally satisfied with hyperopic PRK up to 3 D, the pain, prolonged re-epithelialization with large treatment zones, slow visual recovery, and some loss of contrast sensitivity that persisted meant we were keen to pursue hyperopic LASIK.

The Summit Apex Plus laser is an expanding aperture laser using 193 nm emission at a fluence of 180 mJ per cm^2 and a repetition rate of 10 hz. Hyperopic ablations are performed with an erodible disc cassette that is placed in the down rail of the laser followed by a nondisposable Axicon lens ablation to a zone of 9.5 mm. Ablations are performed in a two-stage procedure. The hyperopic erodible disc allows removal of tissue at the periphery of the 6.5 mm ablation zone, starting at 6.5 mm and ablating toward the visual axis. There is virtually no energy delivered at the central zone. The laser is reprogrammed for the Axicon portion of the procedure, and the number of Axicon pulses delivered varies with the hyperopic correction. The Axicon lens diverges the laser beam, and despite the aperture only opening to 6.5 mm, the ablation extends as far as 9.5 mm. Furthermore, the properties of the Axicon lens allows maximum energy delivery at 6.5 mm, and this tapers off as the beam approaches 9.5 mm. The result is a blend zone over the mid peripheral cornea.

The ablation profile was modified for LASIK. An L disc was created to treat from 6.5 mm into the visual axis. Between 5.75 mm and 6.5 mm, the disc aimed to create a trough mimicking the Axicon lens pulse ablation that had been used for surface treatments. In our early cases, we combined this with a small number of Axicon pulses between 6.5 mm and 9.5 mm using only 20% of Axicon pulses that would have been used for surface hyperopic treatment. We used this method between April and November 1997; and since November 1997, we have abandoned the use of the Axicon pulses entirely, relying purely on the disposable L disc to perform the ablation.

OPERATIVE TECHNIQUE

Preoperative preparation involves instillation of 2%
Pilocarpine drops 20 minutes prior to the procedure. Once positioned on the laser bed, 1% Amethocaine eye drops are used three times. The patient practices fixating on a green flashing fixation light. A speculum is inserted, and a Chiron automated microkeratome is used to create a hinged flap 180 microns in thickness. The flap is retracted and excess fluid is removed from the stromal surface. The hyperopic erodible disc is inserted into the down rail of the laser. A special interlock device ensures that the cassette is properly located and the disc is aligned in the optical beam path. The operating microscope light is turned off and the patient takes up fixation. Patient fixation and cooperation can be assessed by the surgeon via the operating microscope aided by two HeNe aiming beams positioned at 3 and 9 o'clock on either side of the visual axis. With the patient satisfactorily positioned, the hyperopic ablation is performed. The ablation commences at the 6.5 mm ablation zone and works towards the visual axis. Unlike a myopic LASIK procedure, most of the ablation occurs in the mid periphery and very little in the visual axis centrally.

The operating light is turned on, and the hyperopic erodible disc is removed from the down rail of the laser and replaced by the Axicon lens in its own cassette. The laser is re-programmed for the Axicon portion of the procedure. The number of Axicon pulses delivered varies with the hyperopic correction. After the corneal surface is checked, the operating light is again turned off and the patient takes up fixation. The Axicon lens ablation then commences. It is important at this stage to protect the under surface of the reflected flap from the diverged laser pulses. The property of the Axicon lens allows maximal energy delivery between 6.5 mm and 7.5 mm and tapers off as the beam approaches 9.5 mm. This creates a blend zone at the treated area of the cornea.

Following the laser treatment, the stromal bed is irrigated and the flap repositioned. Extensive irrigation underneath the flap is performed, and correct flap position is assessed with the gentian violet markers. The flap edge is also assessed. The patient is left for 2 to 3 minutes to ensure adherence of the flap while the epithelium is hydrated as necessary. A drop of Ofloxacin and Prednefrin Forte is instilled into the eye and the patient is reviewed 30 minutes later to ensure correct flap position.

RESULTS

We treated 80 eyes with hyperopic LASIK in this manner. The mean preoperative spherical equivalent was +3.2 D (standard deviation [SD] = 1.69). At 1 month, the mean spherical equivalent was +.25 (SD = .76). Sixty-three percent of eyes at 1 month were within .5 D of emmetropia, and 92% were within 1 D of emmetropia.

At 2 months, the mean spherical equivalent was +.65 D (SD = 1.11). There was no statistically significant regres-

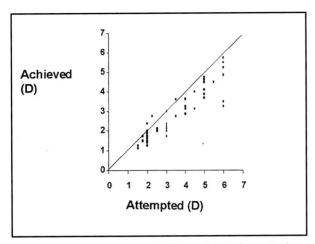

Figure 27-1. Hyperopic LASIK: spherical equivalent, attempted versus achieved.

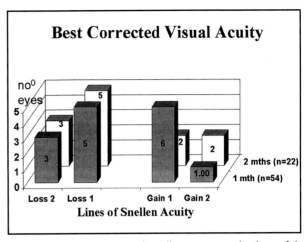

Figure 27-2. Best-corrected Snellen acuity at the latest follow-up.

> Sixty-three percent of eyes at 1 month were within .5 D of emmetropia, and 92% were within 1 D of emmetropia.

> Uncorrected visual acuity of 6/12 or better was achieved in 87.3% of patients at 1 month, and 77.3% of those followed at 2 months.

sion between 1 and 2 months. Astigmatism was not treated in this series of patients, and the average preoperative cylinder was 1.01 D. There was no statistically significant change at 1 and 2 months. Uncorrected visual acuity of 6/12 or better was achieved in 87.3% of patients at 1 month, and 77.3% of those followed at 2 months.

The attempted versus achieved graph (Figure 27-1) shows a degree of undercorrection with more marked in the higher hyperopic attempted treatments. At last follow-up, changes in the lines of BCVA are seen (Figure 27-2) with some patients gaining best-corrected and some patients losing best-corrected vision. No patients lost more than two lines of BCVA. For this study, a line was defined as 20/20, 20/25, 20/30, 20/40, and 20/60.

Three patients complained of night halos, although the incidence of this is less than in our routine myopic LASIK corrections. There were no cases of clinical or topographic decentration, which may be related to the fast ablation time—generally less than 30 seconds. In some patients there does appear to be a multifocal quality to the cornea, whereby their reading vision is better than predicted given their age and refractive outcome. This may be a mixed blessing in that any multifocal quality may detract from best-corrected vision overall while allowing simultaneous uncorrected distance and reading vision in presbyopic patients. It will take some time to determine the visual quality in these patients, however this study is already under way in analyz-

> In some patients there does appear to be a multifocal quality to the cornea, whereby their reading vision is better than predicted given their age and refractive outcome.

ing high and low contrast acuity with and without glare and contrast sensitivity with and without glare. This analysis, which will be performed over the next 6 to 12 months, will determine the real visual outcome of these patients and whether the corneal shape is of appropriately good quality.

CASE REPORTS

Two examples represent the normal pattern of correction and visual recovery expected in hyperopic LASIK with this system.

Mr. PT, age 44, had a cycloplegic refraction of right +3.25/-.5 at 80°, and left +4/-.5 at 110°. Both eyes were best-corrected 20/20.

A +3 D right hyperopic LASIK using an L disc was performed, and a +3.5 D left was performed as a simultaneous procedure on September 3. The following day, his unaided acuity was 20/30 right and 20/25 left. His 1-day topography is shown in Figure 27-3a and 27-3b.

At 3 months, his unaided acuity was 20/20 right and 20/20 -2 left. His residual cycloplegic refraction was +1/-.75 at 90° right and 1/-.75 at 111° left. He did not feel the need to wear either distance or reading correction, but his topography at 3 months (Figure 27-4a and 27-4b) shows some irregularity across the visual axis with a multifocal effect within the central cornea, although his visual quality subjectively is extremely good.

Mrs. MD, a 54-year-old woman, was scheduled for bilateral simultaneous hyperopic LASIK. Her preoperative refraction was right +5.75/-1.75 at 15° with corrected 20/20,

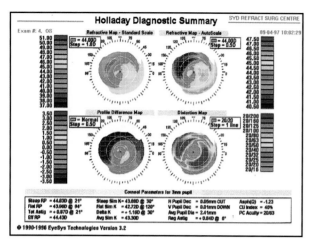

Figure 27-3a. Topography 1 day after +3 D hyperopic LASIK.

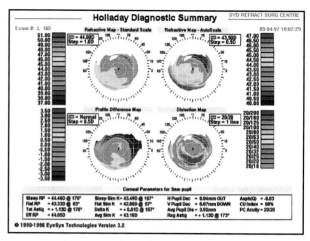

Figure 27-3b. Topography 1 day after +3.5 D hyperopic LASIK.

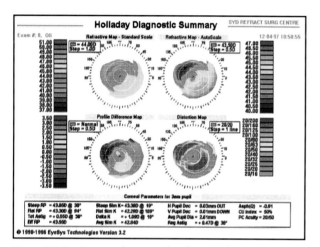

Figure 27-4a. Topography 3 months after +3 D hyperopic LASIK.

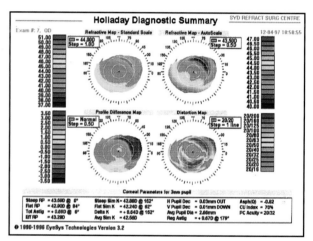

Figure 27-4b. Topography 3 months after +3.5 D hyperopic LASIK.

and left +6.75/-2.75 at 157° corrected 20/20.

The right eye was performed first using a customized L disc to allow for an astigmatic correction as well, and a slight undercorrection in the spherical equivalent was aimed for. There were no technical problems with the right eye, although when it came time to do the left eye, it was not possible to obtain adequate suction. We have found that with using the Chiron automated shaper, hyperopic eyes suffer from inadequate suction more commonly than myopic or astigmatic eyes. The reasons for this are unclear, although it may be related to scleral curvature or the overall smaller size of these eyes. This has not resulted in any free caps, as all cases unable to obtain suction were recognized prior to the microkeratome pass. These patients were rescheduled for different days and suction has been able to be obtained.

With Mrs. MD's right eye, her day 1 unaided acuity was 20/25 with topography as shown in Figure 27-5. At 1 week, she had regressed unaided 6/12 and cycloplegic refraction of +1.75. This has remained stable at 1 month. There was no loss of BCVA. Her topography at 1 month is shown in Figure 27-6.

SUMMARY

Hyperopic LASIK with the Summit Apex Plus laser is an effective means of treating hyperopia. In our hands, it is superior to hyperopic PRK and the level of patient satisfaction is high. The erodible disc technology is evolving with customized discs that are able to provide more appropriate mid peripheral corneal shape transfer. They also have the ability to treat hyperopic astigmatism and can be custom designed with an ablatable disc based on topographic patterns.

Centration, which has been a problem with some hyperopic treatments in the past, has not been a significant problem in our cases to date. This may be partly due to surgeon experience but is more likely to be related to the short ablation period and the fact that there is no tissue removed over the visual axis. Longer term follow-up of these cases is required to ensure stability and better analyze corneal shape and its effect on visual quality.

Hyperopic LASIK with this system is our current method of choice for treating hyperopia up to 5 D. We feel

LASIK after Penetrating Keratoplasty

Michiel Kritzinger, MD
Louis E. Probst, MD

Despite the refinement of our microsurgical techniques, penetrating keratoplasty (PKP) continues to be associated with significant postoperative ametropias. A recent study found that the average residual astigmatism following PKP was often over 3 D.[1] Significant myopic refractive errors have commonly been produced from the increased post-PKP corneal curvature, which is associated with the placement of an oversized donor corneal graft in the recipient bed.[2] Spectacle correction of these refractive errors can induce anisometropia and image distortion. Contact lenses are often difficult to fit and maintain on these corneas or may be poorly tolerated due to peripheral edge touch.

Many surgical techniques have been proposed to address the induced astigmatism following PKP. Lindstrom and co-workers have described the use of relaxing incisions, astigmatic keratotomy, compression sutures, and wedge resections to correct the varying degrees of postoperative astigmatism.[3] In older patients with cataracts, cataract extraction with intraocular lens (IOL) implantation can be done a few months after PKP in order to allow better prediction of the correct IOL diopter power and reduce the final refractive error.[4] Unfortunately, these techniques have been unable to provide consistent predictable results, leaving many patients with significant residual refractive errors following PKP.[5]

Photorefractive keratotomy (PRK) has been reported for the treatment of refractive errors following PKP.[6-10] Unfortunately, the published reports of this technique are limited to low myopia and have short follow-up. Corneal graft rejection has been reported following PRK after PKP, which may have been induced by the ultraviolet irradiation or irritation of the transplanted cornea.[11,12] PRK has been associated with haze when it is performed in eyes with previous ocular surgery and particularly if PRK is performed after laser in situ keratomileusis (LASIK) on the corneal flap.[13] Kritzinger has found that significant persistent corneal haze commonly occurs when PRK is used following PKP. Since the peripheral graft interface healing and corneal sutures continue to induce a corneal haze response long after PKP, further surface manipulation with PRK would appear to be undesirable in most cases.

> Kritzinger has found that significant persistent corneal haze commonly occurs when PRK is used following PKP.

Lamellar keratoplasty has recently been reported as a successful method of correcting the ametropias following PKP.[13-17] When the precision of LASIK is applied to the post-PKP cornea, the results appear to be reasonably predictable, particularly for the correction of spherical myopia.[13-15,17] Along with the obvious advantages of rapid visual rehabilitation and a pain-free postoperative course, the intrastromal ablation reduces the incidence of postoperative corneal haze. The decreased necessity for epithelial healing after LASIK reduces the risk of a postoperative bacterial keratitis, which could be detrimental to the post-PKP cornea.

The disadvantages of LASIK following PKP are mainly focused on the mechanical effects of this procedure on the tenuous graft-host interface of the post-PKP cornea. There is a definite risk of inducing graft dehiscence during LASIK with the pneumatic suction ring when the intraocular pressure is applied and rapidly increased to over 65 mm Hg. Since spontaneous corneal graft dehiscence has been observed decades after PKP, there is a definite risk of this complication during the mechanical manipulation of the post-PKP eye during LASIK. Graft dehiscence during LASIK with intraocular pressure (IOP) over 65 mm Hg would likely result in extrusion of the intraocular contents with sight-threatening complications (Figure 28-1).

Although less serious, the application of the suction ring may induce a shift in the astigmatism, which could decrease the predictability of the LASIK correction. The continued endothelial cell loss following PKP [18,19] places the cornea at a potential risk for failure after LASIK, which has been associated with endothelial cell loss in some studies.[17] The peripheral corneal neovascularization commonly associated with the healing of the graft-host interface after PKP can produce postoperative bleeding if these vessels are cut by the microkeratome.[15] Finally, all sutures must be removed from the cornea prior to LASIK, as retained sutures can block the movement of the microkeratome.[15]

> The application of the suction ring may induce a shift in the astigmatism, which could decrease the predictability of the LASIK correction.

Martiz and co-workers[14] reported the results of LASIK following PKP on six eyes with 1-month follow-up. The mean spherical error was reduced from -3.25 diopters (D) to -.7 D and the mean astigmatism was reduced from -4.2 D to -2.35 D. Arenas and co-workers[15] presented the results of four cases of LASIK following PKP with an average follow-up of 7 months. The mean spherical error was reduced from -10.75 D to -2.37 D. The astigmatism changed from -2.87 D to -3.5 D. Parisi and co-workers[13] described one eye that had LASIK after PKP. The preoperative refraction of -7 -1.25 X 60 was reduced to +1. − .75 X 80 at the 11-month follow-up visit. All of the cases described above had LASIK performed more than 1 year after PKP. None of the cases reported a loss of best-corrected visual acuity (BCVA) or graft dehiscence and no sight-threatening complications were observed. These studies illustrate that LASIK following PKP seems to be particularly effective for reducing spherical myopia but less effective for treating astigmatism. This may be due to the somewhat irregular astigmatism that often occurs following PKP, which is not well-treated by the current generation of excimer lasers. Topography-assisted LASIK should offer a more refined method of correcting the complex refractive errors induced by PKP.

> These studies illustrate that LASIK following PKP seems to be particularly effective for reducing spherical myopia but less effective for treating astigmatism.

THE KRITZINGER SURGICAL TECHNIQUE FOR LASIK AFTER PENETRATING KERATOPLASTY

After nearly 100 cases of LASIK following PKP, the following protocol has been adopted.

PREOPERATIVE ASSESSMENT
1. All corneal sutures are usually removed by the end of 1 year postoperatively.
2. After the last suture is out, wait an additional 4 months for the cornea to stabilize.
3. After 4 months, a full LASIK work-up is done, which includes corneal topography, pachymetry, and a corneal orbscan (elevation topography).
4. Auto refraction.
5. Cycloplegic refraction.
6. Subjective refraction.

SURGICAL TECHNIQUE
This is a two-step technique. The microkeratome cut is made into the transplanted cornea. The flap is *not lifted* and the interface is *not irrigated*. The surface of the flap is gently wiped and then allowed to seal into the stromal bed. The cornea is then allowed to stabilize for 2 to 3 weeks after this cut. A repeat preoperative assessment is then performed. In approximately 50% of patients, the refraction will change—particularly the amount and axis of the cylinder. The excimer laser ablation is then performed on the new refractive error after gently lifting the corneal flap. The flap is then replaced and allowed to stabilize in the usual manner.

If the LASIK ablation is immediately performed on the transplanted cornea, postoperative results are highly unpredictable with the fluctuating axis and diopters of the cylinder and sphere. This can result in the need for several LASIK enhancements, which may lead to a thin cornea with an unstable refraction. When the microkeratome cut is performed first and the cornea is allowed to stabilize, the number of enhancement procedures can be significantly reduced and the postoperative refraction is more predictable.

The other risk of performing multiple enhancements following PKP is that a wound leak may be created at the graft interface. This has happened to one of us (M. Kritzinger) on two occasions. In both cases, PKP was performed more than 25 years previously (when microsurgical techniques were still evolving). With the significant improvements in PKP techniques, including the use of fine suture material along with the improvements in quality corneal donor material, we believe that the risk of this complication is greatly diminished.

When we consider the horrible refractive errors patients are often forced to contend with after PKP, LASIK can make a dramatic improvement in uncorrected vision. LASIK can often reduce an extremely visually disabling

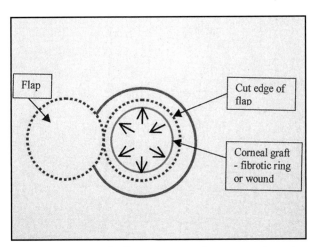

Figure 28-1. Once the flap is cut, new forces come into play within the grafted tissue that alter the refractive error. The microkeratome cut should be performed, and then the excimer laser ablation should be performed 2 to 3 weeks later, after the new refractive error has been measured.

refractive error to one that can be corrected with a small spectacle correction and even produce good uncorrected vision in many cases. Kritzinger has found that postoperatively the BCVA is maintained and the uncorrected visual acuity was 20/40 or better in approximately 80% of eyes. Preliminary experience with LASIK following PKP suggests that it can play a major role in the visual rehabilitation of the ametropic eye following PKP.

The new hyperopia PlanoScan software uses the optical zone size of 6 mm with a transition zone of up to 9 mm.

REFERENCES

1. Gross RH, Poulsen EJ, Davitt S, Schwab IR, Mannis MJ. Comparison of astigmatism after penetrating keratoplasty by experienced cornea surgeons and cornea fellows. *Am J Ophthalmol.* 1997;123(5):636-643

2. Kaufman HE. Corneal transplant optics and visual disability. *J Refract Corneal Surg.* 1989;5:213-215.

3. Lindstrom RL, Lindquist TD. Surgical Correction of postoperative astigmatism. *Cornea.* 1988;5:213-215.

4. Geggel HS. Intraocular lens implantation after penetrating kerato-plasty. Improved unaided visual acuity, astigmatism, and safety in patients in patients with combined corneal disease and cataract. *Ophthalmology.* 1990;97(11):1460-1467.

5. Lavery GW, Lindstrom RL, Hofer LA, Doughman DJ. The surgical management of corneal astigmatism after penetrating keratoplasty. *Ophthalmic Surg.* 1985;16:165-169.

6. John ME, Martines E, Cvintal T, et al. Photorefractive keratectomy following penetrating keratoplasty. *Journal of Refractive Surgery.* 1994;10(suppl):S206-S210.

7. Nordan LT, Binder PS, Kassar BS, Heitzmann J. Photorefractive keratectomy to treat myopia and astigmatism after radial keratotomy and penetrating keratoplasty. *J Cataract Refract Surg.* 1995;21:268-273.

8. Cheema D, Desschemes J, Galazsi G, Mullie M, Guibault N, Burnier M. Photorefractive keratectomy for correction of astigmatism after penetrating keratoplasty. *Invest Ophthalmol Vis Sci.* 1995;36(Suppl):S715.

9. Amm M, Duncker GIW, Schroder E. Excimer laser correction of high and astigmatism after keratoplasty. *J Cataract Refract Surg.* 1996;22:313-317.

10. Campos M, Herzog L, Garbus J, et al. Photorefractive keratectomy for severe post-keratoplasty astigmatism. *Am J Ophthalmol.* 1992;114:429-436.

11. Hersh PS, Jordan AJ, Mayers M. Corneal graft rejection episode after excimer laser phototherapeutic keratectomy (letter). *Arch Ophthalmol.* 1993;111:735-736.

12. Epstein RJ, Robin JB. Corneal graft rejection episode after excimer laser phototherapeutic keratectomy (letter). *Arch Ophthalmol.* 1994;112:157.

13. Parisi A, Salchow DJ, Zirm M, Stieldorf C. Laser in situ keratomileusis after automated lamellar keratoplasty and penetrating keratoplasty. *J Cataract Refract Surg.* 1997;23:1114-1118

14. Martiz JR, Slade SG, Baker RN. LASIK to treat myopia and astigmatism after penetrating keratoplasty. *Invest Ophthalmol Vis Sci.* 1997;38(4) (suppl):1960-B753.

15. Arenas E, Maglione A. Laser in situ keratomileusis for astigmatism and myopia after penetrating keratoplasty. *Journal of Refractive Surgery.* 1997;13:27-32.

16. Kremer F, Kremer I. Post-keratoplasty myopia treated by keratomileusis. *Ann Ophthalmol.* 1993;25:370

17. Pallikaris IG, Siganos DS. Excimer laser in situ keratomileusis and photorefractive keratectomy for correction of high myopia. *J Cataract Refract Surg.* 1994;20:498-510.

18. Bourne WM. One-year observation of transplanted human corneal endothelium. *Ophthalmology.* 1980;87:673-79.

19. Culbertson WW, Abbott RL, Forster RK. Endothelial cell loss in penetrating keratoplasty. *Ophthalmology.* 1982;89:600-604.

LASIK After Corneal and Intraocular Surgery

Jose L. Güell, MD, PhD
Ana de Muller, OPT
Oscar Gris, MD
Felicidad Manero, MD
Mercedes Vazquez, MD

LASIK AFTER OTHER SURGICAL PROCEDURES

During the last 4 years, we have been using LASIK for correcting myopia, astigmatism, and hyperopia in eyes with previous surgery. In this chapter, we will first discuss our experience with a control group of eyes, which has been previously published in other sources.[3,5] Second, we will discuss our experience with LASIK in previously operated eyes, as well as the advantages and disadvantages of LASIK compared to the other options for the correction of residual ametropias in these cases.

MATERIALS AND METHODS

Between March 1994 and August 1996 we performed LASIK to correct residual myopia and astigmatism on 87 eyes (62 patients) that were previously operated on by means of other surgical techniques. The distribution of the cases according to the previous surgery resulted in six separate groups. There were 26 eyes with previous phacoemulsification with IOL implantation (Figure 29-1), 20 eyes with previous penetrating keratoplasty (Figure 29-2), 22 eyes with previous RK (Figure 29-3), 10 eyes with previous PRK (Figure 29-4), four eyes with previous penetrating ocular trauma (previous corneal suture with or without additional intraocular surgery) (Figure 29-5), and five eyes with a previous insertion of a phakic IOL implantation (Figure 29-6 and Table 29-1). All patients had a stable refraction over a minimum of at least a 6-month period. Sutures that were still present were removed at least 8 weeks prior to pro-

ceeding with LASIK in all cases. All patients were fully informed about the advantages and disadvantages of LASIK, and they all had an unsatisfactory correction with glasses or contact lenses due to medical, professional, or personal reasons.

The average patient age was 33.15 years (±5.3 standard deviation [SD]) and ranging between 21 and 52 years. We corrected myopia (.5 D and 9.75 D) and astigmatism (.75 D and 6 D).

A complete ophthalmological examination was carried out, which included evaluation of uncorrected visual acuity (UCVA), spectacle-corrected visual acuity (SCVA), subjective and cycloplegic refraction, keratometry (Javal), videokeratography (EyeSys Corneal Analysis System, Houston, Tex), slit lamp biomicroscopy including tear film break-up time and Schirmer test without topical anesthesia, endothelial cell count with specular noncontact microscopy (Conan), Goldmann applanation tonometry, indirect ophthalmoscopy, as well as ultrasonic pachymetry and axial length measurement (Omega Biometer, Storz).

As with any LASIK case, we based our refractive corrections on the subjective refraction, although the final decision was slightly modified according to the cycloplegic refraction if there was any discrepancy. For our results, we used the spherical equivalent of the subjective refraction in both pre- and postoperative data. For the visual acuity results, the decimal fraction of visual acuity is used.

SURGICAL TECHNIQUE

The main surgical techniques used in this study have been previously published.[6] The basic steps of the surgical

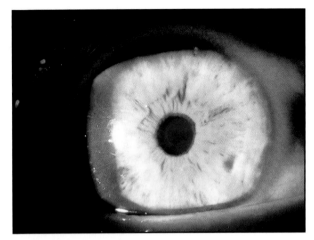

Figure 29-1. LASIK after radial keratotomy.

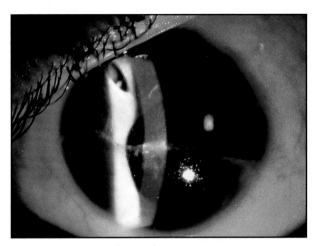

Figure 29-2. LASIK after ocular trauma.

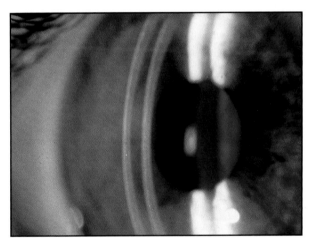

Figure 29-3. LASIK after PRK.

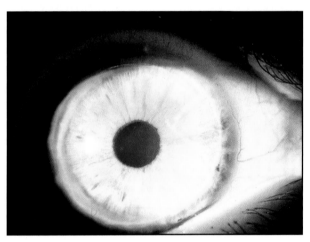

Figure 29-4. LASIK after penetrating keratoplasty.

procedure were consistent, although small modifications have been included in our LASIK experience during the last few years. Refractive data was collected and analyzed with D-Base III software.

RESULTS

Refraction

Mean preoperative spherical equivalent was -5.25 D (± 2.1 SD). Mean refraction, as a spherical equivalent at 6 months, was -.7 D (± .65 SD). At 6 months, we had 49 eyes between plano and -.5 D, representing 56.32% of the patients. Between plano and -1 D we had 66 eyes, representing 75.86%. Between plano and -2.25 D, we had 86 eyes, representing 98.85%. We only had one patient overcorrected whose residual refractive error at 6 months was +.5 D.

In terms of stability over the 6-month follow-up period, there was less than ±.5 D change in 94.3% of patients. An important exception was a patient who regressed over 6 months to 2 D of astigmatism originally present after pene-

trating keratoplasty. Follow-up differences existed in the different groups, different cases, and different times of surgery (eyes operated on in March 1994 as opposed to eyes operated on by mid 1996).

Visual Acuity

Preoperatively, the SCVA was 10/10 or better on 21 out of 87 eyes (24.13%), 5/10 or better in 78 of 87 eyes (89.65%), and less than 5/10 in 9 cases (10.34%). Six months postoperatively, including all the eyes in a same group, 23 out of 87 eyes (26.4%) achieved 10/10 or better SCVA, 83 of 87 eyes (95.40%) achieved 5/10 or better SCVA, and 4 of 87 eyes (4.59%) were less than 5/10 SCVA (Table 29-2). Safety of the procedure appeared to be excellent with no loss of SCVA during the follow-up period.

Preoperatively, UCVA was count fingers or worse in all cases except three eyes in which it was 1/10. At 6 months time, UCVA was 10/10 or better in a single case out of the 87 eyes (1.14%), 61 of 87 (70.11%) eyes achieved 5/10 or better UCVA, and 25 of 87 eyes (28.62%)

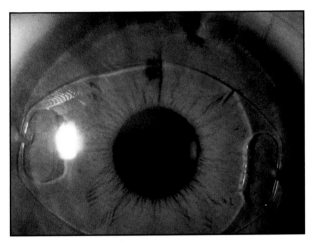

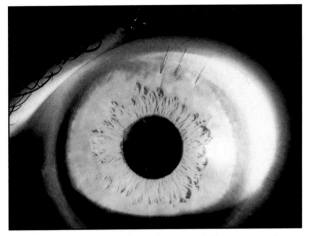

Figure 29-5. LASIK after phakic IOL.

Figure 29-6. LASIK after phacoemulsification and 1OL implantation.

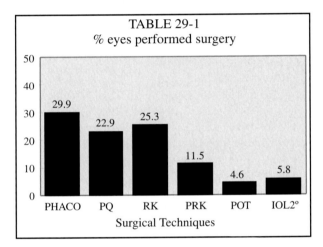

TABLE 29-1
% eyes performed surgery

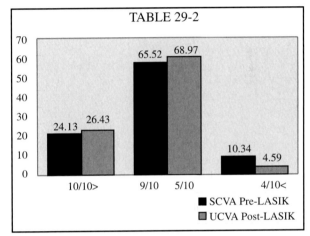

TABLE 29-2

achieved UCVA worse than 5/10. Stability of visual acuity results was excellent during the follow-up period.

Astigmatism

Based on keratometry (irregular mires) and videokeratography (irregular patterns), no postoperative irregular astigmatism was observed.

Analyzing the entire group, 61 of 87 eyes did not present any residual refractive astigmatism, 16 of 87 eyes had less cylindrical component though on the same axis, and most of these eyes (11 eyes) had undergone previous penetrating keratoplasty. We found that 10 of 87 eyes had less astigmatism than preoperatively, however this was on a different axis.

Slit Lamp Examination

Twelve to 24 hours after surgery, the flaps were either clear or demonstrated slight edema. Flap beds and edges were difficult to discern and flap interface was clear, except in some cases in which small areas with conjunctival debris were noted, which reabsorbed over several weeks of follow-up.

Complications

There were no complications related to the microkeratome in our patients. In the first case of reoperation for undercorrected LASIK after an undercorrected 8-incision radial keratotomy, an important complication occurred. During our standard flap dissection with our iridodialysis spatula, the old radial incisions came apart. The procedure was completed without any further complication, yet the patient developed symptoms of recurrent corneal erosion over a 3-month period after the operation. Application of topical hyperosmotic agents controlled these symptoms.

We did not observe clinically significant epithelial ingrowth in any of our cases, although small epithelial islands at the edge of the flap less than 1 mm in diameter were observed. Contrary to our LASIK experience on virgin eyes, night vision was not a special problem in this patient group (subjective analysis). However, daytime visual fluctuations were noted in those eyes with previous RK (three

Daytime visual fluctuations were noted in those eyes with previous RK (three eyes) and with greater residual myopia (more than 6 D).

eyes) and with greater residual myopia (more than 6 D). These day time fluctuations of the refractive correction are a new complication on our LASIK experience. This was probably related to instability of the cornea from the previous aggressive RK.

The main complication in this series was a slight undercorrection as in our normal LASIK series.

Reoperations

We did not have to reoperate on any patient due to interface problems, though we did reoperate for undercorrections. Five of the 26 (19.2%) previous phacoemulsification cases, 9 of the 20 (45%) previous penetrating keratoplasty cases, 4 of the 22 (18.8%) previous RK cases, and one of the 10 (10%) PRK cases required reoperation (Table 29-3). No penetrating ocular trauma or phakic IOL case for high myopia was reoperated. Therefore, the overall LASIK enhancement rate for this group was 19 of 87 eyes (21.8%).

DISCUSSION

LASIK was originally introduced by Ioannis Pallikaris and co-workers in 1990.[7] Initially, the technique comprised the standard free cap in situ keratomileusis with the excimer laser used for the corrective ablation. Later, Pallikaris and co-authors[8,9] described the hinge technique in which the resection of the anterior corneal disc with the microkeratome was incomplete. LASIK combines the advantages of laser ablation (high accuracy and flexibility with corneal tissue ablation) with the advantages of intrastromal or lamellar surgery (preservation of the epithelium-Bowman's membrane complex with reduced risk of haze on enhanced refractive stability). Several studies[6,10] have demonstrated the efficacy of LASIK in correcting low, medium, and high myopia with outstanding predictability and stability. At present we are using LASIK to correct myopia with or without astigmatism, from 1 D up to 14 D as long as the corneal thickness is adequate for full correction.[11]

Most refractive surgery specialists agree that further incisional surgery for undercorrected RK is only effective if the refractive error is less than 1.5 D,[12,13] and in most cases further incisional surgery is best avoided.[14] Over the last few years we have observed a growing interest in treating undercorrected RK with PRK with good results reported by a large number of researchers[15,16,17,18,19,20,21] even when two-stage treatments are used for high myopia.[22] However, other groups have noted a clear deviation towards hyperopia[23] and a lower predictability with a higher incidence of haze[24,25] when PRK is performed after RK as compared to the results of PRK on a virgin eye. Surgeons have proposed other techniques to correct residual myopia after RK, including LASIK[26] and phakic IOL implantation.[27] We have successfully used LASIK as our standard technique to treat undercorrected RK eyes.

Most researchers concur that PRK undercorrections

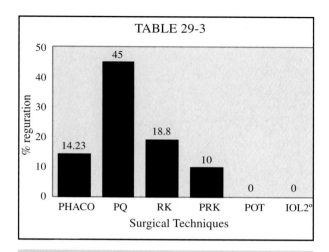

TABLE 29-3

should be treated with enhancement PRK, although some groups have utilized RK in these cases. Once Bowman's membrane has undergone laser ablation, it is generally preferable to perform PRK in these cases. LASIK treatment also achieved excellent results in these cases of undercorrected PRK without the problems of haze or regression, however some cases may not be suitable for lamellar surgery because of an extremely flat or thin residual cornea.

Despite the postoperative methods of controlling the residual cylinder, including suture manipulation and/or removal, astigmatism after penetrating keratoplasty is the most common complication. Techniques such as wedge resection[28,29] or relaxing incisions[30,31,32] can be used to reduce post-penetrating keratoplasty astigmatism, however these techniques tend to have a low predictability and may need to be repeated. Mechanical lamellar surgery has also been used[33] to correct myopic spherical residual defects, although predictability has been poor and there was no correction of astigmatic errors. PRK has also been used to treat these patients with good results for both the correction of spherical as well as cylindrical defects;[34,35,36] however significant complications have been published, including regression, haze,[37,38] and graft rejection.[39,40] This corneal rejection could be explained by the traumatizing nature of PRK after de-epithelializing and laser impact on the stroma with the subsequent corneal tissue recovery.

We have used LASIK to correct the residual refractive errors following penetrating keratoplasty (spherical and cylindrical) with very good results. Although the surgical principles are different in LASIK as compared to PRK, and the risk of graft rejection is theoretically smaller, we prophylactically treat our patients with topical steroids for several weeks prior to LASIK. With the use of prophylactic

> LASIK treatment also achieved excellent results in these cases of undercorrected PRK without the problems of haze or regression, however some cases may not be suitable for lamellar surgery because of an extremely flat or thin residual cornea.

> Although the surgical principles are different in LASIK as compared to PRK and the risk of graft rejection is theoretically smaller, we prophylactically treat our patients with topical steroids for several weeks prior to LASIK.

preoperative steroid drops, we have not encountered graft rejection after LASIK. The entire refractive error was corrected when the astigmatism was equal or less than 6 D. In those cases with more than 6 D of astigmatism (not included in this series), we initially performed relaxing incisions to reduce the cylinder and when stability of the resultant refractive error was confirmed (3 to 4 months), we used LASIK to correct the remaining refractive error. If the spherical equivalent is plano after penetrating keratoplasty, relaxing incisions may be sufficient, however even in cases with low cylinder we prefer to treat with LASIK because of the higher predictability. In our experience, the predictability of LASIK for treating astigmatism after penetrating keratoplasty has been as successful as with virgin eyes. We have always used the PlanoScan software (25 or 50 Hz) with our Chiron Technolas excimer laser for the cylinder correction and this may be the reason that Arenas and coworkers,[41] who used the Chiron Multizone software (10 Hz), had different results in their four patients.

There is a paucity of information in the literature regarding treatment of refractive errors after anterior segment ocular trauma. Most descriptions have focused on the insertion of the correct IOL, with rigid contact lenses for the corneal astigmatism, and the eventual need to carry out penetrating keratoplasty. These techniques were intended to correct high refractive errors rather than to adjust small residual errors that can be successfully treated with LASIK.

Phakic IOLs are one of the most exciting new refractive surgical techniques. Although there is a high degree of predictability with this procedure, an enhancement procedure is often required to correct the small residual spherical defects and, most importantly, the astigmatic errors that are not corrected by the phakic intraocular implant. The surgical correction of these refractive errors has not been previously described. We have used LASIK in these cases, and the results have also been excellent. We are now combining phakic IOL implantation with LASIK to correct high myopia so that we can use larger ablation zones with the LASIK to improve the quality of postoperative vision.

Similarly, it is relatively common to find residual defects after cataract surgery in highly myopic or hyperopic eyes despite improvements in the IOL power calculation formula and standardization of the surgical techniques. Many surgeons have suggested the use of corneal refractive surgery to correct smaller defects. Both RK[42] and PRK can be useful in these cases, however the potential limitations and complications of these procedures must be considered. An IOL exchange or a second piggy back IOL can also be performed to correct the residual refractive error, however this may induce excessive ocular trauma, particularly if the IOL has been in place for a long time. These techniques will also require incisional surgery, which may actually increase the residual astigmatism. We have found LASIK to be an excellent procedure for the correction of small refractive errors after cataract surgery, as it allows the simultaneous correction of spherical and astigmatic refractive errors in a safe and predictable manner.

> We have found LASIK to be an excellent procedure for the correction of small refractive errors after cataract surgery, as it allows the simultaneous correction of spherical and astigmatic refractive errors in a safe and predictable manner.

THE WORST IRIS CLAW PHAKIC IOL AND LASIK FOR THE CORRECTION OF HIGH MYOPIC ERRORS

Our preliminary data for this new approach to the correction of high myopia is available with 12 months of follow-up. We have operated on 61 eyes with this double technique and the results are extremely encouraging. First, we will review the results of 18 eyes, and then we will discuss the main advantages and disadvantages of this approach.

The goal of this study was to prospectively analyze the efficacy, safety, stability, and optical performance of phakic IOL implantation followed by LASIK in high myopic eyes. The results were also compared to phakic IOL alone or LASIK alone.

METHODS

Eighteen eyes of 18 patients between 25 and 36 years old were included in the study. All the eyes had an spherical equivalent refraction between -14 D and -24 D and an SCVA of 20/40 or better. The phakic IOL was the standard -14 D Worst iris claw lens with a 6 mm optical zone diameter that was inserted through a superior capillary corneal incision. Four months later, all the sutures were removed. LASIK was performed to correct the residual spherical and cylindrical error.

The preoperative ophthalmological examination was normal in all cases. Pre- and postoperative examinations (1, 3, 6, and 12 months) included slit lamp examination, laser flare meter measurements, Goldmann applanation tonometry, spec-

> We are now combining phakic IOL implantation with LASIK to correct high myopia so that we can use larger ablation zones with the LASIK to improve the quality of postoperative vision.

ular microscopy with the noncontact Conan microscope, indirect funduscopy, UCVA, SCVA, videokeratography, automatic and subjective refraction, contrast sensitivity testing, and subjective night vision scale testing. These results were compared with those previously obtained with LASIK alone (18 of JL Güell's best LASIK cases) and with the phakic IOL alone (18 uncomplicated cases published by other investigators).

RESULTS

Our 12-month preliminary optical performance analysis found that 82.5% of the eyes were within .5 D of spherical equivalent (SE) residual refraction and 100% within 1 D. Eleven percent of the eyes gained three lines of SCVA, 55% gained two lines, and 100% gained one line. During the 12-month follow-up period, 93.5% of the eyes had a change equal to or less than .5 D in their SE refraction, demonstrating good stability.

Specular microscopy data was statistically better 12 months after surgery—probably because the patients were not using contact lenses. Laser flare meter measurements showed no progressive changes over this short follow-up period. IOP was elevated 1 mm Hg in 27% of the eyes at the 3-month follow-up and in 5.5% of the eyes at the 12-month follow-up. The subjective analysis of night vision found an increase in night vision difficulties in 11% of the eyes. There were no other clinical or surgical complications.

As would be expected, UCVA was better in all the eyes with the double-procedure approach. Ten eyes in the double approach group and eight eyes in the single approach group gained two lines of SCVA (seven phakic IOL and one LASIK). None of the treated eyes lost any lines of SCVA. Although a detailed evaluation of the contrast sensitivity is not available, most of the eyes with both procedures had no night vision problems from the 1-month follow-up (two patients had subtle problems), and all of the eyes from the single approach group had moderate problems.

CONCLUSIONS

This preliminary data suggest that the combined technique of phakic IOLs with a LASIK enhancement procedure can produce excellent results with minimal complications. While the final UCVA is the most important parameter, the small optics necessary for the treatment of high myopia result in significant night vision problems. It is probably best not to treat our highly myopic patients with LASIK alone because of the small optical zone that is required to maintain adequate corneal thickness. Extremely flat corneas (LASIK in very high myopia) and a small opti-

> Extremely flat corneas (LASIK in very high myopia) and a small optical zone (LASIK or phakic IOLs alone) are the main causes of poor postoperative night vision.

cal zone (LASIK or phakic IOLs alone) are the main causes of poor postoperative night vision.

After our preliminary experience in high myopia surgery with LASIK and with several phakic IOLs (anterior chamber Baikoff-style phakic IOL, posterior chamber Staar phakic IOL and the Worst Iris Claw phakic IOL), we decided to use the Iris Claw IOL because it provides the largest optical zone due to its location on the eye (far from the endothelium and anterior capsule—pigmentary epithelium complex). Myopic correction with this phakic IOL is performed up to -15 D in order to avoid peripheral endothelial damage.

With these concepts in mind, we developed the double-procedure approach to avoid the small optical zone required for a single-procedure approach with the currently available technology. The long-term follow-up results of our work, along with that of other investigators, will show us if the combined procedure concept produces safe and stable results.

THE ADJUSTABLE REFRACTIVE SURGERY CONCEPT

Both intraocular and corneal refractive surgery techniques have undergone a remarkable evolution over the last 15 years. One of the most important advances of refractive surgery has been the excimer laser. Photorefractive keratectomy (PRK) revolutionized corneal refractive surgery in the 1980s and laser in situ keratomileusis (LASIK) has had a similar effect in the 1990s.

At the same time, demands from both the refractive surgeon's perspective as well as the patient's are becoming more exacting. The primary goal of refractive surgery is to achieve the smallest residual refractive error along with preserving contrast sensitivity and the same visual capacity under bright and dim illumination conditions.

Although we do not know the absolute limits of LASIK, it has become clear that LASIK cannot be used to treat extreme myopias or hyperopias. With LASIK, between 10 and 14 diopters (D) is the limit of myopic correction, and between 4D and 6 D is the limit of hyperopia correction in a spherical equivalent form. Intraocular refractive surgery (both clear lens extraction with intraocular lens [IOL] and phakic IOL surgery) is a much better option for higher corrections. Improvements in biometry measurements and nomograms for phakic IOL power calculation have reduced the final refractive error in most of these cases.

In the past, several corneal refractive surgery techniques have been used to refine the final refraction after penetrating keratoplasty (PKP) and intraocular refractive surgery, such as radial keratotomy (RK), arcuate and transverse keratotomy and photorefractive keratectomy (PRK).[1,2] For the last 4 years, we have been using LASIK to correct myopia from .5 D up to 18 D. Since March 1994 we have also been

The increased IOP during the LASIK procedure can result in a change in the contour of the cornea, which can result in endothelial touch to the IOL.

using LASIK to correct residual ametropia after intraocular surgery. LASIK has been performed after cataract/clear lens extraction with IOL implantation, PKP, pars plana vitrectomy, PRK, radial and arcuate keratotomy, and phakic IOL implantation.[3]

In order to achieve emmetropia, LASIK has been extremely useful for us in highly myopic or hyperopic eyes with lens surgery or phakic IOL implantation. Up to 60% of our very high ametropic patients treated with intraocular surgery are, as a second step, referred for LASIK surgery.

There are several potential complications related to the increase of intraocular pressure (IOP) during the LASIK procedure in pseudophakic eyes or in eyes with phakic IOLs, especially those eyes with angle or iris-supported IOLs. The increased IOP during the LASIK procedure can result in a change in the contour of the cornea, which can result in endothelial touch to the IOL. This could result in significant endothelial cell trauma with potential corneal endothelial cell loss.

In order to avoid this problem as well as allow for some adjustability of the refractive procedure,[4] we started to proceed with the practical concept of adjustable refractive surgery (ARS). In all our highly myopic and hyperopic candidates for intraocular surgery with lens surgery and IOL implantation or those with phakic IOL implantation, we now perform the lamellar cut at the time of the first surgery. After our retro-peribulbar block or under topical anesthesia (15% of our intraocular cases), we first make our flap with the microkeratome. Once we consider the flap is adhered (between 30 and 120 seconds), we proceed with the intraocular surgery in the standard manner. Between 2 and 4 months after the intraocular surgery (depending on the incision size and location, we may wait a few more weeks), we can easily correct the residual refractive error with the excimer laser by lifting the corneal flap in the same manner as any of our other post-LASIK retreatments. The main advantage of such an approach is that we are avoiding the possible risks related to the microkeratome use in these operated eyes. The enhancement procedure also becomes simple to perform for any surgeon, even without training in lamellar surgery, if he or she has accessibility to an excimer laser and experience with PRK.

Although refractive predictability in IOL implantation

In all our highly myopic and hyperopic candidates for intraocular surgery with lens surgery and IOL implantation or those with phakic IOL implantation, we now perform the lamellar cut at the time of the first surgery.

in phakic and pseudophakic eyes will be much better in the near future, ARS can be extremely useful in young patients with high ametropias. In these cases, we need to use both intraocular and corneal procedures to completely correct the error. By using the techniques in combination, we can avoid the small optical zone we would need for a single procedure LASIK approach. Long-term follow-up is required to evaluate the safety and stability of this approach.

SUMMARY

LASIK has been shown to be a safe and effective procedure with regard to improving UCVA with minimal complications such as endothelial trauma. LASIK has been shown to have a high degree of efficacy, predictability, and stability for corrections of up to 12 D of spherical myopia and up to 6 D of astigmatism. The refractive results of LASIK are also titratable with a relatively simple enhancement procedure. LASIK is our current technique of choice to correct this type of refractive defect both on virgin eyes and on eyes that have undergone other surgical procedures.

Several special situations require the alteration of our LASIK technique. LASIK enhancements on eyes with previous RK must be performed with a new cut and not with flap dissection, which is generally performed during the 12-month postoperative period. In our experience, flap dissection can result in flap fragmentation when previous RK has been performed. Despite reports at international meetings of epithelial ingrowth after LASIK in these complex cases, we have not observed clinically significant ingrowth in any of our cases. Even in the cases of high astigmatism when arcuate keratotomy was performed only 3 to 4 months prior to LASIK, none of the cases had significant epithelial ingrowth.

Regarding LASIK after PK, we presently treat our patients with topical steroids for several weeks preoperatively and no case of rejection has been observed to date. The slight improvement in SCVA results is due to the reduction in cylinder in post-PKP eyes. The low rate of surgical complications with LASIK after other corneal or intraocular surgery, in our experience, is probably related to our extensive experience with LASIK and the precautions adopted for this particular group.

From the surgeon's viewpoint, it is a great advantage to be able to use the same procedure to correct different refractive errors in different clinical cases. Our results have demonstrated that with a careful and cautious approach, LASIK can achieve excellent results in eyes with previous ocular surgery.

LASIK enhancements on eyes with previous RK must be performed with a new cut and not with flap dissection.

REFERENCES

1. Agapitos PJ, Lindstrom RL, Williams PA, Sanders DR. Analysis of astigmatic keratotomy. *J Cataract Refract Surg.* 1989;5:13-18.
2. Maloney RK, Chan WK, Steinert R, Hersh P, O'Connell M. Summit Therapeutic Refractive Study Group. A multicenter trial of photorefractive keratectomy for residual myopia after previous ocular surgery. *Ophthalmology.* 1995;102(7):1042-52. Discussion.
3. Güell JL, Gris O, Muller A. LASIK over other refractive surgery procedures. *Ophthalmology.* In press.
4. Waring GO III. Lans distinguished refractive surgery lecture. *Journal of Refractive Surgery.* 1987;3:140-141.
5. Güell JL, et al. LASIK enhancement following previous surgical procedures. In: Lucio Buratto, ed. *LASIK: Principles and Techniques.* SLACK Incorporated: Thorofare, NJ; 1997.
6. Güell JL, Muller A. Laser in situ keratomileusis for myopia from -7 to -18 diopters. *Journal of Refractive Surgery.* 1996;22:222-228.
7. Pallikaris I, Papatsanaki M, Stathi E, Frenschock O, Georgiadis A. Laser in situ keratomileusis. *Lasers Surg Med.* 1990;10:463-468.
8. Pallikaris IG, Papatzanaki ME, Siganos DS, Tsilimbaris MK. A corneal flap technique for laser in situ keratomileusis human studies. *Arch Ophthalmol.* 1991;145:1699-1702.
9. Pallikaris I, et al. Technica de colgajo corneal para la queratomileusis in situ mediante laser: estudios en humanos (in Spanish). *Arch Ophthalmol.* 1992;3:127-130.
10. Pallikaris IG, Siganos DS. Excimer laser in situ keratomileusis and photorefractive keratectomy for the correction of high myopia. *J Refract Corneal Surg.* 1994;10:498-510.
11. Güell JL, et al. Correction limits with LASIK. In: Pallikaris I and Siganos D, eds. *LASIK.* SLACK Incorporated: Thorofare, NJ; 1997.
12. Coulon P, Poirier L, Williamson W, Verin P, Roques JC. Results of reoperation for undercorrection of radial keratotomies. Apropos of 25 cases. *J Fr Ophtalmol.* 1993;16(2):95-102.
13. Montard M, Piquot X, Bosc JM, Posposil A. Reoperation after radial keratotomy. When is it indicated? *J Fr Ophtalmol.* 1991;14(3):177-80.
14. Poirier L, Coulon P, Williamson W, Barach D, Mortemousque B, Verin P. Effect of peripheral deepening of radial keratotomy incisions. *J Refract Corneal Surg.* 1994;10(6):621-4.
15. Nagy ZZ, Suveges I, Nemeth J, Fust A. The role of excimer laser photorefractive keratectomy in treatment of residual myopia followed by radical keratotomy. *Acta Chir Hurg.* 1995-96;35(1-2):13-9.
16. Kwitko ML, Gow JA, Bellavance F, Woo G. Excimer photorefractive keratectomy after undercorrected radial keratotomy. *Journal of Refractive Surgery.* 1995;11(3suppl):s280-3.
17. Durrie DS, Schumer DJ, Cavanaugh TB. Photorefractive keratectomy for residual myopia after previous refractive keratotomy. *J Refract Corneal Surg.* 1994;10(2suppl):s235-8.
18. Epstein D, Fagerholm P, Hamberg-Nystrom H, Tengroth. Twenty-four month follow-up of excimer laser photorefractive keratectomy for myopia. *Ophthalmology.* 1994;101:1558-1564.
19. Machat JJ, Tayfour F. Photorefractive keratectomy for myopia: preliminary results in 147 eyes. *J Refract Corneal Surg.* 1993;9(suppl):16-19.
20. Gallinaro C, Cochener B, Mimouni F, Colin J. Treatment by refractive photokeratectomy of undercorrections after radial keratotomy. *J Fr Ophthalmol.* 1994;17(12):746-9.
21. Seiler T, Jean B. Photorefractive keratectomy as a second attempt to correct myopia after radial keratotomy. *J Refract Corneal Surg.* 1992;8(3):211-4.
22. Lee YC, Park CK, Sah WJ, Hahn TW, Kim MS, Kim JH. Photorefractive keratectomy for undercorrected myopia after radial keratotomy: 2-year follow-up. *Journal of Refractive Surgery.* 1995:11(3suppl):s274-9.
23. Meza J, Perez-Santonja JJ, Moreno E, Zato MA. Photorefractive keratectomy after radial keratotomy. *J Cataract Refract Surg.* 1994;20(5):485-9.
24. Ribeiro JC, McDonald MB, Lemos MN, et al. Excimer laser photorefractive keratectomy after radial keratotomy. *Journal of Refractive Surgery.* 1995;11(3):165-9.
25. Hersh PS, Shah SI, Durrie D. Monocular diplopia following excimer laser photorefractive keratectomy after radial keratotomy. *Ophthalmic Surgery and Lasers.* 1996;27(4):315-7.
26. Lyle WA, Jin GJ. Initial results of automated lamellar keratoplasty for correction of myopia: 1-year follow-up. *J Cataract Refract Surg.* 1996;22(1):31-43.
27. Choyce DP. Residual myopia after radial keratotomy successfully treated with Baikoff ZB5M IOLs. *J Refract Corneal Surg.* 1993;9(6):475. Letter.
28. Frucht-Pery J. Wedge resection for post-keratoplasty astigmatism. *Ophthalmic Surg.* 1993;24(8):516-8.
29. Lugo M, Donnenfeld EO, Arentsen JJ. Corneal wedge resection for high astigmatism following penetrating keratoplasty. *Ophthalmic Surg.* 1987;18:650-653.
30. Seit B, Haumann GO. Limbus parallel keratotomies and compression sutures in excessive astigmatism after penetrating keratoplasty. *Ger J Ophthalmol.* 1993; 2:42-50.
31. Jacobi PC, Hartmann C, Severin M, Bartz SK. Relaxing incisions with compression sutures for control of astigmatism after penetrating keratoplasty. *Graefes Arch Clin Exp Ophthalmol.* 1994;232:527-32.
32. Kirkness CM, Ficker LA, Steele AD, Rice NS. Refractive surgery for graft-induced astigmatism after penetrating keratoplasty for keratoconus. *Ophthalmology.* 1991;98:1786-92.
33. Roholt PC. Automated lamellar keratoplasty after penetrating keratoplasty. American Society of Cataract and Refractive Surgeons. Symposium of Cataract IOL and Refractive Surgery. San Diego, Calif; April 1995.
34. Nordan LT, Binder PS, Kansar BS, Hetzmann J. Photorefractive keratectomy to treat myopic and astigmatism after radial keratotomy and penetrating keratoplasty. *J Cataract Refract Surg.* 1995;21:268-273.
35. Lampos M, Hertzog L, Gardus J, et al. Photorefractive keratectomy for severe post-keratoplasty astigmatism. *Am J Ophthalmol.* 1992;114:429-436.
36. Amm M, Dunker GW, Shröder E. Excimer laser correction of high astigmatism after keratoplasty. *J Cataract Refract Surg.* 1996;22:313-317.
37. John ME, Martines E, Cvintal T, et al. Photorefractive keratectomy following penetrating keratoplasty. *J Refract Corneal Surg.* 1994;10(2suppl):s206-10.
38. Tuunanen TH, Ruusuvaara PJ, Uusitalo RJ, Tervo TM. Photoastigmatism keratectomy for correction of astigmatism in corneal grafts. *Cornea.* 1997;16(1):48-53.
39. Hersh PS, Jordan AJ, Mayers M. Corneal graft rejection episode after excimer laser phototherapeutic keratectomy. *Arch Ophthalmol.* 1993;111:735-736.
40. Epstein RJ, Robin J. Corneal graft rejection episode after excimer laser phototherapeutic keratectomy. *Arch Ophthalmol.* 1994;112:157
41. Arenas E, Maglione A. Laser in situ keratomileusis for astigmatism and myopia after penetrating keratoplasty. *Journal of Refractive Surgery.* 1997;13:27-32.
42. Au YK, Lucius RW, Granger B. Radial keratotomy in an elderly patient after ECCE/IOL. *J Cataract Refract Surg.* 1993;19(3):415-6.

SECTION NINE
LASIK Complications

LASIK Complications

Lucio Buratto, MD
Stephen Brint, MD
Massimo Ferrari, MD

INTRODUCTION

Laser in situ keratomileusis (LASIK) complications can be divided into the categories of preoperative, intraoperative, and postoperative (Table 30-1). This chapter is a comprehensive review of the various complications.

PREOPERATIVE COMPLICATIONS

ANESTHESIA COMPLICATIONS

General anesthesia is rarely used in the United States, as the large majority of lasers are housed in physician's offices or laser centers where it is not available. Internationally, excimer lasers are often used in the hospital setting where general anesthesia is more available. General anesthesia should be considered only in extremely anxious patients or doctors performing their very first cases with the microkeratome.

Anesthesia by retrobulbar or peribulbar injection is preferable to general anesthesia as soon as the surgeon is reasonably comfortable with the microkeratome. Retrobulbar injections should be reserved only for special cases such as to increase exposure in patients with sunken eyes or very narrow interpalpebral spaces. The retrobulbar injection must be performed carefully and correctly, as there is always a danger of globe perforation and retrobulbar hemorrhage especially in highly myopic eyes. The injection may also cause conjunctival chemosis, especially peribulbar injections. Conjunctival chemosis makes the use of the suc-

tion ring more difficult because of the poor grasp on the suction ring on the conjunctiva and sclera and the inability to maintain necessary intraocular pressure (IOP).

As soon as a comfort level with the microkeratome and laser are achieved by the surgeon, topical anesthesia is the technique of choice, as it avoids all of the problems previously mentioned. Topical anesthesia is also preferable to the patient, as it eliminates the need for a patch (a clear shield is normally used). With LASIK under topical anesthesia, the patient usually appreciates the immediate improvement in vision and the continued improvement over the next few postoperative hours.

Topical anesthesia, however, should be applied sparsely. Three to four instillations of anesthetic drops during the 15 minutes prior to the procedure are more than sufficient. Excessive or prolonged application of the anesthetic drops is toxic to the epithelium and may cause epithelial edema or sloughing, especially as the microkeratome traverses over the cornea.

If a corneal abrasion is encountered from the microkeratome pass, the visual recovery is significantly delayed and can even possibly impact the quality of the cut. Epithelial defects may also increase the incidence of epithelial ingrowth. Therefore, attention to the timing of the topical

> Excessive or prolonged application of the anesthetic drops is toxic to the epithelium and may cause epithelial edema or sloughing, especially as the microkeratome traverses over the cornea.

TABLE 30-1.
COMPLICATIONS OF KERATOMILEUSIS

Preoperative

Induced by anesthesia

Induced by application of the
  drape and/or speculum

Induced by an excess of fluids

Induced by corneal marking

Conjunctival chemosis, poor suction

Corneal abrasions, epithelial defects

Interferes with good suction

Toxic changes to the epithelium

Interference with the pass of the microkeratome

Contamination of the interface

Dispersion of the dye

Intraoperative

Corneal perforation (absence or incorrect insertion of the plate in the microkeratome)

Incomplete primary cut

Incorrect primary cut (superficial, decentered, with irregular surfaces)

Thickness of cut that differs from section to section

360° cap resection and the lack of hinge formation ("free-cap")

Damage or destruction of the cap

Incorrect replacement of the cap

Physical alterations of the cap

Poor adhesion and anchoring between the lenticle and the stroma

Intraoperative contamination of the surfaces

Loss of the cap (in the sutureless technique)

Dislocation of the lenticle in the hinge technique with a corneal flap

Intraoperative Specific to the Use of the Laser

Incorrect ablation (myopic, astigmatic, or mixed)

Decentration of the ablation

Interruption of the laser treatment for technical problems

Damage to the hinge through poor protection during astigmatic photoablation

Changes to or contamination of the cap during the transference between the microscope and the laser and vice-versa (only in reference to LASIK on the cap)

Ablation of the hinge stroma during the in situ ablation

Poor ablation when liquid and/or impurities are present

Postoperative

Epithelial trauma

Induced topographical alterations (central island)

Epithelialization of the interface

Debris in the interface

Irregular astigmatism

Distortions of the optic zone

Traction folds on the flap

Haze at the interface

Stromal melting

Undercorrection

Regression

Overcorrection

Induced astigmatism (regular or irregular)

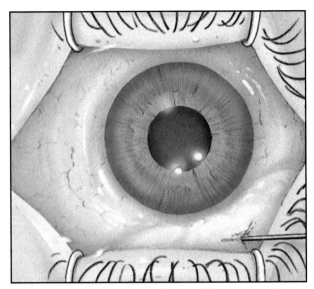

Figure 30-1. Complications from infiltration anesthesia: chemosis of the conjunctiva.

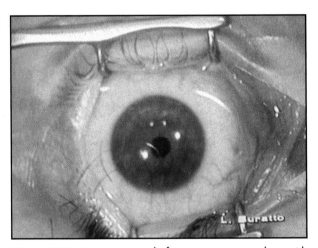

Figure 30-3. Eye exposure before surgery: speculum with optimal opening of the margins.

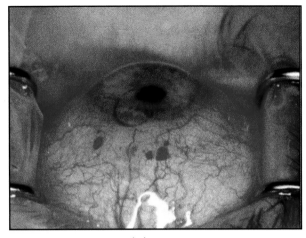

Figure 30-2. Conjunctival chemosis.

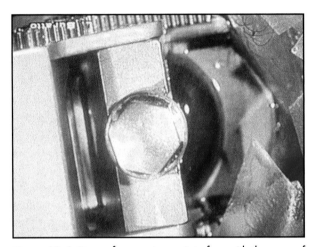

Figure 30-4. Drape fragments can interfere with the pass of the microkeratome: excessive magnification of the microscope restricts the overall view of the surgical procedure.

anesthetic drops and remembering to moisten the cornea with balanced salt solution (BSS) just prior to the microkeratome pass is critical to minimize corneal epithelial trauma.

DRAPE AND SPECULUM COMPLICATIONS

The drape should retract the margin of the eyelids and cover the eyelashes (Figures 30-1 through 30-3). It serves two functions: removal of the lashes from the operating field and retraction of the eyelids to increase globe exposure. Preventing the lashes from being accidentally engaged between the gears and track of the suction ring allows for a smooth, complete cut. The drape also helps to provide a sterile operating field.

Care needs to be taken so that the drape does not interfere with the pass of the microkeratome or interfere with the stop mechanism of the microkeratome (Figure 30-4). The drape rubbing on the cornea itself should also be avoided, as this can induce a small abrasion.

The same considerations apply to the lid speculum, which should not only provide good exposure, but must be carefully handled so that it does not produce a corneal abrasion during its insertion or removal. It should also allow a clear path for the microkeratome progression.

Just before engaging the microkeratome, our practice is to have the assistant on one side and the laser operator on the other side to aid the surgeon in checking that the lashes, drape, and speculum are all clear of the path of the microkeratome.

COMPLICATIONS FROM TEAR FILM AND CONJUNCTIVAL SECRETIONS

Prior to the patient entering the laser room, the cul de sac of the eye should be irrigated to remove debris and the oily tear film, and provide a more aseptic operating field.

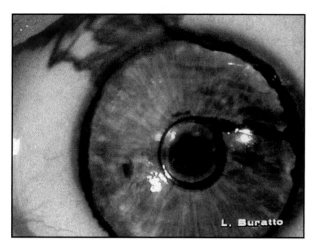

Figure 30-5. Excessive dye is toxic to the cornea and can seep into the interface.

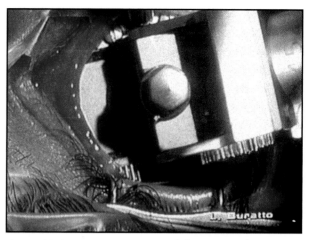

Figure 30-6. Excessive pressure of the ring on the eye can induce conjunctival chemosis, which will interfere with the progression of the microkeratome. The microkeratome path is also poorly directed.

After draping and placement of the lid speculum, the cul de sac should be dried so that no fluid is aspirated by the suction ring, which results in poor suction. Any remaining conjunctival debris should be removed with a Merocel sponge to decrease the potential for this debris to find its way into the flap interface.

CORNEAL MARKING COMPLICATIONS

The gentian violet used to mark the cornea prior to the keratectomy is toxic to the epithelium, therefore a minimal amount should be placed on the corneal marking instrument (Figure 30-5). If a marking pen is used alone, it should be moist and fine so that it does not cause a corneal abrasion.

Aggressive indentation of the cornea by the marking instrument should be avoided, as this induces an irregular surface that can be a source of potential problems with the microkeratome resection.

> The gentian violet used to mark the cornea prior to the keratectomy is toxic to the epithelium, therefore a minimal amount should be placed on the corneal marking instrument.

INTRAOPERATIVE COMPLICATIONS

CORNEAL PERFORATION

By far, the most serious intraoperative complication is corneal perforation with entrance into the anterior chamber. This may have devastating consequences on both the anterior and posterior segments. The damage occurring in the anterior segment is magnified by the high IOP (60 to 65 mm Hg) induced by the suction ring during this surgical phase and the unanticipated immediate drop in eye pressure following perforation.

Damage may be a simple corneal perforation with aqueous leakage, which may be sutured. This is rarely seen, though, as only a very experienced surgeon who is controlling the microkeratome pass himself would be quick enough to notice the aqueous leak and be able to stop the microkeratome pass in time to prevent more serious problems. More commonly, the microkeratome can enter the anterior chamber, cut the iris and lens, and induce potential vitreous loss or an expulsive hemorrhage with possibly irreversible blindness.

> This devastating complication is avoidable by double checking that the thickness plate of the microkeratome is present and securely positioned prior to every LASIK case.

This devastating complication (Figures 30-6 and 30-7) is avoidable by double checking that the thickness plate of the microkeratome is present and securely positioned prior to every LASIK case. We advocate a double check system in which the assistant states that both the plate and stop are present and secure, and the surgeon confirms this under the microscope, noting that the hexagonal head of the plate screw is visible at all times through the microscope. Fortunately, this problem will be reduced in the future with the use of new microkeratomes that have fixed plates that do not require disassembly and reassembly, eliminating the possibility of forgetting the plate or not assembling the microkeratome correctly.

> The best course of action if perforation with appearance of aqueous occurs is to immediately deactivate suction to stop all pressure on the globe and the microkeratome.

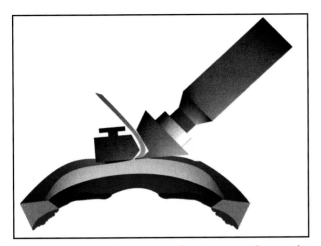

Figure 30-7. Complications: perforating cut. Observe the depression into the anterior chamber.

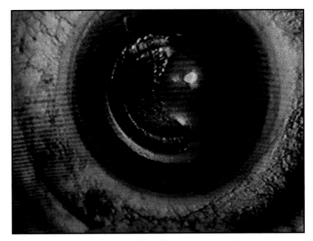

Figure 30-8. Incomplete lamellar cut secondary to suction loss.

With the present generation of microkeratomes, it is important that the plate is not only present but inserted completely as it is being positioned into its groove. Pushed into position by the index finger of the surgeon, it snaps into place and is flush with the front of the microkeratome. It should then be tightly screwed into place with the hex wrench. Firm tightening of the nut with the hex wrench is essential, as vibrations during the cutting phase can potentially loosen the plate, causing the gap to increase and possibly cause corneal perforation.

The best course of action if perforation with appearance of aqueous occurs is to immediately deactivate suction to stop all pressure on the globe and the microkeratome. Unfortunately this is difficult to perform, as the microkeratome pass occurs quickly and the surgeon's lack of visibility may hinder him or her from detecting the perforation in time.

Slit lamp examination, corneal topography, and pachymetry are mandatory preoperative tests to detect any unexpected cases of irregular or thin corneas and thin corneas associated with keratoconus. In these cases, a lamellar cut is definitely not recommended. Only procedures of corneal addition, such as epikeratophakia, should be considered.

This most serious complication of corneal perforation may be avoided by both careful preoperative screening and diligent attention to intraoperative detail.

INCOMPLETE PRIMARY CUT

An incomplete primary cut (Figure 30-8) may result from:
- electrical failure
- blockage of the foot pedal or accidental interruption of its motion
- blockage of the microkeratome pass by obstruction
- suction loss, resulting in complete or incomplete detachment of the suction ring
- mechanical obstruction caused by lids, lashes, drapes,

lid speculum, and conjunctiva
- debris along the track, such as conjunctival debris, salt crystals, eyelid make-up, and eyelashes
- obstacles on the microkeratome's edge

How to Proceed with an Incomplete Flap

If the keratectomy leaves adequate space for the refractive ablation, one may proceed. Consideration should be given to reducing the optic zone of the ablation to fit this smaller space. Always keeping in mind that smaller optic zones may induce visual difficulties. We feel that an optic zone smaller than 4.5 mm should not be considered. In this case, if the keratectomy extends past the anticipated optic zone, it may be possible to complete the keratectomy manually with lamellar dissection. A lamellar dissection blade, such as a #69 Beaver, may be used, taking great care to maintain the same lamellar plane. The ablation may then be performed with the originally planned optic zone or one that is slightly smaller. In these cases, it is difficult to maintain the exact cleavage plane of the microkeratome.

If the keratectomy does not allow room for the ablation, a manual dissection is contraindicated and it is mandatory to abort the refractive ablation and replace the flap, taking care to ensure that the interface is free of debris (as one would with a normal flap) (Figure 30-9 and 30-10). A suture may be necessary to secure the irregular flap. After the postoperative recovery, the keratectomy can be repeated 3 to 4 months later, ideally using a 180-µm plate if there is adequate stromal tissue for laser ablation.

If the flap is excessively thin and/or decentered, the excimer ablation should also be aborted and the flap

> If the keratectomy does not allow room for the ablation, a manual dissection is contraindicated and it is mandatory to abort the refractive ablation and replace the flap.

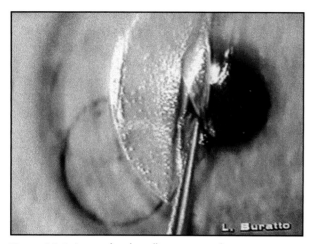

Figure 30-9. Incomplete lamellar cut secondary to premature release of the foot pedal.

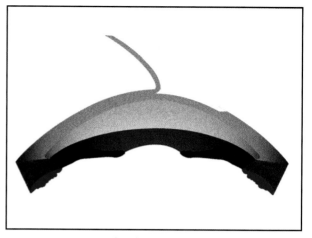

Figure 30-10. Incomplete lamellar cut in cross section.

replaced, checking the interface and adhesion in the normal manner. If there are any doubts about flap stability, the flap should be resutured with 10-0 nylon and a repeat keratectomy performed after a period of no less than 6 months.

> If the flap is excessively thin and/or decentered, the excimer ablation should also be aborted and the flap replaced.

POOR PRIMARY CUT

This is a cut with an irregular surface resulting from alterations in the speed of advancement of the microkeratome along the track (the so-called "plow-up" phenomenon) (Figure 30-11). To prevent this, the guides of the microkeratome track should be meticulously clean and smooth. The corneal and track surfaces (not the gears) should be moistened with BSS, and the pathway of the microkeratome should be unobstructed. Preoperatively, the voltage and motor function must also be checked.

It is important to remember that all surface irregularities in the visual zone modify the transmission of light, causing symptoms for the patient such as glare, diplopia, triplopia, and poor visual recovery. If the cut is highly irregular, the procedure should be aborted, no laser ablation performed, the flap should be replaced, and the procedure repeated 3 to 4 months later, possibly with a slightly deeper keratectomy.

> If the cut is highly irregular, the procedure should be aborted, no laser ablation performed, and the flap should be replaced.

In an even more complicated situation, a homoplastic keratectomy may be required and the refractive procedure must then be delayed at least 6 months.

Thin cuts are the result of:

- choosing the wrong plate

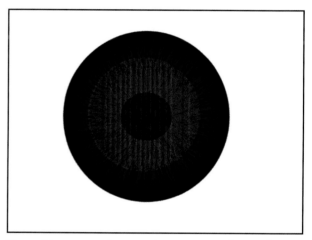

Figure 30-11. Complications: keratectomy with irregular surfaces (plow-up phenomenon).

- excessively rapid advancement of the microkeratome
- poor suction
- insufficient elevation of IOP, therefore lack of firmness of the globe
- epithelial sloughing

In the event of an excessively thin keratectomy, the flap should be replaced (with or without sutures, as needed) and the procedure repeated after 3 to 4 months. If the flap is sufficient, however, the ablation can be performed as planned with great attention to detail in replacing the flap, monitoring alignment, and avoiding wrinkling of the flap.

Decentered cuts are usually due to:

- surgeon error in marking the pupil and pararadial mark
- incorrect centration of the suction ring
- poor patient cooperation

If the resection is decentered slightly but allows for the ablation to be carried out with an adequate size in the corneal bed, the ablation can be continued, possibly considering the reduction of the optic zone (Figures 30-12 and 30-13). If this is not possible, the flap should be replaced with-

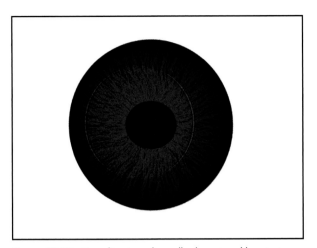

Figure 30-12. Complications: laterally decentered keratectomy.

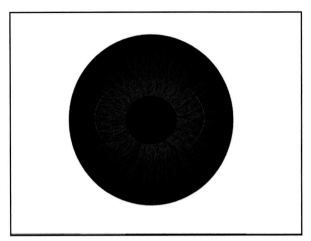

Figure 30-13. Complications: keratectomy with oval shape.

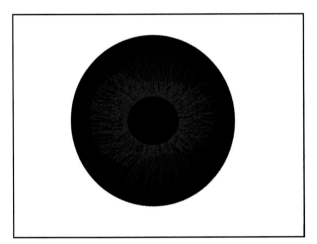

Figure 30-14. Complications: pyriform keratectomy.

out performing the refraction ablation, allowed to heal, and the procedure rescheduled for 3 to 4 months later (Figure 30-14).

IRREGULARITY IN THICKNESS OF THE RESECTION

The original suction rings had only one groove present, which caused nonparallel face resections to occasionally occur. This may also occur in situations in which the scleral surface is irregular, such as with cysts, folds, and filtering blebs. A keratectomy without perfect parallel faces may occur (Figures 30-15 through 30-17). This may not present a serious problem if the refractive cut is to be made with the excimer laser. If the refractive cut is to be made mechanically with the microkeratome (automated lamellar keratoplasty [ALK]), this takes on a greater significance.

COMPLETE CUT AND ABSENCE OF THE HINGE OR FREE CAP

Free caps can occur in several situation (Figure 30-18):
• in very flat corneas (mean keratometry less than 41 diopters [D])

• reduced intraoperative IOP
• lifting of the suction ring with the dehydrated flap adherent to it and with subsequent detachment
• incorrect stop setting

When this occurs, the free cap should be placed in the closed antidesiccation chamber, epithelial side down, on one drop of BSS. The ablation in situ is then performed in the routine manner. The cap is then transferred from the antidesiccation chamber to the corneal bed with the use of the Barraquer perforated spatula, taking care to reposition it in exactly the previous orientation. The pararadial marks should be aligned correctly, and the epithelial side should be up. The surgeon should also take care that the gutter is symmetrical for 360°. The often irregular resection may be of some advantage, as it helps to align the free cap.

A free cap is more of a nuisance than a significant complication—this is the way keratomileusis was performed for years. In most situations, the cap will adhere without the need for sutures, although the patient should be monitored for approximately 2 hours in the laser area before being discharged.

If one is unsure about the adhesion of the cap, a continuous 8-bite antitorque suture should be placed or an external compression-type suture may be needed.

> A free cap is more of a nuisance than a significant complication—this is the way keratomileusis was performed for years.

DAMAGE TO THE FLAP

During the cut, the flap tissue may fold over on itself, come in contact again with the blade, and be irreversibly damaged. This is an extremely rare complication and usually occurs when the cut is performed on a dry corneal surface. During the ablation, the hinge of the cap may be damaged to such a degree that the surgeon may need to replace it with a homoplastic cap.

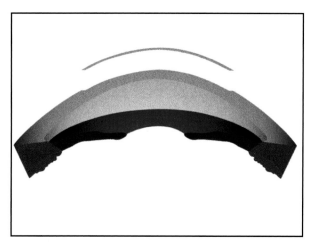

Figure 30-15. Complications: free cap keratectomy with reduced thickness over the entire cut surface.

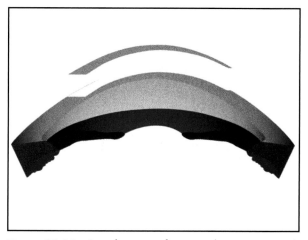

Figure 30-16. Complications: free cap keratectomy with greater thickness in the final part of the cut.

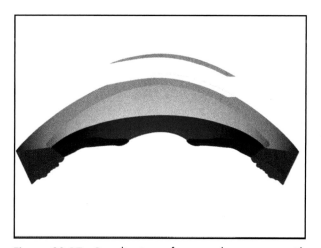

Figure 30-17. Complications: free cap keratectomy with reduced thickness in the final part of the cut.

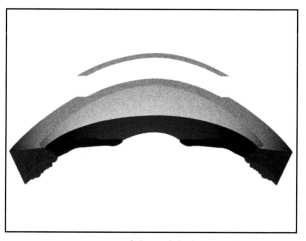

Figure 30-18. Free cap of desired thickness: side view.

With laser in situ keratomileusis (LASIK), this may be due to either accidental decentration of the photoablation with excessive ablation of the hinge area or lack of protection of the hinge during ablation with particularly large optic zones, such as in the correction of hyperopia or astigmatism.

In the original Buratto technique in which the ablation was performed on the stromal surface of the flap or cap, the damage to the cap may be caused by:
- incorrect centering
- excessive ablation on an overly thin flap
- poor distention of the flap prior to ablation
- ablation of a flap that is not uniform from such physical conditions as variable thickness due to variable hydration with dry areas and wet areas due to BSS instillation on the flap in irregular areas

LOSS OF FLAP/CAP

This may occur in cases in which a 360° disc (free cap) is achieved either intentionally or unintentionally. It may also occur in those cases in which the flap has a very minimal and fragile hinge, where the flaps/caps are replaced without sutures. Energetic rubbing of the operated eye, movement of the eye underneath a pressure patch, excessive force of the lids against the corneal/flap surface, epithelial abrasions, or accidental trauma may dislodge the unsutured corneal cap or poorly adherent flap. Rarely is the cap completely lost in these situations.

If the lost cap can be detected immediately and the undersurface of the cap and stromal bed are meticulously cleaned to prevent debris or epithelial ingrowth, the cap can usually be realigned to its original position. Prolonged observation in the office should take place before allowing the patient to be released. When in doubt, an 8-bite antitorque suture can be placed. When the flap has been off for

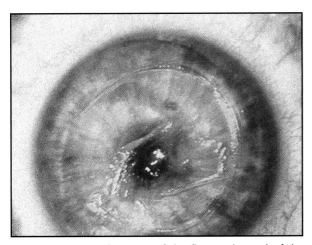

Figure 30-19. Displacement of the flap at the end of the operation due to incorrect removal of the speculum.

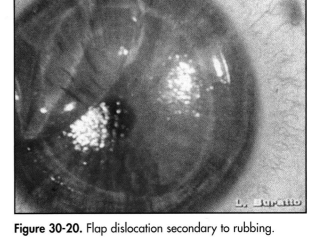

Figure 30-20. Flap dislocation secondary to rubbing.

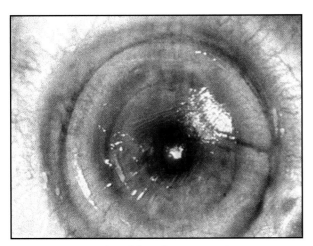

Figure 30-21. Displaced flap due to immediate postoperative trauma.

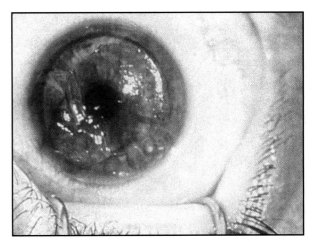

Figure 30-22. Many folds on the flap due to bad repositioning.

a prolonged period of time it will become edematous. Clearing the epithelium that begins to encroach over the stromal bed is very important and should be done aggressively along with cleaning the undersurface of the flap. The flap will be too edematous to adhere without sutures, and a single or double 8-bite antitorque suture is required.

If the flap has been irreversibly damaged, the surgeon has two options. One is to remove the flap completely and allow the cornea to re-epithelialize, as if surface photorefractive keratectomy (PRK) had been performed. Amazingly, a significant number of these eyes actually heal well and require no further treatment. However, they are more prone to haze development, as usually a significant amount of myopia has been corrected with a large ablation. If excessive haze develops, consideration must be given to debridement of the epithelium, phototherapeutic keratectomy, and then covering the bed with a resected homoplastic cap. If homoplastic material is available immediately, this can be used to replace a lost cap as well.

DISLOCATION OF THE FLAP

With the hinge technique it is almost impossible to lose the flap. It is usually partially attached to the underlying bed. Decentration or irregularity in the surface of the flap is usually the first clue to poor flap adherence (Figures 30-19 through 30-25). In this case, the flap should be lifted as soon as it is detected, and the undersurface and bed should be meticulously cleaned of debris and epithelium. The flap is then replaced and carefully stroked to completely distend it to avoid microstriae. This requires more than the usual 3 to 4 minutes of drying observation time to ensure good flap adherence.

If the surgeon delays treatment of these cases, the striae will become more difficult to remove with a higher instance of visual and functional problems postoperatively. If adherence of the flap is not assured, two to three equally spaced interrupted sutures may be used to stabilize the flap position. The sutures should be rotated, otherwise the knots will generate tearing, which may once again interfere with flap adhesion.

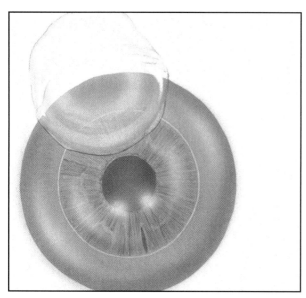

Figure 30-23. Intraoperative complication: dislocation or sliding of the free cap from its original position.

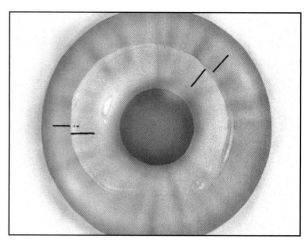

Figure 30-24. Intraoperative complication: twisting of the flap and loss of correct centration with respect to the bed.

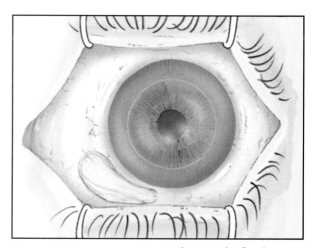

Figure 30-25. Intraoperative complication: the flap has separated from the corneal hinge and is dislocated on the conjunctiva.

Usually if the flap has been displaced either partially or totally, epithelium will already be extending underneath the flap, which may be detected either with direct visualization or after fluorescein staining. In this case, it is again mandatory to lift and carefully clean both surfaces of the flap before replacement. The epithelium must be completely removed from the stromal bed. For severe flap problems, consideration should also be given to flap replacement with homoplastic tissue.

IRREGULARITIES IN THE FLAP

During the LASIK procedure, the flap should be handled with care to avoid traumatizing it or inducing debris on its undersurface or in the bed. Any irregularities resulting from poor handling can affect the final refractive result; therefore, it is better not to grasp the flap with forceps, especially toothed forceps. A blunt spatula should be used to elevate the flap, and one should take care that the spatula is extremely clean and free of debris from the autoclave, which may adhere to the undersurface of the flap.

Excessively prolonged operating times, which allow excessive dehydration of the flap, should be avoided. Rubbing of either the undersurface or the bed with swabs or other instruments should also be avoided, as this also induces microtrauma.

IRRIGATION COMPLICATIONS

While it is important to irrigate the interface following flap replacement to not only remove potential interface debris and epithelial cells but also to float the flap into the correct alignment position, it is also possible to irrigate excessively, inducing edema of the flap, which reduces the ability for good tissue adherence.

A little drop of fluid may also be left behind in the inter-

> It is also possible to irrigate excessively, inducing edema of the flap, which reduces the ability for good tissue adherence.

face. This may be avoided by stroking the surface of the flap with a cannula or spatula from the nasal hinge temporally and then superiorly and inferiorly to squeegee the flap down. A better alternative is to take a slightly moistened Merocel sponge and "paint" the flap into its bed with gentle, but strong, painting movements nasal to temporal, then central to superior and inferior, once again making sure that the flap is extremely smooth and the width of the gutter is equidistant throughout the resection curvature.

DEBRIS IN THE INTERFACE

The cap/stromal interface may contain debris from:
- particles in the air of the operating room
- secretions deposited in the interface, originating from

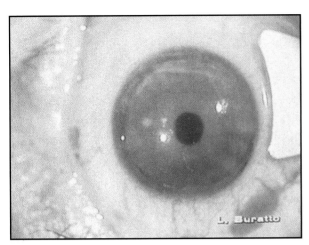

Figure 30-26. Blood in the interface at the end of the operation due to corneal neovascularization secondary to long-term contact lens wear.

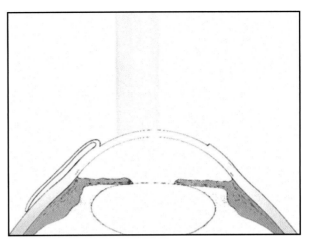

Figure 30-27. Decentration of photoablation.

pooling of the tear film in the conjunctival fornix

- debris deposited from instruments during various manipulations of the flap
- material floating in the operative field, such as talc from surgical gloves, lint from gauze, cotton swabs, sponges, and fabric drapes
- friction in the components of the microkeratome may induce metallic debris in the interface
- blood or epithelial cells and inorganic matter floating (Figure 30-26) in the area of the operating room are also possible sources

Usually this interface debris is of no clinical significance and does not affect the functional recovery of the eye. On rare occasions, however, the debris may actually interfere with the optical quality of the result and require lifting of the flap and removal of the debris. If the debris is seen in the immediate postoperative period, the patient should be returned to the laser suite and the debris removed.

One should always ensure that the laser room is as free of debris as possible with the use of HEPA air filtration in the laser room, avoidance of debris-producing material such as towels, sponges, and gauze. In addition, meticulously clean the instruments following their removal from the autoclave, as rust particles and other debris from the autoclave may deposit on the instruments.

LASER COMPLICATIONS

An incorrect ablation is usually due to an incorrect setting of the surgical parameters of the laser's computer, affecting either the optic zone or amount of diopter correction. Errors may also occur with a poor nomogram during the surgeon's learning curve of adjusting the PRK algorithm to LASIK. Technical faults in the laser may occur during the ablation. The laser is a very fragile device and problems resulting from inadequate gases (nitrogen, helium, argon, fluorine) or defects in the optics or mirrors of the laser may occur, resulting in a nonhomogenous laser beam. All of these problems may contribute to a poor quality ablation with a poor result, such as induced regular or irregular astigmatism.

Decentration of ablation is an eccentric ablation that is usually the result of either poor patient fixation or lack of attention to detail by the surgeon (Figure 30-27). This is a difficult problem with visual disturbances related to the decentration and its topographical position.

POSTOPERATIVE COMPLICATIONS

EPITHELIAL INGROWTH

Epithelial ingrowth may manifest itself by small islands of epithelial cysts or ingrowth from the periphery of the lamellar resection (Figure 30-28 through 30-30). There is some controversy involving this terminology, as some (Draeger) feel that true seeding of the epithelial interface with epithelial cells is the etiology, and others (Maloney) feel that this situation occurs only when the epithelium truly grows in from the periphery of the resection under a poorly adherent flap margin. Isolated islands of centrally located epithelial cells can occasionally be seen, and they may reduce visual acuity by induction of irregular astigmatism. In this situation, the flap should be lifted and these cells mechanically removed as quickly as possible. Surgeons should not wait while the ingrowth progresses because of the potential for melting the corneal flap.

Epithelialization of the interface may take many forms. Occasionally, multiple small sites may occur that do not involve the visual axis and do not affect the corneal surface, refraction, or keratometry (either regular or irregular). These may be left but should be observed and possibly photographed to monitor potential enlargement.

On the other hand, the epithelium may also be observed at the margins of the flap and remain constant and nonpro-

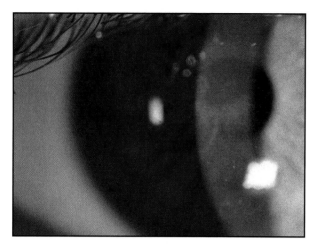

Figure 30-28. Small epithelial clusters at the interface.

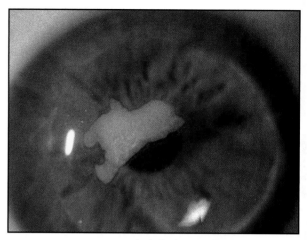

Figure 30-29. Large epithelial cluster of the interface 6 months after the operation.

gressive. In some situations, it may appear at the flap margin and continue to enlarge and begin to affect the visual axis, in which case prompt removal is mandatory.

Rarely, spontaneous regression and disappearance of epithelial islands from the periphery are seen. There is no histological explanation for this phenomenon. However, it is thought that this epithelial material may suffer from inadequate nutrition, which prevents further development and in some cases actually causes regression.

Treatment of Epithelial Ingrowth

1. Raising the flap: The patient is normally seated at the slit lamp following adequate topical anesthesia. The edge of the flap may be difficult to identify. However, with high magnification and depression of the cornea, the edge can usually be seen. After breaking the surface of the epithelium with an instrument such as a Sinskey hook or the end of jeweler's forceps, the patient is moved to the operating microscope. The edge of the flap is teased up, and then using two blunt forceps to grasp the periphery of the lenticle, it is gently elevated without grasping the central portion.

Using a spatula or chalazion curet (Figures 30-31 and 30-32), the epithelial island is removed. It is usually round—similar to an encapsulated cyst. If performed carefully, it can usually be removed in a single step, and it is unlikely that any cellular debris will remain or reoccur. If multiple passes of the removing instrument are necessary, it is likely that some residual cells may persist, and the two surfaces should be carefully debrided and washed and the interface rinsed thoroughly with BSS to remove residual cells.

In general, when irrigating the interface with BSS, it is advisable to direct the jet of irrigation obliquely to the surface, taking advantage of the waterfall effect to remove any trapped impurities. Irrigation in one direction with removal of the fluid helps to remove the deposits and impurities without recurrence.

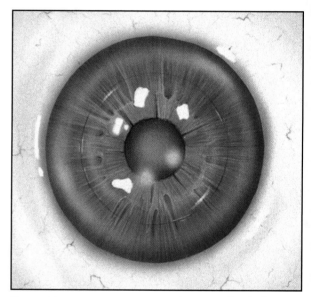

Figure 30-30. Postoperative complication: island of epithelialization at the interface.

Many surgeons prefer to lift the entire flap as opposed to only the area where the epithelial ingrowth has occurred, as they feel that repositioning the entire flap allows for a more regular postoperative surface without the induction of a ridge created by only partial elevation. When the flap is replaced, the surgeon should monitor flap adherence and determine whether sutures are required.

2. Incision and squeezing: Another technique that has been advocated to eliminate the peripheral island of epithelial cells is to cut down through the corneal surface into the interface over the island with a diamond radial keratotomy (RK)-type knife and squeeze the liquefied epithelial cells out. This is a simple, easy procedure; unfortunately, there is a high incidence of recurrence.

3. Laser removal: The use of the Nd: YAG laser or the ISL laser has been advocated for ablation of epithelial islands in the periphery. With the YAG laser, powers of 1.2 to 1.3 mJ

T A B L E 30-4.
TREATMENT OF POST-LASIK OR ALK MYOPIC OVERCORRECTIONS

Slight or moderate residual hyperopia (1 to 4 D)	Retreatment with excimer laser directly onto the stromal bed once the flap has been raised (lifting of the flap and re-ablation). LTK: treatment of the peripheral cornea with Holmium laser 6 months after LASIK or ALK (oz 7 to 8 mm). Hyperopic PRK: on the epithelial surface of the flap
Severe residual hyperopia (> 4 D)	Hyperopic LASIK: to be done when refraction is stable but at any rate at least 3 months from the first primary LASIK. There are 2 possibilities: • lifting of the flap and ablation of the stromal bed • a new keratectomy with the microkeratome with equal or greater thickness cut

OVERCORRECTION

Overcorrection is defined as hyperopia seen with refractive (manifest as well as cycloplegic) evaluations performed 1 month postoperatively (Table 30-4).

Etiology:

* incorrect preoperative refractive evaluation—the preoperative refraction measures more myopia than actually exists. This can be prevented by using cycloplegic refractions in young patients.
* incorrect entry of operative parameters into the laser— excessively low humidity in the laser suite, allowing dehydration of the corneal tissue, results in overablation. This can be managed by controlling the humidity in the operating suite and adjusting the algorithm of the laser appropriately

Overcorrections are generally unpleasant for the patient, and the level of dissatisfaction is usually higher than with undercorrections. Overcorrections are also more difficult to retreat. It is therefore better to err on the side of undercorrection when performing LASIK, particularly in the presbyopic age group.

> It is better to err on the side of undercorrection when performing LASIK, particularly in the presbyopic age group.

Treatment of Overcorrection

1. LASIK enhancement with lifting of the flap and reablation is done in a manner similar to that done with myopic undercorrection. It is usually done 2 to 3 months after the initial treatment to allow for possible regression. The flap is raised and a hyperopic ablation is performed in the bed if the surgeon is fortunate enough to have an excimer laser capable of hyperopic ablation.

2. Hyperopic PRK could be an alternative for overcorrection, as opposed to undercorrection, because the treatment is peripheral rather than central. If haze develops it does not impinge on the visual axis. The haze, however, is generally greater than in corneas undergoing primary hyperopic PRK. Hyperopic PRK in general can correct only up to approximately 4 D to 5 D.

3. Contact or noncontact holmium laser thermal keratoplasty (LTK) (for overcorrections up to 3 D to 4 D) produces localized corneal coagulation, which increases the central corneal curvature with reduction of hyperopia. It may be performed after 3 months postoperatively and should be done peripheral to the lamellar resection. Overtreatment is necessary with holmium LTK because of the marked tendency for regression.

4. Hexagonal keratotomy has been largely abandoned because of unpredictability. When performed, the hexagonal incisions are done at approximately 90% corneal depth as determined by pachymetry and on the basis of the corneal topography using the Mendez nomogram.

5. Hyperopic automated lamellar keratoplasty (ALK) is rarely performed but may be considered an alternative method of treating overcorrections. The hinge/flap technique is performed in the same manner used with primary hyperopic ALK. The optic zone is small with a depth of approximately 75% of the central pachymetry. The correction is determined by the diameter and thickness of the cut. This is a single cut weakening procedure with no secondary refractive cut.

LASIK Complications and their Management

Ioannis G. Pallikaris, MD
Dimitrios S. Siganos, MD
Vikentia I. Katsanevaki, MD

When compared to photorefractive keratectomy (PRK), laser in situ keratomileusis (LASIK) is a more complex procedure that requires a skilled surgeon. Based on 7 years experience with this procedure, some of the most common LASIK complications will be presented along with their management. In this chapter, the complications of LASIK are divided into those related to the use of the microkeratome and those resulting from the use of the excimer laser. Complications from both these categories can occur in the same patient.

It must be emphasized that changes in the shape and form of the cornea as well as changes related to the corneal structure and properties as a refractive medium will influence the final optical result. Certain patients with satisfactory topography, manifest refraction, and slit lamp examination still complain of poor vision. This is mostly related to light distortion at the interface that, unfortunately, cannot be detected from the common examination.

KERATOME-RELATED COMPLICATIONS

Apart from the initial keratome problems that can occur during the surgeon's LASIK learning curve, the operation can always be complicated by inappropriate preoperative preparation since flap-making depends on a very sophisticated instrument—the microkeratome. Trained and reliable personnel must be responsible for its assembly and maintenance. The microkeratome should be cleaned with a sterile hard brush and properly assembled before use. Dirty gears will result in intermittent advancement of the blade, pro-

> Dirty gears will result in intermittent advancement of the blade, producing a flap of irregular thickness.

ducing a flap of irregular thickness (Figures 31-1 through 31-4).

The quality of the blade is crucial for good, consistent results. With the Chiron microkeratome, a new blade must be used for each eye. A poor quality blade will result in a flap that is thinner than expected, with irregular borders and/or thicknesses (Figures 31-5a through 31-8). Regarding Figure 31-8, the following points should be considered:

1. In case of PRK over phototherapeutic keratectomy (PTK), after transepithelial removal of the initial 40 µm, add +1 diopter (D) for every 20 µm removed to the final PRK correction (for 5 D of residual myopia and 60 µm of PTK prior to PRK, the attempted correction should be only 4 D).

2. In case of PRK over PTK with the use of a smoothing agent or masking material and epithelial debridement, add 1 D to 2 D to the final PRK correction.

Ideally, flap thickness must range between 130 and 170 µm. Thicker flaps may not leave enough residual corneal stroma for the correction, while thinner flaps are difficult to manipulate when repositioned (Figures 31-9a through 31-9d).

A poor quality blade can leave metal particles in the stroma (Figure 31-10). These can be detected under the flap at slit lamp examination postoperatively. Metal particles must be removed immediately, as they can induce scar formation.

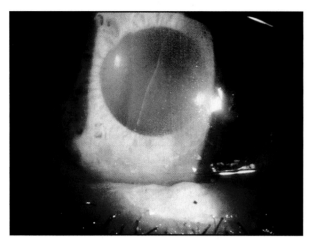

Figure 31-1. Intermittent advancement of the keratome.

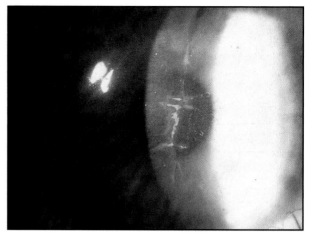

Figure 31-2. Scar formation.

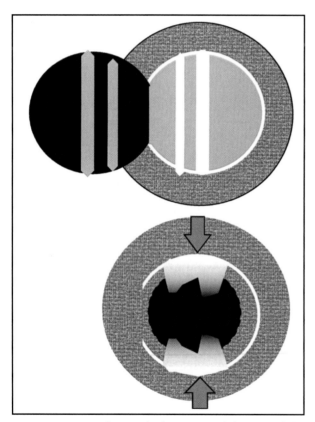

Figure 31-3. *Irregular cap thickness:* vertical direction of the thinner part, very often multiple parallel lines consisting only of stromal tissue, irregular cap edges respectively to the thinner areas. *Cause:* intermittent advancement of the blade (gear problems). *Early:* intrastromal epithelial ingrowth (occasional stromal melting). *Late:* scar formation.

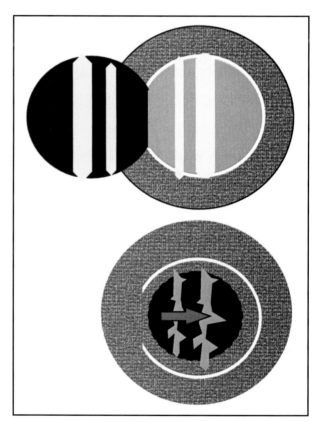

Figure 31-4. *Irregular cap thickness:* vertical direction of the thinner part, multiple parallel lines consisting of epithelial only. *Cause:* intermittent advancement of the blade, along with low IOP (gear and suction problems). *Early:* intrastromal epithelial ingrowth (occasionally due to stromal melting). *Late:* scar formation.

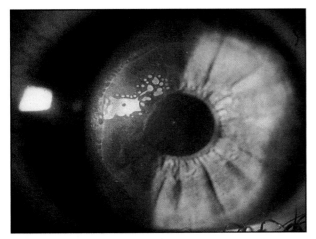

Figure 31-5a. Corneal scar and intrastromal island.

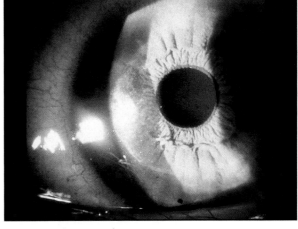

Figure 31-5b. Corneal scar.

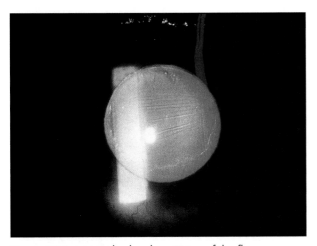

Figure 31-6a. Irregular borders. Striae of the flap.

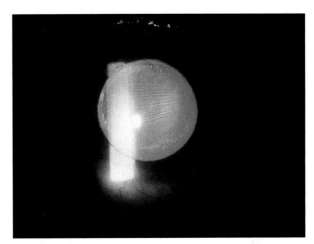

Figure 31-6b. Irregular borders. Striae of the flap.

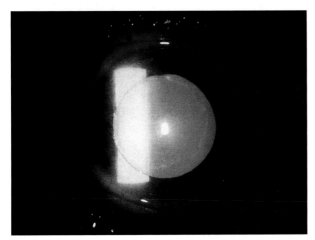

Figure 31-6c. Irregular borders. Striae of the flap.

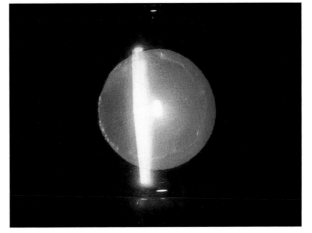

Figure 31-6d. Irregular borders. Striae of the flap.

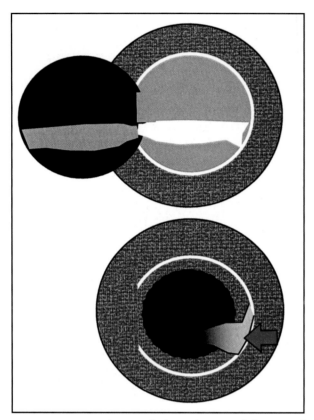

Figure 31-7. *Irregular cap thickness:* horizontal direction of the thinner part (thinner part consists of epithelial and stromal tissue). *Cause:* blade cutting edge irregularities. *Early:* intrastromal epithelial ingrowth, very often cornea melting. *Late:* scar formation.

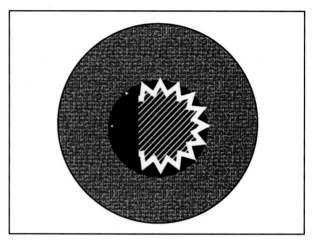

Figure 31-8. Small cap or flap. Size: < 5 mm. Thickness: < 100 µm. Eccentric flap or cap borders within the 5 mm central optical zone. Abnormal border with epithelial ingrowth or scar and central striae. (A) BCVA loss of two or more lines. (A1) Smooth anterior corneal surface (no irregular astigmatism) = transepithelial PTK, 60 µm in depth and 8 mm in diameter, centered at the pupil center, plus PRK for residual refractive error (7 mm tapered transition zone recommended). (A2) Irregular corneal surface (with irregular astigmatism) = epithelial debridement (using beaver, not brush) and PTK with smoothing agent (depth of the ablation will be optically estimated from the quality of the surface), plus PRK for residual refractive error (7 mm tapered transition zone is recommended). (B) Loss of BCVA of one line or less. (B1) Intense glare and halos = transepithelial PTK 50 µm in depth with a 7 mm zone, plus PRK. (In case of myopic refraction up to 3 D, additional 30 µm PTK in a 7 mm zone). (B2) Minimal glare = secondary LASIK (second cut) for residual refractive error with the flap thicker than 160 µm and wide ablation zone.

Should particles of a different origin (glove powder, sponge remnants, etc) affect best-corrected visual acuity or induce astigmatism or hyperopia, the stroma must be cleaned (Figures 31-11 through 31-13g).

The intraoperative intraocular pressure (IOP) measurement should never be neglected. Inadequate IOP (less than 65 mm Hg) can result in a small or total cap with/or irregular cap thickness (Figures 31-2, 31-4, 31-14 through 31-17). Whatever the reason, irregular cap thickness will result in intrastromal epithelial ingrowth and eventually corneal scarring.

> Whatever the reason, irregular cap thickness will result in intrastromal epithelial ingrowth and eventually corneal scarring.

OPTICAL COMPLICATIONS

The optical result of the photoablation can be evaluated by three main factors that can be detected on the patient's postoperative topographic map:

1. The diameter of the central ablation (S): This is defined as the size (in millimeters) of the area, including 1.5 D of steepening, from the flattest value of refractive power on an autoscaled topography map. A small-sized central ablation can induce glare or "ghosting" around headlights, especially at night. There are three sizes of central ablation. Size S1 refers to a central ablation larger than 5 mm (Figure 31-18). These patients are not expected to experience any glare or halos. Size S2 (see Figure 31-18) refers to a central ablation measuring 3 to 5 mm, and size S3 (see Figure 31-18) refers to a central ablation that is smaller than 3 mm. The halo effect of these ablations will vary according to their maximal pupillary dilation.

2. Ablation pattern (P): Asymmetrical ablation patterns (Figure 31-19) can result in an irregular astigmatism and, in extreme cases, the patient complains of multiple images due to corneal prismatic effects. Ideally, the corneal refractive power should normally be increased from the center to the periphery of the ablated zone. This means that in each meridian, symmetrical points from the center of the ablation should have the same refractive power and thus be represented with the same color on an autoscaled topographic

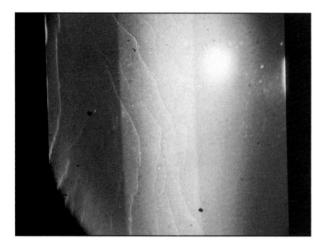

Figure 31-9a. Thin flap with striae and regular borders.

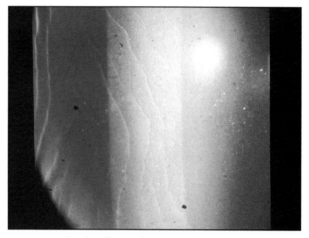

Figure 31-9b. Thin flap with striae and regular borders.

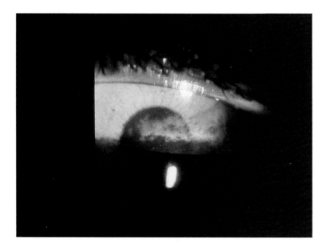

Figure 31-9c. Thin flap with striae and regular borders.

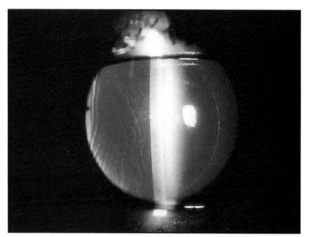

Figure 31-9d. Thin flap with striae and regular borders.

map. In Figure 31-17, consider A as the smaller and B as the greater distance (in millimeters) between the flattest (deep blue) and the mean refractive power (middle green) area on the autoscaled topographic map. We define R as the ratio of A:B. In order to assess the extent of the irregular pattern, we classify irregularity into three patterns with respect to R. P1 (see Figure 31-19) refers to ablation patterns in which R is greater than one third. This case is within normal range, and the patient may not suffer from subjective symptoms. On the other hand, in cases classified as P2 (see Figure 31-19) (R between one third and one fifth) and P3 (see Figure 31-19) (R less than one fifth), severe complications exist and need to be treated.

3. Centration of the ablation: When the ablation center does not correspond to the center of the map, the ablation is considered to be eccentric (E). This is a severe complication that needs to be treated since it induces a multifocal effect in the optical zone that could result in blurred images, glare, ghost images, poor visual acuity, or poor contrast sensitivity. Eccentricity is evaluated on an autoscaled topographic map in which, ideally, the flattest (deep blue) area must include the center of the map. For treatment purposes,

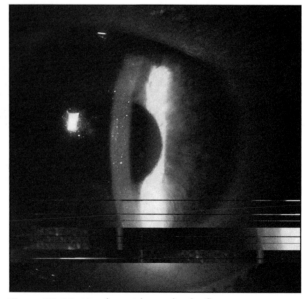

Figure 31-10. Metal particles under the flap.

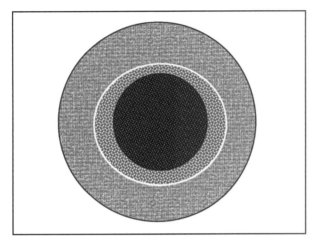

Figure 31-11. Fine interface remnants. (1) Smooth corneal surface, no striae, no BCVA loss at 1 month = wait. (2) Loss of BCVA greater than or equal to one line, or no loss of BCVA but induced cylinder greater than 1 D = immediate cleaning. (3) Metal particles = immediate cleaning.

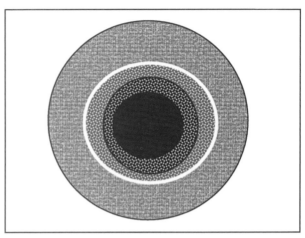

Figure 31-12. Peripheral interface remnants or particles. (1) Not affecting BCVA or inducing irregular astigmatism, no hyperopic shift = wait. (2) Not affecting BCVA or inducing astigmatism, hyperopic shift (hyperopic effect due to the elevation of the periphery of the flap) = remove. (3) Affecting BCVA or inducing irregular astigmatism = remove. (4) Metal particles = remove.

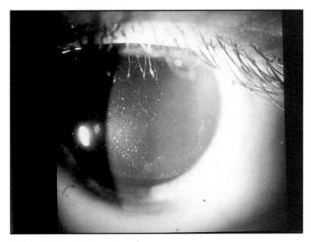

Figure 31-13a. Fine interface remnants.

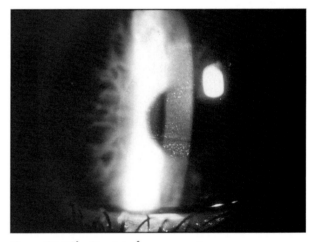

Figure 31-13b. Fine interface remnants.

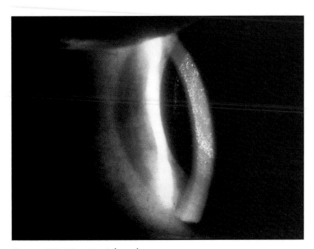

Figure 31-13c. Peripheral remnants.

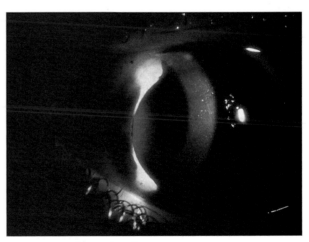

Figure 31-13d. Peripheral remnants.

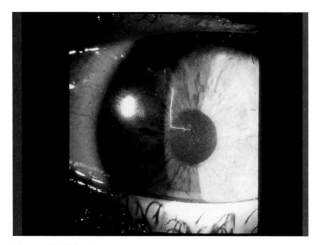

Figure 31-13e. Sponge remnants.

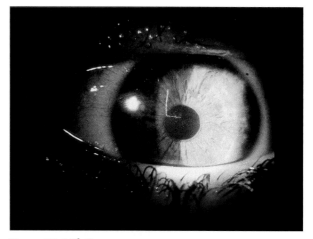

Figure 31-13f. Sponge remnants.

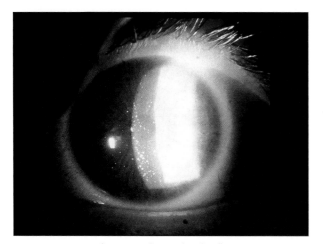

Figure 31-13g. Glove powder under the flap.

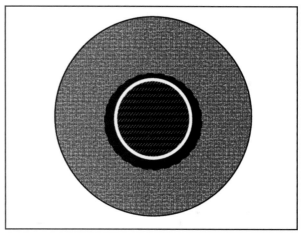

Figure 31-14. Small flap or cap: 5 mm < size < 7 mm. Thickness: 100 μm, well-centered, faint striae. (1) No BCVA loss, no induced astigmatism = wait. (2) BCVA loss or induced irregular astigmatism = early (within 1 month) repositioning and cleaning of the flap or cap. In case of a total cap, do not remove the cap, leave a small epithelial hinge, preferably where the cap is better fitted to the stroma, to prevent cap loss.

eccentricity is classified as E1 if the center of the map is situated within the area of the mean refractive power (middle green) and E2 if elsewhere (Figures 31-20 and 31-21). Both categories have subdivisions regarding the 3 mm optical zone. Subcategory A is defined as that having one quadrant of the 3 mm zone out of the green encircled area; subcategory B is defined as that having more than one quadrant of the 3 mm zone involved. Therefore, four eccentricity patterns can be identified as E1A, E1B, E2A, and E2B (Figures 31-20 through 31-23).

If the topography of a complicated case reveals a combination of the above regarding the size, pattern, and centration of ablation, the treatment aims to restore a normal topographic map either by enlargement of the central ablated area using arcuate cuts (in milder cases) or with supplemental ablation that can be diagonal or masked. Diagonal ablation is centered at a distance equal to the smaller radius of the initial ablation on an imaginary line passing from the center of the cornea to the center of the initial ablation (3 mm away from the center of the map diagonally placed to the previous ablation of the 6 mm zone). Diagonal ablation

applies to cases with small-sized (S3) ablation combined with a mild (P1), moderate (P2), or severe (P3) irregularity pattern and moderate (E1B or E2A) eccentricity (Figures 31-24 and 31-27).

Masked ablation is a procedure during which the surgeon covers the flattest part of the initial ablation with Vinciguerra or other customized masks while keratectomy takes place. Smart masks (under patent) are silicone or plas-

> The treatment aims to restore a normal topographic map either by enlargement of the central ablated area using arcuate cuts (in milder cases) or with supplemental ablation that can be diagonal or masked.

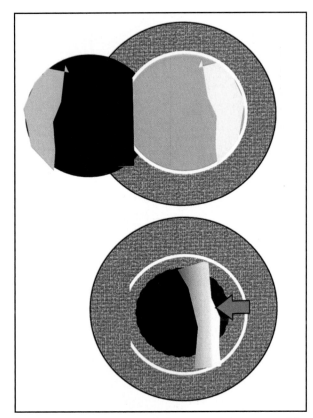

Figure 31-15. Irregular cap thickness: vertical direction of the thinner part located at the temporal edge of the flap consisting only of epithelium. *Cause:* inadequate suction, low IOP. *Early:* intrastromal epithelial ingrowth. *Late:* scar formation.

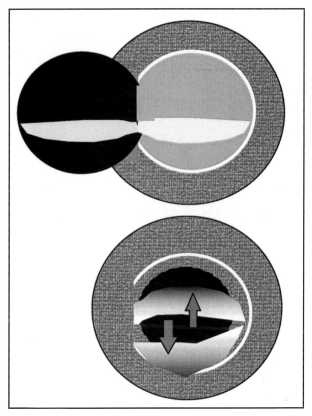

Figure 31-16. Irregular cap thickness: horizontal direction of the thinner part or half cut flap (thinner part consists of epithelium only). *Cause:* low IOP by inadequate suction. *Early:* intrastromal epithelial ingrowth. *Late:* scar formation.

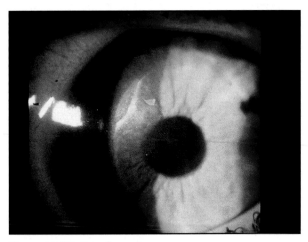

Figure 31-17. Scar formation.

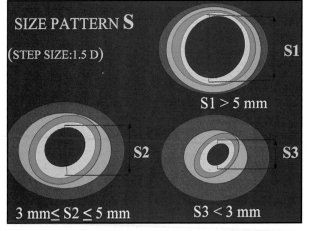

Figure 31-18. The diameter of the central ablation (S) is defined as the size (in mm) of the area including 1.5 D of steepening, from the flattest value of refractive power on an autoscaled topography map (S1: 5 mm or more; S2: 3 to 5 mm; S3: 3 mm or more).

LASIK Complications

Jeffery J. Machat, MD

There is a definite surgical learning curve to laser in situ keratomileusis (LASIK) that is filled with many nuances that require hundreds of procedures to fully grasp. Experience with automated lamellar keratoplasty (ALK) and other lamellar procedures are clearly beneficial in shortening the learning curve. Experience with photorefractive keratectomy (PRK) is another important prerequisite to fully understanding all that encompasses LASIK. With respect to photoablation dynamics, it has been stated by Stephen Slade that LASIK is 90% keratectomy and 10% laser, and I believe this is true for the beginning LASIK surgeon. Once the LASIK surgeon is more experienced, the keratectomy and photoablation have a more equal importance. The number of procedures required to feel comfortable enough with LASIK to handle truly difficult cases is dependent upon the individual surgeon. I have found that I continue to learn, despite having performed more than 15,000 LASIK procedures. The first 40 procedures were associated with a 25% complication rate, varying from minor problems to quite serious ones. At present, the complication rate has dwindled to 1% to 2% for minor complications, such as epithelial ingrowths and irregular astigmatism, and .1% or less for truly severe complications relating to loss of flap integrity from microkeratome performance and stromal melts.

With proper training, education, and caution, LASIK complications should not be feared, but rather understood. Understanding the mechanisms that produce LASIK complications is the first step in prevention, followed by the second step of complication management. Most complications are related to lamellar dissection or flap management.

Errors in refractive predictability and topographical abnormalities are a result of the LASIK nomogram and ablation profiles but remain within the influence sphere of individual healing patterns. Newer scanning excimer lasers should reduce many of these ablation problems, as the ablation profiles are more encompassing, flexible, and refined.

Complications can be divided into three categories:
* Intraoperative
* Early postoperative (within the first month)
* Late postoperative (beyond the first month)

INTRAOPERATIVE COMPLICATIONS

The primary intraoperative complication is that related to creation of the corneal flap. The proper assembly and preparation of the microkeratome is fundamental in avoiding corneal flap complications. Surgeon and staff training in nuances of the care of the unit is the cornerstone to achieving reproducible high-quality lamellar incisions.[1] Corneal flap complications can essentially be divided into five major problems:
* A lamellar incision that is too short
* An incision that is too long
* An incision that is too superficial
* An incision that is too deep
* An irregular incision or one of poor quality

PUPIL BISECTION

Clinical

If the microkeratome stops prior to completing the

Figure 32-1. Clinical appearance of a corneal flap complication following ALK during the initial access pass of the microkeratome. The pupil was bisected with a short corneal flap by the referring surgeon due to either an encountered obstacle or unit malfunction resulting in linear vertical scarring across the visual axis, which was more pronounced superiorly. Refractive error remained unchanged at -8 D with reduced best-corrected vision of 20/25 with qualitative visual distortion. The patient was treated with multizone PRK with a 7-mm blend zone with a transepithelial approach to remove scarring and re-establish a smooth contour. The patient required two surface ablation procedures achieving 20/25 uncorrected vision and improving best-corrected vision back to 20/20 with elimination of the scar.

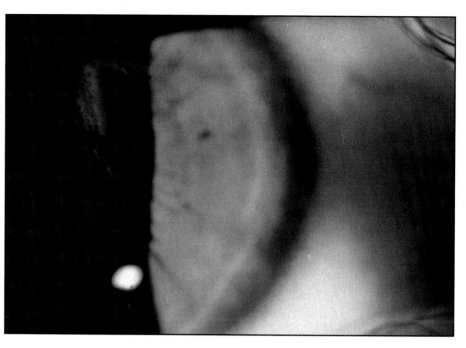

lamellar incision due to jamming of the unit or because an obstacle has been encountered (such as draping, redundant conjunctiva, or the speculum or lids of a tight orbit), an inadequate size flap will be fashioned. It is important to check that the microkeratome travels smoothly within the tract and the passage of the unit is clear prior to advancing the corneal shaper head. If the hinge bisects the pupil, it is impossible for an adequate ablation zone to be treated (Figure 32-1). The point at which the hinge is fashioned determines whether the laser application can be continued safely and without clinically significant glare nasally. Even if the hinge is more temporal than anticipated, so long as at least a 6 mm treatment area is available, the procedure can be continued by utilizing a flap spatula or expanded spear to protect the hinge. A PRK zone marker can be placed over the pupil to determine if an adequate area exists for ablation. Induced cylinder may also result from a short flap, and distortion may be perceived by the patient with or without ablation. If the undersurface of the flap is ablated, two problems occur:

- The area along the hinge will be doubly treated once the flap is closed, disturbing normal topography
- It is possible to damage the integrity of the flap and hinge

Management

There are three approaches to managing a short flap bisecting the pupil. The first is to close the flap and wait at least 3 months for it to adequately solidify, then repeat the LASIK procedure. This is clearly the recommended approach. I explain to patients that the flap is short and unacceptable night glare is likely, and that it is best to let the flap heal and recut a new larger flap in 3 to 4 months. Most patients are quite understanding and accepting. Too often the surgeon wishes not to disappoint the patient and proceeds, leaving the patient with an asymmetric ablation pattern, poor qualitative vision, and night glare, which is very difficult to repair.

Alternatively, once the eye has healed, a transepithelial PRK may be indicated if there was a specific difficulty with the problem, like a small, deep-set, or crowded orbit. The risk of corneal haze is far greater in these cases, and sometimes referral to a more experienced LASIK surgeon is preferable. The PRK technique must be transepithelial because any manual debridement will disrupt the corneal flap. In addition, PRK should not be performed without allowing for an adequate healing time of at least 4 to 6 weeks—to allow the eye to settle—as the risk of haze and irregular astigmatism are even higher initially. The last and more complex approach is to extend the flap manually with a freehand lamellar dissection. This approach definitely entails more risk and should only be attempted by very experienced lamellar surgeons, as corneal perforation and serious flap irregularities may occur.

In summary, the safest method is to reposition the corneal flap and create a new flap. Ideally, the new corneal flap is thicker by at least 20 microns, the eye has been allowed to settle for at least 4 months and the new cut is started temporal to the first.

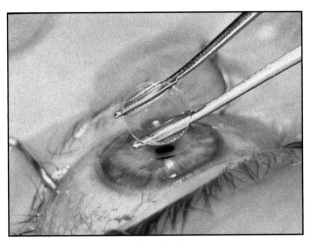

Figure 32-2. Free corneal lenticle from inadvertent resection of the corneal flap hinge. It is most commonly associated with flat corneas. There is an increased risk of irregular astigmatism, delayed visual recovery, epithelial ingrowth, and lost corneal caps. Must maintain hydration status of lenticle within the antidesiccation chamber then tape the eyelid shut postoperatively once the flap adheres. Sutures are not required.

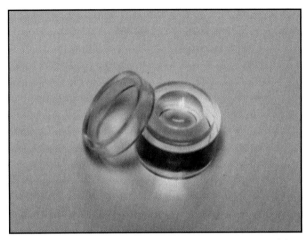

Figure 32-3. Antidesiccation chamber used in cases of free corneal caps to maintain the hydration status of the lenticle. A drop of filtered BSS is dropped in the chamber and the lenticle is placed epithelial side down. The stromal side is not rehydrated until it is replaced on the ablated stromal bed. Placement of the lenticle in excess fluid or stromal side down will result in considerable swelling of the cap.

FREE CAP

Clinical

A free cap is not a complication in the true sense, since free caps were the standard technique by which LASIK was performed when developed. As well, free caps should theoretically not occur if the corneal shaper hinge stop is built-in or is assembled and set properly to create a hinge; however, certain corneal dimensions will predispose certain eyes to this occurrence. It is important to recognize these corneal parameters preoperatively and be familiar with the proper management of a free cap, should it occur intraoperatively. Patients with flat corneas and mean keratometry below 41 D are at a higher risk of encountering a free cap. Insight into the mechanism is important, as it allows the surgeon to anticipate and thereby avoid surprises. A flat cornea will protrude relatively less into the suction ring compared to a steep cornea and present a smaller cap diameter to the microkeratome blade. The applanation lens meniscus will appear smaller with flat corneas. The Chiron Hansatome has a much wider range of acceptable keratometry and even virgin corneas as flat as 36 D will not result in a free cap. It is also important to recognize that the important keratometry value in a retreatment in which a new cut is planned is the original keratometry value since it is the peripheral cornea that is first presented to the microkeratome blade. That is, a postoperative LASIK cornea with a mean central keratometry value of 36 D treated for -10 D with an original preoperative keratometry measurement of 43 D will not be at higher risk for developing a free cap. Furthermore, with both Chiron units, flat corneas will produce smaller corneal

flaps and narrower hinges. An eye that is flat with a small diameter cornea may be suspect for developing a free cap; however, when the eye is placed within the suction ring, the cornea sits higher because the ring is seated on the surrounding limbus. This placement essentially presents an effectively steeper and larger cornea for the microkeratome blade, typically producing a larger flap relative to the corneal diameter. Peripheral neovascularization may be encountered in these cases.

In summary, free caps are more likely to occur with the classic Chiron Corneal Shaper than the Hansatome, and more likely to occur in cases in which a large diameter (> 14.5 mm) and flat cornea (< 41 D) are to be treated.

Management

Free caps occur with most, if not all, surgeons at one time or another, typically earlier in the learning curve (Figure 32-2). Anticipation and preparation are the first steps in management. Once a free cap is inadvertently produced, the cap must be placed in an antidesiccation chamber. The key principle to managing a free cap is to prevent excessive drying and swelling of the cap while preserving the epithelium. The cap is placed epithelial surface down on a drop of balanced salt solution (BSS) to help preserve the epithelium (Figure 32-3). No fluid is placed on the stromal surface, as corneal edema is a function of time rather than a function of the amount of fluid. Therefore, even a small amount of fluid left on the stroma during the procedure will result in considerable edema and prolong proper re-adhesion. The antidesiccation chamber will prevent excessive drying of the cap, but if the ablation is brief and the surgeon is experienced, the cap can be placed on the conjunctiva near the medial canthus, epithelial side down.

Once the cap is prepared, the ablation is performed and the stromal bed is kept dry. The free cap is then removed from the chamber, and at this point the stroma can be rehydrated with one or two drops of BSS. The cap is then placed on the stromal bed, stromal surface down, with the alignment markings coinciding. The importance of the alignment markings is most easily recognized when one encounters a free cap, as the markings not only become paramount to correct placement but in distinguishing the epithelial side from the stromal undersurface of the cap. It can be more difficult to assess the epithelial surface from that of the stroma with a free cap than one would expect, especially if stromal swelling or loss of the epithelium occurs. The classic alignment marking is the paraxial line extending from the central cap to the peripheral cornea. It is impossible to align the paraxial line unless the corneal cap is oriented properly, but the double circle markings provide easier four-point alignment. The two different sized circles only coincide if the correct orientation is achieved with the epithelial side up. Even minor misalignments are more readily observed with the four-point alignment system with hinged flaps. The Kritzinger-Updegraff marking system or other similar systems with multiple radial and pararadial lines also work extremely well in these cases. It is important for the beginning surgeon to always prepare the anti-desiccation chamber and place alignment markings for orientation, especially in cases in which the corneal diameter is large(> 14.5 mm) or the mean central keratometry value is flat (< 41 D). It is also important in cases of large flat corneas not to place the markings too peripheral so as to be outside the small free cap.

In cases in which no alignment markings have been made or the markings have been lost, alignment can often be made based upon three key elements:

- The orientation of the cap can be made based on how the cap is removed from the microkeratome unit (the orientation of the cap is the same as it will be in the unit with the temporal side extending out of the unit).
- Chatter marks from the oscillating blade along the bed margins are often helpful in determining the precise rotation of the cap.
- If the epithelium has been denuded, using fine forceps, the presumed undersurface of the flap can be depressed and will dimple inward, whereas Bowman's layer will be smoother and dimple somewhat outward.

Once the corneal cap has been replaced and aligned, it is important to give adequate time for a strong adhesion to develop. I typically wait 8 minutes then tape the eyelid closed. No bandage contact lens is used unless the epithelium is denuded, as this may act to displace the cap. After 1 hour, the cap is assessed for displacement then retaped overnight. Patients are asked to sleep for several hours and are provided with sedation. Pressure patching is not recommended. The eye is taped so that there is less friction from blinking on the cap. More importantly, if the cap becomes dislodged, it will remain in the fornices and be lubricated and available for replacement.

THIN AND PERFORATED CORNEAL FLAPS

Clinical

The incidence of clinically significant corneal flap problems is estimated to be approximately .2% once the initial learning curve is passed, and perhaps approximately .1% for severe corneal flap complications (Figures 32-4 through 32-5b). Although thin flaps may be produced from a lack of blade sharpness, and occasionally are observed in very flat corneas, perforated flaps likely occur primarily as a result of inadequate intraocular pressure (Figures 32-6 through 32-7b). A perforated or button-holed flap may also be produced by placing BSS on the cornea and then drying the central cornea. Central perforations have also been noted with a higher than expected frequency in very steep corneas, although the mechanism remains unclear. One theory is that the advancing depth plate pushes the steep central apex, creating a small valley just as the blade reaches the apex and thus forming a central perforation. The difficulty with this theory is that inferior, or even superior, flap perforations are not encountered in cases of forme fruste keratoconus as would have been predicted. The mechanism by which loss of suction creates a centrally perforated flap stems from an understanding of the balance of forces that operates when a lamellar incision is made with the microkeratome. The depth plate pushes down on the cornea as it advances, which is balanced against the suction pressure pushing up on the cornea, resulting in a flattened cornea that allows a planolamellar flap to be cut. If the depth plate is absent or incompletely inserted, the suction pressure continues to push up unopposed, causing the cornea to essentially "bulge" upward, becoming perforated by the advancing oscillating blade. If the suction pressure is low or absent, the depth plate force is not counterbalanced and the cornea essentially "sags," resulting in a centrally thin or perforated corneal flap. While there may be other mechanisms and factors leading to the development of button-holed flaps, they are clearly more common in eyes with an increased risk for poor suction, such as those with a history of retinal detachment, low scleral rigidity due to high myopia, vitrectomy, and those with conjunctival scarring or chemosis.

Each patient should be treated with a new blade. LASIK results, unlike ALK, are dependent upon laser ablation rather than the resection; therefore, bilateral cases may be performed safely with one blade. It does not appear from the large collective experience of high volume LASIK surgeons worldwide that bilateral infections are a realistic concern when using the same blade for both eyes of the same patient during the same operative session. In fact, a stronger case

to the microkeratome blade; therefore, care should be taken to avoid producing a free cap. It is recommended that a 180- or 200-micron depth plate be inserted when treating a flat cornea, as the hinge will be slightly wider and more secure. Experienced surgeons can also stop the microkeratome 1 mm earlier to create a wider hinge but slightly shorter flap. The Chiron Hansatome has a much wider range of acceptable central mean keratometry values and can safely treat virgin corneas with keratometry values as low as 36 D without risk of a free cap. In repeat LASIK in which a new cut is fashioned, it is the original keratometry values that are important since it is the mid-peripheral cornea that is presented to the microkeratome blade. A thicker depth plate is still recommended for retreatment if adequate tissue is available.

If a patient has a very steep cornea with mean keratometry greater than 47 D, occasionally it may make advancing the microkeratome into position slightly more difficult by obstructing the depth plate, and it may result in a large flap encroaching on peripheral blood vessels. In the case of superior macropannus, one may wish to decenter the flap inferiorly up to 1 mm. Care must be taken with decentration in cases of very steep corneas since the corneal flaps created are usually large, and decentration may result in encroachment of limbal vessels inferiorly. Very steep corneas are also associated with button-holed flaps through an unclear mechanism.

Diameter

Small corneas are similar to steep corneas in that the pneumatic suction ring is seated on the limbus or limbal conjunctiva, thereby placing the corneal vertex at a much higher plane relative to the suction ring. Occasionally, greater height can impede advancing the microkeratome into position so that the gears are engaged. The suction ring should be centered about the cornea and then decentered nasally, in a two-thirds to one-third ratio. A commonly encountered difficulty is the encroachment upon peripheral corneal neovascularization or limbal blood vessels, which can produce significant intraoperative bleeding. The Chiron Hansatome creates a 9.5 mm flap at present, which is problematic for small diameter corneas and leads to excessive bleeding from limbal vessels. Small flat corneas are typically acceptable with the Hansatome, as flaps smaller than 9.5 mm are fashioned. By raising the height of the plane at which the Hansatome head pivots, an 8.5 mm flap can be hinged superiorly with a revised suction ring. A 7.5 mm Hansatome flap will also be released at a later date.

Large corneas, alternatively, behave like flat corneas and are more likely to produce smaller flaps with narrower hinges or free caps. Thinner flaps may also be observed. Since the suction ring adheres to the peripheral cornea, it is more difficult to maintain adequate suction, so flap perforations can also occur, as can epithelial abrasions and broken limbal blood vessels. The Hansatome is ideal for large diameter corneas, whether flat or steep, and the problems encountered with flat large corneas with the Chiron Corneal Shaper are avoided with the Hansatome. Hyperopic eyes are more likely to have larger, flatter corneal configurations.

It is important to be able to apply alignment markings appropriately, especially in cases of flat corneas, so that if a free cap is produced, proper alignment can be achieved. Alignment markings on large and flat corneas if made too peripheral may remain on the peripheral cornea and be of no help. Additionally, care must be taken to mark out to the limbus in cases of small or steep corneas.

SUBCONJUNCTIVAL HEMORRHAGES

The pneumatic suction ring produces considerable vacuum pressure, which can produce subconjunctival hemorrhages (Figure 32-11). This is more common with prolonged suction pressure, excessive eye manipulation, patients on blood thinners such as aspirin or other anti-arthritic medication, or with recent alcohol consumption. There are typically no sequelae and the most important aspect is to explain to the patient that they he or she has a bruise, that these changes are common, may get worse before they get better, may change color, and clear up over approximately 3 weeks.

The only clinical note of significance is that a large subconjunctival hemorrhage or significant conjunctival edema during manipulation of the suction ring may prevent adequate suction pressure from being achieved and/or maintained. There are two means by which this may be managed:
- The blunt side length of forceps may be utilized to milk the edema or subconjunctival heme into the fornices (Figures 32-12a and 32-12b).
- The procedure may be postponed for several hours to days, which is preferable. It is important to recognize that any question of achieving adequate pressure should always be treated conservatively and surgery canceled.

IMPROPER POSITIONING

If the pneumatic suction ring is improperly positioned, the vacuum pressure must be released immediately or repositioning is impossible. Within seconds, a scleral ridge is formed from the vacuum pressure and reapplication of the suction ring, regardless of the new position, will immediately return to the initial application site. Therefore, it is essential to align the suction ring carefully and seat it firmly in position prior to application of the vacuum pressure and to immediately determine if the position is correct. The surgical assistant should be in position to control the vacuum pressure both to engage and disengage suction at the time the pneumatic ring is positioned. If the suction ring is more than 1 mm decentered or improperly decentered and the scleral indentation precludes proper placement, the procedure should be postponed by as little as 15 to 30 minutes and re-application attempted. If there is edema or excessive

Figure 32-11. Subconjunctival hemorrhage observed following an uncomplicated LASIK procedure. No clinical or visual significance.

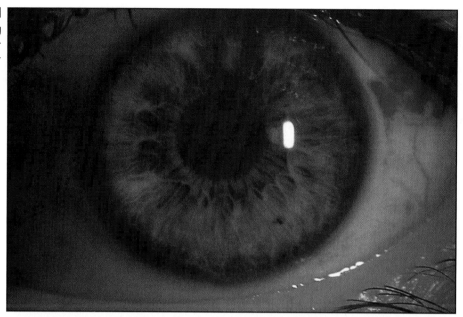

Figure 32-12a. Management of conjunctival edema by milking the edema away from the perilimbal area and toward the fornices so that adequate suction can be obtained. Pseudosuction may be obtained if the conjunctiva occludes the suction ring without elevating the potentially serious corneal flap complications. If there is clinically borderline pressure, delay surgery by 1 to 24 hours and apply frequent topical steroids to reduce inflammation during the interval (courtesy of Stephen Slade, MD).

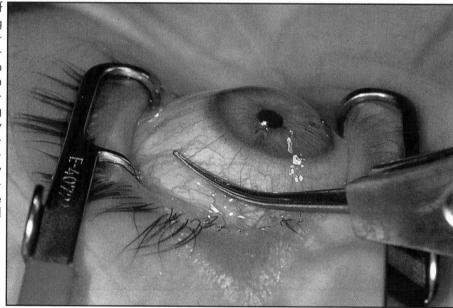

subconjunctival heme, the surgery should be postponed to the following day.

NEOVASCULARIZATION

Clinical

Many patients have a history of extensive contact lens wear and have developed superior and, occasionally, inferior macropannus. Bleeding from the area of neovascularization may occur when the corneal flap involves the vessels, which is common with either large corneal flaps or extensive corneal neovascularization. Large flaps are associated with steep corneas. In addition, corneal flaps from small diameter corneas are relatively large and encroach upon the peripheral vessels.

Preoperative examination should specifically note not only the presence, but the extent to which the vessels encroach upon the peripheral cornea so that technique modification may be considered. Intraoperative bleeding complicates the procedure with respect to intraoperative visualization, changes in stromal hydration, asymmetric blockage of laser pulses, and postoperative interface opacification (Figure 32-13). Bleeding can be very extensive and difficult to control if the corneal vessels are numerous and lysed proximally at the limbus. It is also important to remember that the excimer laser beam consists of far ultraviolet radiation and is essentially nonthermal in nature; therefore, it is incapable of coagulating these vessels. Fortunately, despite the clinical appearance of bleeding blood vessels at the edge of the flap, the sequelae are typically minimal.

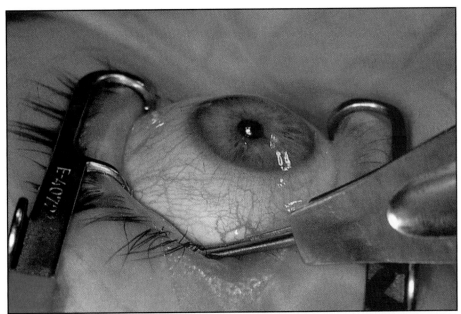

Figure 32-12b. Management of a conjunctival edema by milking the edema toward the fornices, away from the perilimbal area, so that adequate suction can be obtained (courtesy of Stephen Slade, MD).

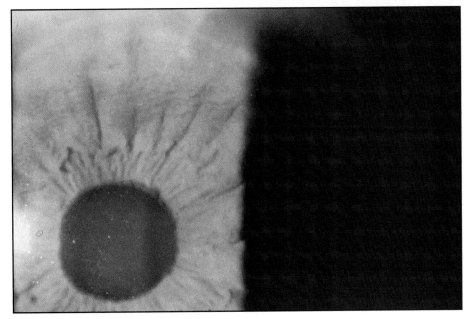

Figure 32-13. Interface blood observed during the early postoperative period from corneal neovascularization bleeding intraoperatively. Interface heme cleared gradually over months without treatment. There were no visual sequelae associated (courtesy of Stephen Slade, MD).

Management

The most important aspect of managing intraoperative bleeding from corneal neovascularization during LASIK is prevention. The pneumatic suction ring should be placed on the eye such as to avoid the vessels upon creation of the corneal flap. If the suction ring is somewhat decentered inferiorly, superior macropannus can be avoided with the lamellar incision. There are two risks with this approach:
1. The inferiorly decentered corneal flap will involve inferior vessels.
2. Excessive decentration will result in a poor quality flap. An argon laser can even be used preoperatively to coagulate the vessels in preparation. In general, no precautions need be taken with corneal neovascularization, as closing the flap with active bleeding will typically begin to tamponade the vessels and result in external bleeding outside of the interface. Interface blood that has been entrapped will spontaneously clear over weeks to months and is outside the visual axis.

If bleeding from corneal neovascularization does occur, management involves a host of options. Typically no intervention is required, as the bleeding is minimal and will arrest once the flap is closed. Any red blood cells within the interface can be irrigated out under a closed flap. Usually any further bleeding will occur externally and can be siphoned away using a dry surgical spear as a wick along the flap margin. Pharmacological agents can also be used to reduce or arrest blood flow. Although phenylephrine is the most well-known agent for constricting blood vessels, it will also result in pupil dilatation, which is disconcerting to patients. Therefore, we prefer to utilize topical steroids, which also have a blanching effect on vessels. The topical steroid dexamethasone .1% has significant vasoconstricting action and can be soaked into a surgical spear and applied along the limbus for several seconds. Phenylephrine can be a more effective option, but patients should be warned that their eye appearance may be altered and more glare and blur may initially be present. Additionally, phenylephrine concentrations of 10% should be avoided, as they may have systemic cardiovascular effects, with amplified risks in patients with a history of beta-blocker use. Only phenylephrine 2.5% should be considered and, again, is best applied with a surgical spear locally for maximum effectiveness and safety.

Occasionally, bleeding cannot be arrested or pharmacological agents are not available and management includes blowing compressed air, which constricts and coagulates the vessels, or the suction ring is applied with or without suction. Simply placing the suction ring over the eye, either prior to or after the flap is opened, and placing downward pressure will blanch the limbal vessels mechanically and stem blood flow. The patient will feel pressure, but this technique is effective in maintaining fixation. In cases in which the bleeding is so profuse that it cannot be controlled either for the ablation, which is rarely the case, or once the flap is closed to keep the interface clean, the suction pressure can be activated. If the suction pressure is adjustable, it should be lowered to a minimal level. The suction ring should not be activated if the ring is placed over an open flap, as it may damage the flap. Suction should also not be activated for longer than 30 seconds at a time to avoid the potential for ischemic events.

What often occurs is controlled vessel bleeding, but once the flap is closed and the interface irrigated, further bleeding develops into the interface. Irrigation or any disruption of the vessels, even if bleeding has been previously controlled, will cause them to rebleed. Since it is often only a matter of obtaining control for several seconds to allow the flap to seal and have the bleeding occur externally, applying the suction ring manually or with active suction for 30 seconds or so may be adequate. Fortunately, the cut edge of the vessels is along the flap edge. Rebleeding will then ensue within the peripheral gutter and externally—not within the interface beneath the flap. As stated earlier, a small amount of blood beneath the flap need not be disconcerting or necessitate further intervention.

DECENTRATION

Clinical

This intraoperative complication is usually not apparent until the patient is examined in follow-up (Figure 32-14). Pupil centration is more appropriate than visual axis fixation as symptoms occur chiefly from an expanded pupil in dim light extending beyond the treatment area. If there is a large angle kappa, the treatment should be shifted toward the visual axis. The incidence increases when the pupil is pharmacologically altered. Topographical appearance consists of a superior ablation if the patient looks down in an effort to get away from his or her surgeon during the procedure, and an inferior ablation if the patient squeezes his or her eyes to induce Bell's phenomenon. Nasal decentration is more common with the use of miotics and temporal decentrations with subconscious efforts to avoid hitting the nasally hinged flap. Dilatation makes centration more difficult and may obscure proper centration, usually resulting in superotemporal decentrations. Self-fixation is optimal, but once the flap is open and the stroma begins to dry, patients are often unable to accurately pinpoint target fixation light, so it is important for the surgeon to ensure proper alignment during ablation.

When evaluating a postoperative map, it is also important to distinguish between a preoperative asymmetric cornea and true decentration of the ablation zone by either assessing the preoperative corneal videokeratography or a difference map. A large angle kappa or eccentric fixation, more commonly encountered with high myopes, will give the clinical appearance of decentration.

Decentration may produce asymmetric night glare or ghosting of images and tilting or distortion of images related to induced cylinder. Decentration may produce both a reduction of best-corrected vision secondary to irregular astigmatism and a reduction of UCVA from the associated undercorrection and cylinder since the maximally treated area is not aligned. Decentrations greater than 1 mm are usually symptomatic, and those greater than 2 mm typically induce severe qualitative and quantitative visual symptoms.

Management

Until only recently there have been no effective means of retreating these patients; management involved either rigid gas permeable lenses or artistic attempts at re-establishing improved topography. The introduction of custom corneal ablations with topography-assisted LASIK has offered new hope to these patients. The most difficult case to correct would be one with a significant decentration, asymmetric night glare but plano refractive error, and excellent daytime visual acuity. If the patient is undercorrected, which is common in these cases, he or she can be retreated with proper centration with emphasis on simultaneously correcting the original topography. That is, the untreated area may be kept more dehydrated to increase the refractive effect in that area. In general, treating the undercorrection and expanding the optical zone maximally with the enhancement procedure reduces patient symptoms dramatically since the flap will blend the new treatment. Unlike PRK, in which there is significant concern for creating an edge effect inducing haze, the essentially inert stroma can be manipulated more safely to improve corneal topography. Most patients improve subjectively with time and treatment

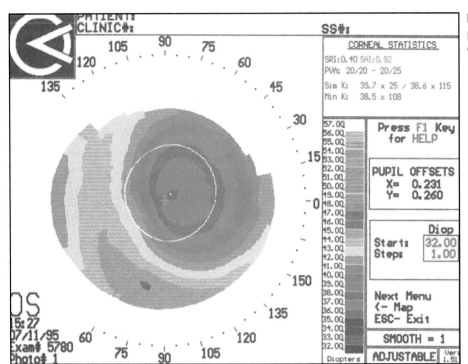

Figure 32-14. Videokeratography of a decentered LASIK ablation.

of their second eye. Artistic attempts to reconfigure the ablation pattern involved properly centering a new ablation, usually 25% to 50% of the preoperative correction at the maximal optical zone or the last two zones of a multizone ablation while protecting the adequately treated area. It remains to be seen if similar cases of poorly centered PRK treatments can be corrected intrastromally as well. Kritzinger has also described surface PTK for the correction of decentered intrastromal ablation with significant improvement observed upon videokeratography.

EARLY POSTOPERATIVE COMPLICATIONS

PAIN

Clinical

Most patients remarkably do not experience any discomfort; however, a foreign body or gritty sensation is commonplace. Some patients complain of both eye pain and orbital discomfort, which may be related to the pressure exerted by the eyelid speculum and suction ring rather than the lamellar incision itself. Most patients do not require postoperative narcotic analgesia, although sedatives and non-narcotic agents may be helpful. Infrequently, some complain of severe pain, and the patient is examined for a short differential diagnosis consisting of a displaced corneal flap or an epithelial defect. Very rarely infection may be the problem and the interface should be examined carefully for any infiltrates. As with all procedures, patient variability plays a large role in the amount of discomfort experienced.

Management

The most important aspects in management include ensuring that the flap is in place and epithelium intact. Most patients are simply concerned that any pain or discomfort is indicative of a healing complication, and simple reassurance is an essential part of management. Non-narcotic agents, especially sedatives, are routinely prescribed postoperatively for LASIK patients. Sleep is the most effective management, as even a 2-hour nap can dramatically reduce discomfort and improve visual performance. Narcotic agents are rarely indicated. Topical nonsteroidals and bandage contact lenses may be useful adjuncts to control pain, especially in cases of epithelial breakdown. All patients are given Voltaren (diclofenac sodium .5%, CIBA), two drops immediately preoperatively and two drops immediately postoperatively. Voltaren has been found in a randomized clinical study at our clinic to dramatically reduce postoperative symptoms of pain, burning, and irritation. Lubrication is another important element, as these eyes may have an associated superficial punctate keratitis in which lubricating agents should be strongly encouraged. Although Celluvisc (methylcellulose, Allergan) is viscous and highly effective in promoting epithelial health, it may crystallize on the lashes. GenTeal (hydroxypropyl methylcellulose, CIBA) is our lubricating agent of choice. Although GenTeal is not preservative-free, it acts similarly because of the enzymatic breakdown of the sodium perborate preservative upon contact with the patient's own tears. This avoids the noncompliance issues associated with single dose unit minums since GenTeal is available in 15 ml bottles. Punctal plugs are also recommended to keep the eye well-lubricated and promote

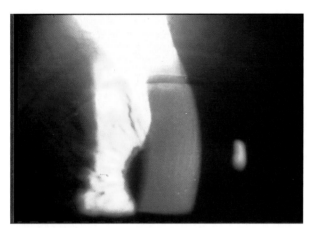

Figure 32-15. Superior gap along the flap edge, indicating flap displacement.

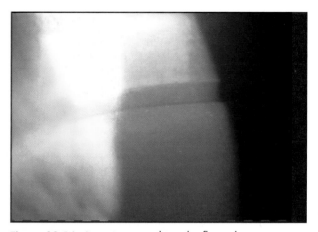

Figure 32-16. Superior gap along the flap edge.

comfort. While night glare is the most common visual complaint, dry eye is the most common postoperative nonvisual symptom of refractive surgery patients.

DISPLACED FLAP

Clinical

Patients with a displaced corneal flap can typically be diagnosed upon entering the examination room, as these patients have their eyes covered, are tearing profusely, are quite photophobic, and are in considerable pain (in direct contrast to most LASIK patients who have white, quiet eyes). The vision is extremely blurry, in the counting fingers range, as would be expected.

The introduction of the hinged flap technique by Ioannis Pallikaris, MD, originally conceived by Jose Barraquer, dramatically improved the safety and even the results of LASIK. The corneal flap reduced the concern of a free or lost corneal cap and improved realignment, thus reducing the incidence of irregular astigmatism.

It is highly unusual for the corneal flap to displace if the striae and blink test are normal without incurring trauma. Occasionally, however, the corneal flap will displace postoperatively, especially during the first 6 to 12 hours. Typically, displacement is 1 mm or less, producing corneal striae peripherally or centrally (Figures 32-15 and 32-16). Rarely will the flap become completely free and attached only by the hinge. If the procedure had been complicated, the flap allowed to become edematous, or excessive irrigation was utilized, the risk of displacement is greater. Movement of the flap to smooth or extend the flap edges during intraoperative positioning can break the adhesion and increase the chance of displacement if not allowed to re-adhere properly. The utilization of Celluvisc (methylcellulose, Allergan) or other viscous agents to coat the epithelium intraoperatively increases the time required for full adhesion and the vulnerability for displacement. Also, free caps are not only more likely to become dislodged but

require that the eyelid be taped shut so that if dislodged, the loss of the cap would not further complicate management. Even if the cap is lost, it is important to recognize that it has no direct refractive effect on the eye and that it should be managed with PTK of the bed margins and a topical steroid regimen as with PRK (as described earlier in this chapter).

Management

Once again, prevention of corneal flap displacement is the primary form of management by ensuring the flap is secure at the conclusion of the procedure. Testing the flap with the striae and blink tests are essential steps in the procedure. Waiting an adequate amount of time after the corneal flap has been properly realigned, usually in the range of 1 to 3 minutes, and avoiding excessive interface irrigation allows for a strong seal to form.

If the corneal flap becomes displaced either completely or partially, it must be replaced as soon as possible to not only avoid infection and reduce pain but to avoid permanent striae and damage to the flap. The incidence of epithelial ingrowth increases with both displacement and free caps (Figure 32-17). If the flap has been displaced, anesthetize the eye for examination. Management until the flap is replaced involves lubrication every 30 minutes with sterile preservative-free artificial tears. It is important to keep the displaced flap hydrated, as the flap is more vulnerable to damage when desiccated. In addition, striae and various irregularities will form more easily in the flap and be more difficult to remove when repositioning the flap if the flap dries. Patients usually keep their eye closed due to discomfort; alternatively, the eye can be taped shut until treated.

The technique by which the flap is replaced involves the same principles by which the flap is first secured. Exposure and fluid management are important elements to all lamellar procedures. Once the stromal bed and flap are cleaned of debris and any epithelium ingrowth on the stromal bed is debrided, the flap is closed and realigned into position.

If there are any striae (Figures 32-18 through 32-22e),

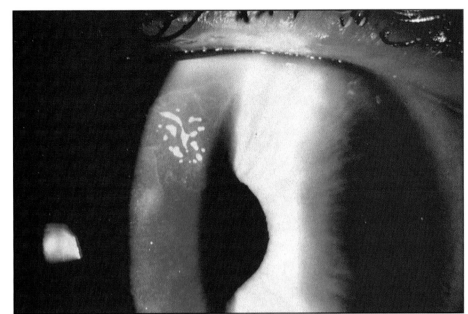

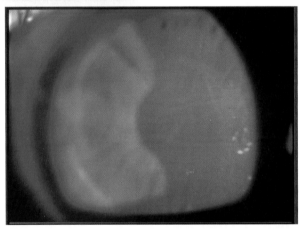

Figure 32-17. Epithelial ingrowth following inadvertent resection of the corneal flap hinge during a LASIK procedure resulting in a free cap. Preoperative mean keratometry was 40. Induced irregular and regular astigmatism gradually resolved over 11 months, improving best-corrected vision from 20/50+ to 20/25+ without treatment. At 11 months, astigmatic keratotomy was performed for regular mixed astigmatism reducing cylinder from 1.75 to .75 D.

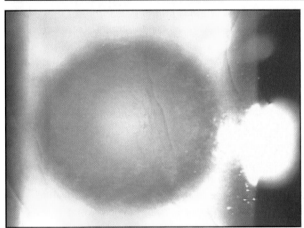

Figure 32-18. Fine, significant, vertical flap striae through the visual axis.

Figure 32-19. Fine, horizontal flap striae are highlighted with fluorescein staining.

the flap should be smoothed with wet surgical spears and allowed to settle for 2 minutes. Persistent striae can be ironed using the blunt side of forceps over a dry corneal surface, stretching the flap toward the peripheral gutter. Residual striae may still be evident and the flap should be ironed as smoothly as possible with the underlying objective of approximating the flap edges and the stromal bed margins as closely as possible. One will not observe elimination of the corneal striae until the next morning even if the flap is stretching into proper alignment; therefore, the goal should not be to eliminate the striae during the session. If however it is apparent that the peripheral gutter is asymmetrical, and then the flap should be stretched further or lifted and refloated and the process started again (Figure 32-23).

The concept behind my technique is that the corneal flap is elastic; the corneal flap and stromal bed should approximate one another. Therefore, any corneal flap striae

are indicative of tenting of the flap preventing the flap from filling the peripheral gutter. Thus, if the flap can be stretched to fill the gutter, the striae should be substantially reduced or eliminated. Once again, it is not possible to observe the complete smoothing of the flap striae; however, if the flap is taut, it should be recognized that many of the striae will clear by the next morning. With a dry corneal flap surface, striae can often be eliminated by stretching and ironing the edges of the corneal flap outward to fill the peripheral gutter over 8 to 10 minutes. This is a very tedious, but potentially successful, technique. Although it is best to treat displacement and striae as soon as possible, this technique can be used even many months postoperatively.

EPITHELIAL DEFECTS

Clinical

Epithelial defects only occur in a small percentage

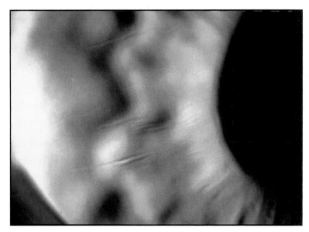

Figure 32-20. Peripheral fine radial flap striae.

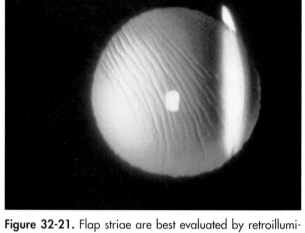

Figure 32-21. Flap striae are best evaluated by retroillumination.

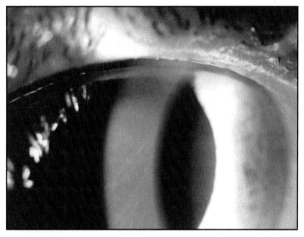

Figure 32-22a. Corneal flap striae secondary to displacement.

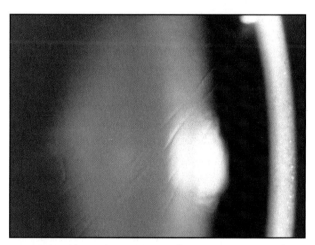

Figure 32-22b. High power view demonstrating corneal striae with reduced BCVA and UCVA.

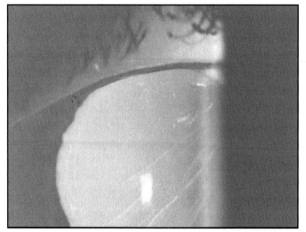

Figure 32-22c. Retroillumination of the corneal flap with a dilated pupil is the best technique to assess striae.

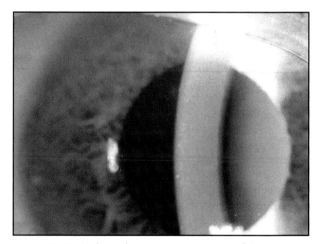

Figure 32-22d. Three days postoperative view following correction of flap striae.

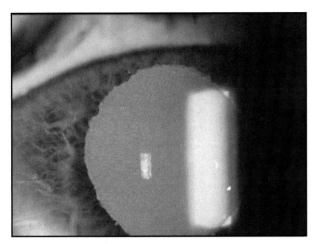

Figure 32-22e. Day 3: no striae visible on retroillumination.

(< 3%) of patients, with large defects being more common early in the surgical learning curve and secondary to drying of the flap surface. The most frequent site of epithelial defects is along the flap incision edge, related to manipulation of the flap or the microkeratome pass (Figure 32-24). Certain patients have very loose epithelial adherence and the microkeratome head may pull the epithelium rather than incise it cleanly. The epithelium beneath the upper eyelid is the most vulnerable, perhaps related to hypoxia or edema. Central or peripheral epithelial defects may occur with excessive use of topical anesthetic related to epitheliotoxicity, or in second eyes of bilaterally treated cases, owing to dehydration if the fellow eye is not taped shut. Additionally, it is not uncommon for a superficial punctate keratitis to be observed in the area of the alignment markings associated with the use of gentian violet. Avoiding alignment markings of the central 3 mm of epithelium provides for faster visual recovery.

Maintaining the epithelial integrity improves comfort, safety, and visual rehabilitation. Epithelial defects can be associated with tremendous pain, especially when large. Photophobia and tearing are commonly associated. There are two potential complications that may ensue with epithelial effects:

- The risk of infection is increased
- The incidence of epithelial ingrowth is also higher

The theoretical advantages of LASIK over PRK are reduced when an epithelial defect is produced. A clinical history of anterior basement membrane dystrophy or severe recurrent corneal erosion syndrome are the primary indications to consider PRK as the procedure of choice over LASIK.

Management

The importance of maintaining adequate hydration of the epithelium and reducing manipulation of the flap is immediately apparent from the preceding clinical discussion in order to reduce the incidence of epithelial defects.

Patients with anterior basement dystrophy should be avoided, as significant sloughing of the epithelium is commonly encountered and visual recovery is often very prolonged with associated significant irregular astigmatism.

Topical anesthesia should be applied sparingly in all LASIK patients and should be instilled only just before the procedure is to begin. The epithelium can also be insulated from anesthetic toxicity through direct application of the topical anesthetic to the bulbar conjunctiva and fornices with an anesthetic-soaked surgical spear. The eye should not be allowed to sit for any length of time once the lid speculum is inserted and exposure is attained to prevent desiccation of the epithelium. The cornea should also be wet with BSS prior to advancing the microkeratome in order to reduce surface friction.

If an epithelial defect occurs, there are several principles to maintain:

1. During the LASIK procedure, care should be taken to ensure that epithelium has been cleared from the interface and irrigation should be directed from the opposite axis.

2. The patient must be observed daily, as with PRK, for evidence of infection.

3. Although routinely recommended, a prophylactic antibiotic should be used postoperatively in cases of an abrasion. Some surgeons recommend double coverage such as a fluoroquinolone (Ocuflox, Allergan or Ciloxan, Alcon) and an aminoglycoside (tobramycin).

4. Pain management is quite variable and dependent upon the patient and the size of the epithelial defect. For small epithelial defects, it may simply involve reassuring the patient that he or she will experience some discomfort associated with a foreign body sensation.

Frequent lubrication is always advocated. For larger epithelial defects, a bandage contact lens is recommended and is inserted sterilely at the conclusion of the procedure. The bandage contact lens must be carefully inserted so as not to disturb the flap. A bandage contact lens with a base curve of 8.4 or fit on preoperative mean keratometry is recommended, as excessive movement will increase patient discomfort and slow epithelial healing. The fit of the contact and re-examination of the flap should be performed after instillation of the lens. If observed to be too tight rather than snug, the contact should be replaced with a flatter base curve of 8.8. The patient is placed on a topical nonsteroidal anti-inflammatory preparation such as Voltaren (diclofenac sodium, CIBA). Topical nonsteroidals can delay epithelial healing and should be used twice a day as needed but not beyond 48 hours. Patients are maintained on a full-strength topical steroid as well with a four times daily regimen. Oral agents such as a sedative, non-narcotic, and even a narcotic agent may all play a role in maintaining patient comfort during the epithelial healing process. Pressure patching is contraindicated, as patient eye movement against the firmly applied eyelid may create excessive shearing forces and displace the flap.

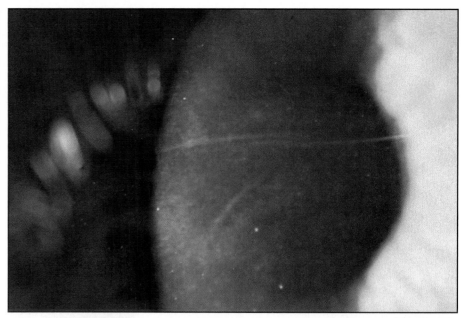

Figure 32-23. Late corneal flap striae in association with mild interface haze after LASIK for extreme myopia correction. It is difficult, if not impossible, to correct misalignment at this late stage, several months postoperatively. BCVA was reduced from 20/25 to 20/30 postoperatively, with minimal subjective qualitative visual disturbance.

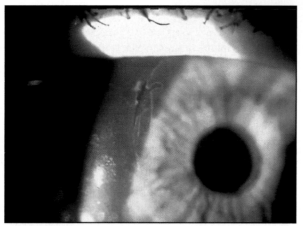

Figure 32-24. Peripheral epithelial defect along the flap edge.

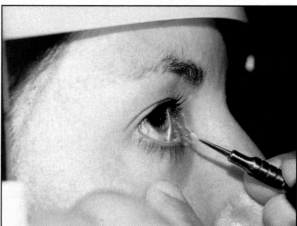

Figure 32-25. Removal of a bandage contact lens with fine nontoothed forceps. The therapeutic lens is hydrated and topical anesthetic instilled. Patient gaze is elevated and the inferior aspect of the lens is grasped and drawn down and away from the eye.

The bandage contact lens should be removed in the same manner as that for a patient following PRK, ensuring that the contact lens is well-lubricated with artificial tears and a topical anesthetic such as proparacaine .5% instilled, as it is the least epitheliotoxic. The preferred technique is to have the patient look up while at the slit-lamp biomicroscope. In this manner the inferior aspect of the bandage lens is visible and may slide down. Using fine nontoothed forceps, the inferior aspect of the contact lens is firmly grasped and the lens pulled down and away from the eye (Figure 32-25). This is the most gentle and precise technique for bandage contact lens removal with least risk of flap displacement. It is always important to anesthetize the eye first, then copiously lubricate the contact lens to literally float it prior to removal.

INFECTION

Clinical

The incidence of infection is rare, likely in the order of 1 in 5000 to 10,000, based on international experience. However, keratitis and endophthalmitis have been reported after LASIK.[2,3] The nature of the procedure, when properly performed with an intact epithelium, makes the stroma only vulnerable to bacterial inoculation for a very brief period of time intraoperatively. However, operative trauma or breakdown of the epithelium increases the risk of surface infection. Prophylactic antibiotics and sterilization of the microkeratome between procedures dramatically reduces the risk. The risk can further be reduced with proper lid hygiene and antiseptic eyewash such as poviodine preoper-

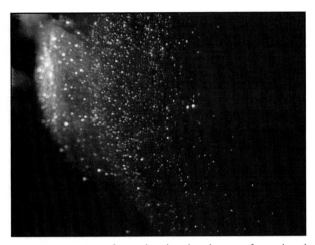

Figure 32-26. Interface talc related to the use of powdered gloves. Greater risk involves microkeratome malfunction secondary to talc within the gears and oscillating blade mechanism. In general, about half of all surgeons use powderless gloves and half perform the procedure without gloves (courtesy of Stephen Slade, MD).

atively. Gloves are used by roughly half the surgeons performing the procedure, and, if utilized, are of the talc-free variety, as the talc can damage the microkeratome gears and accumulate in the interface (Figure 32-26).

Clinical Note

Infiltrates can rarely be observed within the interface and may be in response to infection, but may also be inflammatory in reaction to foreign matter. The stromal interface is typically inert and does not elicit any reaction to entrapped foreign debris. One such case I encountered was managed by lifting the flap and debriding the infiltrates, then irrigating the infiltrates with antibiotics. The patient remained pain-free postoperatively and was observed to have two pinpoint infiltrates upon routine follow-up on the first postoperative day. The patient was placed on frequent fluoroquinolone and aminoglycoside topical antibiotics, and within 24 to 48 hours of this course of therapy had a clear and quiet interface with no sign of infection or infiltration.

Clinical Note

Another much more unfortunate postoperative course involved a 35-year-old woman who underwent LASIK for extreme myopia correction of -14 D. On the first postoperative day, the patient was completely comfortable with a quiet white eye and clear cornea with intact epithelium. Uncorrected vision was a remarkable 20/60. On the second postoperative day the patient was re-examined and had unaided vision of 20/40, but the patient returned late in the afternoon complaining of pain and tearing. Examination revealed two small epithelial defects at 5 and 6 o'clock, just within the area of the flap. Both

denuded areas contained small infiltrates, and the patient was cultured and placed on hourly tobramycin and Ocuflox (ofloxacin, Allergan) by her ophthalmologist, a corneal specialist, then referred back the following morning for follow-up at our facility. No bandage contact lens was inserted. Despite an acute increase in pain, redness, and swelling of the eye within hours, the patient did not seek further assistance until her appointment the following morning. Copious purulent discharge was evident in the morning, although frequent antibiotics had been instilled throughout the night. From 5:00 pm to 9:00 am the following morning the eye had dramatically worsened. The two .5 mm superficial infiltrates described by the co-managing physician had increased to a single 3 mm arcuate infiltrate along the inferior aspect of the flap with a 2-mm hypopyon. There was a mild to moderate degree of conjunctival injection and chemosis. Vision had reduced to counting fingers and the patient was quite photophobic. A tentative diagnosis of Pseudomonas aeruginosa or possibly pneumococcus was made. The patient was started immediately on hourly fortified cefazolin 50 mg/cc alternating with fortified tobramycin 14 mg/cc in addition to hourly Ocuflox. Cycloplegia was also maintained. After discussion with the co-managing corneal specialist, it was decided to admit the patient to the hospital for the initial management of the corneal ulcer in light of the rapid deterioration. The patient received subconjunctival injections of tobramycin and cefazolin. Within hours, the flap had become necrotic and dislodged with the stromal bed also infiltrated (Figure 32-27a). The flap was removed and treatment in the hospital continued (Figure 32-27b). Initial culture indicated a gram negative organism, possibly Hemophilus, sensitive to cefazolin. After 48 hours of hourly broad spectrum coverage with topical fortified antibiotics and twice daily subconjunctival antibiotic injections, final cultures yielded Serratia marcescens sensitive to tobramycin. After 5 days, the patient was discharged, as the infection appeared under control with a resolution of the hypopyon. The surface epithelium healed over 3 to 4 weeks (Figure 32-28a) and the corneal scarring reduced over months (Figure 32-28b). The patient ultimately required PTK for corneal scarring and later lamellar keratectomy with homograft tissue, which was performed by Stephen Slade, MD with excellent results. The patient impressively recovered full best-corrected vision of 20/25; however, a posterior subcapsular cataract developed, which ultimately required extraction.

There are a few unusual features of this case in that the infection was incredibly virulent and occurred 2 days postoperatively. The epithelium was initially intact. The postoperative prophylactic antibiotic was tobramycin, which the bacterium had been sensitive to. The infection was superficial rather than within the interface. No other patients had developed

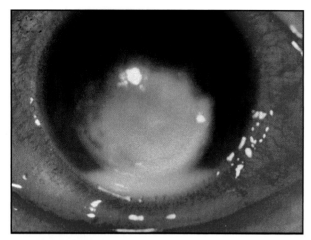

Figure 32-27a. Acute *Serratia marcescens* corneal ulcer following superficial infection of the corneal flap. Postoperative inferior corneal abrasion on the second postoperative day with rapid deterioration and infection of the corneal flap. High magnification clinical appearance of the corneal ulcer and hypopyon observed less than 24 hours after focal infiltrates were first noted.

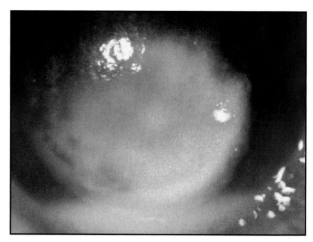

Figure 32-27b. Severe conjunctival infection and associated chemosis.

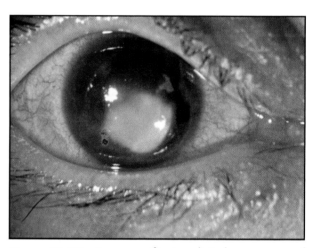

Figure 32-28a. Low magnification clinical appearance of the treated corneal ulcer after 3 weeks with loss of the corneal flap. No hypopyon was evident and ocular inflammation was reduced.

an infection. The only conclusion to draw was that the procedure had merely made the patient vulnerable to an epithelial breakdown. The inoculation of bacterium had likely occurred postoperatively. The patient's only risk factor was a history of very dry eyes for many years with intolerance to contact lens wear. Lindstrom describes three cases of Serratia marcescens seen in consultation and determined infected make-up (eyeliner) to be the underlying etiology (personal communication). The primary conclusion is that the epithelium provides an important barrier to infection and measures such as frequent postoperative lubrication are critical elements in preventing infection.

Nonspecific Diffuse Intralamellar Keratitis

Clinical

Nonspecific diffuse intralamellar keratitis (NSDIK) was originally referred to as *Sands of the Sahara* and depicted an early postoperative condition marked by the development of interface haze. The haze appears much like mild to moderate PRK haze, with a granular appearance (Figures 32-29 through 32-40). Bobby Maddox, MD coined the original name of Sands of the Sahara, which best describes the "sifted sand" appearance of this powder-like material. The material can be observed to delineate the ablation steps and even the keratectomy chatter markings (see Figure 32-31). Occasionally, it is interpreted as a severe diffuse epithelial keratitis, but careful examination reveals it is at the level of the interface and that the flap stroma is unaffected. While

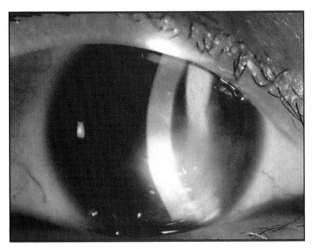

Figure 32-28b. Clinical appearance of a corneal ulcer after 9 weeks demonstrating residual stromal scarring.

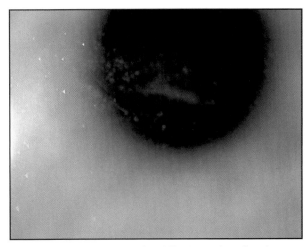

Figure 32-29. Nonspecific diffuse intralamellar keratitis with a fine granular appearance in the flap interface (courtesy of Kerry Assil, MD).

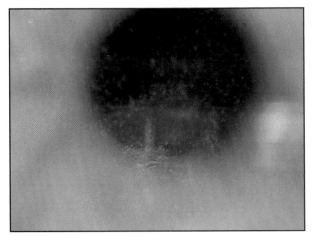

Figure 32-30. Nonspecific diffuse intralamellar keratitis with a fine granular appearance in the flap interface (courtesy of Kerry Assil, MD).

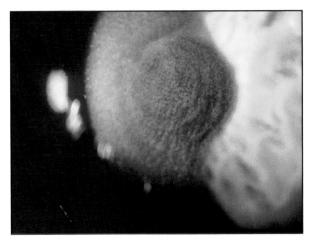

Figure 32-31. NSDIK in a radial pattern following the ablation zones and the chatter marks of the microkeratome (courtesy of Stephen Slade, MD).

the haze is often diffuse, it is typically more dense centrally but may be sectoral and can be evident only peripherally. It is of unclear etiology and usually presents on the first postoperative day but may develop, or at least is recognized, anytime within the first week. It has been described to occur with various microkeratome manufacturers. In addition, NSDIK, although more common following primary LASIK, can develop following LASIK retreatment in which a new cut was not made but the original corneal flap has been lifted. Although typically unilateral, it has been described to occur bilaterally. Even in bilaterally treated patients, the condition typically develops in only one eye—usually the first eye treated—but it can also be limited to the second eye treated, leaving the first eye with a clear interface. These cases typically occur sporadically, but surgeons have described multiple cases occurring on a single day. The condition is classically a one-time event, but we have encoun-

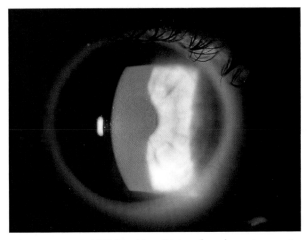

Figure 32-32. NSDIK with mild interface haze in a quiet white eye following LASIK.

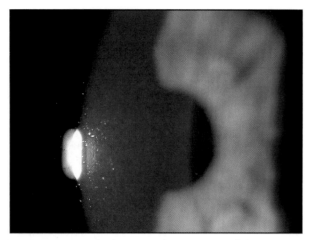

Figure 32-33. A higher magnification view of the eye with NSDIK in Figure 32-34.

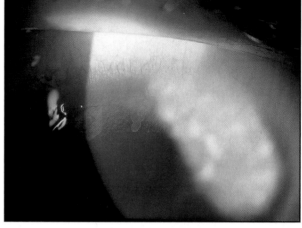

Figure 32-34. NSDIK with interface keratitis under a healing superior epithelial defect 1 day after LASIK.

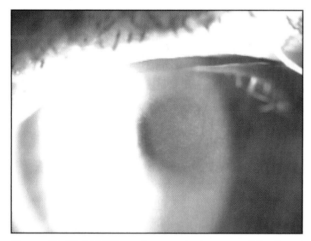

Figure 32-35. NSDIK can be seen in the area of the flap 4 days after primary LASIK.

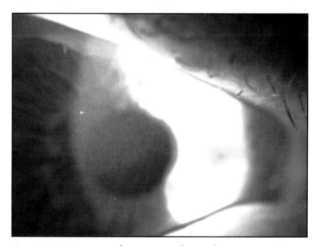

Figure 32-36. NSDIK has occurred over the superior portion of the flap and has extended into the visual axis.

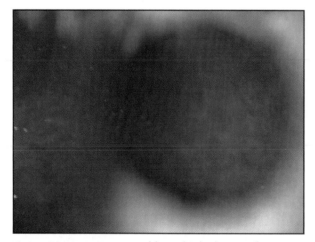

Figure 32-37. NSDIK is visible under high magnification as interface haze. The patient's visual acuity was still 20/20.

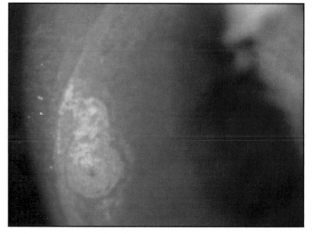

Figure 32-38. Another high magnification view of NSDIK.

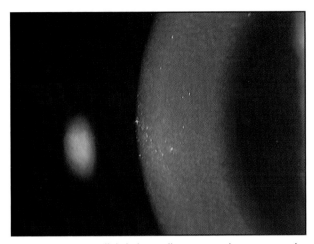

Figure 32-39. Parallel slit lamp illumination demonstrates the depth of NSDIK. The NSDIK was first noted inferiorly on the first postoperative day and by the second day, the NSDIK had extended to involve the entire interface. The UCVA remained at 20/20. Topical steroid therapy resulted in 50% resolution by the fourth postoperative day (courtesy of Jonathan Woolfson, MD).

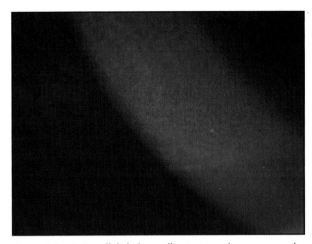

Figure 32-40. Parallel slit lamp illumination demonstrates the termination of NSDIK at the edge of the corneal flap (courtesy of Jonathan Woolfson, MD).

tered at least one case that was definitely recurrent.

The condition remains enigmatic to date, and the underlying etiology remains unclear. Scrapings of the interface material have demonstrated neutrophils, but no bacteria. It is felt that the acute polymorphnuclear reaction is an inflammatory reaction in relation to some unknown antigen or antigens. As most of these cases follow uneventful and uncomplicated LASIK procedures, it is unclear what the trigger may be. Possible antigens include blood from neovascular vessels, various drops of microkeratome cleaning agents or fluids, various bacterial toxins from the lids, or sebaceous debris found within the fornices. Latex from surgical gloves, which may intermittently come into contact with instruments, is also suspect, but surgeons who do not use gloves have also seen NSDIK. Jon Dishler, et al have questioned thermal energy as the cause; however, high myopes are not more likely to encounter this condition and enhancements typically involve very small corrections. The only common element is the BSS used for irrigation. Occasionally, the irrigation cannula will be noted to have crystalline deposits and some have recommended disposable cannulas be used. Trauma and epithelial defects appear to be associated with the development of NSDIK and should be considered risk factors. There appears to be more cases of NSDIK recognized within the past year, even though rare cases were noted previously but not recognized. The question remains as to whether there is a true increase in incidence or simply more LASIK cases being performed, thus more recognition of NSDIK. It is my personal feeling that the true incidence is rising and is approaching .2%. I have examined approximately 15 cases of NSDIK to date, ranging from very mild to very severe cases. Most occurred within the past year to myself and other TLC surgeons, the

majority within the past few months. I continue to feel that some aspect of our evolving LASIK technique and patient preparation has promoted the development of NSDIK. Clearly, there has been no consensus as to the underlying mechanism of NSDIK, but management has become better defined.

Management

NSDIK can vary considerably in presentation from very mild cases of interface haze to very severe cases that are difficult to distinguish from infection. Management varies with severity, but topical steroids remain the mainstay of therapy. It may simplify management to define a simple grading system in which grade 1 represents very mild cases that typically resolve spontaneously over 1 month and may be diffuse or peripheral. The clinical appearance is that of trace or very mild PRK reticular haze, and both vision and refraction remain unaffected. Patients are asymptomatic and grade 1 NSDIK is typically noted on routine day 1 or week 1 examination. When detected, even mild cases should be treated with high potency and high frequency topical steroids to ensure successful resolution and prevent progression of severity.

Grade 2 NSDIK, according to my grading system, would be the more diffuse variety commonly described by LASIK surgeons, which is comparable to mild to moderate PRK haze, and again may appear more dense centrally. It is these cases that are often confused with a superficial punctate keratitis. Vision is typically affected and best-corrected vision may be reduced by one to two lines. The refractive error in these cases may be slightly hyperopic. Patients are commonly symptomatic and will experience a worsening of their vision over the first week unless aggressive steroid therapy is started. The recommended steroid regimen is Maxidex (dexamethasone phosphate .1%, Alcon) hourly for the first day while awake, then every 2 hours while awake the second day, then every three hours while awake the third day, followed by qid dosing for 3 weeks. Ciloxan (ciprofloxacin .3%, Alcon) is maintained qid for 4 to 7 days only. There is considerable improvement within the first few days in the intensity of the interface reaction, often demonstrating a 50% reduction in severity, usually clearing peripherally first. Even if NSDIK is diagnosed late after 1 or more weeks, the same steroid regimen is recommended. Often by 1 month, complete resolution is noted and most cases return to their preoperative best-corrected vision. Early detection and treatment will considerably improve the visual and refractive prognosis. Failure to demonstrate considerable improvement in 1 week requires surgical intervention (as described for grade 3 NSDIK).

The most severe and rare form of NSDIK, grade 3 according to my grading system, results in a dense central infiltrate that is quite disconcerting upon initial examination and can easily be confused with an active stromal infection or grade 4 PRK haze. The eye, however, is once again white and the patient, although complaining of blur and irritation, is for the most part comfortable. No purulent discharge, anterior chamber reaction, or hypopyon is typically evident. The infiltrate is limited to the interface, and although the bed may be minimally involved, the undersurface of the flap appears uninvaded. The central flap typically appears to have striae centrally over the infiltrate. Epithelial breakdown may even occur centrally and an AC reaction with keratitic precipitates may even be observed. Uncorrected vision is typically 20/200 or worse, and best-corrected vision is less than 20/60. Refraction is difficult but manifests several diopters of hyperopic astigmatism. The typical presentation is on day 5 with the patient looking essentially normal on day 1 and returning because of worsening vision. The patient is typically on little or no topical steroids.

Management involves both the topical steroid therapy described and surgical intervention. Patients can be placed on high-dose steroid therapy for 1 to 2 weeks then evaluated and treated, or the flap can be lifted immediately and the interface cleaned, then the steroid therapy initiated. The corneal flap lifts very easily, as there is no fibrosis despite the clinical haze appearance. The inflammatory material appears as a thin milky fluid, whitish gray in appearance and can be easily debrided. Caution should be taken when cleaning the interface, as aggressive debridement produces increased hyperopia; therefore, the stromal bed and flap undersurface are carefully and gently wiped with a dull blade, spatula, or surgical spear, followed by 5 microns of PTK applied to both the stromal bed and flap undersurface. The final step involves flap closure and thorough irrigation. Utilizing this technique with PTK gives the best results and the eyes look surprisingly good even the next day. Hourly topical steroids are started immediately postoperatively.

Debridement alone or debridement with irrigation has produced less impressive results, and interface haze is often diminished but still evident. I have attempted to lift corneal flaps in these NSDIK patients and irrigate on 1 day, at 1 week, and at 1 month. The primary benefit to delaying surgical intervention is that the associated hyperopic astigmatism can be treated simultaneously. The hyperopia is related primarily to the stromal bed melt from the inflammatory reaction but also due to irregular astigmatism, so 75% of the measured hyperopia is typically targeted. With this approach, we have treated two grade 3 NSDIK patients who manifested 4 D to 6 D of hyperopia with 1 D to 2 D of hyperopic astigmatism. Both patients lost four to six lines of best-corrected vision, and both are now correctable to 20/20 and manifest 1 D to 1.5 D of residual hyperopia. Although both seem to be doing equally well, one patient was treated immediately upon detection at day 5, the second patient was first seen at 2 weeks postoperatively and was treated at 1 month after 2 weeks of intensive topical steroids.

In summary, nonspecific diffuse intralamellar keratitis is likely an inflammatory toxic-based reaction that is very steroid responsive but of unknown etiology. Early recognition and proper management is essential to achieving a good visual prognosis.

IRREGULAR ASTIGMATISM

Clinical

Virtually all patients immediately postoperatively have some degree of irregular astigmatism and will complain of poor qualitative vision, despite excellent quantitative vision. Patients should be counseled that this is a normal part of the healing process, especially for those requiring higher degrees of myopia correction. High myopes typically complain of what can best be termed "Vaseline vision." The qualitative disturbance is compounded by any residual refractive error. Most irregular astigmatism clears over 2 to 4 weeks, and virtually all by 3 months, although some cases will continue to improve over 12 months. Approximately 1% to 2% of patients have a significant degree of irregular astigmatism resulting in a permanent loss of BCVA of two or more lines. During the early stages of the surgical learning curve and in complicated cases such as those resulting in a free cap, the incidence of irregular astigmatism of any degree resulting in loss of best-corrected vision is likely in the order of 5% to 10%.

Management

Surgical technique is important in reducing the incidence and severity of irregular astigmatism. A certain degree of irregular astigmatism, however, is unavoidable with lamellar surgery. Specific aspects of flap replacement constitute the greatest step at which the eye is vulnerable to the creation of irregular astigmatism. The corneal flap must

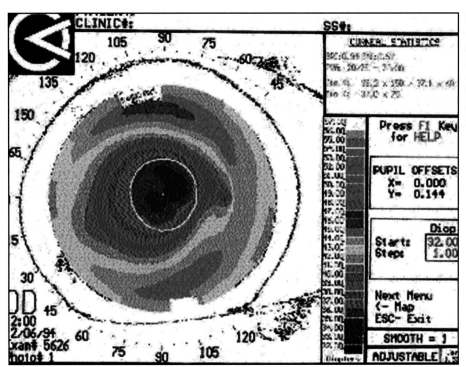

Figure 32-41. Corneal videokeratography demonstrating a small effective optical zone following a LASIK procedure. Clinically significant night glare is generated postoperatively, especially in high myopes secondary to spherical aberation.

be floated back into position in as smooth a maneuver as possible. The size of the hinge and thickness of the flap may also have relevance in that a broader hinge and thicker flap typically have greater memory and resiliency to return to the natural alignment, making placement easier. Smoothing the flap into position with a wet surgical spear helps to reduce any flap irregularities and gently stretch the flap into position. The corneal flap tissue is elastic and hydrated, therefore it tries to contract, producing fine virtually invisible microirregularities. Any drying effect will only serve to exacerbate these irregularities. It is unknown what impact various ablation profiles have on the development of irregular astigmatism, however, central island formation may produce irregular astigmatism in itself. Higher refractive corrections produce greater degrees of irregularity both in relation to the ablation profile and, more importantly, in relation to the healing pattern of the eye.

Night Glare

Clinical

Night glare is another seemingly unavoidable side effect experienced by many corrected high myopes. Night glare is a result of a pronounced form of spherical aberration, with the pupil diameter in dim light exceeding that of the effective optical zone created (Figure 32-41). Efforts to increase the diameter of the optical zone utilized are complicated by the greater depth of ablation, and in the case of broad beam excimer lasers, the formation of central islands. Patients complain of halos, starbursts, and a general reduction of qualitative vision in conditions of reduced illumination. Night glare can virtually disable extremely myopic individ-

uals preoperatively and especially postoperatively for night driving. The longer daylight hours of summer reduce visual complaints during that season; therefore, summer is the preferred season of patients and surgeons alike. Any residual refractive error will exacerbate night glare, especially residual myopia.

Management

Fortunately, most patients improve with time and bilateral treatment as a result of cortical integration. Simply stated, they learn to ignore the visual disturbances that surgery produces under low light conditions. Various ablation algorithms have been attempted to achieve superior visual results both quantitatively and qualitatively, but all must sacrifice diameter for reduced depth of ablation when treating high myopia. With broad beam excimer delivery systems, a multizone technique or aspheric profile can be utilized to reduce depth of ablation in high myopia correction, but the effective optical zone is less than that created with single-zone techniques. Scanning excimer lasers have more flexible and complex profiles and are very effective at reducing night glare, as they can expand the optical zone to 9 or 10 mm, but if stromal depth is limited, smaller transitions zones must be used.

Another essential principle is that unlike ALK, whereby the corneal flap actually acts to increase the effective optical zone relative to the resected area, in LASIK, the corneal flap acts to decrease the effective optical zone. That is, the second refractive pass of ALK removes a plano lenticle, but the corneal flap drapes over the area of excision and enlarges the effective optical zone. In LASIK, the removed tissue is a myopic lenticle with tapered edges, which allows

Figure 32-42. Postoperative clinical appearance of advancing epithelial ingrowth detected with fluorescein staining 10 days postoperatively, demonstrating a nonadherent flap edge. Advancing edge or wave border of epithelium is commonly visible without staining. Epithelium within ingrowth can be thick, easily observed, and possibly commonly requiring treatment, or it is very thin, more difficult to detect, and usually stable without treatment.

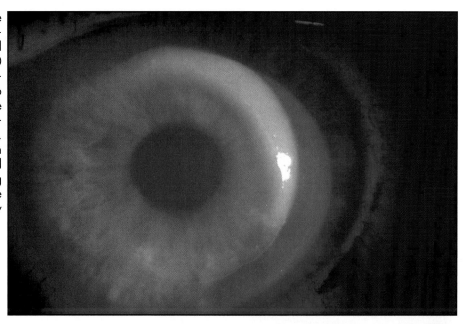

the flap to actually mask the peripheral area of ablation. In addition, not only does the flap appear to mask the extent of the treatment area, but the increased hydration of the deeper stroma reduces the effectiveness of the peripheral ablation curves. This fact becomes readily apparent when one examines the postoperative LASIK topography and compares it to that of PRK performed with the same nomogram. The circular area of flattening representing the treatment area of LASIK is reduced, indicating a smaller effective optical zone than that programmed.

In PRK, one requires well-blended peripheral curves to avoid inciting haze formation—such is not the case within the stroma. Another approach to LASIK is to ablate a larger optical zone within the stroma, but limit the peripheral blend to reduce the overall depth of ablation. This is the approach currently utilized for the high myopia PlanoScan program with the Chiron Technolas 217. This program, which utilizes flying spot technology, enables us to improve both qualitative and quantitative vision for high myopes even when illumination is not optimal. The limiting factor remains the minimum thickness of the stromal bed needed to maintain long-term stability—a minimum of 200 microns but ideally 220 microns.

While night glare is often improved by treating any residual myopia with a maximal optical zone, some patients are fully corrected but have significant night visual disturbances. Currently in these patients, glasses or contacts that overminus the patient by -1 D are the mainstay of conservative therapy. Pilocarpine is avoided in high myopes due to the small potential for retinal pathology to develop. Custom cornea software from TopoLink with the Chiron Technolas 217 or ScanLink with the Lasersight LSX is evolving for enlarging optical zones even when the refractive error is plano by performing PTK centrally and PRK peripherally. Residual corneal thickness once again determines candidacy.

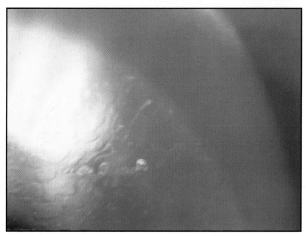

Figure 32-43. Early epithelial ingrowth extending from the flap edge.

EPITHELIAL INGROWTHS AND STROMAL MELTS

Clinical

The incidence of epithelial implantation and ingrowths is roughly 2% and is usually observed within the first few weeks of surgery. With experience and improved technique, our incidence of epithelial ingrowth has reduced to less than 1%. Epithelium within the interface may occur in nests that have been implanted and are usually nonprogressive or more commonly grow peripherally beneath the flap edge.[4] The epithelial ingrowth may be progressive in nature or self-limited, rapid in onset or slow in development. The natural history is variable in that the epithelial ingrowth may be static or precipitate a stromal melt of the overlying cap. The stroma is sandwiched between epithelium within the interface and on the surface and may experience necrosis as collagenase is released from the necrotic epithelium. The pri-

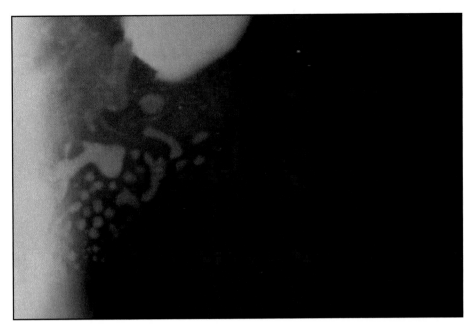

Figure 32-44. Epithelial ingrowth growing within the corneal interface, usually extending from the periphery although it can have implanted nests of epithelium. It has a gray clinical appearance with white pearls forming a whorl pattern within the epithelial peninsulas. The thicker the epithelial ingrowth, the darker gray in appearance and the more likely it will be associated with white geographic patterns or pearls. These white areas most likely represent necrotic islands of epithelium within the ingrowth.

mary risk factors for an epithelial ingrowth are a peripheral epithelial defect, poor flap adhesion, free cap, or a perforated corneal flap. Poor or improper adhesion of the corneal flap will encourage migration of epithelial cells into the interface (Figures 32-42 and 32-43). The clinical appearance of an epithelial ingrowth is typically a tongue or peninsula extending from the cap edge with a whorl or finger-like pattern (Figures 32-44 through 32-46). Patients who exhibit considerable blepharospasm are at higher risk for developing ingrowth, which usually develops superotemporally or inferotemporally owing to the eyelid action. Patients with anterior basement membrane dystrophy are at highest risk for developing epithelial ingrowth. Patients over 50 years of age also exhibit weaker epithelial adherence patterns and carry a slightly elevated risk of ingrowth. The flap edge may be gray and rolled or necrotic (Figures 32-47 through 32-52). The visual acuity, topography, and refraction may all be affected since the epithelium extends beneath the flap and encroaches on the visual axis. Regular and irregular astigmatism may be induced, reducing BCVA and UCVA, even if a stromal melt is not clinically evident.

Management

Prevention is again an important part of management and care should be taken to preserve the flap epithelium intraoperatively and approximate the peripheral gutter to create a narrow seam. If there is any epithelial defect noted intraoperatively, weekly visits during the first month should be scheduled. If there is no epithelial ingrowth developed by 4 weeks, then the risk is negligible thereafter. In general, an epithelial ingrowth of 2 mm or greater usually requires treatment to prevent a stromal melt. The presence of epithelium itself does not indicate that treatment is warranted, but size, progression, and clinical appearance of the epithelial ingrowth determine the predicted natural history and man-

agement. While various subclassifications are possible, this grading system simplifies identification and management of epithelial ingrowths. The most important elements of the Machat epithelial ingrowth grading system are that it is management-based with classic clinical hallmarks identifying each grade. The system is designed to categorize ingrowths into three grades to indicate the urgency of treatment required and risk that flap integrity will be permanently lost, with grade 3 epithelial ingrowths having the greatest risk.

The clinical hallmark of grade 3 is the presence of white geographic nests that represent necrotic epithelial cells within the interface, which release collagenase, resulting in active flap melting and indicating urgent treatment. The classic hallmark of a grade 2 is the presence of translucent vacuolated cells that may be accompanied by early flap edge erosion, indicating that epithelial cells are dying and are imbibing fluid in the precursor stage of cell death, therefore treatment within 1 to 2 weeks is needed. Grade 1 epithelial ingrowths demonstrate no evidence of cell necrosis or loss of flap integrity and usually have a white advancing line along the proximal edge, indicating stability and no treatment is required.

An epithelial ingrowth requiring treatment should be performed as soon as possible to avoid progression with stromal melting, which complicates treatment and usually results in a worse prognosis. Flap melting results in an irreversible loss of qualitative and potentially quantitative vision. Treatment of grade 2 and grade 3 epithelial ingrowths involves lifting the flap and removing the epithelium from within the interface. Typically, these flaps are much easier to lift due to the presence of the epithelium itself within the interface and the fact that management usually occurs within the first month. The corneal flap edge should be marked preoperatively and an alignment marking

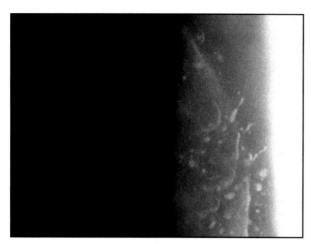

Figure 32-45. Strands of epithelial ingrowth extending from the flap edge to the central cornea (Machat grade 2).

placed as described later under LASIK retreatments (see Chapter). The flap edge should be lifted with a Suarez spreader or equivalent to expose the undersurface of the flap and stromal bed. The flap edge can often be grasped temporally with nontoothed forceps and gently reflected back.

Although epithelium is typically adherent to the undersurface of the flap, both stromal surfaces should be debrided. Sharp debridement is preferable to improve the probability that all residual epithelial cells have been removed. The epithelium can often be dissected off in a single sheet. A dry surgical spear is useful to scrub the stromal surfaces but may leave fragments and must be discarded after each pass to avoid re-implanting epithelial cells. The edges of the corneal flap and along the periphery of the stromal bed are the primary sites to clear of epithelial remnants. Do not use alcohol or cocaine within the stromal bed or other such toxic agents, as they will cause irreparable damage. If there is any concern for additional epithelial nests, irrigation and brushing can be used. Epithelial cells will also fluoresce in a dark room with no microscope illumination if five to 10 pulses of PTK are placed over the bed and flap. This is not routinely recommended but is effective at clearing these cells. Once the epithelium has been adequately debrided, the flap is replaced, as for any retreatment. It is important to irrigate beneath the flap to clear any residual epithelial cells from the interface, aiming in the direction of the ingrowth from the opposite side. Wet surgical spears are used to smooth the flap into alignment. A bandage contact lens may be required if the surrounding epithelium has been denuded during the debridement.

Another technique that can occasionally be helpful for small peripheral growths with no flap abnormality is to use a spreader at the slit lamp when ingrowths are small and try to milk the cells out under direct visualization. If it does not work, lie the patient down and lift the flap. Prepare the patient with two drops of anesthetic and antibiotics. The lashes are cleaned. The entire flap is not lifted or disturbed. A speculum is not usu-ally needed when treating at the slit lamp. A dry surgical spear is used to smooth the edge back into position and clean any loose epithelial debris away. Fine tiers are used to pull any loose pieces of ingrowth away. Patients look at it as less surgery, less disruption of the flap, and you have direct visualization. Sometimes the ingrowth is a sheet that gets into the interface and can be removed easily, other times the cells are necrotic and can be milked out. Wait approximately 30 seconds after smoothing the flap back with the eye open and it will seal since there has been no irrigation.

STROMAL MELTS

Clinical

The patient with an aggressive epithelial ingrowth—grade 2 or 3, especially if associated with a thin corneal flap—will develop a stromal melt within 1 to 4 weeks. These are often very rapid in onset, noted within 1 to 2 weeks of the primary procedure but typically asymptomatic or associated with a foreign body sensation due to edge lift. Occasionally, blurred vision, photophobia, or pain may be associated but only if it is very advanced with surface epithelial breakdown. The flap is seen to lose its integrity and alter its shape, with the flap edges becoming blunt, squared off, or eroded (Figures 32-56a through 32-56c, see Figures 32-50 through 32-52). The flap edge itself usually appears gray and rolled. Small focal nests of epithelial cells are often visible in the area of the stromal melt (Figures 32-57a and 32-57b). An epithelial erosion may be evident, producing discomfort and placing the patient at risk for infection. The appearance is radically different from a normal flap with scarring along the cut edge of Bowman's layer at the periphery of the flap, which appears white with smooth flap edges.

Management

Management is difficult at best and involves determining first if the epithelial ingrowth is active or if the melt is stable. The appearance of necrotic cell nests indicates that treatment is warranted. If scarring is evident with cell nests, no surgical intervention is indicated and the patient should be checked at 1 to 2 weeks, then at 1 month to ensure stability. If there is considerable melting involving the central visual axis and affecting best-corrected vision, the flap is typically not viable and requires removal to improve visual symptoms. An attempt should be made in all but the most damaged flaps to preserve the tissue as best as possible. The earlier these flaps are treated, the more likely they will remain viable. The initial steps of surgical management are to lift the flap, even if fragmented, and debride the flap undersurface and stromal bed. Care should be taken to remove all the epithelial nests without further damaging the flap. The flap should then be replaced and allowed to settle. A bandage contact lens can provide comfort if the surface

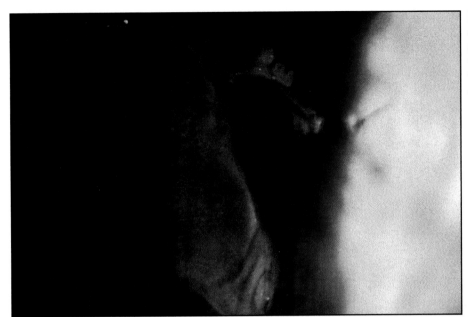

Figure 32-57a. Stromal melt secondary to epithelial ingrowth encroaching upon the central visual axis. Qualitative vision was reduced with significant glare inferotemporally and monocular diplopia.

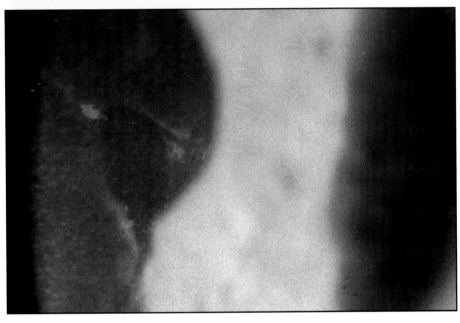

Figure 32-57b. Management consisted of debridement of the interface and smoothing of the corneal flap. Removal of the corneal flap increases haze formation but does not alter refraction.

hemorrhages following bilateral surgery. No surgical details are available. A review of more than 10,000 LASIK procedures in our clinic and a further 10,000 LASIK procedures in South America failed to disclose any other cases. The history is highly suggestive that the macular hemorrhage was indirectly related to the procedure and that the patient was predisposed to develop a break in Bruch's membrane with a secondary choroidal neovascular net, and that the surgery merely precipitated the occurrence at an earlier date.

LATE POSTOPERATIVE COMPLICATIONS

Late postoperative complications are those which either occur over time or are independent of time, typically observed at or after 1 month. Errors in refractive pre-

dictability are included in this section in concert with regression and central islands.

ERRORS IN REFRACTIVE PREDICTABILITY

Overcorrections

Clinical

An overcorrection with any refractive procedure is more difficult to manage. Although there is no ability to induce LASIK regression through steroid withdrawal as in PRK, consecutive hyperopia with LASIK can be easily managed with hyperopic LASIK ablation patterns using scanning technology. Holmium laser thermokeratoplasty can also be effective, but treatment should not be attempted ideally for

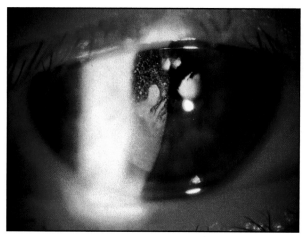

Figure 32-58a. Clinically aggressive epithelial ingrowth.

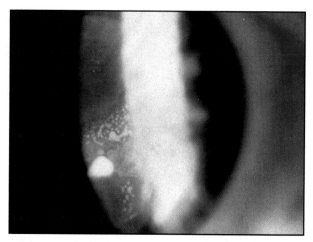

Figure 32-58b. Epithelial ingrowth resulting in rapid deterioration with a corneal flap melt necessitating flap removal in a secondary procedure.

6 months to ensure that the flap is completely stable (Figures 32-61a and 32-61b).

Management

Our preferred management of consecutive hyperopia post-LASIK is to lift the corneal flap at 2 to 4 months (once stability is evident) and ablate 70% of the hyperopic refractive error measured. As always, although younger patients may cope well with mild hyperopia, pre-presbyopic and presbyopic patients are immediately disconcerted by the loss of reading ability and distance blur imposed. Some patients will gradually improve with regression, but a number of these overcorrected LASIK patients must be treated. Patients can be fit with a disposable contact lens as early as 1 week to ease the accommodative strain and improve their vision pending enhancement. The hyperopic lenses are typically of a lower power than measured. Patients with reduced best-corrected vision likely have a degree of irregular astigmatism present, and the flap and topography should be assessed for other problems. It is best in patients with reduced best-corrected vision to wait longer, as improvement is often observed over several months and the associated hyperopia may improve spontaneously.

Undercorrections

Clinical

Undercorrections are common in higher attempted corrections, especially those above -10 D or 12 D. Creating a tight nomogram is optimal; however, reality dictates that overcorrections will occur with greater frequency in high myopia correction as the standard deviation increases with increasing correction. Since it is far easier to correct residual myopia than hyperopic overcorrection, the nomogram should always be developed conservatively and undercorrections anticipated as the attempted correction increases. Undercorrected patients complain of poor distance vision and night glare but have functional vision at near.

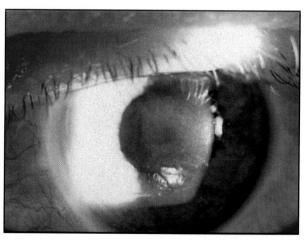

Figure 32-58c. After topical steroid treatment and repeat PRK, UCVA returned to 20/40 after 9 months, although BCVA remained reduced to 20/25 with residual stromal haze.

Management

Patients should be prescribed temporary glasses by the end of the first week after surgery or fit with disposable contact lenses. We have been fitting patients with disposable contacts routinely at 1 week for more than 3 years without any difficulties. Patients are fit on their preoperative keratometry, as the contact lens sits on the midperipheral cornea. Disposable contact lenses are recommended because further regression is easily and inexpensively corrected with a new pair of lenses. The contact lens power is typically much higher than what we may refract due to the positive tear meniscus and lens vaulting. Patient symptoms dramatically reduce once some form of temporary correction is obtained pending additional surgical treatment. Fluctuating vision and loss of best-corrected vision experienced frequently by highly myopic patients early in their healing are much better tolerated when corrected with lens-

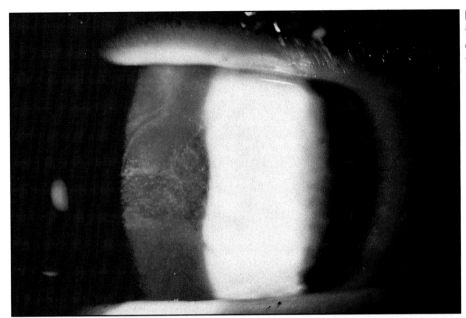

Figure 32-59a. Central corneal flap perforation with central epithelial ingrowth and haze formation. Intraoperative loss of suction was experienced.

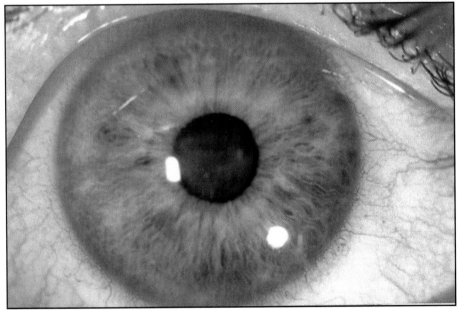

Figure 32-59b. Following removal of a nonviable corneal flap, PTK retreatment was performed to reduce central scarring. Residual haze and myopia required further PRK enhancement after 6 months. BCVA was still reduced to 20/30, with UCVA at 20/60 and +.25 -1.25 x 60 refraction. Time will likely restore one additional line of BCVA and no further surgery would be attempted for the residual refractive error.

es. Night visual disturbances, although reduced, continue to remain a problem for many highly myopic patients, but they do improve with retreatment.

Regression

Clinical

Somewhat surprisingly, some LASIK patients experience considerable myopic regression despite the fact that the deep stroma is considered to be virtually inert with respect to wound healing. It is unclear precisely what occurs physiologically, but there appears to be multiple factors affecting regression observed with LASIK. More severe degrees of myopic correction have a greater likelihood of

myopic regression, as is the case with PRK. Both epithelial hyperplasia and stromal remodeling appear to be factors in regression and are more active in deeper ablations. Regression also appears to occur much more rapidly than with PRK and is clearly much less responsive to topical steroid manipulation.

It may very well be that the initial baseline refraction and unaided visual acuity measured on day 1 or 2 is not always representative of the achieved refractive endpoint but is altered by early edema, irregular astigmatism, and dehydration effects of the procedure. A hyperopic refraction can mean irregular astigmatism, and a myopic refraction can indicate the presence of a central island, which is often visible at day 1 on videokeratography in a majority of

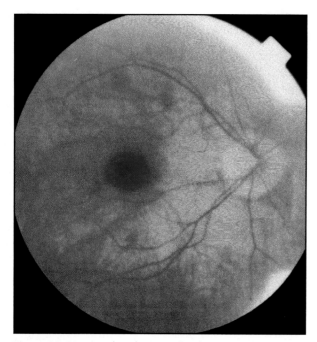

Figure 32-60a. Fundus photography demonstrating a superficial macular hemorrhage following LASIK in a highly myopic patient. Suction time was approximately 30 seconds. The role of the procedure in precipitating hemorrhage was unclear and surprisingly was felt to be coincidental by the patient's retinal specialist, who observed macular changes several months preoperatively.

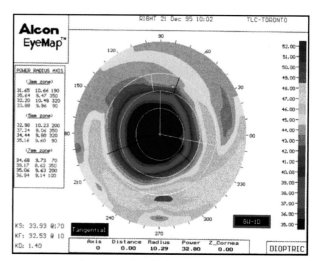

Figure 32-60b. Corneal videokeratography demonstrating excellent central flattening following a LASIK procedure for -12 D. The patient remained 20/80 uncorrected at 6 weeks due to macular hemorrhage, although vision slowly improved both subjectively and objectively.

LASIK patients. The multifocal nature of the corneal contour produced can create a poorly defined refractive endpoint.

Although there are multiple problems in defining the true residual refractive error early in the healing process, it does appear that a certain amount of myopic regression is inevitable in the correction of severe myopia. Myopic regression in severe myopes (-6 to -9 D) may be as great as 1 or 2 D, and in extreme myopia (-9 to -15 D) as high as 3 or 4 D. Regression of several diopters may be seen to occur in patients treated for over 15 D to 20 D of myopia. Treatment of these patients is ideally performed with a combination of phakic implants and LASIK, rather than LASIK alone. Smaller optical zones used in high myopia treatments to preserve stromal tissue also demonstrate more regression.

As stated, the cause of myopic regression appears to be a combination of epithelial hyperplasia and stromal remodeling. It is evident that the epithelium will increase in thickness in response to a significantly flattened cornea. Stable central mean keratometry below 33 D is difficult to achieve and below 30 D is rarely obtained. Larger optical zones blending into the periphery may reduce or eliminate the cause for epithelial hyperplasia centrally by creating a smoother, more acceptable contour to the anterior corneal curvature. Additionally, upon lifting the corneal flap of highly myopic patients, some fibrosis is usually evident centrally over the area of ablation, indicating some degree

of active stromal remodeling. In some eyes treated for high myopia, a significant stromal reaction at the site of the ablation becomes evident with reticular haze observed within the interface. The only association observed in these cases is the correction of at least 10 D of myopia and excessive drying of the interface intraoperatively. These patients have an aggressive healing course with myopic regression, and elevation of the flap for retreatment is very difficult even early in the healing process once the clinical appearance is noted. It is unclear as to what degree stromal remodeling may occur within the interface and to what extent it may contribute to myopic regression in LASIK.

Rarely, highly myopic patients post-LASIK will develop interface fibrosis over several weeks, which should not be confused with NSDIK, which develops over 1 to 2 days. The haze develops in less than .1% of cases and appears reticular or even somewhat confluent in some cases. It may reduce quantitative and qualitative vision. These very rare cases occur in extremely severe myopes with aggressive wound healing responses. Treatment of myopic regression and ablation of the fibrosis must occur early, usually at 4 weeks, if the flap is to be elevated and the interface ablated and cleared. Excessive force will result in tearing or damaging the flap. Topical steroids are helpful in controlling haze in these cases.

One particularly disturbing cause of myopic regression is iatrogenic keratoconus, when an inadequate amount of stromal tissue remains after the primary procedure. It is vital to maintain the stability of the cornea by leaving an adequate amount of tissue in the stromal bed, ideally 240 microns with a minimum of 200 microns.

Management

Management for myopic regression is unchanged from

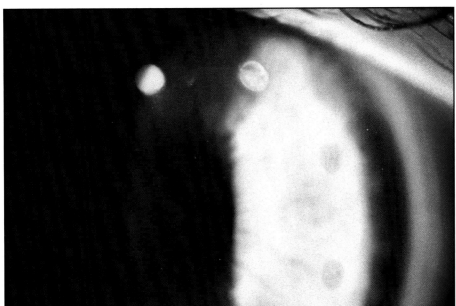

Figure 32-61a. Sunrise holmium laser thermokeratoplasty for hyperopic overcorrection following a LASIK procedure for severe myopia. The patient measured +1.75 D 6 months postoperatively with a very stable refractive pattern observed from 3 months. Following LTK application, no corneal flap shrinkage was observed.

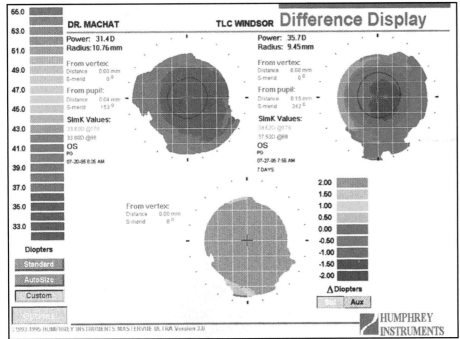

Figure 32-61b. Humphrey MasterVue Ultra corneal videokeratography demonstrating the corneal steepening effect of holmium LTK. Preoperative mean keratometry was 31.4 D, which improved to 35.7 D 1 week following Sunrise LTK. Refractive error measured -.75 D at 1 week, regressing to +.25 D at 5 months following LTK for LASIK overcorrection.

that for myopic undercorrection and is discussed in the Chapter 20. Fitting with contact lenses for the residual PRK procedure over the LASIK flap for the correction of residual myopia is not recommended as the risk of haze is high. A postoperative steroid regimen similar to that used for PRK has not been found to be effective at controlling infection in our experience.

Jose Güell proposed intra-epithelial ablation for the correction of low degrees of residual myopia. Repeat LASIK utilizing a lift and ablate technique or a new lamellar cut is recommended once stability is achieved between 1 to 4 months.

ABNORMAL INDUCED TOPOGRAPHY

Central Islands

Clinical

The most common topographical abnormality observed postoperatively with LASIK patients is central island formation. The incidence of central islands is actually increased relative to PRK unless nomogram and/or technique alterations are made to compensate for the pronounced hydration of the deeper stroma. Although small optical zones are not associated with central island formation, optical zones of 6 mm or greater have an extremely high incidence, approaching 100%, if no internal or external compensation is made with a broad beam excimer laser. Symptoms of central island formation include blurred vision, ghosting, and monocular diplopia. Objectively, they are difficult to refract and have a disproportionately high degree of residual myopia relative to their UCVA. For example, a typical central island patient post-LASIK may have an uncorrected visual acuity of 20/30 with a measured refraction of -2 D, far greater than would have been predicted based on the unaided vision. Unlike central islands observed with PRK, the topographical abnormalities observed with LASIK do not seem to resolve with time, as there is no epithelial remodeling. Topographically, a central island appears as a central steepening red or a light shade of blue-green in color, 2 to 3 mm in diameter, and relative to the surrounding area, which is notably a darker green or more typically blue. Clinically, it is impossible upon corneal examination to determine the presence or absence of a central island.

Management

The management of central islands focuses on both prevention through modification of software algorithms and techniques and retreatment, the latter of which is covered in Chapter 20. Furthermore, it is important to recognize that scanning excimer lasers are not associated with central island formation.

Understanding the cause of central islands is essential in developing appropriate measures to prevent their formation. Central islands are multifactoral and related to both hydration and plume effects. Hydration effects are related to differential hydration of the corneal stroma—both naturally occurring (Lin) and from acoustic shockwave (Machat) effects of photoablation. The plume created with each pulse is theorized to block successive pulses centrally by creating a vortex pattern (Klyce) and a shielding effect on the stromal surface (Neuhann). Although the cornea itself is 70% water, the distribution is not homogeneous. Central stroma is more hydrated than the peripheral cornea, making the central tissue more resistant to photoablation and less compact (Lin). Scanning lasers, as mentioned, do not produce central islands as would be expected with the differential hydration model alone. Therefore, a mechanism peculiar to broad beam lasers must be operational. The plume models both depict the pattern of blockage as different when broad beam and scanning lasers are used. The acoustic shockwave model notes that the pulses produced by broad beam lasers produce circular acoustic shockwaves during myopic correction. These drive stromal fluid both centrally and peripherally, which is visible intraoperatively. Central fluid accumulation produces a relative central undercorrection or central island. The increased incidence of central island formation at the deeper layers of the stroma are simply related to the increased hydration level of the deeper stroma. As previously stated, central islands typically resolve with PRK over 6 months but typically do not with LASIK because of the absence of epithelial remodeling.

Intraoperatively, it is very evident that central fluid accumulation occurs during the ablation process, as the iris diaphragm expands for myopia correction. The central stroma appears translucent or black relative to the expanding gray ring demarcating the extent of the treatment zone. Management, therefore, centers around compensating for the central undercorrection and controlling stromal hydration. Compensation for the central undercorrection is made by altering software algorithms. Hydration is controlled through the application of compressed air, drying with surgical spears, or wiping fluid accumulation with a spatula.

As discussed in earlier sections, the pretreatment technique consists of the application of pulses to the central 2 to 3 mm of cornea above and beyond what is required for the full refractive effect. The pretreatment technique compensates for the central undercorrection produced when applying a theoretical lenticular curve to the hydrated stroma. Pretreatment not only reduces the incidence and size of central islands but improves qualitative vision. The amount of pretreatment required is increased for both higher degrees of correction and for intrastromal ablation, as the deeper layers are more hydrated. The pretreatment nomogram for PRK and LASIK is dependent upon the laser system utilized, the specific technique, and the number and size of the optical zones.

All broad beam excimer laser systems produce central islands when a large optical zone is utilized, unless a small optical zone or gaussian energy beam profile is used. The gaussian beam profile that is much hotter or of higher energy centrally will remove a greater proportion of tissue centrally and/or drive fluid peripherally. The Summit Apex series has a somewhat gaussian beam and will produce a central island if the optical zone is 6 mm or greater. The aspheric multizone program of the Summit Apex series places the majority of the treatment in the central 4.5 mm and blends out to 6 or 6.5 mm, thereby reducing the incidence of central island formation. The VISX Star algorithm currently includes pretreatment with a central island factor based on my initial work in July 1992. Summit Apex international software also includes the pretreatment step but is pending US Food and Drug Administration approval. In the United States at present, surgeons utilize Patient Training A, approximately 1 micron per diopter to compensate for central islands. The Chiron Technolas 116 multizone programs have a pretreatment step within the software to reduce central island formation. Scanning excimer laser delivery systems such as the Chiron Technolas 217 PlanoScan program do not require pretreatment, as they produce minimal acoustic shockwave.

Treatment of a central island is fully explained in Chapter 20 and involves lifting the flap and concentrating the treatment in the area of the topographical island. The amount of treatment required is based on the diameter and dioptric height of the island of topography and is calculated using the Munnerlyn formula.

Long-term Corneal Striae

My approach to long-term corneal striae involves the same techniques and principles I described for an early displaced corneal flap in this chapter; however, the issue of flap fibrosis and the more permanent nature of the folds must be addressed. Only corneal striae that affect best-corrected vision should warrant treatment, as fine wrinkles are often present in eyes treated for high myopia as the radius of curvature of the stromal bed is reduced.[5,6] The critical element is that once the flap is carefully dissected open, which can be performed even at 1-year postoperatively, the undersurface of the corneal flap is treated with 10 microns of PTK. If any residual myopia is present, the corneal bed is ablated with a refractive profile to eliminate any fibrosis, otherwise 10 microns of PTK are applied to the stromal bed as well. Consecutive hyperopia can be treated in the bed, however caution should be exercised as irregular astigmatism that is always evident in these cases may be the cause of the hyperopia rather than a true refractive error. That is, we have treated patients with long-term corneal striae without treating the associated hyperopia, and the reduction in striae alone resulted in a reduction in the associated hyperopia. The use of PTK on the undersurface of the flap serves to free the folds and allow stretching and smoothing techniques to reduce and sometimes eliminate them. The objective behind treating patients with long-term corneal striae should always be improvement rather than resolution.

Once the corneal flap has been dissected open and the associated fibrosis ablated, the technique mirrors that performed for early striae—the corneal flap is floated back into position and stretched toward the peripheral gutter over 8 to 10 minutes. The epithelial surface is left dry and the side of fine forceps or the Machat striae spatula can be used to stretch the flap edges, approximating them to the stromal bed margins. Others have recommended corneal sutures for 3 days to stretch the flap, and while they can be effective in these cases, they are associated with both irregular and regular astigmatism and may create striae of their own. Therefore, suturing should be used as a final approach, and I have yet to find this approach necessary. In some cases, the epithelium will be denuded peripherally and this cannot be avoided.

A bandage contact lens, Voltaren twice a day for 1 day, Ciloxan qid for 4 days, and Maxidex (dexamethasone phosphate .1%, Alcon) every 1 to 2 hours for 2 days, then qid for 4 days comprise the postoperative drug regimen. With this technique we have been able to improve best-corrected vision from 20/100 to 20/40 after 14 months and 20/60 to 20/25 after 9 months. In cases less than 6 months, we have been able to restore best-corrected vision to 20/20 in more than a dozen cases.

REFERENCES

1. Gimbel HV, Basti S, Kaye GB, Ferensowicz M. Experience during the learning curve of laser in situ keratomileusis. *J Cataract Refract Surg*. 1996; 22(5):542-550.

2. Perez-Santonja JJ, Sakla HF, Abad JL, Zorraquino A, Esteban J, Alio JL. Nocardial keratitis after laser in situ keratomileusis. *Journal of Refractive Surgery*. 1997;13(3):314-317.

3. Mulhern MG, Condon PI, O'Keefe M. Endophthalmitis after astigmatic myopic laser in situ keratomileusis. *J Cataract Refract Surg*. 1997; 23(6):948-950.

4. Helena MC, Meisler D, Wilson SE. Epithelial growth within the lamellar interface after laser in situ keratomileusis. *Cornea*. 1997; 16(3):300-305.

5. Pannu JS. Incidence and treatment of wrinkled corneal flap following LASIK. *J Cataract Refract Surg*. 1997; 23(5):695-696 .

6. Probst LE, Machat JJ. Removal of flap striae following laser in situ keratomileusis. *J Cataract Refract Surg*. 1998;24:153-155.

MANAGING THE PATIENT WITH A LASIK COMPLICATION

Jeff Machat, MD

Nick Nianiaris, MD

Rhonda Kerzner, OD

The most difficult aspect to co-managing PRK and LASIK patients is managing poor outcomes. In fact, it is the primary reason that many doctors do not wish to perform refractive surgery or co-manage at all. That is truly a shame, as laser refractive surgery is overwhelmingly rewarding on an emotional level, for both the surgeon and the co-managing doctor. The information below will give a little insight into how we manage the 1% of mild to severe complications rather than discuss the wonders of the 99% who call the laser a "miracle machine." There is truly a philosophy that we advocate at TLC, as we consult and treat literally dozens of severe complications from centers across North America each month. Below is the TLC Toronto philosophy.

PATIENTS ARE SEEKING YOUR COMFORT AND CONFIDENCE, NOT GUARANTEES WITH PRK AND LASIK

We begin with the premise that "no one would knowingly have an elective procedure that is considered high risk; however, patients do recognize that some element of risk is expected." What patients are looking for is the *comfort and confidence* of their doctor and surgeon to say they are not having a high risk procedure, and specifically, that the patients will not be doing something foolish. Considering that TLC surgeons have performed more than 80,000 procedures and treated more than 800 doctors, laser refractive surgery today would certainly not be considered high risk or foolish.

Patients are seeking information, not guarantees— there is both tremendous awareness and desire. It is our responsibility preoperatively to provide information about available options, outlining the risks and benefits of various techniques. Many doctors, unfortunately, feel that if they refer a patient to our clinic and that patient develops a complication, they are responsible, which is absolutely not the case. Although as surgeons we feel the same commitment to the patients we care for as our co-managing doctors, we recognize that complications do and will occur. All that patients are seeking is that we do our best, communicate to them throughout the process, and not abandon them. The entire TLC model of co-management was developed with only one essential element in mind: to ensure that someone is always overseeing the quality of our patient care. TLC was the first to advocate this model for refractive surgery worldwide and time has proven that patients advocate this model as well.

TALKING TO PATIENTS WITH REFRACTIVE SURGERY COMPLICATIONS

Even prior to any discussion with his or her co-managing doctor or surgeon, each patient recognizes that surgery has risks. So it is important to appreciate that all patients who consent to surgery come in with expectations of a positive outcome and a primary belief that they will not have a complication. Those patients who believe a complication will occur will never even consider surgery. All patients receive a detailed informed consent prior to their procedure, so problems, although infrequent and unwelcome, are not truly a surprise. The incidence of complications for both PRK and LASIK in experienced hands is about 1% for a mild problem and .1% for a serious problem with associated significant visual impairment. Therefore, approximately 99% of refractive surgery patients have an uneventful procedure and recovery, however, to the one patient in a thousand with a serious complication, the incidence is immaterial. With this background, one sets out to manage patients with undesirable outcomes following refractive surgery.

Each patient who experiences a complication wishes to know two things:
1. What happened
2. What will happen

Each patient wishes to understand what is the specific problem and how is that problem going to affect his or her vision. Secondly, what is the treatment plan, recovery time, and final prognosis.

Explaining these issues to each patient allows him or her to better handle the problem and recovery. Communication is the cornerstone to managing these difficult patients, and information helps resolve fear of the unknown and provide a means of coping for patients. Often the explanation is time-consuming and requires repetition, as patients attempt to assimilate these new facts. Most patients are not looking to ascribe blame contrary to the fears of most co-managing doctors or surgeons unless they specifically feel they have been misled during the preoperative phase. The most important element is to acknowledge that there is a problem so the patient is not defensive and concentrate any discussion on what occurred and what will occur.

Patients wish to understand the type of problem they have, how it develops, whether they did something wrong, and whether they can do something now to improve the situation. It is important for them to remain participants in their care, understanding the medications that are prescribed, and what procedure, if any, may be required to improve their condition, as well as when it would be performed. It is important to appreciate that they need to plan their recovery time with respect to their lives at work and home.

Lastly, although guarantees should never be made, an educated guess concerning the visual outcome following treatment and adequate healing time should be made. In most complicated cases, the prognosis is explained to the patient by the surgeon or center director.

SURGICAL PROBLEMS: HOW TO TALK TO A PATIENT WHO HAD A CORNEAL FLAP COMPLICATION

Probably one of the most difficult aspects to refractive surgery is managing a patient with a surgical complication. When a patient has a poor flap, we inform the patient intraoperatively, then talk to the patient again 15 minutes postoperatively with his or her family in attendance to explain the problem and the plan. This is often a very emotional time for the patient, and he or she often absorbs very little. It is important to always be honest and direct in explaining the problem that occurred, the cause, and the range of possible outcomes. Surprisingly, most flap complications resolve with proper treatment without affecting the final visual outcome; however this is impossible to know immediately. The first postoperative day examination is the most informative. It is at this time that one begins to assess the prognosis for full visual recovery.

CARE OF THE LASIK FLAP COMPLICATION

The important aspects to explain are that despite our best efforts, poor corneal flaps can and do occur and that vision will be very blurry immediately and perhaps uncomfortable for a few days. Patients are often placed on steroid drops every 1 to 2 hours to reduce swelling, antibiotics to prevent possible infection, and often a bandage contact lens may be inserted for comfort. The patient cannot insert a contact lens for refractive correction for at least 1 week and only soft disposable lenses thereafter, which may not provide full visual correction if cylinder or irregularity exists. Patients with severe flap complications are usually examined every 1 to 3 days during the first 1 to 2 weeks, then every 2 to 4 weeks for 3 months. Frequent examinations (such as weekly) throughout the 3-month recovery period are excessive and only serve to undermine treatment efforts. Numerous visits are actually disconcerting for patients since any measured improvement is minimal on a weekly basis and the frequent need to return only serves to increase patient anxiety. LASIK retreatment is typically performed after 3 to 4 months, not earlier. Switching to PRK provides less optimal results. Clinical

results are still impressive in most cases. Best-corrected vision may or may not return, depending on severity of the flap complication, management of the complication, and individual healing patterns. Without giving false hope, more than 50% of all serious corneal flap complications we have cared for returned to their best-corrected vision, and virtually all others returned to within two lines of the preoperative best-corrected vision. Thus, with proper management, experience, and time, an overwhelming majority of serious flap complications can be managed to an excellent and acceptable outcome.

Our considerable LASIK experience enables us to enjoy a very low incidence of such complications and manage them not only appropriately, but more effectively than virtually any other center. For the record, neither one of us have ever had a corneal perforation or other sight-threatening surgical complication to occur in any of our patients at any time.

TALKING TO YOUR PATIENT WITH A CORNEAL FLAP PROBLEM

It is important not to guarantee that everything will be okay, which is a common tendency both preoperatively to make a patient feel more secure about having the procedure and postoperatively to comfort a patient who had a complication. The only guarantee is that everyone will continue to do their best. Do not apologize for complications or even feel guilty—another common tendency. The patient is a responsible adult who was well-informed and accepted the risk, the matter at hand is optimizing the outcome, not deflecting blame. These procedures work extremely well, giving most patients a feeling that a minor miracle has occurred. We personally speak very directly with patients and inform them of the problem, how it will affect them, what will happen, and that 3 to 6 months time for recovery will be needed.

The co-managing doctor should not be alarmed or fearful. He or she should recognize that complications are an integral part of surgery and that he or she is in partnership with the surgeon not just when all goes well, but especially when complications occur. The co-managing doctor should work hand-in-hand with the center, center director, and surgeon to provide the patient with optimal care and a consistent message. Communication between the center, co-managing doctor, and the patient must be well-executed. The co-managing doctor must continue to express confidence and trust in the surgeon and the center. Often, the patient will need to be seen more frequently, including more shared care and visits with the center. In the TLC system, the center director is the co-managing doctor's primary support and should be utilized extensively.

Key points:
- Acknowledge complications
- A letter and call will outline the complication and plan

- Re-explain the complication
- Avoid blame and guilt
- Explain that unfortunately these problems are rare but do occur and occurred to your patient
- Emphasize the treatment plan and expected recovery time
- Ensure that the co-managing doctor does not feel abandoned
- Recognize that the patient is simply looking for your continued reassurance, not guarantees
- Do not lose the primary belief that these procedures work well, as the patient may require more surgery at a later date and will look to his or her co-managing doctor once again for comfort and confidence
- Lastly, recognize that most complications do exceedingly well with time and treatment

HEALING PROBLEMS: HOW TO TALK TO A PATIENT WHO IS EXPERIENCING AN ABNORMAL HEALING PATTERN

Healing difficulties are more common than surgical complications but less severe in general. Patients and co-managing doctors are usually more fearful of surgical complications, but as we explain preoperatively, the final outcome is based on two elements: *how well the surgery proceeds and how well the patient heals.* It is the latter factor that is often forgotten and not given adequate weight.

With each patient who does not heal as expected we begin with a simple statement, "You are not healing as we hoped." It is important to emphasize that the problem with the patient's vision is related to his or her unique healing pattern and not the procedure. Corneal haze is a good example of how a patient's healing pattern can affect the surgical outcome, despite even a flawless procedure.

CORNEAL HAZE

In the case of corneal haze, we would state:
1. You are developing corneal haze.
2. Haze is related to your healing pattern, your genetics.
3. Your vision may get worse, so do not be alarmed.
4. If your vision does get worse we will need to retreat you.
5. For now, we just want you to stay on your drops and return in a month. we state there is a problem even before the patient may notice his or her vision is affected.

We state it is related to his or her healing and simply tell the patient what to expect and what we will do.

UNDERCORRECTIONS AND OVERCORRECTIONS

A more common example would be related to residual refractive errors affecting postoperative visual results:

overcorrections, undercorrections, and residual astigmatism. It should always be recognized that the correct treatment parameters that provide an ideal 20/15 outcome in one patient may result in an overcorrection in another patient because of the patient's healing pattern. That is, it is not that the patient was overcorrected but that the patient over-responded. When talking to patients with undercorrections and overcorrections it is important to specify that their outcome was based on their healing and not a surgical planning error, and that their need for enhancement is also necessitated by their healing pattern and not because the surgeon targeted incorrectly. The wording of these explanations is very important to maintain patient trust, confidence, and ease of managing these patients.

LOSS OF BEST-CORRECTED VISUAL ACUITY

Loss of BCVA may also occur because of irregular healing. This is most common in the treatment of high myopia, as these individuals must heal to a greater extent. Once again, when a patient experiences a loss of BCVA, it is important to emphasize the role of the individual healing pattern when speaking to the patient. We usually start with, "you are not healing as we had hoped." This is to acknowledge that we recognize the patient is having a problem. Second, we explain that he or she is "healing irregularly." This is usually evident with either topography mapping or keratometry mires in which the mires appear distorted. We explain that "all surgery messes with Mother Nature and about 1% to 2% will heal irregularly, as he or she has." We explain that it can take "weeks or even months in some cases for the irregularity to smooth itself out and retreatment surgery too early can worsen the irregularity, but some improvement over time is likely." In cases of hyperopia or high myopia treatment, we emphasize that a "slower visual recovery is more common and we do not become concerned until at least 3 months after the primary procedure." Use of a soft contact lens for any residual correction is helpful and helps provide better quality of vision in some cases. Rigid gas permeable lenses, while ideal for correction of irregular astigmatism, can adversely affect the healing and should be avoided. Unless corneal striae, haze, or a central island is present, waiting 6 months for nature to take its course is best.

EPITHELIAL INGROWTH

Epithelial ingrowth is another healing-based complication that is related primarily to the corneal epithelial adherence pattern of the patient. That is, patients with strong basement membrane complexes that bond firmly to the overlying epithelium usually do not develop epithelial ingrowths. Certain surgical aspects can promote epithelial ingrowths in susceptible individuals, such as excessive topical anesthetic, which weakens the epithelium. When discussing an epithelial ingrowth with a patient, it is important not to worry the patient as most ingrowths do not require treatment, and for those that do, so long as the ingrowth is treated relatively rapidly (within the first 2 to 4 weeks) no sequelae will result.

DRY EYES AND NIGHT GLARE

Other common side effects that may require discussion include dry eyes and night glare. Both are common preoperatively but become more pronounced in the immediate postoperative phase and improve over several months. With respect to night glare, we explain the cause of halos as being derived from the pupil size enlarging at night and exceeding the size of the treatment area. We explain that myopic eyes are longer than normally sighted eyes, therefore the peripheral light rays scatter in the eye and produce halos, starbursting, and degradation of overall night vision. For most patients, simply understanding the cause of their symptoms makes them feel better.

Treatment of the second eye is essential for improvement over time. Short-term prescription of night-driving glasses over-minused by –.75 D is very effective. If the patient is significantly undercorrected, scheduling an enhancement is indicated. Lastly, emphasizing that improvement over 6 months is common reduces the concern of the patient. Once again, acknowledging the problem, explaining the problem, and providing short-term solutions and the long-term prognosis is what the patient is expecting. In other words, explain what happened, what is happening, and what will happen.

Similarly, on the issue of dry eyes, we explain that the patient always had dry eyes, but the surgery simply made them symptomatic, just as contacts may have done preoperatively. We describe the symptoms of dry eye as being related to losing your windshield, after a lifetime of wearing glasses or contacts, so now wind and dust directly irritates your eye, like sticking your head out the window of a moving car. Lubricants and punctal plugs are advocated short-term treatments. We use the analogy of a sink with a faucet and two drains for the eye. We explain dry eye as being produced by a faucet turned too low, with lubricants trying to fill the sink externally and the punctal plug blocking one drain, both acting to increase the water level in the sink to improve comfort. Most patients identify with these analogies to understand their condition and the suggested treatment regimen.

In general, unless a surgical complication is identified, it is important to emphasize the individual healing aspect of any visual problem or symptom that develops. Most healing problems will fortunately resolve or improve with time.

CONCLUSION

In summary, most patients do well with current laser refractive surgery techniques, but problems may and do occur with all surgeons. Co-management is a partnership that involves mutual support of the center and co-managing doctor for the clinical benefit of the patient. Never is that partnership more important than the management of patients with complications. Patients who develop complications require information to help them cope. Provide information about what happened, what is happening, and what will happen to the eye. Answer these questions directly and completely. Do not alarm the patient and do not guarantee that everything will be perfect. Do not become alarmed yourself. Do not accept blame or feel responsible. This is the most difficult aspect, as we all have a tendency to feel responsible and become defensive. Simply explain that the problem, explain it will take time, it may take further surgery, and most patients experience improvement. Communicate with your patients, but do not see them more than necessary since little improvement is noted between frequent examinations and your patient may become even more discouraged. Be sure the patient does not feel abandoned. Demonstrate confidence while supporting the patient in concert with the center director and surgeon.

CHAPTER 33

LASIK:
Complications and Management

Stephen G. Slade, MD
John F. Doane, MD

INTRODUCTION

Although lamellar surgery techniques appear to be devoid of complications associated with intraocular surgery,[1-13] they are critically dependent on the use of the microkeratome and complete understanding of the excimer laser. The inspection, set-up, and preoperative testing of these instruments is critical. Careful attention to minute detail is essential to minimize and avoid potential complications as well as to obtaining an excellent result. Postoperative optical complications for lamellar surgery are analogous to those seen following many corneal procedures, including glare, halos, problems with night driving, and decreased contrast sensitivity. Complications of laser in situ keratomileusis (LASIK) include all the potential complications associated with ocular surgery in general, such as infection and loss of vision, as well as complications specific to lamellar corneal surgery like flap/cap-induced irregular astigmatism and stromal interface epithelialization. Unusual complications such as vascular occlusion, macular hemorrhage, perforated globe, and microbial infection can all be seen with these techniques.

The advent of LASIK represents a tremendous advance in the field of refractive surgery. It has several positive attributes that many eyecare providers have come to appreciate and from which an ever-growing number of patients benefit. These beneficial aspects include the ability to simultaneously treat a large range of myopia or hyperopia and associated astigmatism, relatively quick return of visual function, minimal pain or discomfort, and rapid, if not

uninterrupted, return to preoperative lifestyle. Continued evaluation of the efficacy, predictability, safety, stability, and quality of vision following LASIK are ongoing and have shown extremely encouraging results. Nevertheless, as with any surgical discipline, vision correction surgery will likely never find a procedure that anyone would call perfect, and LASIK is no exception.

There is a tremendous amount of technology involved in LASIK, including the laser, the microkeratome, and such examination instruments as phoropter, trial frame, topography, and pachymetry. All must be appreciated for their impact on operative results. Each instrument should be compulsively tested and calibrated prior to use. Complications during and after LASIK can result from improper preoperative evaluation directly attributed to instrumentation, surgeon-related factors, or the result of postoperative factors.

COMPLICATIONS RELATED TO PREOPERATIVE FACTORS

Complications resulting from pre-existing conditions or improper preoperative evaluation are largely preventable. A thorough patient history and examination will alert the surgeon to potential complicating factors such as recurrent erosion or dry eye syndrome. If the refraction is unstable, improperly obtained, the cornea is too thin, or there is evidence of keratoconus, LASIK should not be considered. Lamellar corneal surgery should not be performed if active corneal or intraocular inflammation exists.

LASER-RELATED COMPLICATIONS

Complications directly related to the excimer laser are numerous but can largely be eliminated if the laser is in proper working order and its beam centration, energy level (fluence), and beam quality (homogeneity) are critically evaluated before each case. It is important to understand that the laser is an ever-fluctuating instrument that is highly dependent on room temperature, humidity, and air purity. An improperly centered laser beam can result in a decentered ablation with induced irregular astigmatism and disabling visual side effects. Improper fluence can result in either over- or undercorrections, and poor homogeneity can result in an irregular ablation with associated irregular astigmatism and visual side effects. Decentered ablations (Figure 33-1) are uncommon with an experienced surgeon and are caused by poor technique or a misaligned laser beam. Decentrations can be avoided or minimized by a preoperative check of laser centration, proper patient fixation, centration on the entrance pupil, and frequent monitoring of the beam position during the ablation by the surgeon. If a significant decentration does occur, the best approach is the use of topographic-assisted flying or scanning spot laser correction. In this technique, the data acquired from topography is interfaced with the excimer laser computer to customize the ablation and enlarge the ablation zone to optical quality over the entrance pupil. By doing this, unwanted visual symptoms like glare or halos should be markedly decreased, if not eliminated.

As with any operation, prevention is the easiest and most desired solution to complications. A basic review of the laser step of the LASIK technique is appropriate. Prior to lifting the flap and beginning the ablation, the surgeon and staff should confirm proper laser settings and position the patient's head so the corneal surface is perpendicular to the ablation beam. The flap is then lifted and folded out of the ablation field. The ablation is centered over the entrance pupil. As the ablation proceeds, centration should be monitored diligently. If significant patient head or eye movement occurs, the surgeon should stop the ablation, reorient the patient, and proceed when aligned. During the ablation, fluid can accumulate on the corneal surface and should be wiped dry with a single pass of a sponge or blunt spatula. As the largest diameter treatment zones are completed, the corneal hinge should be covered with a blunt instrument to prevent ablation of the back surface of the corneal flap. This prevents a "double ablation" with resultant induced irregular astigmatism.

CENTRAL ISLAND FORMATION

A central island is one of the most common irregular ablations encountered and consists of a small steep area in the central cornea. In most cases, it can be demonstrated by

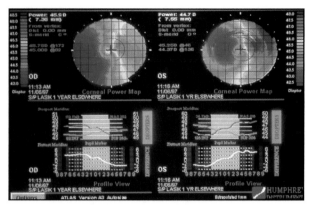

Figure 33-1. Topography of the right and left eye of a patient treated with a large area ablation laser in which the laser treatment beam misaligned from the patient fixation target. The center of the ablation zone is shifted toward the 180° meridian with the transition area of the ablation passing through the pupillar axis. The patient had marked subjective visual complaints of glare and halos that were exacerbated in scotopic conditions. Note in the lowest profile view of each eye, the power changes horizontally across the pupillary space.

videokeratography within 1 hour after surgery and usually regresses over time. A central island can occur as a result of a cooler central beam, irregular hydration during the ablation with central accumulation of fluid, or delayed clearance of ablation debris from the central cornea. In the latter two circumstances, the fluid or debris accumulation masks the central stroma from the ablation. Scanning lasers largely avoid the problem of central islands.

Typically, a patient with a significant central island complains of visual disturbances, has a best spectacle-corrected visual acuity of 20/30 or worse, and may have a few diopters of residual myopia. The diagnosis is surmised by clinical suspicion and confirmed with videokeratography, in which there will be an isolated area of relative steepening compared to the overall ablation zone (Figure 33-2a).

Central islands are best avoided but are treatable. They occur more frequently when there is a large single ablation zone treatment and can be prevented or minimized by proper software modifications (anti-central island algorithms), increased wiping of the central cornea to dry the stroma, or by additional ablation of the central 2.5 to 2.7 mm of the cornea if they occur with the primary procedure. If a central island occurs and causes symptoms, two possible approaches can be taken: no treatment with expectant observation or early treatment. The central island will lessen over the ensuing months; however, early treatment can be taken by lifting

> Typically, a patient with a significant central island complains of visual disturbances, has a best spectacle-corrected visual acuity of 20/30 or worse, and may have a few diopters of residual myopia.

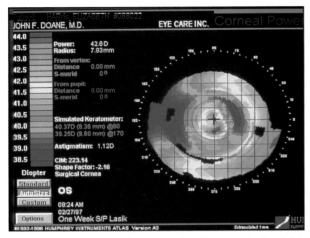

Figure 33-2a. Topographic example of a central island following LASIK defined by an area of central steepening with associated subjective visual complaints.

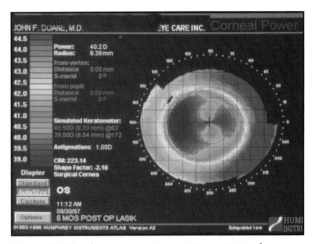

Figure 33-2b. The same patient as Figure 33-1 after treatment of the central island with flap lifting and additional laser ablation in the central 2.7 mm optical zone.

the flap and ablating a spherical 2.7 mm diameter central zone (Figure 31-2b). With early treatment, the patient is likely to notice immediate and marked reduction of symptoms at the 1-day postoperative visit.

UNDER/OVERCORRECTING MANAGEMENT

Missing the refraction target with LASIK should be defined and discussed based on degree and chronicity. With LASIK, it is not uncommon for the refraction and topography to change with time. With myopic LASIK, refraction and topography are typically stable by at least 3 months postoperatively. With hyperopic LASIK, this time frame can extend for another 2 to 3 months. In effect, what may be perceived as an overcorrection early on (1 week and 1 month examinations), may be a perfect refractive result over time (3 months). On the other hand, an early (1 week postoperatively) undercorrection may hearken a significant undercorrection by the 3-month postoperative examination.

Undercorrections are not uncommon, and the necessity for more surgery (5% to 10 % of all eyes) often depends on the patient's requirement for best unaided visual acuity. The patient record and laser treatment parameters should be evaluated to rule out error. Prior to retreatment, the refraction should be stable (the overwhelming majority of patients are stable by 3 months) and videokeratography should be obtained to rule out a central island with residual myopia or abnormal ablation pattern. Reoperation can be accomplished by lifting the flap, or after 3 months from the original surgery, a new keratectomy can be performed and additional laser ablation of the stromal bed completed. The same nomogram used for the initial procedure can be used in the retreatment.

Primary overcorrections of myopic LASIK with an experienced surgeon and tested nomogram are infrequent.

Refractions tend to regress over the first 1 to 3 months after LASIK, so the vast majority of early overcorrections are "on target" at the 3-month postoperative examination. If the overcorrection persists, videokeratography and pachymetry should be checked and compared with preoperative values. The surgical record and laser parameters should be checked to make certain a typing error or data entry error are not the cause. If the overcorrection is chronic and disabling, the best surgical option is hyperopic LASIK completed no sooner than the 3-month postoperative visit.

> Refractions tend to regress over the first 1 to 3 months after LASIK, so the vast majority of early overcorrections are "on target" at the 3-month postoperative examination.

TIMING AND TECHNIQUE OF ENHANCEMENT SURGERY

Enhancement surgery can be completed very early after LASIK (weeks after surgery) or after an extended period of time (years). The vast majority of patients undergo enhancement by 3 to 4 months postoperatively, since their decision for enhancement is driven by uncorrected visual function requirements that are less than acceptable. The most important point to be made is that the refractive status and topography should be stable whenever the enhancement surgery is performed. LASIK enhancement can be completed by lifting the flap or passing the microkeratome to create a second keratectomy. Each approach has relative advantages and disadvantages. The perceived advantage of lifting the flap is the lack of potential microkeratome-related complications. The perceived disadvantage of lifting the flap is the difficulty in finding the previous surgical plane and excessive disruption of the epithelium at the keratectomy edge. Additionally, some surgeons have anecdotally reported a higher incidence of epithelial ingrowth with lifting the flap for enhancement surgery. This is presumed to occur because the keratectomy edge epithelium is not as regular as that created with the microkeratome cut. It is recommended that the epithelium be minimally disrupted, and the stromal edges be properly repositioned and then irrigated to remove any residual epithelial cells. In general, the advantage of repassing the microkeratome is the fact that it is a quick procedure; and the disadvantage is the potential for creating a second interface layer of stroma. It is advisable to wait at least 2 months, but preferably 3 months or longer, before repassing the microkeratome for enhancements since good adhesion of the initial interface is required to achieve a smooth keratectomy.

The actual technique of enhancement surgery with repassing the microkeratome is identical to the initial operation. In the event a second interface is created anterior to the initial interface, one can encounter a thin layer of stromal tissue that can be continuous or, on occasion, multiple hinged filament-like layers that should be anatomically repositioned before beginning the ablation. Doing this will minimize inducing irregularities in the stromal bed.

Lifting the flap for enhancement surgery can be a challenging task intraoperatively. The excellent magnification and clarity that the surgeon is accustomed to at the slit lamp while observing the keratectomy and interface is not present with the optics of most excimer laser surgeon microscopes. In practice, what is clearly seen with a slit beam is simply not evident with broad illumination at low or high magnification with the operating microscope. Clinical appearance of the keratectomy edge can be predictive of how easy a flap will be to lift. Patients can be divided into two distinct groups: those with visible fibrosis or haze at the gutter edge in which flaps will be more difficult to lift, and those who have completely clear gutter edge in which flaps will be easier to lift. This can be the determining factor as whether to lift the flap (clear keratectomy edge) or repass the microkeratome (fibrotic ring at keratectomy edge). If the surgeon elects to bring the patient directly to the laser for lifting the flap, a mental note of the keratectomy edge location should made. Frequently, once under the operating microscope the surgeon must work from memorization of the slit lamp appearance. If the surgeon cannot identify the edge while under the laser, a blunt instrument or dry cellulose sponge can be used to depress the peripheral cornea and help highlight the anatomic position of the keratectomy border. Some surgeons elect to mark the keratectomy edge at the slit lamp by scoring the epithelium at the edge with a sharp instrument (hypodermic needle) or using a marking pen to highlight the keratectomy edge.

The actual lifting of the flap requires the proper instrumentation and technique to not only perform the procedure but also to minimize complications. A cyclodialysis spatula with certain specifications or any commercially available LASIK flap-lifting instrument will work. It is best for the lifting spatula to have a thin tip that is not too sharp. If the tip has too much bulk or is extremely blunt, it will make entry into the interface difficult. If the tip is too pointed or sharp there is potential for shearing or perforating the flap. After the surgeon identifies the keratectomy edge, a short, quick stab of the tip at a 30° angulation will penetrate the interface. Once in the interface, the spatula should be advanced with lateral sweeping motion to dissect the interface. To avoid damage to the flap, care should be taken to not excessively lift the tip of the spatula. Once the interface is dissected, the epithelium can be broken at the keratectomy edge. The flap is then carefully reflected to expose the stromal bed for ablation. The surgeon's standard nomogram can be used without modification. Repositioning the flap and epithelium in proper anatomic location and irrigating the interface with balanced salt solution (BSS) should be performed as in the original surgery.

POSTOPERATIVE MANAGEMENT OF ENHANCEMENT SURGERY

The postoperative management of LASIK enhancement procedures is identical to the initial surgery. Prophylactic antibiotics, an orbital shield, and early postoperative physical limitations should be reiterated to the patient. Re-evaluation should be done 1 day postoperatively to make certain the flap is well positioned. Anecdotal reports of increased incidence of epithelial ingrowth after enhancement LASIK have been reported, and its appearance should be ruled out by careful slit lamp examination at each postoperative visit.

DECENTRATION OF THE ABLATION

Centration of the ablation is separate from centration of the flap and depends on the technique of the surgeon and the alignment of the laser. Decentration of the ablation (See Figure 33-1) may be minimized by making sure the patient is fixating, carefully checking the laser beam position, and monitoring the ablation. Some laser systems have stereo reticle-type centering devices to assist the surgeon (ie, VISX Star), while others have paired HeNe beams (Summit, Schwind), and yet others have automated eye tracking systems whereby a reference point is set with respect to the pupil before surgery. If decentration occurs, the best approach to correction is the use of a scanning laser with topographic interface.

ALTERED ABLATIONS

Bleeding from incised vessels associated with contact lens-induced micropannus can complicate the ablation by hydrating the stroma or directly blocking the incident beam, leading to an asymmetric ablation. Blood should be sponged at the keratectomy edge prior to and during the ablation to avoid this problem. Attention should also be given to the outer extent of the treatment zone to avoid ablation of the back surface of the flap at the hinge. This problem tends to occur more frequently with larger zone scanning lasers.

MICROKERATOME-RELATED COMPLICATIONS

Perhaps the most serious complications of LASIK are those resulting from an improper keratectomy. Although lamellar surgical procedures appear to be devoid of the complications associated with intraocular surgery, they are critically dependent on proper use of the microkeratome. It takes only 3 to 6 seconds for the microkeratome to make the cut (whether automated or manual), and very little can be done during this time to correct a problem, even if one is recognized. Preoperative inspection, proper assembly, and thorough testing of the microkeratome are critical, as are the education and skill of the surgeon and staff. Careful attention to minute detail is essential while this instrument is in use.

Much like phacoemulsification, properly executed lamellar corneal surgery builds on the success of the previous step in the operative sequence. That being said, the keratectomy is the most important component of the LASIK technique. Appropriate placement of the suction ring as well as consistent suction throughout the procedure and the smooth movement of the microkeratome across the cornea are all essential elements of adequate lamellar resections. Interruption of the movement and/or suction during the resection can result in irregular resections and may necessitate abortion of the procedure. In this circumstance, the flap should be repositioned and left to heal. If this is done, the patient should not experience any permanent impairment in vision since no corneal volume has been removed. Reoperation 3 months later can be completed if the patient desires.

Exposure is the key to any surgical endeavor. The need for proper draping to keep eyelashes and redundant tissue out of the path of the microkeratome passage and laser beam should not be undervalued. The speculum selected should also achieve the stated goal of maximal exposure without impeding access of the LASIK suction ring to the anterior globe surface. Head and chin position should be such that the amount of sclera showing superiorly and inferiorly is equal. This allows for proper placement of the suction ring without undue torque of the speculum or LASIK ring. The cornea should be properly marked in case of a free cap.

> Head and chin position should be such that the amount of sclera showing superiorly and inferiorly is equal.

After application of the suction ring, appropriate elevation of intraocular pressure should be confirmed before completing the keratectomy. Just prior to passage of the microkeratome, the corneal surface should be irrigated with saline solution to minimize epithelial disruption; the path of the microkeratome should be cleared to avoid blockage of a complete pass.

When the ablation is completed, the backside of the flap and the stromal bed are irrigated with BSS using a syringe and cannula. The flap is then positioned back onto the stromal bed with a blunt-tipped instrument. The cannula is placed underneath the flap and irrigation is completed to clear any remaining debris from the interface. A separate forniceal aspiration system (speculum or cannula) can also be used to facilitate flow away from the stromal bed. Advocates believe this assures the clearest interface postoperatively. The flap is inspected to ensure proper position by making certain an equal gutter/keratectomy edge distance is present throughout the circumference. The interface is allowed to dry for several minutes. A striae test is completed by depressing the peripheral cornea with closed blunt-tipped forceps. When striae pass well into the flap at 360°, appropriate apposition has been achieved. During the drying phase it is recommended to keep a micro-drop of BSS over the central corneal epithelium to maintain its integrity.

At this point, the case is completed by carefully removing the speculum and drape. The eye is re-examined to make certain the flap is in proper position. A shield is placed over the orbit, but no pressure patch is applied. On the first postoperative day, the uncorrected visual acuity should be 20/40 or better in the low and moderate myopia treatment ranges. On slit lamp examination, the cornea should be clear with an intact epithelium. Proper flap apposition should be checked and stromal edema or interface debris should be documented. The patient can resume normal activities after a normal 1-day postoperative examination. The patient should be cautioned to not rub the cornea and should avoid participating in contact sports without wearing proper eye protection.

IMPROPER KERATECTOMY

Microkeratome-related complications can include a poor keratectomy caused by a used, dirty, or damaged blade. Poor suction can result in an incomplete keratectomy, poor flap, or a free cap. If the microkeratome maintains sufficient stromal depth but does not complete its entire passage, an incomplete flap with a larger than normal hinge can be obtained. The ablation should not be performed if the hinge obscures the ablation zone. The flap should be repositioned and the procedure repeated 3 months later. The use of an improper microkeratome plate, an improperly positioned plate, or no plate at all can result in a disaster from entry into the anterior chamber.

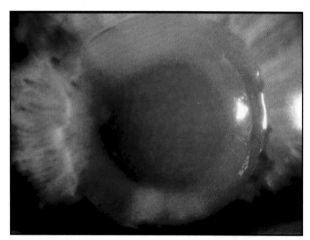

Figure 31-3. Edematous flap/cap. Epithelial ingrowth must be ruled out and may require antitorque suturing.

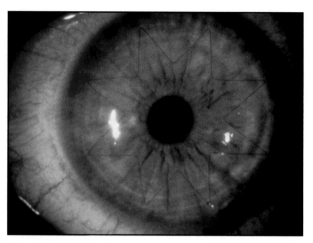

Figure 33-4. Eight-bite antitorque suturing of the lamellar cap.

The ablation should not be performed if the hinge obscures the ablation zone.

A free cap should not present a major problem for the patient or surgeon. If adequate diameter is achieved, it is appropriate to complete the ablation. During the ablation, the free cap should be placed in an antidesiccation chamber and replaced over the stromal bed in proper orientation after the ablation is completed. If a free cap is encountered, most surgeons allow for additional drying time (3 to 5 minutes) and make certain the central epithelium remains moist with BSS. The eyelid is taped shut at the end of the procedure and carefully opened by the surgeon the next day.

Irregular astigmatism associated with the keratectomy has historically been a major problem with keratomileusis in situ but has been markedly reduced with LASIK since only a single keratectomy is performed. Despite this, irregular astigmatism can occur with LASIK and is clinically experienced by the patient in the form of reduced BSCVA. Irregular astigmatism can be diagnosed by keratometry, photokeratoscopy, or videokeratography. Irregular astigmatism as a cause of decreased visual acuity can be confirmed by improvement of vision when a rigid contact lens is placed. In many patients, irregular astigmatism diminishes during the first year post-LASIK and, in some, it continues to decrease throughout the second year after surgery.

When visual acuity does not improve and the patient is unable to wear a contact lens, a thick homoplastic lamellar graft is the only treatment option. One of the advantages of LASIK is that no matter how irregular the keratectomy, when the flap is replaced, it always matches the underlying bed. Specifically, if the keratectomy is of unacceptable quality it should be replaced without proceeding with the ablation. The flap/cap will accurately fit into the stromal bed in jigsaw puzzle-like fashion, and the visual acuity and refraction should return to preoperative levels. If the patient

and surgeon are so inclined, another surgical attempt may be made 3 months later.

MANAGEMENT OF A DISPLACED/DISLODGED FLAP OR CAP

Displacement of the keratectomy flap or cap is relatively rare but can be avoided by placing a shield over the orbit after surgery and instructing the patient to not rub his or her eye postoperatively. The degree of displacement of the flap or cap can vary from subtle wrinkles to a flap or cap that is completely separated from the cornea. Striae that cause irregular astigmatism and decreased visual acuity should be treated as soon as possible by lifting the flap and repositioning it. Flap dislocation can also lead to epithelial ingrowth with the potential for flap melting. In the case of a loose flap, the epithelium is cleaned off the bed and the back surface of the flap, and the flap is repositioned. If the malposition persists due to poor adhesion or flap stromal edema (Figure 33-3) the stromal surfaces should again be cleared of epithelium and the flap secured with 8-bite antitorque suturing (Figure 33-4). If a flap is completely lost, the patient should be treated with prophylactic antibiotics and topical corticosteroids since there will be increased risk of significant haze formation. A lamellar graft may be required if significant haze leads to vision loss.

In LASIK with nasal hinge formation, the flap may be decentered with no visual consequences. Often the flap is intentionally displaced nasally to provide more room for the ablation or inferiorly to avoid an area of vessels from a superior pannus. Likewise, with superior hinge formation, slight superior decentration of the flap may be suggested.

In the case of a loose flap, the epithelium is cleaned off the bed and the back surface of the flap, and the flap is repositioned.

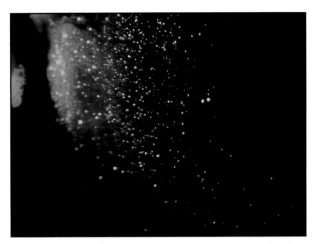

Figure 33-5. Interface contaminant: talc. This typically does not lead to visual complaints.

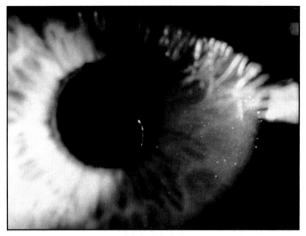

Figure 33-6. Interface contaminant: fiber. This condition rarely requires removal of the fiber since the infection risk is essentially zero and visual degradation is rarely attributed to the fiber.

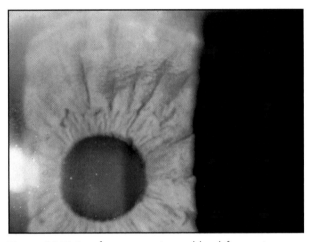

Figure 33-7. Interface contaminant: blood from micropannus. This is usually self-limited.

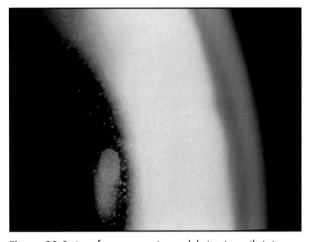

Figure 33-8. Interface contaminant: lubricating oil. It is recommended that no lubrication or instrument milk be applied to the instrument.

If a flap is completely lost, the patient should be treated with prophylactic antibiotics and topical corticosteroids since there will be increased risk of significant haze formation.

INTERFACE EPITHELIAL INGROWTH AND CONTAMINATION

Several contaminants can come to rest in the lamellar interface during the procedure. Good technique and proper irrigation avoid most of these problems. Some contaminants (talc and fibers) (Figures 33-5 and 33-6) are largely avoidable, whereas others (ie, blood from micropannus [Figure 33-7], stainless steel fragments from the blade of the microkeratome, and tear film secretions) are expected and can be removed by proper irrigation. The authors are extremely compulsive in obtaining the clearest interface by proper forniceal irrigation preoperatively to clear conjunctival secretions as well as proper interface irrigation and forniceal aspiration during flap repositioning. Despite these efforts, fibers or secretions occasionally can come to rest in the interface. No lubrication oils (Figure 33-8) or solutions should be applied to the microkeratome since they can also contaminate the interface. Interestingly, most of the above contaminants are of no visual consequence but are aesthetically displeasing to observe at the slit lamp.

Epithelial cyst and ingrowth are a different matter. They can occur by direct implantation during the procedure or ingrowth from the keratectomy edge or previously existing keratotomies (ie, radial or astigmatic keratotomy). Ingrowth can be directly visualized as a sheet with or without white cysts within the interface space (Figures 33-9 through 33-11). Typically, fluorescein staining will highlight the entry

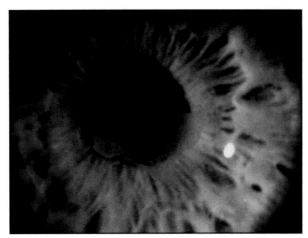

Figure 33-9. Inferior epithelial ingrowth. The central axis is clear, but significant irregular astigmatism and lost lines of best spectacle-corrected vision are due to asymmetric steepening of the flap. Intervention was required.

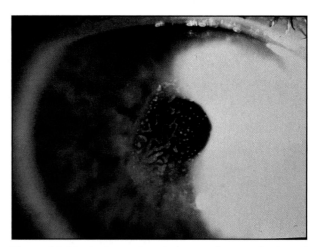

Figure 33-10. A sheet of epithelium with cyst whorls and islands crossing over the visual axis.

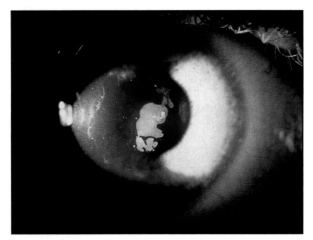

Figure 33-11. Large epithelial cystic inclusion blocking the central visual axis.

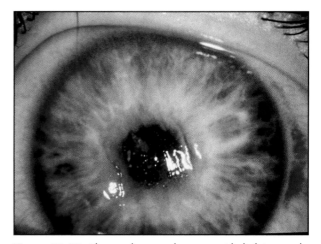

Figure 33-12. Flap melt secondary to epithelial ingrowth. This condition requires emergent intervention.

> Anecdotally, microkeratome blade entry at 25° or greater appears to have a lower incidence of epithelial ingrowth compared to blade entry at or close to 0°.

point of the ingrowth area. Ingrowth from epithelial stem cells outside the keratectomy edge is by far the most common progressive form of epithelial interface growth that requires surgical intervention. Prevention occurs primarily by avoiding epithelial defects and proper replacement of epithelial irregularities. Anecdotally, microkeratome blade entry at 25° or greater appears to have a lower incidence of epithelial ingrowth compared to blade entry at or close to 0°. Epithelium should be removed from the interface if it is progressive, directly blocks the visual axis (see Figures 33-10 and 33-11), causes stromal melting of the flap (Figure 33-12), or induces irregular astigmatism from asymmetric growth (see Figure 31-9).

The epithelium is removed by lifting the flap and manually removing the layer of cells, irrigating the interface with BSS, and replacing the flap. The ingrowth layer may need to be truncated with scissors (Vannas) if it significantly reaches over the gutter of the keratectomy. The patient should be followed closely for recurrence by careful periodic slit lamp examination. Flap melting or necrosis occurs because the flap stroma nutritional support from the aqueous is blocked by the intervening epithelial ingrowth layer. If stromal melting of the flap from epithelial ingrowth destroys the integrity and viability of the flap, the flap may need to be removed and the eye treated as if it had undergone photorefractive keratectomy.

INTERFACE INFECTION

Although incredibly rare, interface bacterial infection is a medical emergency requiring aggressive intervention that

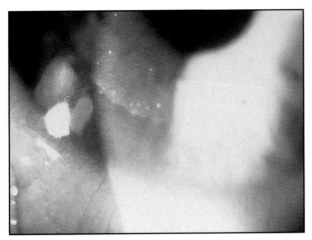

Figure 34-2. Insignificant epithelial ingrowth presenting as a faint white line less than 2 mm under the inferior flap edge 6 weeks after uncomplicated LASIK.

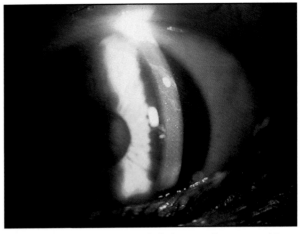

Figure 34-3. Insignificant epithelial ingrowth is just visible as a faint white line central to the superior flap edge 3 weeks after uncomplicated LASIK.

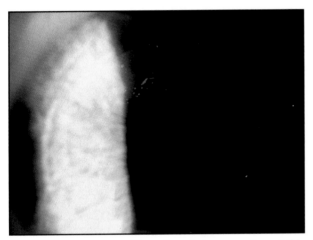

Figure 34-4. Faint speckles of epithelium are just visible under the superior flap 1 week after LASIK.

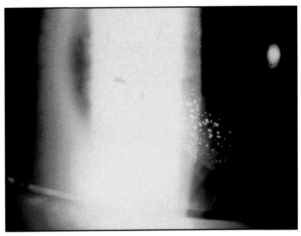

Figure 34-5. Speckles of epithelium are clearly seen on the inferior aspect of the flap interface.

speckles of ingrowth can also be identified under the flap (Figures 34-4 through 34-7), although these rarely progress and often regress by the next follow-up visit. Patients identified with this mild form of ingrowth should be monitored weekly for 1 month with accurate diagrammatic records. The affected area should have slit lamp measurements of extension of the ingrowth from the flap edge. Once the ingrowth has been documented to have stabilized without progression over several visits, the regular postoperative follow-up routine can be resumed.

More aggressive forms of ingrowth that tend to be progressive and often require treatment include epithelial pearls or nests, strands, and sheets. Pearls or nests of ingrowth represent larger collections in epithelial cells that can occur underneath the flap. These do not regress and can be associated with a flap melt over top of the area of ingrowth (Figures 34-8 through 34-12). The most aggressive patterns of ingrowth are characterized strands of epithelial cells streaming underneath the flap towards the visual axis often

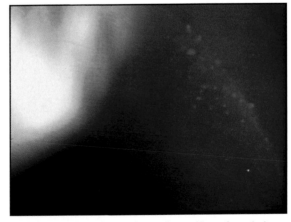

Figure 34-6. Temporally located speckles of epithelium. The flap edge is still intact with no associated melting.

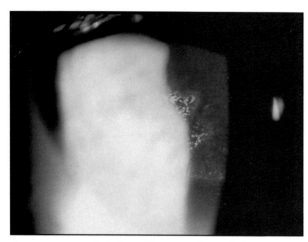

Figure 34-7. Epithelial speckles extending a little more centrally toward the visual axis.

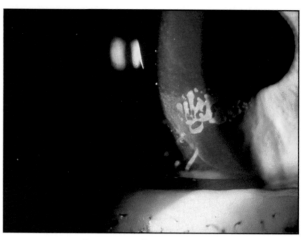

Figure 34-8. A dense nest of epithelial cells present 4 weeks after LASIK in an eye with loose epithelium.

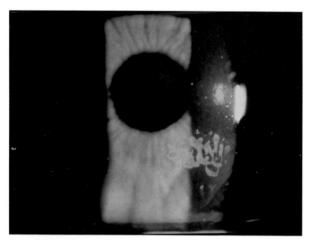

Figure 34-9. The same eye as in Figure 34-8 demonstrating the clarity of the rest of the flap. Removal of the epithelium at this time would lead to an excellent result.

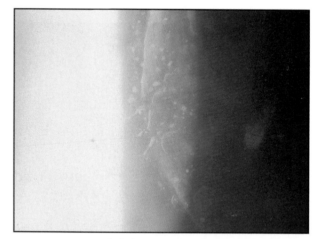

Figure 34-10. Epithelial ingrowth diffusely along the flap edge. Translucent or vacuolated cells are hallmarks of Machat grade 2 classification.

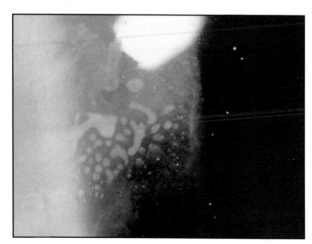

Figure 34-11. Dense nests of the epithelial cells extending toward the visual axis.

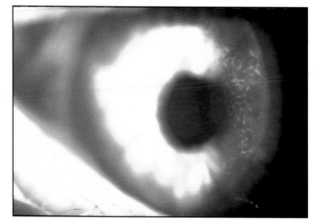

Figure 34-12. Diffuse patches of epithelial ingrowth extending through the temporal aspect of the flap interface.

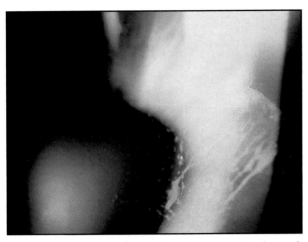

Figure 34-13. Strands of epithelium "streaming" underneath the flap 1 week after LASIK. This aggressive pattern requires immediate treatment.

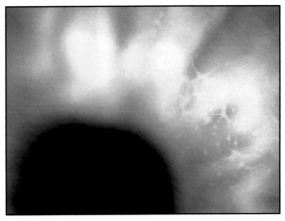

Figure 34-14. Reticular patterns of strands of epithelium in the flap interface 2 weeks post-LASIK. There was an epithelial defect associated with the procedure.

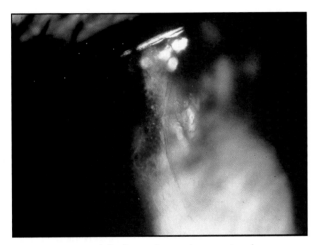

Figure 32-15. Subtle flap edge melt can give the appearance of flap shrinkage. The epithelial ingrowth that caused this peripheral melting has now resolved.

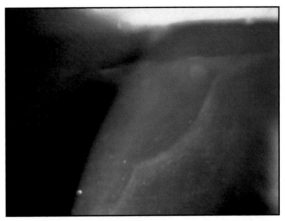

Figure 34-16. Peripheral flap edge melt 3 months after LASIK. The epithelial ingrowth has long since resolved. No treatment is required.

Epithelial ingrowth that has been persistent in the flap interface for several weeks to months can result in a flap melt. Melting can occur in as little as 2 weeks.

as early as the first 2 weeks following LASIK and can precipitate early erosion or melting of the flap margin (Figures 34-13 and 34-14). Obviously, this pattern of epithelial ingrowth requires urgent treatment to prevent further progression. Sheets of epithelium represent the final stage of epithelial ingrowth when the individual nests and strands have expanded and coalesced to form one solid sheet of ingrowth that extends across a large portion of the flap interface.

Epithelial ingrowth that has been persistent in the flap interface for several weeks to months can result in a flap melt that usually begins at the peripheral flap edge that overlies the ingrowth. Melting can occur in as little as 2

weeks. This may be related to a release of collagenase from the hypoxic epithelial cells trapped underneath the flap.[2] The most mild form of flap melt appears as if the flap has slightly shrunk in size. A faint translucent area along a significant portion of the peripheral flap edge is seen representing where the previous epithelial ingrowth had occurred and caused only the peripheral edge of the flap to melt (Figure 34-15 and 34-16). A peripheral flap melt can, however, have a dramatic slit lamp appearance in an asymptomatic patient with excellent uncorrected visual acuity (Figures 34-17 and 34-18). Flap melts can cause a distortion in the corneal surface with an associated disruption in the tear film distribution along the corneal surface, exacerbating dry eye problems following LASIK. Haze and scarring from the ingrowth, which extends near the visual axis (Figures 34-19 and 34-20), can be associated with the visual complaints of glare, ghosting, and halos. These complaints have been identified with other refractive procedures with haze or incision near the visual axis.[10,11]

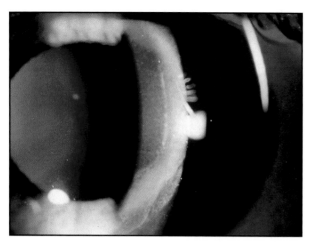

Figure 34-17. Significant epithelial ingrowth associated with a peripheral flap edge melt inferior-temporally. Urgent treatment is required to prevent further flap melting.

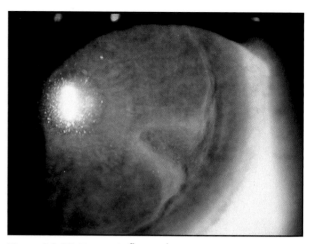

Figure 34-18. Dramatic flap melt presenting in an asymptomatic patient 4 months after LASIK.

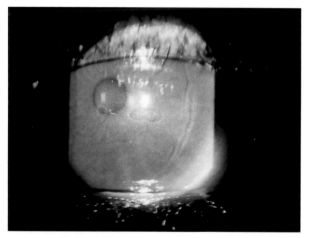

Figure 34-19. Central flap perforation caused by untreated epithelial ingrowth that was allowed to melt through the cornea. The central location of the corneal haze caused visual glare and distortion.

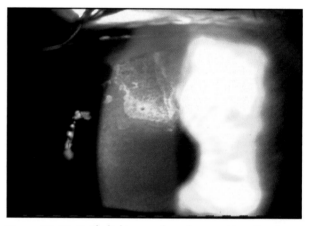

Figure 34-20. Epithelial ingrowth and corneal interface haze extending down towards the visual axis. Urgent treatment is required to preserve the integrity of the flap.

Early identification and treatment of epithelial ingrowth will restore the flap to its original postoperative state and avoid these irreversible flap complications. Once a flap melt has occurred, treatment is often not necessary, as the epithelium trapped underneath the flap has now broken through to the cornea surface so no further progression will occur. LASIK enhancements by lifting the flap after a flap melt are considerably more difficult, as the flap is extremely adherent in the area where the flap melt and stromal scarring occurred.

Machat has devised a system for classifying epithelial ingrowth in terms of severity and treatment options (Table 34-1). Machat grade 1 corresponds to insignificant ingrowth that does not require treatment. Machat grades 2 and 3 correspond to significant ingrowth that requires treatment with different levels of urgency. This grading system has been useful at TLC The Laser Center as a method of standardiz-

> The visual results are excellent and the appearance of the cornea during slit lamp examination can be excellent when the epithelial ingrowth is removed early and the integrity of the cornea flap is preserved.

ing our descriptions of epithelial ingrowth over follow-up visits with different examiners.

Indications for treatment of epithelial ingrowth following LASIK include greater than 2 mm of ingrowth from the flap edge, documented progression, associated flap melting, or a disturbance of BCVA, which can be attributed to the ingrowth. The technique of removal of epithelial ingrowth following LASIK will be described in Chapter 35. The visual results are excellent and the appearance of the cornea during slit lamp examination can be excellent when the epithelial ingrowth is removed early and the integrity of the corneal flap is preserved.

TABLE 34-1.
MACHAT EPITHELIAL INGROWTH CLASSIFICATION

Grade 1: Thin ingrowth, 1-2 cells thick, limited to within 2 mm of flap edge, transparent, difficult to detect, well-delineated white line along advancing edge, no associated flap changes, non-progressive (See Figure 34-1)
No retreatment required.

Grade 2: Thicker ingrowth, discreet cells evident within nest, at least 2 mm from flap edge, individual cells translucent, easily seen on slit lamp, no demarcation line along nest, corneal flap edge rolled or gray, no flap edge melting or erosion, usually progressive (See Figure 34-10).
Requires non-urgent treatment within 2 to 3 weeks.

Grade 3: Pronounced ingrowth, several cells thick, greater than 2 mm from flap edge, ingrowth areas opaque, obvious on slit lamp, white geographic areas of necrotic epithelial cells with no demarcation line, corneal flap margins rolled with thickened whitish-gray appearance. Progression results in large areas of flap melting from collagenase release from the necrotic epithelium. Confluent haze develops peripheral to the flap edge as flap pulls away leaving exposed stromal bed in contact with surface epithelium (See Figure 34-17).
Urgent treatment required with close follow-up, as recurrences are more common due to the altered flap edges.

REFERENCES

1. Probst LE, Machat JJ. Removal of flap striae following LASIK. *J Cataract Refract Surg*. 1997. In press.
2. Machat JJ. LASIK complications and their management. In: Machat JJ, ed. *Excimer Laser Refractive Surgery*. SLACK Incorporated: Thorofare, NJ; 1996.
3. Carr JD, Nardone R Jr, Sulting RD, Thompson KP, Waring GO III. Risk factors for epithelial ingrowth after LASIK. *Invest Ophthalmol Vis Sci*. 1997;38(4):S232.
4. Marinho A, Pinto MC, Pinto R, Vaz F, Neves MC. LASIK for high myopia: one year experience. *Ophthalmic Surgery and Lasers*. 1996; 27(5suppl):S517-S520.
5. Perez-Santonja JJ, Bellot J, Claramonte P, Ismail MM, Alio JL. Laser in situ keratomileusis to correct high myopia. *J Cataract Refract Surg*. 1997; 23(3):372-385.
6. Manche EE, Judge A, Maloney RK. Lamellar keratoplasty for hyperopia. *Journal of Refractive Surgery*. 1996; 12(1):42-49.
7. Kremer I, Blumenthal M. Myopic keratomileusis in situ combined with VISX 20/20 photorefractive keratectomy. *J Cataract Refract Surg*. 1995; 21(5):508-511.
8. Helena MC, Meisler D, Wilson SE. Epithelial growth within the lamellar interface after in situ keratomileusis (LASIK). *Cornea*. 1997;16(3):300-305.
9. Probst LE. Options for refractive surgery. *Journal of Refractive Surgery*. 1997. In press.
10. Probst LE. Haze following PRK. In: Machat JJ, ed. *Excimer Laser Refractive Surgery. Principles and Practice*. SLACK Incorporated: Thorofare, NJ; 1996;182-183.
11. Probst LE. Optical Aberrations following PRK. In: Machat JJ, ed. *Excimer Laser Refractive Surgery. Principles and Practice*. SLACK Incorporated: Thorofare, NJ; 1996;188-189.

Treatment of Epithelial Ingrowth and Flap Melts Following LASIK

Louis E. Probst, MD
Michiel Kritzinger, MD

INTRODUCTION

Laser in situ keratomileusis (LASIK) has become increasingly popular among both patients and refractive surgeons, because of its rapid visual rehabilitation and pain-free postoperative course. However, it has also been associated with a number of complications associated with the creation of the corneal flap including flap striae[1] and epithelial ingrowth.[2-8] Epithelial ingrowth is the most common postoperative flap complication following LASIK. Early recognition of the ingrowth allows for appropriate monitoring and treatment when necessary and can lead to excellent results.

The incidence of significant epithelial ingrowth for more than 10,000 LASIK cases at TLC The Windsor Laser Center and at other centers has been approximately 2%.[2,3] Most commonly, the patient is asymptomatic and the ingrowth is identified on a scheduled postoperative visit as a faint gray line extending less than 2 mm in from the flap edge. Irregular fluorescein staining and pooling is often identified at the flap edge associated with the ingrowth. The visual acuity will be unaffected or drop one line of best-corrected visual acuity (BCVA),[4] except in the most severe cases in which progression occurs into the visual axis. Surface irregularities associated with the epithelial ingrowth can be identified with corneal topography.[4]

PREOPERATIVE ASSESSMENT

Indications for treatment of epithelial ingrowth follow-ing LASIK include greater than 2 mm of ingrowth from the flap edge, documented progression, associated flap melting, or a disturbance of BCVA, which can be attributed to the ingrowth. The clinical presentation of epithelial ingrowth is discussed in Chapter 34.

Epithelial ingrowth is not clearly visible under the operating microscope because of the lack of tangential illumination. Therefore, prior to bringing the patient to the operating microscope, the area of epithelial ingrowth should be clearly identified at the slit lamp. This should be drawn on the operative sheet so the surgeon has a map of the area to be treated.

> Epithelial ingrowth is not clearly visible under the operating microscope because of the lack of tangential illumination.

It is best not to combine myopic enhancement procedures with removal of significant epithelial ingrowth, as the process of epithelial ingrowth itself will induce some refractive change. However, if small insignificant areas of epithelial ingrowth are identified at the time of LASIK enhancement, they should be gently removed from the peripheral edge of the stromal bed just before the excimer enhance-

> It is best not to combine myopic enhancement procedures with removal of significant epithelial ingrowth, as the process of epithelial ingrowth itself will induce some refractive change.

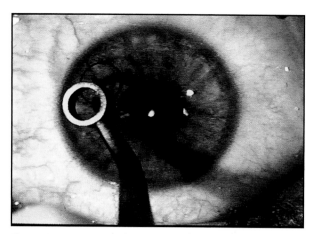

Figure 35-1. Corneal alignment marks are made prior to lifting the flap.

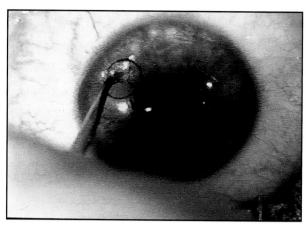

Figure 35-2. The Machat retreatment spatula is used to lift the flap edge.

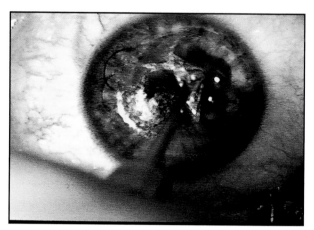

Figure 35-3. The flap is gently peeled back nasally using nontoothed forceps. Note the adherent epithelial ingrowth sticking to the flap and the stromal bed.

ment ablation to prevent further progression of the ingrowth following enhancement. While enhancement procedures have been identified as a risk factor for epithelial ingrowth,[3] our experience has shown that careful meticulous cleaning of the stromal bed and corneal flap can minimize recurrence.[2]

OPERATIVE TECHNIQUE FOR REMOVING EPITHELIAL INGROWTH

The edge of the corneal flap is marked at the slit lamp. This should not be performed under the operating microscope, as the flap edge is often difficult to discern. Under the operating microscope, the patient has peripheral cornea alignment markings placed so that the flap can be accurately repositioned following the enhancement (Figure 35-1). Using a spreading type of instrument, such as the Machat retreatment spatula (ASICO), the flap is then slowly dissected free at its temporal margin (Figure 35-2). The flap can then be lifted using nontoothed forceps and gently peeled back so it is folded over its nasal hinge (Figures 35-3 and 35- 4). If the flap is peeled back in the same manner, a capsulorhexis is carried out during cataract surgery, and a clean, sharp epithelial separation can be created along the flap edge that heals as quickly as the primary LASIK procedure.

Removal of the epithelium underneath the flap must be complete, as residual cells left in the LASIK bed or on the undersurface of the cap will result in recurrence of the epithelial ingrowth. There are three methods of removing the epithelial cells from the flap interface; these are peeling, scraping, and irrigating. If a large sheet of epithelium ingrowth is present in the stromal bed, an edge can be grasped with a fine nontoothed forceps and peeled from the LASIK flap bed (Figures 35- 5 through 35-8). This allows for a large portion of the epithelial cells to be removed with minimal trauma to the stromal bed. A sharp blade is then gently but firmly scraped towards the peripheral stromal

Removal of the epithelium underneath the flap must be complete, as residual cells left in the LASIK bed or on the undersurface of the cap will result in recurrence of the epithelial ingrowth. There are three methods of removing the epithelial cells from the flap interface; these are peeling, scraping, and irrigating.

bed in radial strokes from the central area of the ingrowth (Figure 35-9). The blade is intermittently checked to see if any epithelial cells have been removed and have collected on the blade surface (Figure 35-10). If epithelial cells are present, the blade is wiped clean and gentle scraping of the stromal bed is continued until epithelial cells are no longer identified.

It is important to ensure that there is no epithelium along the flap edge that is hanging into the stromal bed so that when the cap is replaced these epithelial cells will be trapped under the flap edge, which may lead to a further recurrence of the epithelial ingrowth. If epithelium is hang-

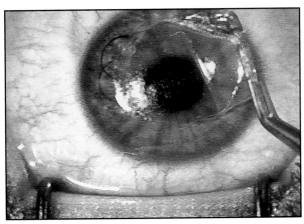

Figure 35-4. The flap is pulled back nasally. Note the edge of epithelium along the inferior flap edge.

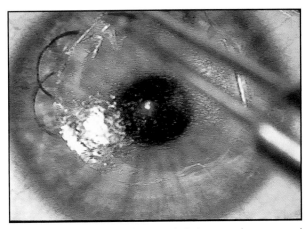

Figure 35-5. The edge of the epithelial ingrowth is grasped with nontoothed forceps.

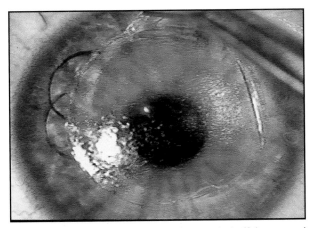

Figure 35-6. The epithelial ingrowth is peeled off the stromal bed.

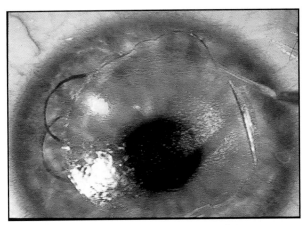

Figure 35-7. Epithelial ingrowth is peeled off the area near the hinge of the flap.

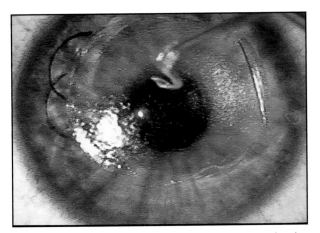

Figure 35-8. The epithelial ingrowth that was removed is displayed over the stromal bed.

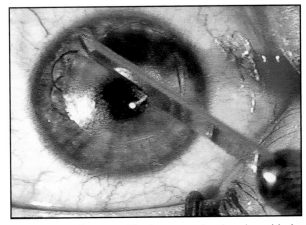

Figure 35-9. The stromal bed is scraped with a sharp blade, moving central to the peripheral bed.

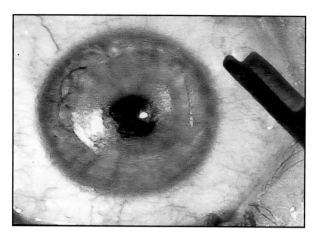

Figure 35-10. The edge of the bed is intermittently checked to identify any epithelium that should be cleaned off before further scraping is performed.

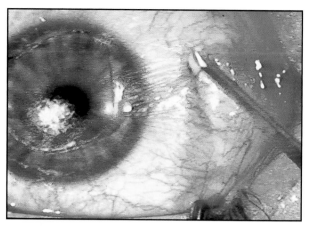

Figure 35-11. The stromal surface of the cap is then scraped in a similar manner. It is helpful at this stage to ask the patient to look temporally.

> Epithelial defects along the flap edge postoperatively will increase postoperative discomfort as well as induce epithelial migration and replication, which will increase the incidence of epithelial ingrowth recurrence.

ing into the peripheral stromal bed, it should be gently pushed back with a sharp blade. While all the epithelial cells must be removed from the stromal bed, it is essential that the epithelial cells on the corneal surface outside of the stromal bed not be removed if at all possible. Epithelial defects along the flap edge postoperatively will increase postoperative discomfort as well as induce epithelial migration and replication, which will increase the incidence of epithelial ingrowth recurrence.

The same scraping maneuver is then performed on the undersurface of the cap. Scraping is performed in a radial pattern going central to peripheral, focusing on the area of ingrowth that must be extrapolated from the preoperative diagram as the flap is now folded over. Once again, the blade is intermittently checked to monitor for epithelial cells that may be present and wiped regularly. While cleaning the undersurface of the flap with a nasal hinge, it is often helpful to have the patient look temporally so that the cap is placed in a more central location (Figure 35-11). The patient should be warned that he or she might feel a pressure sensation when the undersurface of the cap is scraped, as this area of the eye is less anaesthetized with the topical anesthesia.

> While cleaning the undersurface of the flap with a nasal hinge, it is often helpful to have the patient look temporally so that the cap is placed in a more central location.

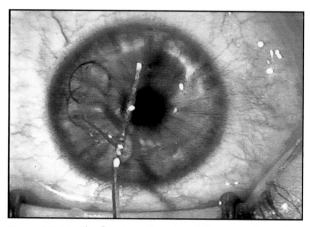

Figure 35-12. The flap is replaced and the stromal interface is thoroughly irrigated to remove residual epithelial cells and to refloat the flap into its correct location.

Once the surgeon is sure that all the epithelium has been completely removed from the flap bed and undersurface of the cap, the flap can be replaced. A few drops of balanced salt solution (BSS) solution are placed on the undersurface of the cap and in the flap bed. The flap can be gently flipped back in place with forceps or a thin spatula slid underneath the nasal hinge, which is then moved nasal to temporal in one fluid motion. The final step of eliminating any residual epithelial cells is thorough irrigation underneath the cap. Using filtered BSS solution on a syringe, the flap interface is irrigated not only to remove debris and refloat the flap as in primary LASIK, but also to remove any residual epithelial cells in the area of the previous epithelium growth (Figure 35-12). The flap alignment is then checked by verifying the realignment of the corneal markings (Figure 35-13) and the gutter test. The flap is left to seal into place for 2 to 3 minutes. The stability of the flap can then be checked with the striae and blink tests as with primary LASIK.[9]

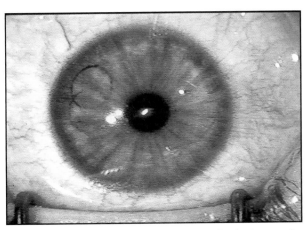

Figure 35-13. The alignment marks are checked once the flap has been refloated and wiped into location. The flap should be left for 3 minutes to seal into the bed.

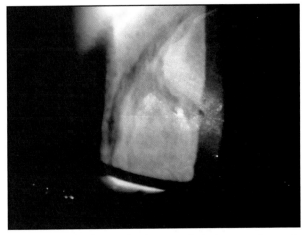

Figure 35-14. Flap melts from epithelial ingrowth rarely extend into the visual axis and cause symptoms of visual distortion.

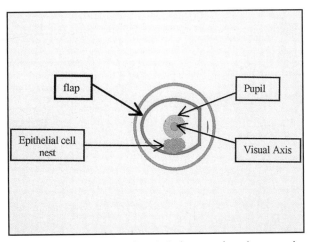

Figure 35-15. The area of epithelial ingrowth is drawn at the slit lamp so it can be easily located under the operating microscope.

OPERATIVE TECHNIQUE OF FREE FLAPS FOR SEVERE FLAP MELTS

Epithelial cell nests underneath the corneal flap as well as flap melts rarely occur with a normal corneal epithelium. Older eyes with loose epithelium or postoperative epithelial defects are at a greater risk for these complications. Approximately .1% of all LASIK eyes will develop a significant flap melt associated with the epithelial ingrowth (Figure 35-14). Flap melts can cause a distortion in the corneal surface with an associated disruption in the tear film distribution along the corneal surface, exacerbating dry eye problems following LASIK. Haze and scarring from the ingrowth that extends near the visual axis can be associated with the visual complaints of glare, ghosting, and halos.

If the melting has advanced close to the visual axis and is associated with visual distortions, treatment should be considered. One option is to simply remove the corneal flap completely. While this may eliminate most of the scarring associated with the flap, it will effectively create a postoperative photorefractive keratectomy (PRK) situation with a high risk of developing haze in the stromal bed. Postoperative steroids will be required to control this haze response. Because the corneal flap is of a uniform thickness, there is very little refractive change induced by the removal of the flap. Phototherapeutic keratectomy or PRK may be required in the future to treat stromal haze or the residual refractive error. PRK should never be applied on top of the corneal flap. This will invariably result in the development of stromal haze that will become difficult to treat without causing further distortion and damage to the remaining corneal flap.

In cases of severe corneal melts in which the flap melt and scarring is approaching the visual axis and a clear flap exists off-center, the technique of a free flap can be used. The area of the epithelial ingrowth and flap melting is first identified and drawn on the operative sheet (Figure 35-15). The flap is dissected along its edge and gently lifted and peeled back nasally (Figure 35-16). The epithelial cells underneath the flap are removed with the techniques previously described. Sometimes it is necessary to remove the epithelial cells from the outside of the flap bed as well, particularly in an eye with very loose epithelium. The hinge of the flap is then cut to create a free flap (Figure 35-17). The free flap is then shifted so that the largest clear area is positioned over the visual axis (Figure 35-18). This will create a

Approximately .1% of all LASIK eyes will develop a significant flap melt associated with the epithelial ingrowth.

The free flap is then shifted so that the largest clear area is positioned over the visual axis.

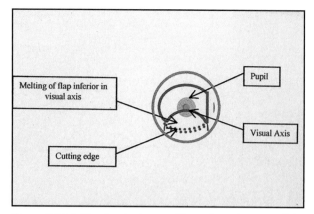

Figure 35-16. The flap is dissected free along the area of the flap melt and the flap edges.

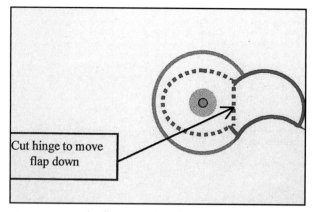

Figure 35-17. The flap is peeled back nasally. The epithelial ingrowth is removed completely. The hinge is cut to create a free flap.

clear area over the visual axis with minimal scarring at the periphery. The flap should be given extra time to secure into its new location. Sutures are generally not required and should be avoided if at all possible, as they will induce astigmatism. The bed from where the flap was shifted is allowed to epithelialize. The patient is asked to keep the eye closed until the next day and a protective shield or glasses are worn while the flap is healing.

POSTOPERATIVE CARE

Postoperatively, patients are warned that they will have a foreign body sensation for the next 24 to 48 hours or until the epithelial defects along the flap edge have healed. We have found the recurrence rate of epithelial ingrowth is approximately 10%, so we suggest that the patient be followed weekly for at least the first month to ensure the epithelial ingrowth does not recur. Patients are placed on a .3% tobramycin/.1% dexamethasone combination and .3% ofloxacin one drop four times a day for 4 days. Patients are encouraged to use copious ocular lubrication. Follow-up is continued daily until the epithelial defects are healed.

While epithelial ingrowth is not uncommon following LASIK, the appropriate treatment will allow the patient to continue to enjoy the excellent uncorrected visual acuity commonly achieved with minimal inconvenience. Visual rehabilitation is usually complete within 2 to 3 days following removal of epithelial ingrowth. The best results are achieved when the integrity of the flap is preserved.

> We have found the recurrence rate of epithelial ingrowth is approximately 10%, so we suggest that the patient be followed weekly for at least the first month to ensure the epithelial ingrowth does not recur.

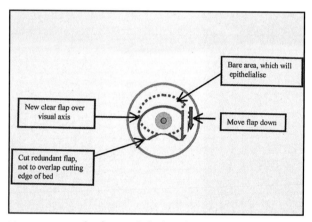

Figure 35-18. The flap is shifted so that the clear area of the free cap is centered over the visual axis. The free flap is then allowed to seal into its new location for at least 5 minutes. Sutures are avoided if possible, as they will induce astigmatism.

REFERENCES

1. Probst LE, Machat JJ. Removal of flap striae following LASIK. *J Cataract Refract Surg.* 1997. In press.
2. Machat JJ. LASIK complications and their management. In: Machat JJ, ed. *Excimer Laser Refractive Surgery.* SLACK Incorporated: Thorofare, NJ; 1996.
3. Carr JD, Nardone R Jr, Sulting RD, Thompson KP, Waring GO III. Risk factors for epithelial ingrowth after LASIK. *Invest Ophthalmol Vis Sci.* 1997;38(4):S232.
4. Helena MC, Meisler D, Wilson SE. Epithelial growth within the lamellar interface after in situ keratomileusis. *Cornea.* 1997;16(3):300-305.
5. Marinho A, Pinto MC, Pinto R, Vaz F, Neves MC. LASIK for high myopia: 1-year experience. *Ophthalmic Surgery and Lasers.* 1996 May; 27(5suppl):S517-S520.
6. Perez-Santonja JJ, Bellot J, Claramonte P, Ismail MM, Alio JL. Laser in situ keratomileusis to correct high myopia. *J Cataract Refract Surg.* 1997;23(3):372-385.
7. Manche EE, Judge A, Maloney RK. Lamellar keratoplasty for hyperopia. *Journal of Refractive Surgery.* 1996;12(1):42-49.
8. Kremer I, Blumenthal M. Myopic keratomileusis in situ combined with VISX 20/20 photorefractive keratectomy. *J Cataract Refract Surg.* 1995;21(5):508-511.
9. Probst LE, Machat JJ. LASIK enhancement techniques and results. In: Buratto L, ed. *LASIK.* SLACK Incorporated: Thorofare, NJ; 1997.

Removal of Flap Striae Following LASIK

Louis E. Probst, MD
Jeffery J. Machat, MD

INTRODUCTION

Laser in situ keratomileusis (LASIK) has recently gained tremendous popularity for the correction of myopia because of the reduced risk of postoperative corneal haze, rapid visual rehabilitation, a pain-free postoperative course, and decreased need for postoperative medications. While LASIK certainly offers a number of advantages over photorefractive keratectomy, the creation of the corneal flap has been associated with a number of intraoperative and postoperative complications.[1-5] The most common postoperative complications associated with the corneal flap include flap striae and epithelial ingrowth.[6] There is a common misconception that flap striae can be eliminated by simply lifting and refloating the corneal flap, however this technique will only be effective for flap striae identified within the first 24 hours after LASIK. In this chapter, we will describe the techniques we have found to be most useful for the removal of flap striae.

PREOPERATIVE ASSESSMENT AND PLANNING

PREOPERATIVE EVALUATION

The first indications of flap striae may include an unexplained reduction in best-corrected visual acuity (BCVA), postoperative regular astigmatism, or postoperative irregular astigmatism. Careful corneal examination with the slit lamp is often all that is necessary to identify significant flap striae passing across the visual axis (Figure 36-1).

There is a common misconception that flap striae can be eliminated by simply lifting and refloating the corneal flap, however this technique will only be effective for flap striae identified within the first 24 hours after LASIK.

Fluorescein staining of the cornea can be useful to demonstrate very fine striae that may not be visually significant (Figure 36-2). Indirect slit beam illumination from the iris may also be useful when peripheral flap striae are suspected (Figures 36-3 and 36-4). Finally, retro-illumination through the dilated pupil is very effective in demonstrating flap striae (Figure 36-5).

INDICATIONS FOR SURGERY

Flap striae result from misalignment of the corneal flap after flap replacement, movement of the corneal flap during the first postoperative day, or a postulated "tenting effect" of the corneal flap over the ablated stromal bed. This tenting effect is most significant in high myopic corrections because of the greater depth of tissue ablation, which alters the original relationship of the undersurface of the flap to the surface of the stromal bed.

Flap striae result from misalignment of the corneal flap after flap replacement, movement of the corneal flap during the first postoperative day, or the "tenting effect" of the corneal flap over the ablated stromal bed.

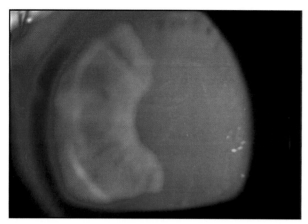

Figure 36-1. Direct focal illumination of the cornea demonstrates fine horizontal flap striae passing directly through the visual axis. This pattern may be asymptomatic or associated with a reduction of BCVA of one to two Snellen visual acuity lines.

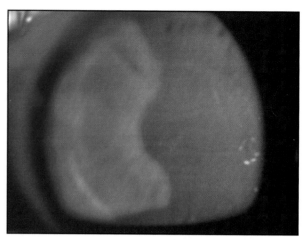

Figure 36-2. Fluorescein staining of the cornea helps to identify horizontal flap striae. The fluorescein will pool in the folds of the flap striae, which creates a more intense green fluorescence along the folds.

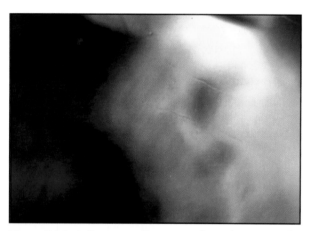

Figure 36-3. Indirect retroillumination from the iris can be useful to locate peripheral flap striae. Fine arcuate peripheral striae are demonstrated, which are not visually significant.

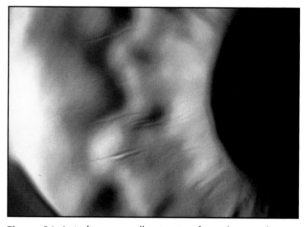

Figure 36-4. Indirect retroillumination from the iris demonstrating radial peripheral flap striae, which are not visually significant.

Flap striae that are peripheral and not affecting the uncorrected vision or the comfort of the eye do not necessarily require treatment. However, flap striae that extend through the visual axis cause a decrease in BCVA or induce irregular astigmatism and should be treated.

> Flap striae that extend through the visual axis cause a decrease in BCVA or induce irregular astigmatism and should be treated.

TIME OF SURGERY

Most flap striae occur within the first hour after LASIK. Flap striae become more difficult to remove as the length of the postoperative course increases, therefore identification of the striae on the first postoperative day is imperative. Even 1 week postoperatively, flap striae become imbedded

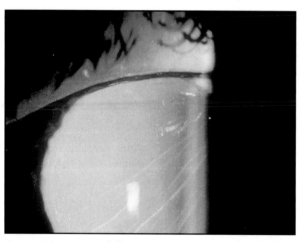

Figure 36-5. Corneal flap striae are most easily identified with retroillumination through the dilated pupil.

Flap striae become more difficult to remove as the length of the postoperative course increases, therefore identification of the striae on the first postoperative day is imperative.

in the corneal flap tissue. Striae that are treated several months after surgery can be very resistant to removal, as they can become permanently molded into the corneal flap. Significant flap striae that are identified within the first postoperative day should be treated the same day. After 1 week, the urgency to treat striae reduces, as the striae are now somewhat imbedded; however, earlier treatment will improve the chances for success.

SURGICAL TECHNIQUE

STEPS OF SURGERY

The first step in treatment is to identify the location and orientation of the striae. Normally, the striae are oriented horizontally when a nasal-based hinge is used. The flap typically rotates counter clockwise for the right eye and counter clockwise for the left eye. The pupil may be dilated preoperatively, as retroillumination of the fixation light and aiming beam of the excimer laser through the dilated pupil provides accurate localization of the flap striae and can allow the surgeon to monitor the surgical success of the various surgical maneuvers. Phenylephrine 2.5% drops provide a rapid and temporary dilation of the pupil, which is quite effective. Retroillumination will also help identify very fine striae in cases of unexplained reduction of BCVA.

Retroillumination will also help identify very fine striae in cases of unexplained reduction of BCVA.

The flap edge is then marked at the slit lamp prior to bringing the patient underneath the operating microscope; identification of the flap edge can be extremely difficult without the tangential illumination of the slit lamp biomicroscope. Once under the operating microscope, the flap alignment markings can be made. Because the flap will be realigned into a more correct position following the removal of the flap striae, the realignment of these corneal markings upon replacing the flap should not be expected. In fact, misalignment is typical and indicates the flap has been repositioned. The flap is then slowly dissected free using an instrument such as the fine tiers, cyclodialysis spatula, or lamellar dissector, which is inserted underneath the flap and the epithelium is carefully cut along the flap edge without disturbing the peripheral epithelium to minimize postoperative epithelial defects and discomfort.

Once the flap is reflected nasally, the stromal surface of

the flap is completely hydrated for a few seconds with several drops of filtered balanced salt solution (BSS). This hydration effect allows the flap to expand and become somewhat edematous, which tends to make the flap more malleable for the removal of the flap striae. The flap is then replaced in the stromal bed and floated into position. The flap is allowed to develop adhesion back to the stromal bed.

This hydration effect allows the flap to expand and become somewhat edematous, which tends to make the flap more malleable for the removal of the flap striae.

After waiting 2 to 3 minutes, the surface of the corneal flap will be relatively dry and the flap will be reasonably adherent to the stromal bed. The side of the blunt forceps can then be placed on the epithelial surface of the flap and gently, but firmly, pushed in a downward and outward motion perpendicular to the orientation of the corneal striae using the Machat stretch and smooth technique.[6] By performing this maneuver on both sides of the corneal striae, the striae can be gradually "stretched" from the flap. The flap edges are stretched away from the central corneal area of the deepest excimer ablation in order to encourage the flap to fill into the ablated stromal bed. It is imperative to stretch the striae for several minutes because stretching occurs incrementally and the flap must be given an opportunity to re-adhere in the new stretched position.

The side of the blunt forceps can then be placed on the epithelial surface of the flap and gently, but firmly, pushed in a downward and outward motion perpendicular to the orientation of the corneal striae using the Machat stretch and smooth technique.

It is imperative to stretch the striae for several minutes because stretching occurs incrementally and the flap must be given an opportunity to re-adhere in the new stretched position.

After several minutes of performing this maneuver, the retroillumination image can be checked through the dilated pupil to monitor the progress of the elimination of the striae. Typically, little or no improvement is noted immediately after stretching the striae. Once the striae have been sufficiently stretched, the eyelid speculum is removed and the eye is taped shut. Patients are given topical ofloxacin .3% and a mild steroid drop to use four times a day for the first 4 postoperative days. If large epithelial defects are present, topical diclofenac sodium .1% used twice a day for the first 2 postoperative days will minimize postoperative discomfort with a minimal risk of sterile infiltrates.[7]

POSTOPERATIVE ASSESSMENT

The status of the corneal flap is checked 20 minutes following the surgery. Commonly, some residual striae are still visible by retroillumination at this time, although the striae often appear less prominent. During the next postoperative day more significant improvement is noted, often with complete elimination of the striae (Figure 36-6). BCVA often improves by one to two lines over the preoperative level. If residual striae persist, this technique can be repeated in 1 month.

REFERENCES

1. Pallikaris IG, Siganos DS. Excimer laser in situ keratomileusis and photorefractive keratectomy for correction of high myopia. *J Refract Corneal Surg.* 1994;10(5):498-510.
2. Marinho A, Pinto MC, Pinto R, Vaz F, Neves MC. LASIK for high myopia: 1-year experience. *Ophthalmic Surgery and Lasers.* 1996;27(5suppl):S512-6.
3. Salah T, Waring GO III, el-Maghraby A, Moadel K, Grimm SB. Excimer laser in-situ keratomileusis under a corneal flap for myopia of 2 to 20 D. *Trans Am Ophthalmol Soc.* 1995;93:163-83.
4. Gimbel HV, Basti S, Kaye GB, Ferensowicz M. Experience during the learning curve of laser in situ keratomileusis. *J Cataract Refract Surg.* 1996;22(5):542-50.
5. Fiander DC, Tayfour F. Excimer laser in situ keratomileusis in 124 myopic eyes. *Journal of Refractive Surgery.* 1995;11(3suppl):S234-8.
6. Machat JJ. LASIK complications and their management. In: Machat JJ, ed. *Excimer Laser Refractive Surgery.* SLACK Incorporated: Thorofare, NJ; 1996.
7. Probst LE, Machat JJ. Corneal Subepithelial infiltrates following photorefractive keratectomy (letter). *J Cataract Refract Surg.* 1996;22(3):281.

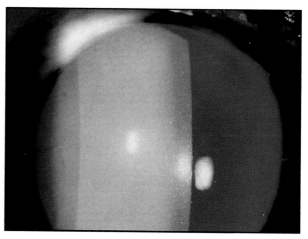

Figure 36-6. Retroillumination 3 days following treatment demonstrates complete removal of the flap striae.

Intraocular Pressure and Central Corneal Thickness Following LASIK

Barry Emara, MD   *Louis E. Probst, MD*
David P . Tingey, MD   *Dennis W. Kennedy, OD*
Lisa J. Willms, OD   *Jeffery J. Machat, MD*

The evaluation of intraocular pressure (IOP) is a cornerstone in the diagnosis and management of many ophthalmic diseases. Although there are many methods of measuring IOP, Goldmann applanation tonometry has proven to be the most accurate and is considered the gold standard of IOP measurement.

When Goldmann first introduced the theory and practice of applanation tonometry, he recognized that IOP measurement would be influenced by central corneal thickness (CCT), however his calculations assumed little variation from a standard CCT of 520 microns.[1,2] With the advent of optical pachymetry, Ehlers and associates described a definite relationship between applanation IOP and central CCT, with elevated readings in thick corneas and lower readings in thin corneas.[3] Sorensen and co-workers reported 15 years of follow-up on patients diagnosed with ocular hypertension with thicker corneas than normal.[4] This relationship between IOP and CCT has since been confirmed using IOP measurements by intraocular cannulation.[3,5]

Recently, a decrease in IOP has been reported following refractive procedures including radial keratotomy (RK), photorefractive keratectomy (PRK), and laser in situ keratomileusis (LASIK). Although the amount of IOP reduction has been correlated to the amount of myopia corrected by PRK,[6] to date there has been no definitive correlation demonstrated between the amount of reduction of CCT and an amount of reduction in IOP. LASIK offers the ideal situation to study this relationship, as corneal pachymetry is an integral part of the preoperative LASIK assessment,[7] and LASIK often results in significant reductions in CCT when correcting high levels of myopia.

In this study, we evaluated the relationship of CCT and IOP measured by Goldmann applanation tonometry in normal myopic eyes and after LASIK.

METHODS

To determine the relationship between IOP and CCT in the untreated myopic population as well as before and after LASIK, a prospective case-control study was conducted. From January to April 1997, consecutive patients were examined at TLC, The Windsor Laser Center. IOP and CCT were measured in three groups:

1. A control group of 120 myopic patients (203 eyes) undergoing evaluation for refractive surgery.
2. A LASIK group of 50 myopic patients (85 eyes) prior to treatment.
3. The same LASIK group of 50 patients (85 eyes) 3 months post-LASIK.

The patient's age and the side of the surgery were recorded for each eye.

All patients had been prescreened by their referring eyecare professional for any eye disease, including glaucoma or previous ocular surgery. None of the patients were taking regular ocular medications. All patients were required to have soft contact lenses out 1 week prior to assessment and hard contact lenses out 4 weeks prior to assessment. Eyes with greater than 2 diopters (D) of astigmatism or irregular corneal surfaces rendering applanation IOP difficult to obtain were excluded. IOP was measured by Goldmann applanation tonometry by two experienced optometrists (LJ Willms and DW Kennedy).

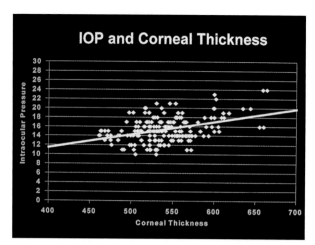

Figure 37-1. Intraocular pressure and corneal thickness.

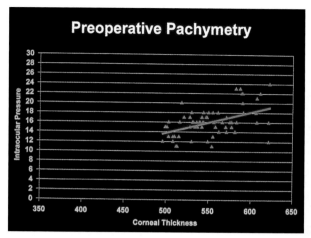

Figure 37-2. Preoperative pachymetry.

CCT was measured by the Sonogage Corneo-Gauge Pulse 2 pachymeter (Sonogage, Cleveland, Ohio). Pachymetry calibration was performed daily according to the instructions provided by the manufacturer. After topical .5% proparicaine had been placed in the eye, the ultrasonic pachymeter probe was placed perpendicular to the corneal surface in the region of the center of the pupil. At least three readings were recorded for each test to the nearest micron and the mean was calculated. All measurements were taken by two experienced optometrists (LJ Willms and DW Kennedy) in the settings of a refractive surgery center completely dedicated to LASIK. In post-LASIK eye cases, the examiners were unaware of the previous IOP and pachymetry readings.

All procedures were performed by two high-volume LASIK surgeons (LE Probst and JJ Machat). LASIK was performed using the Chiron Technolas 116 excimer laser (Chiron Vision, Irvine, Calif) using a partial multizone ablation nomogram. Approximately 50% of the ablation was performed at 5.5 mm and the remainder of the ablation performed between 6 mm and 6.6 mm.[7] The corneal flaps were cut at 180 microns with the Chiron Automatic Corneal Shaper microkeratome. Preoperative calculations were performed in all eyes to ensure that at least 250 microns of posterior corneal stroma would be preserved to maintain the long-term corneal integrity. Postoperatively, a topical corticosteroid antibiotic combination (Tobradex) and a topical fluoroquinolone (Ocuflox) were used with one drop to the operative eye four times a day for 1 week.

Preoperative refractive data and the pre- and post-LASIK corneal keratometry values were not recorded for this study. Data was analyzed with the Pearson correlation coefficient and the paired student's *t* test to compare similar groups of data. A p value of less than .05 was considered significant.

RESULTS

The mean age of the control group was 42.6 ± 7.1 years and the LASIK group was 42 ± 7.6 years. There was no significant difference between the ages of the eyes in either group. In the untreated group there were 95 right eyes and 108 left eyes. In the LASIK group there were 44 right eyes and 41 left eyes. There was no significant correlation detected between the age or side of the eyes and the CCT.

In the untreated group of 288 eyes (control and pre-LASIK eyes), the mean CCT was 544 ± 37.3 microns (range: 461 to 664 microns). The mean IOP was 15.6 ± 2.7 mm Hg (range: 10 to 24 mm Hg). The correlation between the IOP and the CCT was highly significant (r = .44, n = 288, p < .0001). The slope was .032 mm Hg/micron of CCT or an approximate decrease of 1 mm Hg for a reduction of 31.3 microns of CCT (Figure 37-1).

In the pre-LASIK subset of 85 eyes from the untreated group, the results were similar with a mean CCT of 552.2 ± 33.3 microns (range: 496 to 622 microns). The mean IOP was 16.1 mm Hg (range: 11 to 24 mm Hg). A highly significant correlation was found between IOP and CCT (r = .49, n = 85, p < .0001).

Post-LASIK results were obtained 3 months post-treatment. The mean CCT dropped approximately 73 microns to 479.5 ± 41.2 microns (range: 408 to 503 microns). The IOP measurement showed a drop to a mean of 13.6 ± 3.3 mm Hg (range: 7 to 22 mm Hg). A significant correlation between IOP and CCT was found (r = .33, n = 85, p < .002).

When the pre- and post-LASIK mean IOP measure-

When the pre- and post-LASIK mean IOP measurements are compared in the same 85 eyes, there was a significant decrease of 2.5 mm Hg.

TABLE 38-2.
CLINICAL RESULTS OF VARIOUS LTK STUDIES

	Seiler[16]	Ariyasu[20]	Koch[18,19]	Ismail[21]	Ismail[21]	Ismail[25]
1 ring	-	±1.05 D	±1.41 D	±1.8 D	-	-
2 or more	±3.7 D	-	±2.2 D	±2.4 D	±3.7 D	±3.6 D
Follow-up	1 year	6 months	2 years	18 months	12 months	2 years
LTK	Contact	Contact	Noncontact	Noncontact	Noncontact	Noncontact
Hyperopia	Congenital	Congenital	Congenital	Congenital	Post-PRK	Post LASIK

ment of the epithelium layer occurred corresponding to the laser spot area. The underlying stroma presented loss of regular lamellar pattern and increased uptake of the hematoxylin stain. During the first 4 to 8 weeks, epithelial hyperplasia was very evident, also a cone-shape alteration of the stromal tissue corresponding to the spot hardly reached the endothelium in energies below 15 mJ/cm^3. The keratocytic proliferation and new collagen deposition occurs by 3 months after treatment.

In spite of good potential refractive outcomes with LTK, there are two major handicaps for the use of this technique: tissue necrosis and regression of the effect, which in our opinion is due to the existence of a topographic corneal memory.

TISSUE NECROSIS

Thermal collagen shrinkage is directly proportional to age. This relation only occurs inside the temperature range of 58° to 76°C. Higher thermal levels, 78°C or more, will lead to collagen relaxation and complete loss of elasticity. Such temperature profiles induce keratocytic proliferation and significant acceleration of the collagen turnover process. The end result will be a shorter half-life time of the fibers (normally 20 years) and consequently, the deposition of new collagen fibrils.[26-28] With recent advances in laser technology, necrosis is unlikely to be seen in noncontact LTK procedures.

CORNEAL TOPOGRAPHIC MEMORY: BOWMAN'S LAYER

Regression of the obtained effect is the major limitation to thermal keratoplasty. This drawback is a biophysical mechanism that occurs due to the following:
1. It is more often in young adults, as their stroma and Bowman's layer are relatively more elastic.
2. The use of systemic or local anti-inflammatory drugs can increase the rate and amount of regression, especially during the early postoperative period. This occurs because of the alteration of fibroblastic proliferation.
3. Slit lamp examination reveals a gradual increase in the laser spot size after regression, probably because of corneal flattening.

4. After regression, the cornea returns to its exact preoperative topographic image as if it was never touched (ie, it returns according to its own memory).
5. For the same reason, induced hyperopia following myopic PRK and LASIK obtain more effect with stable correction when treated by LTK.

Studying the previous factors for regression, the author deduced a simple formula for the calculation of the amount of regression that can occur after LTK (presented at the second LTK users Pre-American Academy of Ophthalmology meeting in San Francisco, Calif, 1994):[29]

$$\text{Percent of regression} = \frac{\text{keratometry}}{15} \times \frac{\text{central pachymetry}}{\text{age}}$$

The author defends the hypothesis that Bowman's layer is the main topographic memory of the cornea. The alteration of this layer can certainly diminish regression of the obtained effect. This was clearly demonstrated in the study that we realized for the correction of post-PRK hyperopia by noncontact LTK in which the mean postoperative correction was -3.78 D.[21,23] This huge effect might be due to lower central pachymetry and central absence of Bowman's layer in these cases. Both factors can help the cornea remain stable after LTK.

During the LASIK procedure, a lamellar corneal cut is created by the microkeratome before the intrastromal ablation. The cut corresponds to almost 270° of the corneal circumference and usually at 7 to 8 mm of its diameter. The Bowman's layer, once cut, never heals, leading to partial interruption of its continuity. Also, the central corneal thickness following LASIK is significantly reduced.[5,6]

MANAGEMENT OF INDUCED HYPEROPIA AND HYPEROPIC ASTIGMATISM BY NONCONTACT LASER THERMAL KERATOPLASTY

We started a controlled study 2 years ago consisting of 14 patients (eight females and six males) who were operated on for LASIK-induced hyperopia. The Automated Corneal Shaper microkeratome (Chiron), together with the VISX 20/20 excimer laser system (VISX, Inc, Sunnyvale, Calif) were used for the LASIK procedure. The average age was 28.8 ± 3.2 (range 21 to 44 years). The final results were presented at the annual American Academy of

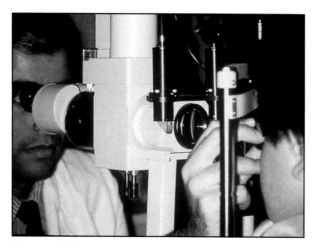

Figure 38-2. Noncontact LTK gLase 210 (Sunrise Technologies).

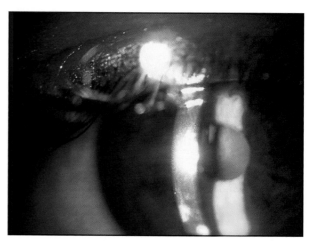

Figure 38-3. LTK spots outside the previous LASIK flap.

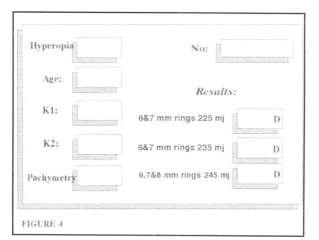

Figure 38-4. Computerized nomogram (Ismail) For LTK treatment. This includes age, pachymetry, keratometry, and a type of hyperopia (congenital, post-PRK, post-LASIK). The computerized simulation, according to three energy/ring profiles, presents results after stability from regression.

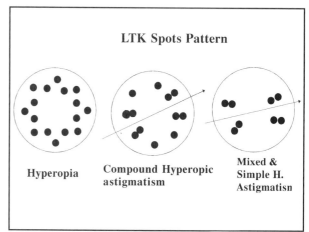

Figure 38-5. A diagram presenting the LTK treatment pattern.

Ophthalmology meeting in San Francisco, Calif, October 1997.[24,25]

Included in the study were motivated patients with significant and stable overcorrection for at least 9 months following the LASIK surgery. Excluded were those eyes with irregular or high astigmatism caused by nonconfluent corneal haze, significant epithelial ingrowth, or flap melting.

LASER THERMAL KERATOPLASTY PROCEDURE

Topical anesthetic was used (tetracaine chlorhydrate .1%, Lab Cusi Barcelona, Spain). We used the noncontact LTK Ho: YAG laser gLase 210 model (Sunrise Technologies, Fremont, Calif) to apply two staggered rings of eight spots for induced hyperopia (spot diameter 600μm)

(Figure 38-2). The spots were placed at 6 mm and 7 mm of the corneal diameter (Figure 38-3), regardless of the previous lamellar cut. The energy used varied between 215 to 245 millijoules and was delivered in eight pulses. The energy was selected according to the author's computer nomogram (Figure 38-4).[29] For hyperopic astigmatism, we applied four spots at 6 mm from the central corneal diameter on the flattest corneal meridian. An additional four spots could be applied at 7 mm if the astigmatism is more than 2 D. However, if a spherical equivalent is associated, an additional eight-spot ring can be added in a radial coherent pattern with the previous astigmatic spots. The laser energy was calibrated before each treatment (Figure 38-5).

The procedure takes only a few seconds, so patients were instructed to fixate on the flickering HeNe beam during the laser application. A plastic lid separator was gently applied for 3 minutes to dry the corneal surface in order to

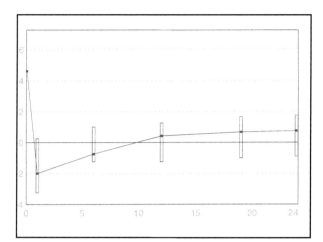

Figure 38-6. Follow-up of the cycloplegic refraction for hyperopia.

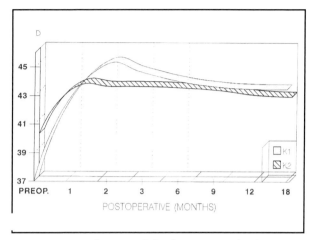

Figure 38-7. Follow-up of the keratometry for hyperopic astigmatism.

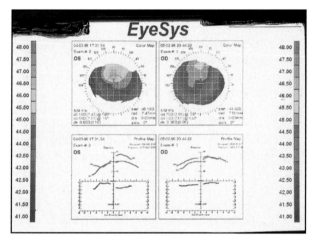

Figure 38-8. Pre-LASIK topography.

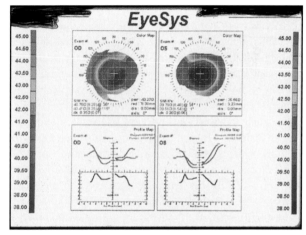

Figure 38-9. Post-LASIK topography: a bilateral induced hyperopia of +4 D with decentrated ablation.

avoid variations that could affect the penetration of the laser beam into the corneal stroma. After the procedure, the eye was rinsed with antibiotic eye drops, and an antibiotic eye ointment was applied. The same topical treatment was continued for 4 days. The patient was sent home with an eye patch for 24 hours. A simple analgesic was prescribed for eye discomfort.

RESULTS

No increase in corneal haze or flap melting was observed in any case. The stability of the corneal flap (of the previous LASIK surgery) was observed in all cases. Immediately after surgery, a myopic shift occurred (Figures 38-6 and 38-7). In the following weeks, most of the patients obtained a stable emmetropic refraction due to partial regression of the effect of the LTK (Figures 38-8 through 38-11). Improvement in uncorrected visual acuity (UCVA) peaked at 3 to 5 months. The BCVA LTK was .69 ± .19

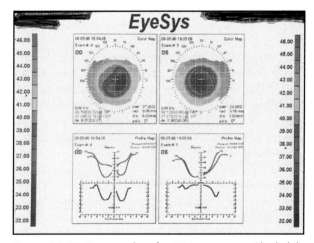

Figure 38-10. Topography after LTK treatment with slightly improved decentration.

(range: .05 to .8 D), while the mean UCVA after 24 months was .61 ± .2 (range: .05 to .8 D). Thirteen patients (68.4%) had a UCVA of .5 or better after 24 months.

The mean cycloplegic refraction before LTK was +4.58 ± 1.4 (range: +2.25 to +7.25 D). After LTK, it was -2.14 ± .7 at 1 month, -.93 ± .13 D at 3 months, +.47 ± .2 at 12 months, and +.78 ± .14 at 24 months. At the end of the study, all patients were within +1.5 D of emmetropia. The mean preoperative keratometry was 37.3 D ± 2.4 (range: 33.5 to 39.75 D); at 1 month it was 44.44 ± 2.1, at 3 months 43.1 ± 2.3, at 12 months 42.08 ± 2.3, and at 24 months 41.7 ± 1.5. A statistically significant difference was obtained (p < .005 student's *t* test) comparing the preoperative status and the 24-month results. There was no statistically significant difference between the results at 12 and 24 months.

CONCLUSIONS

We have to admit that the LASIK technique is rapidly replacing other refractive procedures. Overcorrection following LASIK is considered to be one of the significant complications of this technique. Spectacles or contact lenses can be used to correct LASIK-induced hyperopia, but patients desiring spectacle independence would not welcome such solution. Thus, surgical intervention remains a strong option to treat symptomatic overcorrection following LASIK. Clinical studies regarding noncontact Ho: YAG laser thermal keratoplasty proved its safety and efficacy for the correction of low hyperopia. Regression of the initial effect is the main limitation of this technique. In the early postoperative period, a satisfactory correction up to +6 D may be achieved. However, during the first 3 months, regression occurs and central corneal power returns to previous readings.[18-21] We demonstrated that greater central thickness favors regression.[21,22]

The use of noncontact laser thermal keratoplasty in induced overcorrection after myopic LASIK was satisfactory. The stability of the corneal flap was evident in the treated eyes. A significant improvement of the mean UCVA, central keratometry, and cycloplegic refraction occurred in all eyes (p < .005). No total regression was observed by 24 months. No statistical significantly difference between the results at 12 and 24 months suggests that patients were approaching stability.

In the presence of stromal haze, we recommend the application of the laser spots outside the previous ablation zone to avoid confluent haze. As we obtained a huge myopic shift in the early postoperative period, the application of only eight pulses is sufficient. We concluded that noncontact Ho: YAG laser thermal keratoplasty is a safe and effective alternative for the correction of LASIK-induced hyperopia.

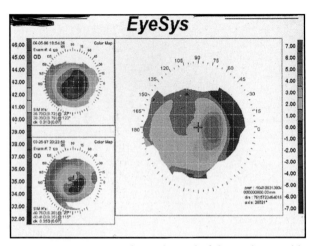

Figure 38-11. Topography at the end of the study: a stable emmetropic refraction.

FUTURE REFINEMENT OF LTK

For fear of regression, the use of LTK is now limited to low hyperopes who have a thin, relatively flat cornea and are over 40 years old. Also, low presbyopia treatment, in a monocular pattern for the nondominant eye, can potentially induce a multifocal corneal topography. Nonetheless, 2% to 5% of myopic patients who undergo LASIK and PRK will suffer from induced hyperopia and hyperopic astigmatism. From our previous experience in these cases, Ho:YAG LTK can be the only choice to undo this complication. What did limit the popularization of this technique is the energy/diopter nomogram that did not include all the variables implicated in the regression. However, the computerized nomogram is a far better alternative for a tailored correction adjusted to the variables of each case.

REFERENCES

1. Pallikaris IG, Papatzanaki ME, Stathi EZ, et al. Laser in situ keratomileusis. *Lasers Surg Med.* 1990; 10:463-468.
2. Lyle WA, Jin GJ. Initial results of automated lamellar keratoplasty for correction of myopia. *J Cataract Refract Surg.* 1996; 22:31-43.
3. Salah T. Waring GO, El Maghraby A, et al. Excimer laser in situ keratomileusis under a corneal flap for myopia of 2 to 20 diopters. *Am J Ophthalmol.* 1996; 121:143-155.
4. Perez JJ, Bellot J. Claramonte P. Ismail MM, Alio JL. Laser in situ keratomileusis to correct high myopia. *J Cataract Refract Surg.* 1997;23:372-385.
5. Arbelaez MC, Perez JJ, Ismail MM, Alio, et al. Automated lamellar keratoplasty and laser in situ keratomileusis. In: *Refractive Surgery Current Techniques and Management.* IGAKU-SHOIN: Tokyo; 1996; 131-150.
6. Rashid ER, Waring GO. Complications of radial keratotomy and transverse keratotomy. *Surv Ophthalmol.* 1989; 34:83-106.
7. Alio JL, Ismail MM. Management of RK overcorrections by

corneal sutures. *J Cataract Refract Surg.* 1993; 19:595-599.

8. Ismail MM, Alio JL, Artola A. Tratamiento de las Hipercorreciones Post-queratotomla Astigmatica. *Archivos de la Soc Espan de Ofta.* 1994; 67:167-172.

9. Anschutz T. Hyperopia: Possibilities and Limitations. *Small Incision Cataract and Refractive Surgery.* Rome; 1996.

10. Anschutz T. Laser Correction of Hyperopia and Presbyopia. In: *Refractive Surgery Current Techniques and Management.* IGAKU-SHOIN: New York-Tokyo; 1996.

11. Lans LJ. Experimentelle untersuchumgen uber entstehung von astigmatismus durch nicht perforirende corneawunden. *Graefes Arch Clin Exp Ophthalmol.* 1889, 45:117-152.

12. Gasset AR, Kaufman HE. Thermokeratoplasty in the treatment of keratoconus. *Am J Ophthalmol.* 1975;79:226-232.

13. Neumann AC, Fyodorov S, Sanders DR. Radial thermal keratoplasty for the correction of hyperopia. *J Refract Corneal Surg.* 1990;6:404-412.

14. Peyman GA, Larson B. Taichand M, Andrews AH. Modification of rabbit corneal curvature with the use of carbon dioxide laser burns. *Ophthalmic Surg.* 1980;11:325-329.

15. Kanoda AN, Sorokin AS. Corneal curvature change using energy of laser radiation. In: *Microsurgery of the Eye.* Moscow: Mir Publishers; 1987.

16. Seiler T, Matallana M, Brinde T. Laser thermokeratoplasty by means of a pulsed holmium: YAG laser for hyperopic correction. *J Refract Corneal Surg.* 1990;63:355-359.

17. Moriera H, Campus M, Sawusch MR, McDonnell JM, Sand B, McDonnell PJ. Holmium laser keratoplasty. *Ophthalmology.* 1992;5:752-761.

18. Koch DD, Abarca A, Villareal R, et al. Hyperopia correction by noncontact holmium laser thermal keratoplasty. Clinical study with two years follow-up. *Ophthalmology.* 1996;103:731-740.

19. Koch DD, Kohnen T, McDonell PJ, Menefee RF, Berry MJ. Hyperopia correction by noncontact holmium: YAG laser thermal keratoplasty. *Ophthalmology.* 1996;103:1525-1536.

20. Ariyasu RG, Sand B, Menefee R, et al. Holmium laser thermal keratoplasty of 10 poorly sighted eyes. *Journal of Refractive Surgery.* 1995;11:358-365.

21. Ismail MM, Perez JJ, Alio JL. Correction of hyperopia and hyperopic astigmatism by laser thermal keratoplasty. In: *Refractive Surgery Current Techniques and Management.* IGAKU-SHOIN: New York-Tokyo; 1996.

22. Alio JL, Ismail MM, Sanchez JL. Noncontact LTK for the correction of hyperopia: 1-year follow-up. *Journal of Refractive Surgery.* 1997;13:17-22.

23. Alio JL, Ismail MM, Artola A, Perez JJ. Correction of PRK-induced hyperopia by holmium laser. Twelve months follow-up. *Journal of Refractive Surgery.* 1997;13:13-16

24. Ismail MM, Alio JL, Perez JJ. Management of Post-LASIK Overcorrection by LTK. Presented at the American Academy of Ophthalmology Meeting; October 26-29 1997; San Francisco, Calif.

25. Ismail MM, Alio JL, Perez JJ. Correction of LASIK-induced hyperopia by noncontact thermal keratoplasty. Eighteen months follow-up. *J cataract and Refract Surg.* 1998. In press.

26. Parel JM, Ren Q. Simon. Non-contact laser photothermal keratoplasty. Biophysical principles and laser beam delivery system. *J Refract Corneal Surg.* 1994;10:511-518.

27. Berry MJ, Fredlin LG, Menefee R. Valderrama GL. Temperature distribution in laser-irradiated corneas. *Invest Ophthalmology and Visual Science.* 1996;103:731-740.

28. Ismail MM, Sanchez-Castro, Alio JL. Efectos histologicos de la termoqueratoplastia con laser de holmio. Estudio experimental. *Archivos de la Soc Espah de Ofta.* 1998; In press.

29. Ismail MM. Analysis of regression after our own nomogram. Presented at Sunrise LTK 2nd Users Meeting. Pre-American Academy of Ophthalmology congress; October 31, 1994; San Francisco, Calif.

SECTION TEN

Innovations and Special Techniques

Topography-Assisted Excimer Laser Techniques

Stephen G. Slade, MD

John F. Doane, MD

Kristian Hohla, PhD

To date, excimer laser refractive procedures have provided tremendous visual benefits to the world's ametropic inhabitants. They have been provided in a noncustomized fashion. In essence, each eye treated has received the same template from the laser algorithm without taking into consideration any specific topographic characteristics for the given eye. Thus far as vision care providers, we have provided functional uncorrected vision improvement to patients with symmetrical corneas. Ideal preoperative corneal shapes have been either spherical (Figure 39-1) or had symmetrical bow-tie astigmatism (Figure 39-2) meaning there are equal areas of steepening or mirror images if a line is drawn perpendicular to the major astigmatic axis. The next phase of laser refractive surgery is to harness all the knowledge gained from computerized videokeratography and use this information along with refractive data to customize the ablation provided to each treated eye (Figure 39-3). This will benefit the entire patient spectrum, from those with symmetric topography to those with marked topographic irregularity or asymmetry. To this end, the customized techniques of topography-linked laser ablations will provide functional improvement for all patients and, importantly, will provide therapeutic correction to improve best-corrected visual acuity (BCVA) and quality of vision in patients with markedly abnormal corneal surfaces.

> The next phase of laser refractive surgery is to harness all the knowledge gained from computerized videokeratography and use this information along with refractive data to customize the ablation provided to each treated eye.

RATIONALE FOR TOPOGRAPHY-LINKED REFRACTIVE LASER TREATMENTS

Traditional excimer laser treatment methods for photorefractive keratectomy (PRK)/laser in situ keratomileusis (LASIK) are based on symmetrical ablation patterns for the correction of refractive errors of the eye. The laser beam emitted from current excimer laser systems is symmetric and assumes the surface that it treats to be symmetric. Hence, if an asymmetric cornea is treated with a symmetric beam, the asymmetric topographic shape will act like a template and result in the creation of the same basic asymmetric pattern deeper in the cornea (Figure 39-4a and 39-4b). Consequently, the laser vision correction can only be as good as the correction with spectacles, as these symmetrical laser treatments are spread out over the whole cornea without taking into account the structure the individual corneal surface.

Vision correction options for eyes with irregular corneal surfaces are limited. Rigid contact lens correction is, in many cases, superior to spectacle correction since corneal surface irregularities are masked by the tear film rigid contact lens surface interface. In reality, a high percentage of

> If an asymmetric cornea is treated with a symmetric beam, the asymmetric topographic shape will act like a template and result in the creation of the same basic asymmetric pattern deeper in the cornea.

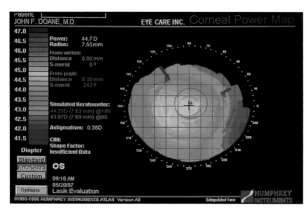

Figure 39-1. Preoperative topography displaying a spherical corneal surface. The refraction was also spherical.

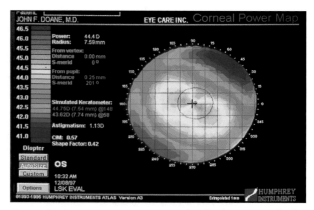

Figure 39-2. Preoperative topography displaying a cylindrical corneal surface. The refraction revealed compound myopic astigmatism with similar amounts of refractive and corneal cylinder at the identical axis.

> In reality, a high percentage of corneas are neither completely regular nor symmetrical.

corneas are neither completely regular nor symmetrical. Bogan, et al have described five basic patterns, including round (22.6%), oval (20.8%), symmetric bow tie (17.5%), asymmetric bow tie (32.1%), and irregular (7.1%)[1] (Figure 39-5). Notably, 40% of the eyes in this study had corneal surface irregularities. For these patients, the postoperative visual acuity theoretically should be improved with topography-linked procedures because the individual surface structure is the basis for the patient/eye-specific laser ablation. This is especially true for patients with irregular astigmatism, non-orthogonal astigmatism (major astigmatic axis being less than 90° apart), or patients who need treatment due to an abnormal corneal surface due to prior laser refractive surgery techniques, trauma, or other causes (Figures 39-6 through 39-9). Treating these types of patients with standard laser correction will not effectively correct their condition, whereas with topography-linked treatments, the custom treatment needed will be provided (Figure 39-10).

PERFORMING TOPOGRAPHY-LINKED EXCIMER LASER ABLATIONS

For topography-linked refractive laser treatments to be performed, there are several hardware and software requirements (Table 39-1). First and foremost, a flying spot excimer laser system is required. The authors have significant experience with the highly advanced Chiron Vision Technolas 217 C-LASIK excimer laser (Figure 39-11). The laser system used has to have the capability to perform off-axis scanning, which means the laser pulse can be placed at any position on the cornea in any order. Chiron Technolas has already successfully created a software version (PlanoScan algorithm) to treat regular corneas that does just that. Another important laser feature is the optimum correlation between laser frequency and laser beam diameter.

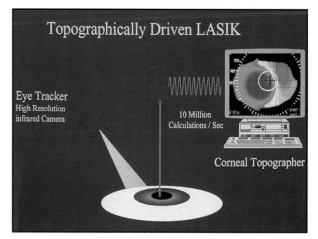

Figure 39-3. Animated view of a topography-assisted excimer laser treatment scenario. Topographic data is use to construct the treatment session. The laser is directed from the refractive and topographic data in conjunction with a high-resolution infrared active eye tracking system to accurately place the incident pulse in the proper location.

The smaller the spot diameter is, the higher the laser frequency has to be in order to complete the treatment in a reasonable time frame. Another essential feature of the laser is a very reliable and stable laser head (like a ceramic laser head) in order to provide a stable energy output during the complete topography-based laser treatment. This is especially important because these treatments require a higher number of laser pulses than standard myopia corrections. Another essential device for performing these treatments correctly is an active eye tracking system, as the laser pulses have to be placed exactly in the proper location to correct

> Without an active eye tracking device, the topography-linked treatments are hardly possible since precise placement of the laser pulse will not be guaranteed.

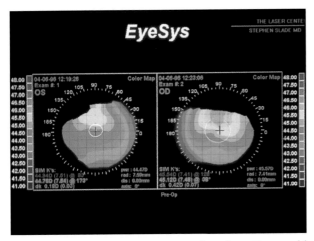

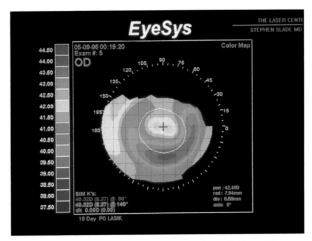

Figure 39-4a. Preoperative topography of a 53-year-old male physicist displaying asymmetric preoperative topography. Note the bilateral superior peninsula of relative steep curvature in comparison to the 270° meridian in each eye. Preoperative refraction was -5.25 - .25 x 180 OD and -5.5 - .5 x 175 OS with best spectacle-corrected vision in each eye of 20/30. He underwent symmetric beam ablation with a large area ablation laser bilaterally. At the 3-month postoperative examination his uncorrected vision was 20/30 in each eye and his refraction was plano -.5 x 180 for 20/30 best spectacle-corrected acuity OD and plano sphere OS for 20/30 best spectacle-corrected vision.

Figure 39-4b. Postoperative topography of the right eye showing a large superior peninsular area of relative steepening, which corresponds to the same area preoperatively. Conceivably with topography-linked laser ablation, this peninsular area could receive extra ablation to make the postoperative corneal curvature uniform and possibly result in improved uncorrected and best-corrected acuity and quality of vision.

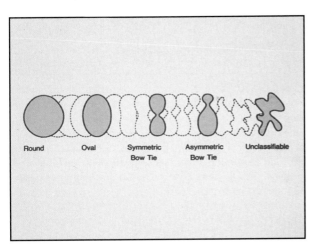

Figure 39-5. Corneal videokeratographic patterns as described by Bogan, et al.[1] Non-Topolink lasers can only accurately treat, in theory, the spherical cornea or the symmetrical astigmatic corneal surface (photo reprinted with permission of *Archives of Ophthalmology*).

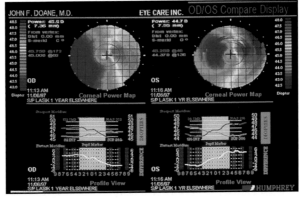

Figure 39-6. Twenty-seven-year-old female who underwent bilateral LASIK. Topography displays ablation decentration toward the 180° meridian in each eye. The patient had residual myopic astigmatic refractive error bilaterally and noted marked scotopic vision complaints. Topography-linked ablation would probably be the best surgical option.

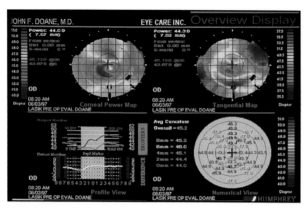

Figure 39-7. Post-PRK 42-year-old female with residual hyperopic astigmatic refractive error. Again, this patient would probably be best treated with topography-linked laser ablation due to the marked topographic irregularity.

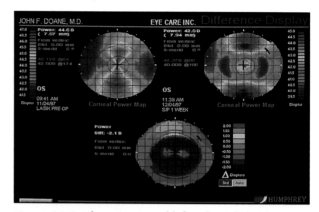

Figure 39-8. Thirty-six-year-old female with preoperative refraction of –6.5 + 5.25 x 090 who has central island postoperatively. Although this can be treated effectively with current laser systems, postoperative results might be improved with topography-linked laser ablation.

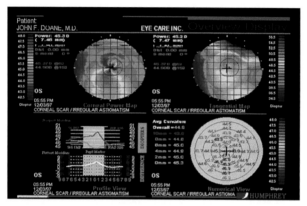

Figure 39-9. Preoperative topography of the left eye of a 42-year-old male who sustained corneal damage without opacity due to corneal infection as an adolescent. His right eye had a round pattern topographically and he underwent LASIK for -3.25 spherical refraction and now has 20/15 uncorrected acuity. Uncorrected vision of the left eye was 20/25 "blurry" with refraction of -2.5 + 2 x 080, his best spectacle-corrected vision is 20/25 "blurry." With topography-linked laser ablation, it is hoped that in circumstances such as this, uncorrected and best-corrected vision as well as vision quality will be improved.

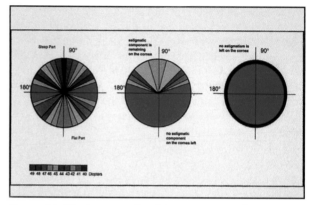

Figure 39-10. An example of the correction of asymmetric astigmatism with the superior hemi-meridian being steeper than the inferior hemi-meridian (left). After standard astigmatic correction, there is residual astigmatism in the superior hemi-meridian (middle). If this type of condition is treated with the topographic-assisted software, the resulting topographic picture is that of the map on the right in which the surface is spherical and of the same dioptric power throughout.

T A B L E 39-1.
REQUIREMENTS FOR TOPOGRAPHY-ASSISTED EXCIMER LASER TREATMENT

Flying spot excimer laser
High hertz pulse repetition rate
Active eye tracking system
Reliable and stable laser head (ceramic tube)
Scanning mirror feedback control
Interface of topography data
Treatment plan to excimer laser hard drive

---

the corneal irregularity. Without an active eye tracking device, the topography-linked treatments are hardly possible since precise placement of the laser pulse will not be guaranteed. An additional welcomed safety feature that the Chiron Vision Technolas 217 C-LASIK laser has is a scanner feedback control, which verifies the correct scanning mirror position before the laser pulse is activated. This device makes certain that the laser pulses are placed exactly at the calculated position referred to by the customized laser ablation.

There are also several requirements of the topography system used to affect accurate topography-assisted ablations. It is essential that the curvature measurements and smoothing algorithms are very precise and the system meets

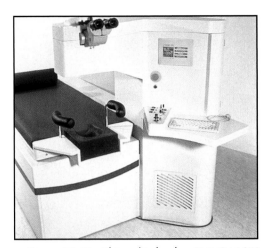

Figure 39-11. Chiron/Technolas 217 C-LASIK Flying Spot excimer laser.

the capability to measure corneal curvatures between at least 30 diopter (D) and 60 D in an effort to cover an exceptionally large range of dioptric powers that are commonly encountered for irregular corneal surfaces. For calculating the exact laser ablation profile on the basis of the topography, the "real" measured topography data is necessary. The initial data calculated by the topography unit typically gives corneal curvature power measured in diopters. It is, therefore, necessary to convert corneal curvature data into height or elevation data. Only with the height data of the corneal surface is the exact calculation of the laser ablation profile possible. With the height data and the spherical and astigmatic refraction, the topography-linked laser treatment is determined by defining the desired postoperative keratometric power reading (k-reading). The postoperative topography is simulated, and finally, the laser ablation is calculated.

Topography-assisted laser ablations can be calculated by entering the desired postoperative k-reading or by making manual adjustments. It is possible to add or subtract laser ablation at any corneal position. This enables the surgeon to design the postoperative cornea individually as desired. The postoperative topography is always calculated. Whether by entering the desired k-reading or designing the cornea by manual adjustments, the postoperative topography calculation becomes the standard for any further changes. Both options (postoperative k-reading and manual adjustments) can be combined for an optimal patient-specific treatment. With this technique, a truly customized treatment becomes reality, which not only treats the refractive error but also has the capability

> A truly customized treatment becomes reality, which not only treats the refractive error but also has the capability to improve the visual acuity of the patient since irregular corneal structure can be removed and a smooth corneal surface can be achieved.

to improve the visual acuity of the patient since irregular corneal structure can be removed and a smooth corneal surface can be achieved.

REAL-TIME TOPOGRAPHY-DIRECTED LASER ABLATIONS

With PRK or LASIK, real-time topography-directed laser ablations are not physically possible at the present time. Topography requires a normal corneal surface to be present for placido ring, raster stereographic, or scanning slit beam topographic systems. Needless to say, with PRK or LASIK, none of these systems can provide useful intraoperative data to direct the active ablation. It is conceivable that if a new technological breakthrough in corneal/intrastromal imaging occurs, this will allow for intraoperative real-time feedback to direct the laser ablation.

TOPOGRAPHY-ASSISTED ABLATION TRIAL CASES

Technolas engineers first tried this technique on polymethylmethacrylate (PMMA) surfaces at the end of 1996 and two examples will be described. The Chiron Vision Technolas 217 C-LASIK laser and the Technomed C-Scan topography system were used. Before the topography-linked treatments were calculated, the topography unit was checked and calibrated on defined regular and irregular surfaces.

Figure 39-12 shows two images: on the right side is the preoperative topography with a steep segment between 0° and 90°. The rest of the surface has a uniform curvature of 43.17 D. With a nonflying spot laser and without a topography link, this irregularity cannot be treated accurately. Only with topography-linked treatments can a uniform curvature be achieved. In this first case, the goal was to smooth the steep area to the same curvature value as the rest of the cornea without changing the overall curvature. Figure 39-13 shows the simulated postoperative topography, which is very close to the real measured one (See Figure 39-12, left map). The desired k-reading after treatment was 43.25 D. The left image, which shows the surface after the laser ablation, illustrates that the treatment was very successful. The surface has a uniform curvature of 43.17 D.

The second example of a topography-linked treatment on PMMA is shown in Figures 39-14 and 39-15. On the right map of Figure 39-14 is the image of a decentered laser treatment. The treatment edge would be inside the pupil in this example. A standard treatment would be very difficult to retreat decentration accurately. For the topography-linked procedure, the target postoperative k-reading was 37.75 D. On the left side of Figure 39-14 is the topography after the laser treatment. Figure 39-15 shows the simulated postoperative topography. Comparing this with the post-treatment

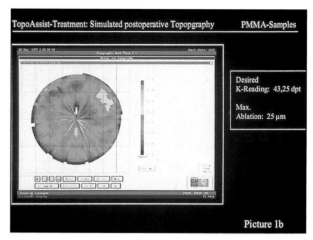

Picture 1a

Figure 39-12. Topography of PMMA irregular surface (right) prior to ablation. Note the steep segment between 0° and 90° on the right topography map. The left-side map reveals topography after topography-assisted ablation.

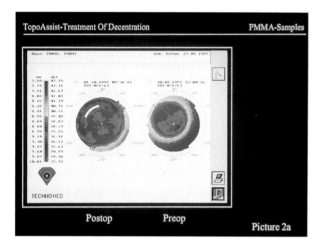

Picture 1b

Figure 39-13. Simulated postoperative topography pre-ablation map planned for Figure 39-12 (right map). It depicts the desired k-reading after treatment as 43.25 and the actual measured k-reading is 43.17 (left map), which is exceptionally close.

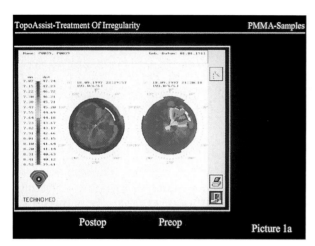

Picture 2a

Figure 39-14. The right map depicts decentered ablation on the PMMA surface with the treatment edge overlaying the pupillary margin. The left map depicts post-treatment topography. The steep edge was moved downward and the central area has a uniform curvature of 37.55 D.

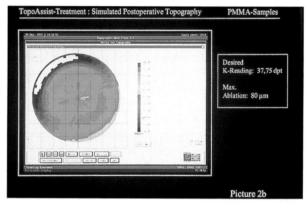

Picture 2b

Figure 39-15. Simulated postoperative topography of the case in Figure 39-14. Target postoperative k-reading was 37.75, and 37.55 was achieved (Figure 39-14, left map).

image, it is evident that they are very close. The edge was completely moved downward and the central area has a uniform curvature of 37.55 D.

TOPOGRAPHY-LINKED PATIENT CASE

Figures 39-16 and 39-17 show the topographies of a human eye treatment done by Prof. Thomas Neuhann of Augenlaserzentrum, Munich, Germany. The patient was a 25-year-old woman. The preoperative topography on the right side shows an irregular surface with a steep section in the lower part of the cornea. She had a refraction of -.75 -1 x 15° and a BCVA of 20/50. Her uncorrected visual acuity (UCVA) was 20/80. Additionally, she had marked subjec-

tive night vision problems. Figure 39-17 depicts the simulated postoperative topography and shows the desired k-reading of 37.5 D. The left side of Figure 39-16 shows the postoperative topography. The irregularity was completely removed and a uniform spherical k-reading of 38 D was achieved with a very small amount of residual topographic astigmatism. Her postoperative UCVA was improved by four lines to 20/40 and her refraction is plano. Her subjective night vision problems have completely resolved.

With these first results, it is evident that the topography-linked refractive laser treatment will be the first treatment type that is capable of improving not only the refractive outcome and UCVA, but also the quality of vision in all patients with marked corneal surface irregularity or in those

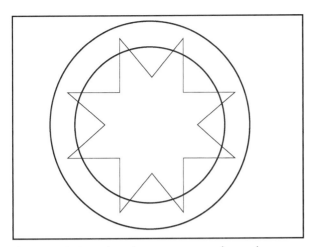

Figure 41-3. A single antitorque suture can be used to secure the disc to the stromal bed; however, this is only used when necessary, as it can induce astigmatism.

lost completely unlike a dislodged flap, which will always be attached to the cornea at the flap hinge.

If the adhesion is considered insufficient, the cap is secured to the corneal bed using a single anti-rotation running suture in 10-0 (Figure 41-3). A protective plastic cup is placed over the eye for at least 24 hours.

ADVANTAGES OF THE REFRACTIVE ABLATION ON THE STROMAL SURFACE OF THE DISC

- The treatment is performed on immobile tissue (no effect from breathing movements or eye-twitching as is the case with LASIK).
- Centering of the photoablative treatment is independent of patient cooperation and is extremely precise because of the preoperative markings.
- Large optical zones can be used because the tissue involved is completely exposed and there are no limits created by the hinge.
- Endothelial damage caused by the laser is avoided because the ablation occurs on the disc.
- In the event of complications, it is possible to perform a lamellar keratoplasty with a homoplastic disc. This is because the complication will usually involve only the disc and not the corneal bed.
- Photokeratomileusis on the disc means that even years later enhancement is possible in eyes that were originally undercorrected. Because of the thickness, it is possible to detach and easily lift the flap; the refractive photoablation can then be performed (in situ or on the stromal face of the disc) to correct any myopic or astigmatic undercorrections.

DISADVANTAGES OF THE TECHNIQUE ON THE FLAP

- The flap must have a certain thickness in order to ensure complete protection of the Bowman's layer from the ablation. The thickness after completion of the ablation must be at least 100 microns in the areas where the ablation is deepest.
- The photoablative treatment is performed on tissue that has been distended artificially and may be unevenly presented. The tissue may be subject to variations in hydration if the operating procedure is prolonged.
- With astigmatic treatment, there is the possibility of errors along the treatment axis because the surgeon has to consider the variation in the axis induced by turning the flap over.
- In the sutureless technique, if the disc detaches postoperatively, it may be lost completely.

INDICATIONS FOR THE BURATTO TECHNIQUE ON THE DISC

The LASIK down-up technique, which Buratto presented in 1996, is currently the most popular procedure for treating refractive defects. As in the LASIK technique with a nasal hinge, the refractive ablation is in situ. The technique with the ablation on the stromal surface of the disc is not often indicated. However, it is a technique that is useful on occasion and therefore provides an option for the refractive surgeon.

- If there is nystagmus or the patient cannot fixate at the laser fixation beam, the surgeon should perform the 360° lamellar cut and the ablation on the stroma of the disc. Alternately, the surgeon can use peribulbar or general anesthesia and ablate in situ without the patient's assistance.
- When a free cap occurs with a cap thickness in excess of 200 microns, a maximal ablation could result in excessive reduction in central thickness of the residual corneal stroma in situ (less than 200 to 250 microns). Free caps, however, are usually associated with thin cuts, and the flap should be replaced. The procedure should then be repeated in 3 months.
- The ablation on the disc can also be used whenever the surgeon feels it is not advisable to perform an in situ ablation, such as when a suitable eye-tracker system is not available or the procedure is prolonged, as in hyperopic LASIK.
- The procedure has great potential in underdeveloped countries, as the ablation can be performed with inexpensive laser machines that are not fitted with an eye-tracker.

- This procedure is particularly useful when superficial corneal opacity involves the superficial 300 to 350 microns of cornea and the eye is also affected by myopia.

  The operation involves a primary cut on the patient's cornea to remove the altered corneal layers; this tissue is then discarded. A second cut is performed on an intact donor bulb (or donor cornea mounted on an artificial anterior chamber) to create a disc of equal diameter and thickness; this is subjected to the refractive ablation on the stromal face to obtain the refractive correction. The homoplastic disc is then sutured into position on the host bulb with a fairly tight anti-torsion suture.

- The operation is also advisable in eyes with abnormally thin corneas and myopia, even though the anatomical shape of the cornea is correct. In this case, Buratto's technique of lamellar keratoplasty of augmented thickness can be used.

  This technique involves the removal of a surface layer from the patient's cornea—about 160 microns for a diameter of approximately 7 mm. This tissue is discarded at the end of the operation. A disc of equal diameter and 300 to 350 micron thickness is then removed from a donor bulb or cornea; this disc is treated on the stromal surface to correct the patient's initial refractive defect. The thick disc then replaces the thinner one (homoplastic keratomileusis with differentiated thickness) and is sutured securely with an anti-rotation suture. This technique can be used to correct even severe myopias without reducing the thickness of the cornea, as the ablation is performed on the stromal surface of the homoplastic disc, which is thick.

- An alternative procedure that gives a better final result involves phototherapeutic keratectomy (a neutral ablation) on the patient's cornea with an optical zone of 7 mm for a depth of 160 microns. Using a disc knife, the cornea is then carved towards the periphery to the depth of the ablation and the homoplastic disc with a thickness greater than the ablation performed (300 to 350 micron) is treated refractively on the stromal surface and applied to the receiving cornea. The periphery of the lamella is undermined into the dissected tissue and sutured. The same procedure can be used with keratoconus in the refractive phase when the cornea is thin, there is superficial opacity, or there is severe myopia combined with intolerance to contact lenses.

CONCLUSION

The results obtained with LASIK for low to severe myopia have created widespread enthusiasm for this technique. As the technique continues to evolve and improve, our techniques of creating the corneal flap have become more consistent and reliable. The most important innovation was the development of the intrastromal refractive ablation using the excimer laser. Buratto was the first to use the excimer laser intrastromally in 1989 and to describe down-up LASIK in 1996. While the application of the excimer ablation in situ is the preferred technique in the vast majority of refractive surgery situations, the technique of ablation on the disc provides some variations on the LASIK technique that can be useful for difficult situations.

CASE 2

Second Cut Complicated with Corneal Resection

Ioannis G. Pallikaris, MD
Theokliti Papadaki, MD
Dimitrios S. Siganos, MD
Crete, Greece

A 19-year-old woman underwent LASIK in OS for the correction of -9.5 -1.75 x 80°. Preoperative BCVA was 20/20. Although the attempted correction aimed at emmetropia, a shift to myopia had been detected throughout the first 3 postoperative months. By 6 months postoperatively, the refractive error had stabilized at -3 -1 x 70°. At the eighth month after the initial operation, the patient sought correction of the residual myopia.

MANAGEMENT

Since retreatment was decided at a relatively late postoperative interval (later than the sixth month), we chose to perform a second flap instead of raising the primary one. Review of the operative data of the initial operation revealed that the Automatic Corneal Shaper (Chiron Vision Corporation, Calif, USA) was used at that time to create an 8.5 mm wide, 133-micron thick, nasally based hinged flap. We decided to use the same microkeratome but to adjust the resection thickness to 200 microns.

INTRAOPERATIVE COMPLICATIONS

The suction ring was placed slightly more nasally than the first time. The microkeratome, therefore, started cutting medially to the borders of the first flap. This resulted in resection of a sphenoid-shaped corneal meniscus approximately .5 mm wide (Figure 42-4). A new hinged flap 8 mm wide and 192 microns thick was created. The operation was completed without any further complications. At the end of the procedure, the flap was repositioned, but the corneal meniscus was too small to be sutured back. An elliptical area of exposed stroma, temporal to the flap borders, had to be left uncovered. A bandage soft contact lens was fitted and the standard postoperative LASIK regime was prescribed.

POSTOPERATIVE COURSE

The contact lens was removed on the fourth postoperative day when re-epithelialization of the exposed area was completed.

Six months after the operation, the patient was satisfied with an uncorrected visual acuity (UCVA) of 20/30. No loss in BCVA was detected. On slit lamp examination, three con-

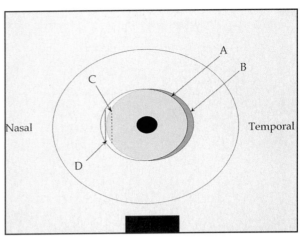

Figure 42-4. Schematic presentation of the intraoperative events. A second deeper, yet not wider, flap was created (yellow). The suction ring was slightly nasally decentered compared to the first time. The microkeratome started cutting medially to the borders of the first flap, which resulted in resection of a sphenoid-shaped corneal meniscus approximately .5 mm wide (blue elliptical area). A = borders of the second flap. B = borders of the first flap. C = hinge of the first flap. D = hinge of the second flap.

centric lines were visible at the temporal corneal periphery. These were, laterally to medially, the scar within the borders of the two flaps corresponding to the area of exposed stroma, the mild punctuate scarring in the area of the sphenoidal corneal resection, and the borders of the ablation (Figure 42-5a). Upon narrowing the beam further, no noticeable corneal thinning was detected (Figure 42-5b), while on retroillumination, the central cornea showed a smooth, even surface (Figure 42-5c).

Computer-assisted corneal topography (Figure 42-6) reveals a steepening of the inferotemporal paracentral zone, probably adjacent to a flatter zone corresponding to the area of corneal resection.

Clinical Note

Unlike photorefractive keratectomy (PRK), regression or undercorrection after LASIK cannot be reversed with steroids. In such cases, a second operation is required. Surgical intervention should be decided as soon as refractive stability is confirmed. The advantage of early retreatment (within 3 to 6 months from the initial operation) is that the flap can be easily raised and manipulated manually. In cases in which retreatment is undertaken later than the sixth postoperative month, we suggest that the most appropriate action is to perform a second thicker and wider cut.

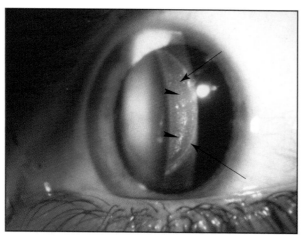

Figure 42-5a. Six months postoperatively. Slit lamp view of the temporal corneal periphery. Three distinct concentric areas are visible: the scar within the borders of the two flaps (long arrow) corresponding to the area of exposed stroma, the mild punctuate scarring in the area of the sphenoidal corneal resection (short arrow), and the borders of the ablation (arrowheads).

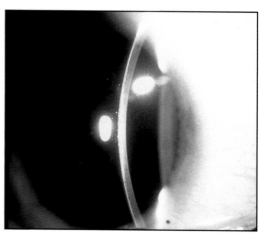

Figure 42-5b. Narrow slit view of the temporal corneal periphery. No noticeable corneal thinning is detected at the area corresponding to the resection.

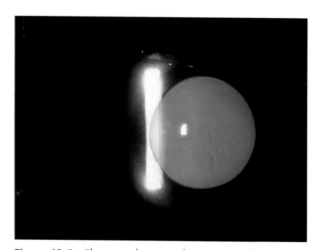

Figure 42-5c. The central cornea shows a smooth, even surface on retroillumination.

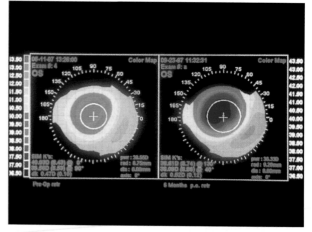

Figure 42-6. Topographic appearance of the cornea prior to retreatment and at 6 months postoperatively.

CASE 3

Free Cap with the FLAPmaker Microkeratome

Ioannis G. Pallikaris, MD
Theokliti Papadaki, MD
Dimitrios S. Siganos, MD
Crete, Greece

A 24-year-old man with a preoperative OD refraction of -10.5 - 4.75 x 25° and a BCVA of 20/30 was scheduled for LASIK.

INTRAOPERATIVE COMPLICATIONS

The FLAPmaker microkeratome was used for the operation. This particular device is adjusted to perform flaps of standard width (approximately 10 mm) and thickness (approximately 160 microns). The shaper head has two sites for connection on its lateral side: a superiorly located opening where the motor that oscillates the blade is locked and an inferiorly located groove for connection with a T-shaped motor that advances the blade (Figure 42-7).

In the present case, the T-shaped motor was inserted but not locked into its site, therefore, as soon as one-third of the actual cut was completed, the motor lost connection to the shaper head and the forward movement of the blade was hindered. This resulted in resection of a corneal meniscus approximately 100 microns thick.

MANAGEMENT

Marking performed prior to the cut helped to properly

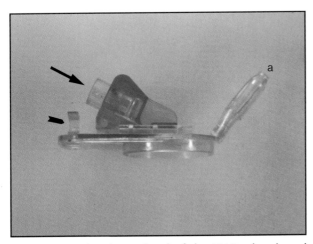

Figure 42-7. The shaper head of the FLAPmaker, lateral view. The arrow indicates the port where the oscillating motor is connected. The arrowhead shows the site where the T-shaped motor is locked once it is connected to the head. In this instance, the motor was unlocked and consequently disconnected from the head during the cut.
a = the connection site of the suction tube.

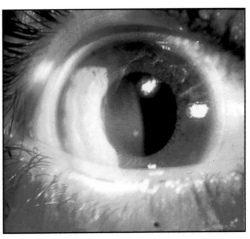

Figure 42-8. On the first postoperative day, the eye, still with the contact lens on, appears white and quiet, and the cornea is clear.

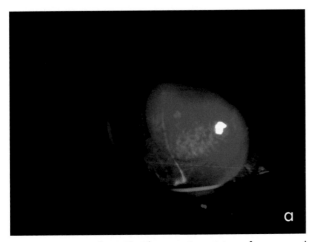

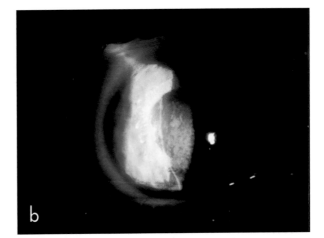

Figures 42-9a and 42-9b. Fluorescein staining after removal of the lens shows a diffuse punctuate epithelial defect and a focal staining at the borders of the half total cap.

align the corneal slice. Dry air was used to enhance attachment of the resected corneal tissue and a bandage soft contact lens was fitted. The routine LASIK postoperative treatment regime was administered.

POSTOPERATIVE COURSE

On the first postoperative day, the eye appeared quiet and the flap was still in position (Figure 42-8). On slit lamp examination, the cornea, when stained with fluorescein, showed a diffuse punctuate epithelial defect and a focal staining at the borders of the free cap (Figures 42-9a and 42-9b). The contact lens was removed on the second postoperative day when the cornea was completely re-epithelialized. Computer-assisted corneal topography revealed almost no alteration of the regular preoperative astigmatic pattern

(Figure 42-10). The patient showed no loss in preoperative BCVA.

A second LASIK was scheduled for 6 months later.

Clinical Note

Marking is the first, and probably one of the most important, steps in LASIK. Not only does it ensure proper repositioning of the hinged flap at the end of the procedure, but it is also crucial in cases of a free cap because it allows for better cap alignment and prevents accidental positioning of the cap with the epithelial side down.

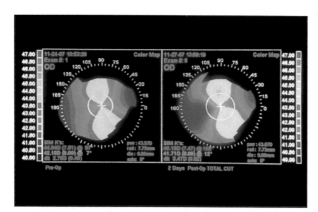

Figure 42-10. Computerized corneal topography shows a minor flattening at the site of the cut, which does not alter the preoperative regular astigmatic pattern.

CASE 4

Thin Cap with the SCMD LASIK TurboKeratome

Ioannis G. Pallikaris, MD
Theokliti Papadaki, MD
Dimitrios S. Siganos, MD
Crete, Greece

A 31-year-old man with a preoperative refraction of -18 -3 x 45° OD underwent myopic LASIK. Preoperative BCVA was correctable to only 20/40.

INTRAOPERATIVE COMPLICATIONS

The SCMD LASIK TurboKeratome System (SCMD, Ariz, USA) was used for the operation. The suction achieved during the cut was inadequate, leading to a resection of a very thin (85 microns) flap with a hinge of only 2 mm. Once the ablation was complete, the flap was repositioned using the dry technique. Air through an air pump was used to enhance attachment to the stromal bed and the cornea was additionally exposed to dry air for 3 minutes. A bandage soft contact lens was placed on the eye and the standard postoperative LASIK regime was prescribed.

EARLY POSTOPERATIVE COMPLICATION

On the first postoperative day, the patient complained of tearing and mild discomfort. The slit lamp examination revealed that, although the contact lens was in place, the flap was detached from the stromal bed and followed the movement of the lens. The flap was also torn from the rest of the cornea so that no hinge could be detected.

An effort was made to suture the total cap back in place, however this was abandoned because the flap was too thin to allow satisfactory alignment. The flap was empirically realigned since the intraoperative markings were no longer visible and the cornea was exposed to dry air for 5 minutes. A bandage soft contact lens was again placed.

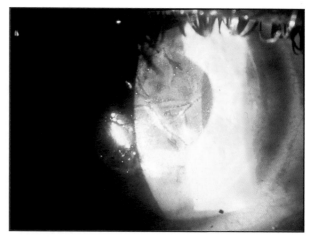

Figure 42-11a. Slit lamp view of the fluorescein-stained cornea 1 week after the operation.

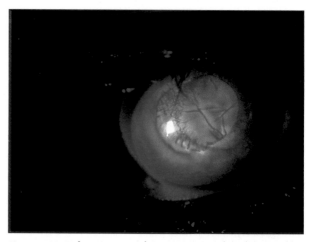

Figure 42-11b. One week postoperatively: the wrinkles became more prominent when the cobalt blue filter was used.

POSTOPERATIVE COURSE

The patient was followed up daily for the first postoperative week. On the seventh postoperative day, the contact lens was removed to reveal a firmly attached, yet extremely wrinkled, corneal cup (Figures 42-11a and 42-11b). A lubricating agent (Tears Naturalle, Alcon) was administered and the patient was followed.

The condition remained stable throughout the first 2 postoperative months. BCVA was reduced to 20/126 with a manifest refraction of -3 -1.75 x 110°. Computer-assisted corneal topography at 2 months postoperatively revealed an irregular induced astigmatism of approximately 7 D oriented at 120° (Figure 42-12).

At the sixth postoperative month visit, the patient reported remarkable improvement in his UCVA (20/80). BCVA had increased to 20/63 (-1.5 -1.5 x 20°) while the central cornea appeared smoother with very few residual wrinkles (Figure 42-13). Comparison of the corneal topog-

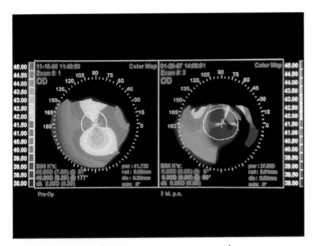

Figure 42-12. Early postoperative topographic appearance of the corneal surface revealed an asymmetrical ablation pattern with nasal steepening of the cornea inducing irregular astigmatism of approximately 7 D oriented at the 120° axis.

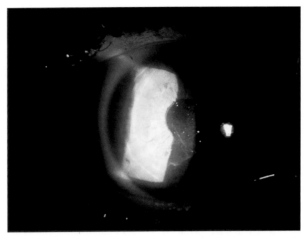

Figure 42-13. Six months postoperatively, a noticeable smoothing of the cornea is detected on slit lamp examination.

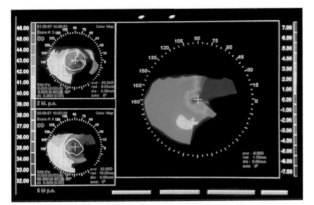

Figure 42-14. The difference map comparing 2 to 6 months postoperatively reveals a shifting of the ablation zone towards the pupil center together with a nasal flattening corresponding to a decrease in induced astigmatism.

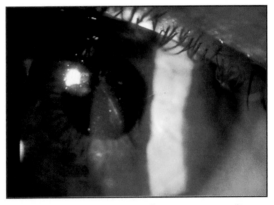

Figure 42-15. Improvement becomes more obvious when the difference between the topographic maps of 2 and 10 months postoperatively is examined. The ablation area becomes more centered and oval, while induced irregular astigmatism can be hardly detected (at least with this scale).

raphy at 6 months to that at 2 months revealed a nasal flattening corresponding to a decrease in irregular astigmatism (Figure 42-14). The cornea became progressively smoother and, at 10 months postoperatively, a round, well-centered ablation area was detected in the corneal topography, while the patient lost only one line of preoperative BCVA (20/63) with a minor residual myopia of -1.5 -1.5 x 20°. The slit lamp appearance of the cornea at 10 months postoperatively is presented in Figures 42-15 and 42-16. Nevertheless, analysis of the Holladay Diagnostic Summary at 10 months postoperatively (Figure 42-17) revealed that distortions ranging from 20/16 to 20/200 are visible within the 3 mm pupil zone (distortion map), indicating a significantly detrimental effect on vision. CU Index = 0%, indicated that the optical quality of the cornea was non-uniform throughout the 3 mm pupil zone. Predicted visual acuity was evaluated as 20/160, which, although not correlating with the patient's actual BCVA, indicated a severely distorted cornea within the 3 mm pupil zone.

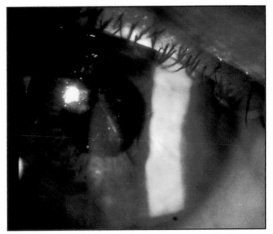

Figure 42-16. At 10 months postoperatively the center of the cornea shows only minor residual wrinkles which, unfortunately, interfere with the visual axis.

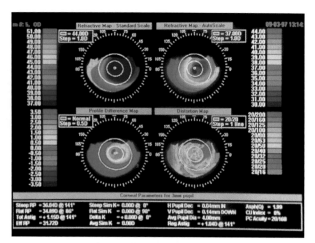

Figure 42-17. The Holladay diagnostic summary at 10 months postoperatively. See text for a detailed analysis.

Clinical Note

Adequate suction must be confirmed prior to the creation of the cut. The cut must not be made unless the suction intraocular pressure exceeds the border level of 65 mm Hg, otherwise the flap created will have a variable and suboptimal thickness because an inadequate amount of tissue will have passed through the suction ring opening.

Flap thickness should ideally range from 130 to 170 microns. Thicker flaps may not leave enough residual stroma for ablation, while thinner ones are difficult to manipulate.

CASE 5

Corneal Cap Soaked in Alcohol

Ioannis G. Pallikaris, MD
Theokliti Papadaki, MD
Dimitrios S. Siganos, MD
Crete, Greece

A 30-year-old woman with a preoperative OD refraction of -14.5 D sph and a BCVA of 20/32 was scheduled for LASIK.

INTRAOPERATIVE COMPLICATIONS

The Automatic Corneal Shaper was used to create an 8 mm wide, 100-micron thick total free cap. The cap was left in the microkeratome slit during the ablation. A member of the operating team, unaware of this, soaked the shaper head into absolute (90°) ethyl alcohol for sterilization purposes. Accidental splash of absolute or nearly absolute ethyl alcohol causes necrosis and opacification of the cornea by inducing protein coagulation and cell death due to abstraction of water.

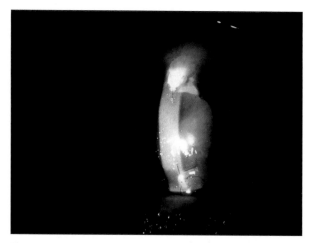

Figure 42-18a. Day 1 postoperatively: the total cap is held in place by two sutures located at 12 and 6 o'clock. Mucin concentration at the site of the sutures is evident.

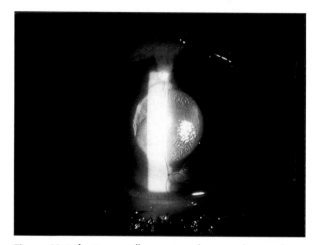

Figure 42-18b. On retroillumination, the central corneal surface corresponding to the cap area appears rough due to a total epithelial defect induced by the chemical burn.

MANAGEMENT

Although the cap was immediately removed from the alcohol and thoroughly irrigated with BSS, severe opacification of the tissue, together with complete epithelial defect, were immediately evident. After the ablation was complete, the damaged corneal tissue was sutured back in place and a bandage soft contact lens was fitted. A lubricating agent was administered along with the routine LASIK postoperative medication, but at a more frequent rate.

POSTOPERATIVE COURSE

The appearance of the cornea on the first postoperative day is shown in Figures 42-18a and 42-18b. Two intermittent sutures were visible at 12 and 6 o'clock, respectively. The sutures were removed at 2 months postoperatively. A noticeable change in corneal topography was detected at 5

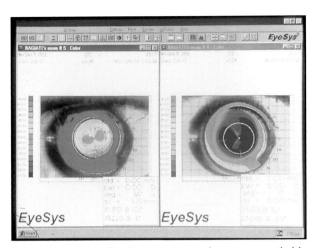

Figure 42-19. The healing process induces a remarkable change in the topographic appearance of the cornea from 1 to 5 months.

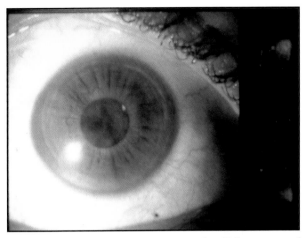

Figure 42-20a. One year postoperatively: slit lamp view of the cornea with direct diffuse illumination barely detects a mild central clouding of the cornea.

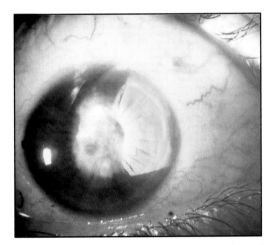

Figure 42-20b. One year postoperatively: a broad slit beam directed obliquely towards the corneal surface helped identify a severe corneal opacification.

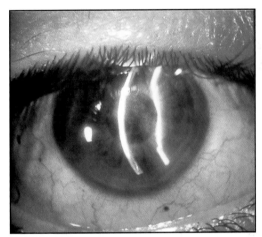

Figure 42-20c. One year postoperatively: a narrow slit beam revealed that the opacification was limited to the anterior stroma (ie, was not extending deeper than the interface).

months (Figure 42-19) .and a steepening of the whole central corneal part of approximately 9 D was detected. This change probably reflects the healing activity in the area of the burned tissue. One year after the operation, the patient still complained of blurred vision. The eye experienced a loss of three lines in BCVA, and slit lamp examination revealed a cloudy central cornea with full thickness opacification of the corneal cap (Figures 42-20a, 42-20b and 42-20c). Analysis of the Holladay Diagnostic Summary at 12 months postoperatively (Figure 42-21) revealed a perfectly centered ovoid 5-mm ablation zone with no irregular astigmatism present. The optical quality of the corneal surface within the 3-mm pupil zone appeared to be excellent (distortion map). Within the 6-mm ablation zone, however, distortions ranging from 20/16 to 20/125 were visible. The CU Index was 40%, indicative of a non-uniform cornea throughout the 3-mm pupil zone, while predicted corneal

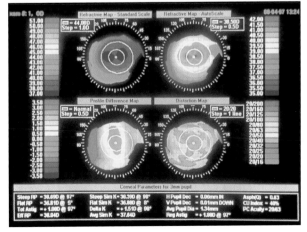

Figure 42-21. The Holladay Diagnostic Summary at 1 year postoperatively.

acuity is evaluated as 20/63, which corresponds exactly to the patient's actual BCVA in this eye.

SUGGESTED FURTHER SURGICAL INTERVENTION

Prior to proceeding to more radical and invasive procedures, such as penetrating corneal keratoplasty, and since the opacification was limited to the anterior 100 microns of the stroma, we suggest that a PRK over a photoablatable lenticular module as a masking agent should be tried in order to restore corneal clarity. Homoplastic lamellar grafting is another option.

CASE 6

Corneal Cap Torn in Half

Ioannis G. Pallikaris, MD
Theokliti Papadaki, MD
Dimitrios S. Siganos, MD
Crete, Greece

A 22-year-old man with a preoperative refraction of -13.75 - .75 x 30° and a BCVA of only 20/63 underwent myopic LASIK in OS.

INTRAOPERATIVE COMPLICATION

The Automatic Corneal Shaper microkeratome was used to resect a total cap 7.5 mm wide and 180 microns thick. To avoid excessive handling and dehydration, the flap was left in the microkeratome slit during ablation. At the end of the ablation, an effort was made to pull the corneal cap out of the slit without hydrating the cap with BSS or disassembling the microkeratome. During this manipulation, the partially dehydrated flap was rubbed against the blade and cut in two.

MANAGEMENT

The operation was completed without any further complications. Proper marking, which was performed prior to the cut, allowed the satisfactory mounting and alignment of the chopped corneal disc. A bandage soft contact lens was placed on the eye and the standard postoperative LASIK treatment regime was prescribed (Figures 42-22a through 42-22c).

SUGGESTED FURTHER SURGICAL INTERVENTION

The most appropriate action is to wait until refraction is stable. It is only then, and never earlier than the third postoperative month, that one should consider reoperation. We propose a second LASIK with an intended flap thickness of

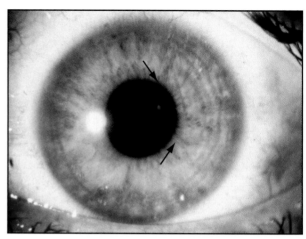

Figure 42-22a. On direct diffuse illumination, linear scarring is just visible at the upper temporal corneal quadrant (arrows).

200 microns. A superiorly hinged flap may prove safer than a nasally based one in order to not accidentally detach the primary cap.

IMPORTANT NOTE

The patient's fellow eye had been operated on 1 year earlier. This operation was also complicated with a small total cap. It is important to notice in the preoperative topography (Figure 42-23) if the cornea is very flat (steepest k-reading: 39.3 D). In the case of a very flat cornea, it is advisable to pre-estimate the diameter of the flap to be resected using applanator lenses. This allows for adjustment of the hinge position so that the risk of a total cap is diminished.

Clinical Note

Excessive handling of a total cap should be avoided. In addition to the defects that excessive handling can produce and the potential of overhydration or dehydration, differentiation of the epithelial and stromal surfaces can become extremely difficult.

The best action when facing a total cap is to leave the cap undisturbed in the microkeratome slit during the laser ablation and have an assistant instill one drop of BSS every 5 seconds in order to prevent dehydration.

Careful inspection of the microkeratome head after every cut and immediately informing the surgical team in cases of a total cap should prevent accidental cap loss or inappropriate handling of the corneal cap.

Applanator lenses used to pre-estimate the diameter of the flap to be resected may diminish the risk of a total cap, especially in eyes with very flat corneas.

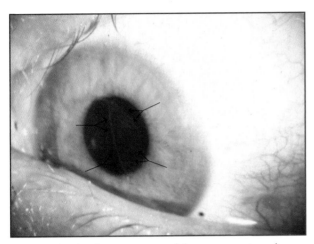

Figure 42-22b. The two pieces of the cap are viewed more easily from the lateral side (arrows demarcating the smaller piece).

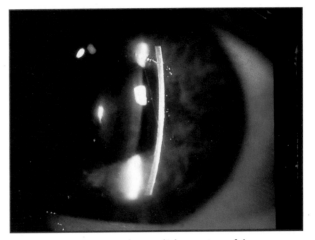

Figure 42-22c. Narrow beam slit lamp view of the area corresponding to the junction between the two corneal pieces indicates no significant alteration in corneal thickness.

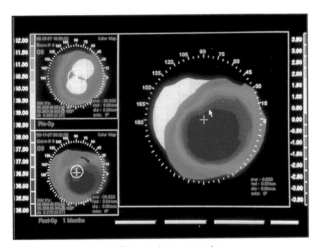

Figure 42-23. The differential topographic map comparing the preoperative pattern to that obtained at 1 month postoperatively.

CASE 7

Flap Striae

Ioannis G. Pallikaris, MD
Theokliti Papadaki, MD
Dimitrios S. Siganos, MD
Crete, Greece

A 25-year-old woman underwent LASIK in OD for the correction of -9.75 - 1.50 x 90°. OS was simultaneously operated with astigmatic PRK for the correction of -7.5 D sph - 1.5 D cyl x 85°. Preoperative BCVA was the same in both eyes (20/25).

OPERATIVE DATA

The procedure was completed successfully. The Automatic Corneal Shaper microkeratome was used to cut a 8.5 mm wide and 160-micron thick flap. This was repositioned using the dry technique. Reattachment was enhanced by exposing the cornea to dry air for a few seconds. The eye was left unpatched.

POSTOPERATIVE COURSE

The corneal topography at the same interval reveals a well-centered flattening of the central cornea of approximately 7 D. (Figure 42-24a and 42-24b).

In the early postoperative period, the patient complained of blurred vision in the LASIK eye, which did not improve with time. At the third postoperative month's examination, achieved correction was within emmetropia (+1.5 - 1.5 x 90°), yet one line loss in BCVA was detected (20/32). The Ast-PRK eye, although presenting the expected hyperopic shift (+4 - .75 x 90°), had reached a UCVA equal to the BCVA (20/25). The difference map between 2 days and 3 months postoperatively in OD revealed nothing but a satisfactorily centered, round 5-mm ablation zone and confirmed a progressive steepening of the central cornea due to a normal healing response (Figure 42-25). On retroillumination, flap striae were prominent and created an uneven corneal surface of poor optical quality (Figure 42-26), when compared to the smooth surface of the fellow PRK eye (Figure 42-27).

MANAGEMENT

The loss in BCVA was attributed to the anterior corneal surface undulations. The decision was made to raise and realign the flap.

The Holladay Diagnostic Summary prior to flap retreatment (Figure 42-28) indicated that the optical quality of the corneal surface within the 3 mm pupil zone was adequate with minimal distortion (distortion map). A CU index of 60%, however, indicated a non-uniform cornea throughout the 3 mm pupil zone, while PC acuity was evaluated as 20/40, which corresponded well to the patient's actual BCVA in this eye.

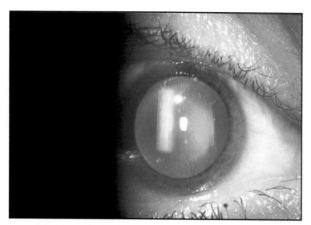

Figure 42-24a. On the second postoperative day fine vertical striae can be detected within the flap area.

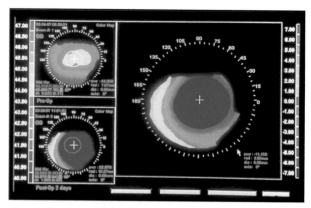

Figure 42-24b. Difference map comparing the preoperative corneal topographic pattern to that obtained immediately postoperatively.

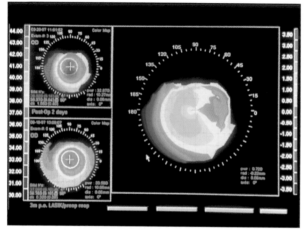

Figure 42-25. Difference map showing the topographic changes throughout the first 3 postoperative months.

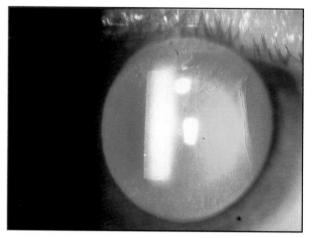

Figure 42-26. Three months postoperatively: flap striae are prominent on retroillumination creating an uneven corneal surface of poor optical quality.

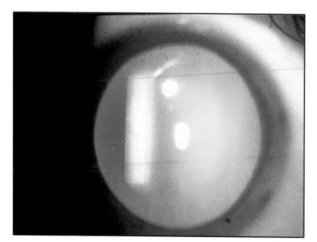

Figure 42-27. Three months postoperatively: compare the previous picture to this one, which presents the smooth, even surface of the PRK fellow eye.

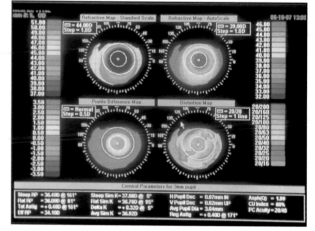

Figure 42-28. The Holladay Diagnostic Map prior to repositioning.

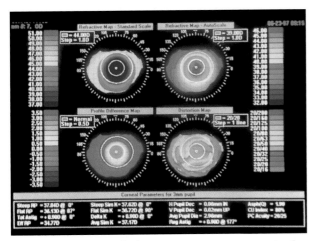

Figure 42-29. The Holladay Diagnostic Map 1 month after repositioning.

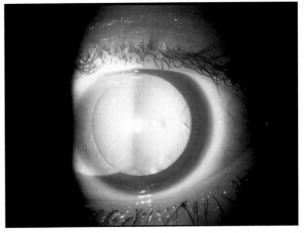

Figure 42-30. Slit lamp view of the corneal surface 1 month after repositioning.

On the first postoperative day after flap repositioning, the Holladay map confirmed that uniformity of the corneal surface had reached normal levels (CU index = 80%), while potential visual acuity had increased to 20/25 (Figure 42-29). One month after reoperation, a BCVA of 20/25 had been achieved with a correction of +1.5 - 1.50 x 80°. A smoother anterior corneal surface was detectable with slit lamp examination (Figure 42-30).

Clinical Note

Flap striae are more common when using the dry technique. The patient should be re-evaluated under the operating microscope 30 to 60 minutes after the operation to ensure proper alignment of the flap. A misaligned or striated flap should be lifted back and repositioned immediately since it may cause loss in BCVA and induce irregular astigmatism.

Postponing repositioning is pointless since flap striation is not a self-limiting condition. On the other hand, delayed intervention may involve permanent damage to Bowman's membrane with subsequent failure of any attempt to realign the flap and eliminate the striae.

CASE 8

Eccentric Ablation and Undercorrection

Ioannis G. Pallikaris, MD
Theokliti Papadaki, MD
Dimitrios S. Siganos, MD
Crete, Greece

A 25-year-old woman underwent LASIK in OD for the correction of -14.5 - 2.25 x 40°. BCVA was 20/40. Preoperative appearance of the eye is presented in Figure 42-31. The Automatic Corneal Shaper microkeratome was used to create a 8.5-mm wide and 150-micron thick flap.

Immediately prior to the ablation, the patient became very anxious and burst into tears. Instead of interrupting the procedure until the patient's composure was restored, the surgeon chose to immediately proceed with the ablation. Ablation was interrupted, and the ablation mask was removed and recentered twice in order to dry the stromal surface with microsponges.

Nineteen months postoperatively, the eye presented an undercorrection of -5.5 - 4.75 x 165° with no loss in BCVA (Figures 42-32a and 42-32b). Furthermore, the patient experienced glare and halos, especially in dim light, and asthenopic symptoms even when corrected with glasses. Computer-assisted corneal topography revealed an eccentricity pattern in which the center of the map was situated outside the area of mean refractive power (middle green) and one quadrant of the 3 mm pupil zone was out of the green encircled area (Figure 42-33). These characteristics correspond to category E2A of Pallikaris' classification.

Management

A second thicker flap (160 microns) was created using the Automatic Corneal Shaper microkeratome. Subsequently, diagonal ablation was applied for correction of the eccentricity. Attempted correction was -6 D with a 6 mm optical zone. The center of the diagonal ablation was placed on the decentration axis 2 mm superiorly from the pupil. A supplementary arcuate cut of 90° radius centered along the decentration axis but situated at 180° opposite the direction of decentration was performed at the borders of the new flap in order to enhance the ablation zone. A bandage soft contact lens was fitted and the routine LASIK postoperative regime was administered.

Postoperative Course

On the fist postoperative day, the eye was quiet (see Figure 42-32b). A noticeable change was detected in corneal topography (see Figure 42-33) in that a new ablation zone 6

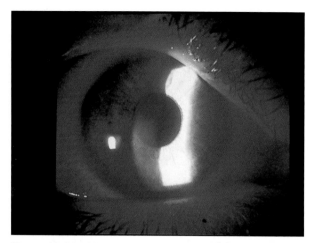

Figure 42-31. Preoperative appearance of the eye.

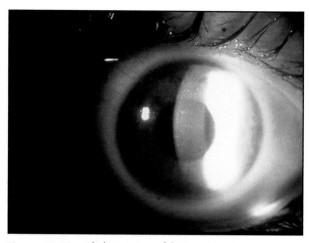

Figure 42-32a. Slit lamp view of the eye prior to retreatment.

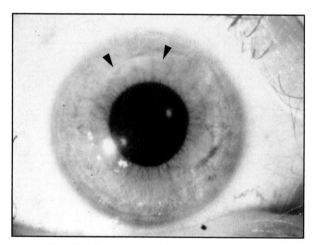

Figure 42-32b. Slit lamp view of the eye on the first day after retreatment. A thin, perfectly arcuate line (arrows) just indicates the area of the cut.

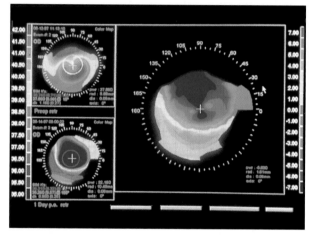

Figure 42-33. Corneal topographic difference map comparing the topographic map prior to retreatment to that obtained at the immediate post-retreatment interval.

D deeper, but perfectly centered, could be seen. The slight shifting of the borders of the zone at the upper temporal quadrant corresponded exactly to the area of the arcuate cut.

At 6 months postoperatively, the patient reported marked improvement in vision. UCVA was 20/50, while BCVA was 20/40 with a correction of +3 - 1.5 x 145°. On slit lamp examination, the cornea showed mild interface opacities and pigment deposits that did not interfere with the visual axis (Figure 42-34a), while on narrow slit beam, a cornea of even thickness was detected (Figure 42-34b). At the upper temporal corneal periphery, three concentric lines can be seen. Superiorly to inferiorly, these are

1. the linear scarring of the cut
2. the borders of the second flap
3. the borders of the diagonal ablation (Figures 42-35 and 42-36)

Corneal topography at the sixth postoperative month showed a slight inferior shifting (Figure 42-37). This alteration represents the expected partial reversal of the relaxing effect of the arcuate cut with time due to healing of the epithelium and scarring within the area of the cut.

Clinical Note

Excessive lacrimation and inability of the patient to follow the surgeon's directions and fixate properly are reasons for interrupting the procedure in order to diminish the risk of undercorrection due to excessive hydration or decentration. In these cases, the most appropriate action is to replace the flap to its original position and proceed as soon as the patient is able to cooperate. With the flap in place, the cornea can be irrigated without affecting stromal hydration.

The same management is also recommended in cases in which there is a time lapse between creation of the flap and laser ablation (ie, temporary laser failure) in order to avoid stromal dehydration, which could result in overcorrection.

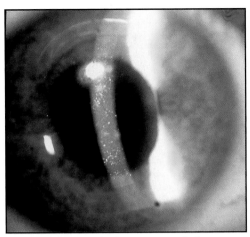

Figure 42-34a. Slit lamp view of the eye 6 months after retreatment. Mild opacities and pigment deposits are detected in the interface though they do not interfere with the visual axis.

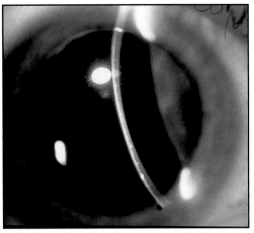

Figure 42-34b. Narrow slit view of the eye 6 months after retreatment. No noticeable corneal thinning is detected.

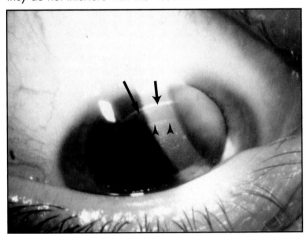

Figure 42-35. At the upper temporal corneal periphery, three concentric lines can be detected. Superiorly to inferiorly, these are: 1.) the linear scarring at the site of the cut (small arrow); 2.) the borders of the second flap (big arrow); 3.) the borders of the diagonal ablation (arrowheads).

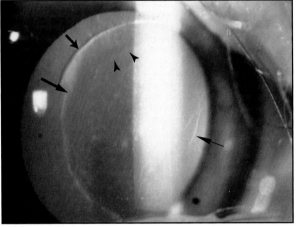

Figure 42-36. View of the upper temporal periphery of the corneal surface on retroillumination. The same three zones can be easily distinguished. Additionally, a few striae radiating from the hinge can be detected (small arrow).

CASE 9

Epithelial Ingrowth Following LASIK

Ioannis G. Pallikaris, MD
Theokliti Papadaki, MD
Dimitrios S. Siganos, MD
Crete, Greece

A 45-year-old woman underwent LASIK in OS for the correction of -16.5 - 0.75 x 75°. The BCVA was 20/20.

The Automatic Corneal Shaper microkeratome was used to create a flap 8 mm wide and 161 microns thick. Apart from a small irregularity at the borders of the temporal edges of the flap, no other intraoperative complications were recorded.

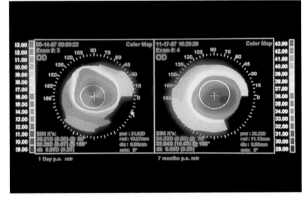

Figure 42-37. Corneal topography at the sixth postoperative month shows a slight shifting of the ablation zone inferiorly. This alteration corresponds with the partial reverse of the relaxing effect of the arcuate cut with time. The latter is caused by the normal healing process that results in sealing the cut.

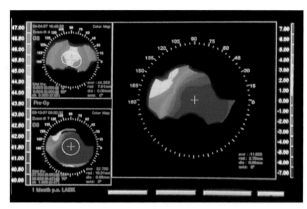

Figure 42-38a. The differential map comparing pre-operative to 1-month postoperative topographic patterns reveals an inferotemporal decentration of the ablation zone.

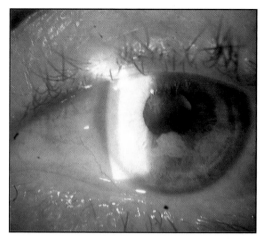

Figure 42-38b. On slit lamp examination, interface accumulation of dense exogenic material is detected in two sites in the central and paracentral zone of the cornea.

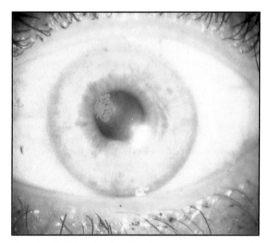

Figure 42-39a. In the third postoperative month, the central focus seems to be growing in size and density, while in the paracentral focus, the cells tend to coalesce and melt.

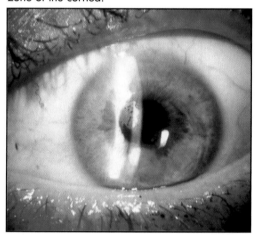

Figure 42-39b. Third postoperative month: narrow beam view reveals that the epithelial accumulation is located within the interface.

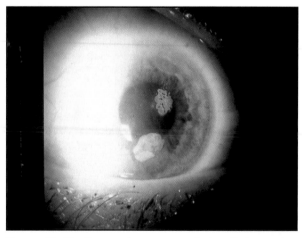

Figure 42-40. Six months postoperatively: slit lamp view shows no further growth of the accumulation. On the contrary, the cells within the ingrowth seem to coalesce, forming a liquid mass demarcated by a surrounding groove.

The preoperative and 1-month postoperative topographic patterns are compared in Figure 42-38a. The wide, dark blue area corresponding to the ablation zone is inferotemporally decentered, while no irregularities within the ablation zone can be detected on this scale. On slit lamp examination (Figure 42-38b), interface accumulation of dense exogenic material was detected in two sites in the central and paracentral zones of the cornea. The patient experienced a loss of two lines in BCVA, which was 20/32 with a correction of +2 -4 x 90°.

At the third postoperative month, refraction remained stable, although on slit lamp examination, the central material seemed to be growing in size and density, while in the paracentral material, the cells tended to coalesce and melt (Figures 42-39a and 42-39b).

Further deterioration in vision was detected at the sixth postoperative month interval. BCVA had reduced to 20/40 with a correction of +3.75 - 4.75 x 130°. Slit lamp view of

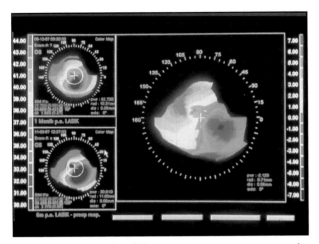

Figure 42-41. On the difference map a steepening at the temporal half of the cornea is detected from 1 to 6 months postoperatively, corresponding to the areas of material accumulation.

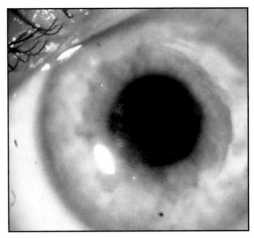

Figure 42-42. Four days after epithelial removal: a mild opacification just indicates the areas where the epithelial accumulations have been located.

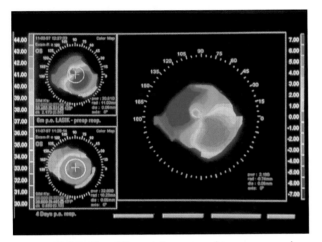

Figure 42-43. The differential topographic map reveals a marked flattening of the area corresponding to the removed material and a simultaneous steepening of the opposite inferotemporal half of the cornea.

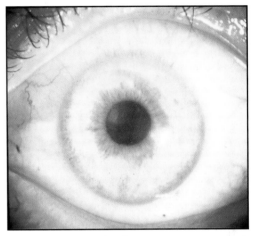

Figure 42-44. In the first postoperative month after retreatment, the cornea appears clear at slit lamp examination.

the cornea at 6 months is presented in Figure 42-40. The change in corneal topography from 1 to 6 postoperative months is presented in Figure 42-41. A steepening at the temporal half of the cornea was detected corresponding to the areas of material accumulation. Steepening was more prominent at the upper temporal quadrant, indicating the location of the growing focus.

MANAGEMENT

In order to prevent further vision loss, we decided to remove the material. The flap was partially detached from the bed until the areas of accumulation were exposed. The exogenic material was then scraped away from the bed and the stromal side of the flap using the aspiration-irrigation cannula. Both surfaces were thoroughly irrigated with BSS, the flap was sealed back using dry air, and a bandage soft

contact lens was applied. Microscopic examination of a smear taken from the material removed showed that the latter consisted mainly of dead epithelial cells.

POSTOPERATIVE COURSE

The appearance of the cornea 4 days after retreatment is presented in Figure 42-42. A mild opacification indicates the areas where the epithelial accumulations were located. The differential topographic map revealed a marked flattening of the area corresponding to the removed material and a simultaneous steepening of the opposite inferotemporal half of the cornea (Figure 42-43).

For the first postoperative month after retreatment, the cornea retained normal clarity (Figure 42-44), while BCVA was restored to 20/25 with a correction of +2.75 D sph -4 D cyl x 110°.

Clinical Note

Epithelial ingrowth at the outer edge of a hinged flap can be left undisturbed unless it induces irregular astigmatism, causes a flap melt, or extends centrally and affects visual acuity, at which time it should be removed.

CASE 10

Corneal Perforation Following LASIK and AK

Michael Lawless, MBBS, FRACO, FRACS, FRCOphth
Sydney, Australia

A 40-year-old man in good health had bilateral corneal transplants for keratoconus in 1976. Both grafts were of a small 7.25 mm diameter. When first assessed in March 1995, the spectacle-corrected vision was 20/30 OD and 20/200 OS; both eyes were contact lens intolerant. The grafts, although of small diameter, were healthy, but the left had a combination of regular and irregular astigmatism. With the best correction of +2 -12 at 120°, the vision could be improved to 20/50 OS. The vision with pinhole was 20/40.

In August 1995, I performed a surface ablation using a disposable disc with a Summit Apex Plus system of -5 at axis 120° using a transepithelial approach. This was combined with two relaxing incisions in the steep axis at 30° just inside the graft/host scar at a depth of 450 microns. This improved his unaided vision to 20/200 and a BCVA of 20/30 with a refraction of -2 -6 at 120°.

In October 1997, nearly 2 years later, the patient presented again requesting further surgery to his left eye. The UCVA was count fingers, and with -2 -7 at 120°, he could achieve 20/30. The cornea was still healthy with no haze from the previous surface ablation and endothelial cell count was good. His topography (Figure 42-45) demonstrated a steep axis on Simulated K at 24° and 11 D of topographic astigmatism with significant irregularity.

The decision was made to proceed with a left toric LASIK in combination with arc incisions in the steep refractive axis at 30°. This was performed in December 1997. A 180-micron plate was used with the Chiron ACS microkeratome to create a flap with a nasal hinge. The laser portion of the procedure was then performed without difficulty with an ablatable disc. The two arcuate incisions were to be at a depth of 450 microns and axis 30° for a length of 45° just inside the old graft/host scar. The first incision was placed without difficulty in the steep axis superotemporally. On placing the blade for the inferonasal incision, a microperforation occurred. The blade was immediately withdrawn. The anterior chamber shallowed with the microperforation and then formed over approximately 1 minute. The incision

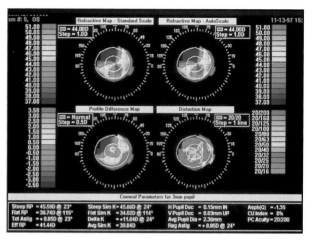

Figure 42-45. Topographic astigmatism with significant irregularity is present after PRK, and AK was used to treat residual astigmatism following a penetrating keratoplasty.

was not completed, but the bed and undersurface of the cap were irrigated, and the cap was repositioned without difficulty. A disposable contact lens was applied because of the microperforation. No patch was used and a shield was placed on the eye overnight.

The next morning the anterior chamber was flat with the iris and lens touching against the cornea. The patient was returned to the operating room, the flap was lifted, and viscoelastic was placed through the microperforation to reform the anterior chamber. Three interrupted sutures were placed in the area of the microperforation, which was just inside the graft/host scar inferonasally. There was no residual leak and the cap was repositioned without difficulty. One hour later, the anterior chamber was formed and there was no leak, so a shield was applied and follow-up was arranged for the next day. The next day, the anterior chamber was formed but slightly shallow; however, there was no detectable leak around the cap.

Two days later, the anterior chamber was flat with no obvious leakage of aqueous. The patient was returned to the operating room that evening. The cap was lifted and again viscoelastic was placed through the previous microperforation. It was not obvious where the leak was occurring. The old graft/host scar was tending to split with an area of ectasia beyond the three interrupted sutures. There was no leak from this area, but because of the ectasia, four more interrupted sutures were placed at either end of the previously sutured microperforation. The anterior chamber remained formed for more than 5 minutes, and the cap was repositioned and secured with two interrupted sutures. The patient was checked 1 hour later showing a deep anterior chamber and no sign of a leak.

The next morning, the anterior chamber was once again flat with the lens and iris touch against the cornea. The patient was taken back to the operating room, the cap sutures were removed and the cap lifted. At this stage, the

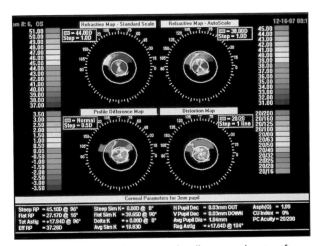

Figure 42-46. Corneal topography illustrates the significant irregular astigmatism after corneal perforation and multiple corneal sutures.

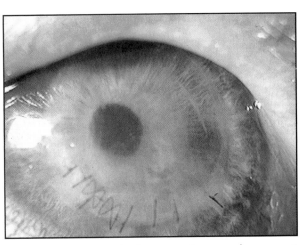

Figure 42-47. Despite the four operative procedures over 1 week, the cap was well-positioned and the anterior chamber deep. The previous AK is visible supranasally. The multiple sutures were required to arrest the wound leak.

anterior chamber was reformed with BSS through the previous microperforation. Once formed, a paracentisis was performed in the host cornea. BSS was then placed through the host cornea and fluorescein applied to detect the area of leakage. There was no obvious leak in the old graft/host scar nor at the site of microperforation. There was a slight suture track leak from one of the interrupted sutures. It was again noted that the area of graft/host scar seemed to have split and was ectatic for about 6 clock hours—more so than it had been on the previous day.

The interrupted suture with the track leak was removed and two overlay cross sutures were placed in this area. Additional interrupted sutures were placed in the area of graft/host scar ectasia. The anterior chamber was formed with BSS through the paracentisis. No leak was observed and the cap was repositioned and again resutured with two interrupted sutures. After a further 5 minutes of observation, there was no obvious leak from beneath the cap.

The next day, the anterior chamber was formed with no leak. The patient was next seen 6 days later. The UCVA was count fingers and did not improve with pinhole. Corneal topography (Figure 42-46) showed significant vertical steepening and irregular astigmatism. The cornea was remarkably clear considering the tumultuous week of four operative procedures. The cap was well-positioned and the anterior chamber was deep (Figure 42-47).

What started out as a relatively minor refractive LASIK procedure with arc incisions in a post-graft setting turned into a series of serious consequences requiring multiple surgeries to restore the corneal integrity. It is not certain that this corneal graft will survive, and even if it does, it may have intolerable regular and irregular astigmatism.

CASE 11

Homoplastic Lamellar Graft for Recurrent Haze After PRK

John F. Doane, MD
Kansas City, Missouri, USA

This 42-year-old caucasian male is a computer software programmer who underwent refractive surgery due to contact lens intolerance and the desire to be less dependent on spectacles. His preoperative refraction was -9 D OU with a BCVA of 20/20 OU. He underwent his initial uncomplicated PRK procedure in September 1995 with target plano OD and -1 sphere OS.

Six months postoperatively, his uncorrected vision was 20/200 OD and 20/60 OS. Manifest refraction revealed -3.5 +1.25 x 120 OD for BCVA of 20/40 and -1 + 1 x 075 OS for a BCVA of 20/30. Slit lamp examination revealed 2+ central corneal haze OD and 1+ paracentral haze OS. Due to his undercorrection and haze, the patient elected to undergo PRK enhancement OD.

Twelve months after the PRK enhancement OD, examination revealed UCVA of 20/200 OD and 20/40 OS. Manifest refraction was -5 + 1 x 115 for a BCVA of 20/70 OD and -1 + .25 x 87 for a BCVA of 20/40 OS. Slit lamp examination revealed 3+ central corneal haze OD (Figures 42-48 and 42-49) and 1+ paracentral haze OS. Central pachymetry was 568 microns OD and 521 microns OS. The patient had been on aggressive topical corticosteroids after the enhancement. Despite this regimen, the patient had recurrent haze that was significantly worse than after the initial operation. He was very unhappy with this situation since his dominant eye had poor BCVA, which made driving a car difficult. He also had significant scotopic visual

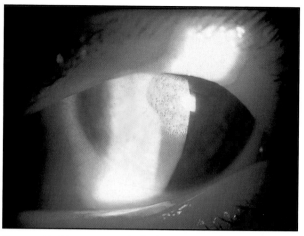

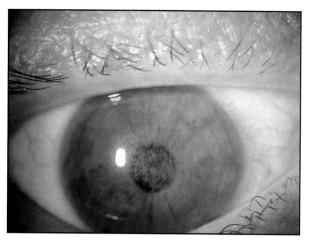

Figure 42-48. Slit lamp biomicroscope view of the right eye prior to lamellar keratectomy after two excimer laser PRK procedures.

Figure 42-49. Tangential slit lamp view of the right eye revealing dense central corneal haze after two excimer laser PRK procedures.

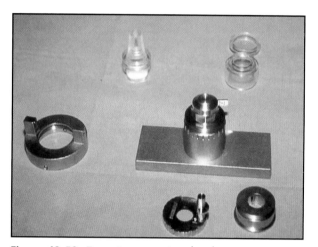

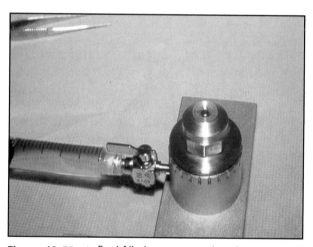

Figure 42-50. Four-piece anterior chamber maintainer set for the Automatic Corneal Shaper. Antidesiccation chamber (left) and Barraquer tonometer (right) are also pictured.

Figure 42-51. A fluid-filled syringe is placed on stopcock and fluid fills the reservoir.

disturbances of glare and halos. He felt he was unable to satisfactorily complete the tasks of his occupation and wanted active intervention to be considered. He was instructed that his three options would be expectant observation for resolution, repeat PRK, or homoplastic lamellar grafting. The patient strongly opposed repeat PRK or expectant observation.

The patient underwent sutureless homoplastic lamellar grafting of the right eye. A 180-micron thick, 7-mm diameter keratectomy was completed with the Chiron ACS. The host tissue was harvested from a donor corneoscleral rim with an anterior chamber maintainer (Chiron Vision, Irvine, Calif) (Figures 42-50 through 42-54). This device is unique because it has a geared track analogous to the geared suction ring that allows for a constant speed of microkeratome passage for donor lenticle harvesting. Postoperatively, a clear shield was placed over the orbit and the patient was prescribed Tobradex (Alcon Laboratories, Fort Worth, Tex) qid for 5 days.

One day postoperatively, the patient was comfortable with 20/200 uncorrected vision. Manifest refraction revealed -6.75 + .25 x 130 for 20/30 acuity. Slit lamp examination revealed a clear cornea and well-positioned sutureless graft (Figures 42-55 and 42-56). Four months post-lamellar grafting, the patient's refraction was -7.5 sphere. LASIK was performed using a standard nomogram with a target refraction of plano. Six months post-LASIK, his uncorrected vision is 20/20 minus, and with refraction of +.25 + .25 x 135, his vision is 20/15. He is fully functional with no visual complaints.

This case highlights several points pertinent to the differences in excimer laser surgical techniques, the utility of lamellar corneal surgical techniques, the management of excimer laser complications, and unmet patient expectations. This patient's personality and lifestyle are quite typical for an elective self-pay surgical procedure. This patient was a classical "type-A" personality that wanted excellent

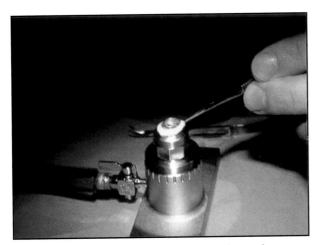

Figure 42-52. A corneoscleral rim is placed over the anterior chamber maintainer reservoir.

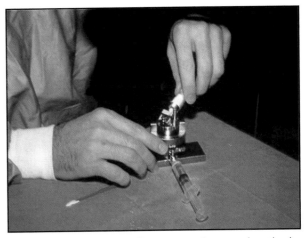

Figure 42-53. The lamellar cap is harvested with the Automatic Corneal Shaper.

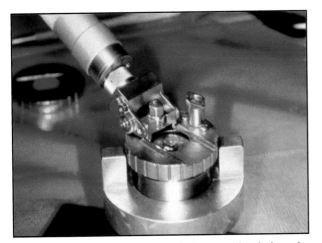

Figure 42-54. Automatic Corneal Shaper is loaded on the geared track stage of the anterior chamber maintainer.

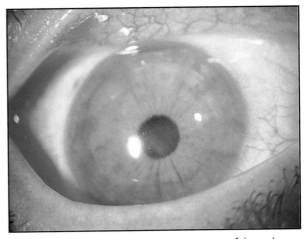

Figure 42-55. Slit lamp biomicroscope views of the right eye 1 day after a sutureless homoplastic lamellar graft.

UCVA. In the end, these became the guiding factors for clinical decision-making.

Visual loss secondary to corneal haze formation with surface PRK tends to be more likely with larger refractive errors treated, although significant visual loss rarely occurs with PRK for low myopia (< 3 D). Visual loss due to haze with lamellar refractive surgical techniques, especially LASIK, is exceedingly uncommon and is one factor favoring a lamellar technique over PRK. Once visually significant haze has formed with PRK, it is quite common for retreatment with a surface excimer laser to be recommended.

This approach requires that the patient instill topical corticosteroids for several months. After the initial surgery, the medical regimen is rigorous. To go through this a second time can be physically and mentally exhausting for the typical patient that has a busy family and professional life. Additionally, since the patient is subject to several more months of topical corticosteroids, there is a potential risk of significant IOP elevation and cataract formation. If haze recurs after the second operation, the patient will be utterly

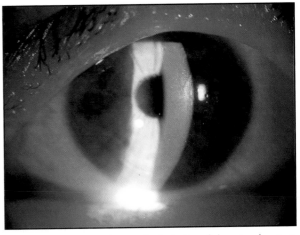

Figure 42-56. Note the marked clarity of the visual axis 1 day following the homoplastic lamellar graft compared to the preoperative figures.

disappointed with what he or she perceived preoperatively to be a relatively hassle-free "high-tech" laser refractive surgical technique that was going to be lifestyle enhancing.

A lamellar graft followed by LASIK for the residual refractive error may not be the choice of many surgeons; however, in this case the options were limited. The patient's preoperative expectations of excellent uncorrected vision have been met. While surface PTK/PRK for haze is relatively simple, it requires considerable effort for the patient to adhere to the postoperative regimen of topical corticosteroids and carries the risk of IOP elevation and cataract formation. Using lamellar corneal surgical techniques, quick visual rehabilitation was achieved without the inherent risks of long-term topical corticosteroids.

CASE 12

Incomplete Flap During LASIK

Lucio Buratto, MD
Milano, Italy

When I started LASIK with the Chiron ACS microkeratome, the microkeratome stopped 2 mm beyond the pupillary center, creating an incomplete corneal flap (tissue available for circular ablation is 4 mm). At that time, I felt that the cut width was sufficient and I performed a multizone refractive treatment for -8 D with a minimum optical zone 4.5 mm and maximum 6 mm on the stroma in situ while protecting the hinge with a spatula.

Performing the refractive treatment in this clinical case was a big mistake. In this situation, the surgeon should always interrupt the operation without performing the ablation, replace the flap, and repeat the operation 3 months later.

In this particular case, the in situ ablation following a cut diameter of 4 mm around the pupil created a number of problems, including irregular astigmatism and considerable night time glare because of the small functional optical zone.

From the outset, topography highlighted a nasal step. Theoretically, this would be more obvious if the ablation is deep and the optical zone wide.

POSSIBLE REASONS FOR AN INCOMPLETE CUT

1. Insufficient run of the microkeratome along the guides because of dust, foreign bodies, eye lashes, or residues from washing (dry soap particles or lubricant)
2. Matter trapped in the teeth of the microkeratome gears
3. The microkeratome progression is blocked when skin from the temporal side of the orbit gets trapped between the stop device and the suction ring
4. The surgeon inadvertently lifts his foot from the pedal before the run is completed

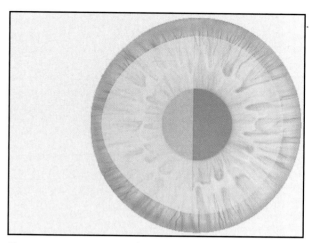

Figure 42-57. An incomplete cut that stops in the pupillary zone: replace the flap and repeat the cut 3 months later.

5. The patient suddenly moves, causing the surgeon to react accordingly with interruption of the cut
6. Power outage
7. Breakdown or blockage of the motor due to rust or other deposits
8. The microkeratome runs into the speculum or surgical drape
9. The surgeon's hand does not follow the movement of the microkeratome. The surgeon can actually oppose the movement because of involuntary emotional tension

POSSIBLE SOLUTIONS

1. Prior to the pupil: replace the flap without sutures and repeat the procedure at least 3 months later.
2. Within the pupillary zone or less than 2.5 mm from the center: replace the flap (Figures 42-57 and 42-58).
3. More than 2.5 mm from the pupillary center: if the myopia is slight, treat with an optical zone of 5 (2.5 + 2.5) (Figures 42-59 and 42-60).
4. If an optical zone wider than 2.5 mm from the pupillary center is required, the cut can be extended by 1 mm using a disc knife.
5. If the cut diameter is less than 5 mm, avoid completing the lamellar cut with the manual method (disc knife, crescent knife, etc), as this would produce an extremely irregular surface with steps and cause serious visual problems.
6. If the cut is incomplete and the quality of the cut is poor, the flap should be replaced and the procedure repeated 3 months later, preferably using a plate that will produce a slightly deeper cut (ie, if a 160 plate was used in the first cut, a 180 plate should be used in the second). Alternatively, the microkeratome used should produce a wider cut or create the hinge in a different position. This is possible with the Chiron Hansatome microkeratome.
7. The hinge must be protected with the spatula during the ablation to avoid a double treatment over the short flap (Figure 42-61).

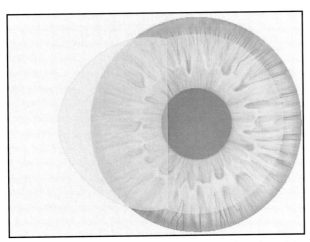

Figure 42-58. An incomplete cut that stops at the edge of the pupillary area: replace the flap and repeat the cut 3 months later.

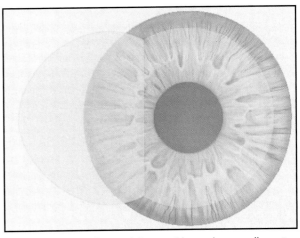

Figure 42-59. Cut beyond the pupil but only a small portion of stroma is exposed: the ablation can be performed with a small optical zone, if not already scheduled, with a large optical zone.

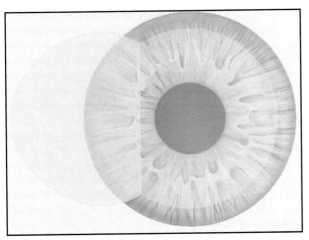

Figure 42-60. The cut is beyond the pupil and the portion of the stroma exposed is quite large: the ablation can be performed.

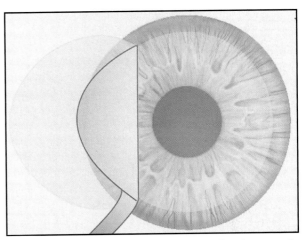

Figure 42-61. The hinge must be protected with a spatula every time the hinge is large, the in situ stromal area exposed for the ablation is small, or when a large area is to be ablated.

POSSIBLE SOLUTIONS FOR THIS CASE

A reasonably tight anti-torsion suture will smooth the flap and allow a certain amount of reshaping by collagen fibers in the untreated area. A contact lens will facilitate distribution of the epithelial cells and try to limit visual disturbances.

Some months later, examine the eye by topography to see how many diopters difference there are between the treated and untreated areas. Then proceed accordingly with one of the methods described below. Wait 2 to 4 months before proceeding.

1. Repeat the cut with the same plate and perform a free cap; then perform a PTK in the area that was not ablated in the first treatment while protecting the previously ablated zone with a shield (piece of plastic, part of a contact lens, viscoelastic substance). Intraoperative control of the surface quality should be done by computerized corneal topography (using artificial tears) and retroillumination. This control should aim to obtain regular keratoscopic patterns.

2. Repeat the cut using the same plate and perform a free cut followed by an ablation using a scanning laser controlled by the topography (Topolink ablation).

3. Repeat the cut with the same plate and perform a free cap. Apply a Nizzola-Vinciguerra shield and perform an in-situ treatment. Consider this situation similar to a decentering of value equal to the difference between the two diameters, then perform the PTK. Alternatively, treat the same optical zone in the untreated area for the same refraction used in the first case or use the difference in topographical values between the treated and untreated zones (the shield will protect and prevent ablation in the area that has already been treated in the primary operation).

4. Perform PRK on the nonablated area while protecting the ablated zone with a shield (a spatula, a specially cut piece of plastic, a metal half moon) or a Nizzola-Vinciguerra shield. In this case, there will still be small steps between the two areas, as there is newly formed tissue. It is better to perform PTK with intraoperative control using a portable Tear Scope Keeler keratoscope.

5. Perform a 360° deeper lamellar cut (220 to 280 microns) with elimination of the superficial free tissue and replace with fresh donor tissue as a homoplastic lamellar graft treated on the stromal face for about half the patient's initial refraction (the first operation will produce a certain amount of the desired refractive result).

CASE 13

LASIK with Forme Fruste Keratoconus

Louis E. Probst, MD
Windsor, Ontario, Canada

A 54-year-old male was originally evaluated for LASIK for high myopia and astigmatism. The preoperative refraction was -8 - 2.75 x 92 OD and -7 -3.5 x 120 OS. Corneal topography performed preoperatively indicated forme fruste keratoconus in the left eye (Figure 42-62). Ocular examination was normal with none of the classic signs of keratoconus (Fleischer's ring, corneal striae, central scarring). Corneal pachymetry found a corneal thickness of 540 and 680 microns centrally and inferiorly respectively OD and 520 and 590 microns centrally and inferiorly respectively OS. The patient had no past history of hard contact lens use and had stopped his soft contact lens use in the left eye 2 weeks prior to assessment.

The unpredictably of LASIK for the left eye was explained to the patient. The patient was also given the option to try additional contact lenses. After two very detailed consultations, the patient elected to try LASIK in the left eye only.

At the 1-month follow-up, the corneal flap position was excellent, the flap and interface were clear, and the flap edge was smooth. The UCVA and BCVA was 20/60 with a refraction of +.75 +175 x 065.

At the 4-month follow-up, the flap was noted to have healed perfectly. The UCVA was 20/100 and the BCVA had improved to 20/25 with -1.5 +4.5 x 27. Corneal topography indicated significant inferior steepening of the left cornea with superior flattening from the excimer laser ablation (Figure 42-63). Corneal pachymetry indicated irregular astigmatism in the same pattern seen preoperatively.

Two months later, the patient was assessed for possible astigmatic surgery. The patient was told that the results would be unpredictable given the irregular nature of the corneal astigmatism. Corneal pachymetry found a central

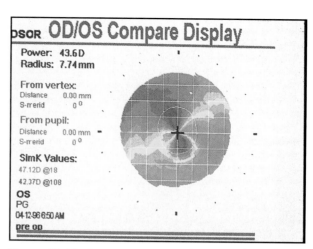

Figure 42-62. Preoperative corneal topography indicates extensive inferior steepening of the cornea with irregular astigmatism, suggesting forme fruste keratoconus.

corneal thickness of 436 microns with an inferior thickness of 631 microns. Corneal topography at this time continued to show irregular astigmatism (Figure 42-64). Two 4 mm straight astigmatic cuts were made at a depth of 550 microns with an 7 mm clear zone.

Three months after the astigmatic keratotomy, UCVA was 20/400 and BCVA was 20/20 with a refraction of -3 + 6 x 22. Corneal pachymetry found the central thickness to be 438 microns and the inferior thickness to be 685 microns. Corneal topography demonstrated significant irregular astigmatism with more than 15 D of cylinder at an axis of 24 (Figure 42-65).

One year and 6 months following the original LASIK procedure, the patient's UCVA was 20/300 and BCVA was 20/30 with a refraction of -4 + 7 x 22. The corneal topography continued to indicate significant astigmatism with more than 15 D of astigmatism at axis 22 (Figure 42-66). Corneal pachymetry at this time found the central corneal thickness was 442 microns and the inferior corneal thickness was 691 microns inferonasally and 502 microns inferotemporally.

Given the visual impairment from the increased astigmatism, a trial with a hard contact lens was attempted in the left eye. This was poorly tolerated. Topography-assisted LASIK was considered, however the central corneal thickness would not allow for further treatment. Further thinning of the cornea would cause further corneal instability.

After considerable discussion, the patient elected to undergo penetrating keratoplasty in the left eye. This was performed without complication with a 8.25 mm donor button. The patient is now in the early postoperative recovery phase of the surgery. The BCVA has remained unaffected.

This case illustrates the unpredictability and instability of the corneas of eyes with forme fruste keratoconus identified on preoperative topography. While refractive surgeons have advocated PRK and LASIK with various treatment modifications for these eyes, this case clearly demonstrates

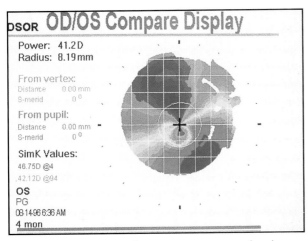

Figure 42-63. Four-month post-LASIK topography demonstrates the superior flattening from the excimer ablation with the same inferior steepening that was observed preoperatively.

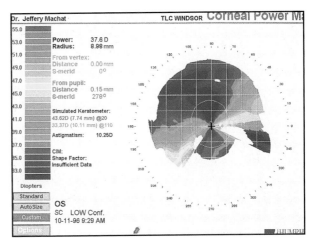

Figure 42-64. At the 6-month visit, the topography found an increasing amount of irregular astigmatism.

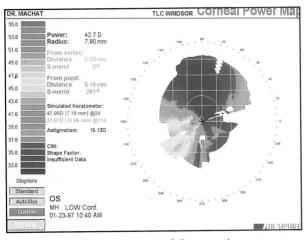

Figure 42-65. At the 18-month follow-up, the astigmatism has increased to SimK values of more than 15 D.

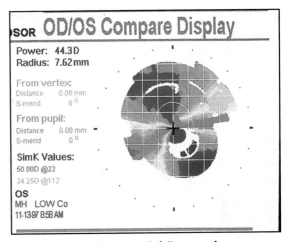

Figure 42-66. At the 9-month follow-up after astigmatic keratotomy, the topography showed no improvement in the astigmatism.

that forme fruste keratoconus should be considered a contraindication for refractive surgery and particularly LASIK.

CASE 14

Free Cap and Epithelial Ingrowth with LASIK

Jonathan Woolfson, MD
Greenville, South Carolina, USA

A 45-year-old female was evaluated for LASIK. The preoperative refraction was -8.5 -.5 x 90 for a BCVA of 20/25 OD and -9 -.5 X 87 for a BCVA of 20/25 OS. The corneal pachymetry indicated adequate corneal thickness, and the corneal topography found regular astigmatism with a curvature flat keratometry value of 41.5 D. LASIK was

performed with the Chiron ACS and a 160 depth plate.

When LASIK was performed in the left eye, a free cap occurred. The free cap was left on the cornea when the microkeratome was reversed rather than left inside the microkeratome. The cap was torn nasally suggesting that adhesion to the microkeratome had occurred. The cut was insufficient for laser to be performed, as the edge of the flap overlapped for more than 1 mm into the ablation zone. The cap was carefully replaced and smoothed onto the stromal bed with interface irrigation. The correct orientation was verified with the preplaced corneal alignment marks. The free cap was then allowed to seal into place for 10 minutes without sutures. Thirty minutes following the procedure, the cap eye was examined and found to be stable. On the first postoperative day, the flap was healing well, the eye was comfortable, and the BCVA was unchanged.

One month later, the patient had significant epithelial

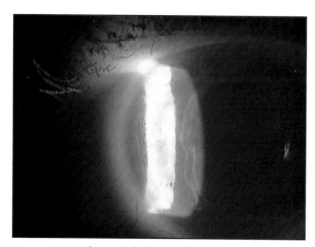

Figure 42-67. The epithelial ingrowth can be seen extending under the small irregular free cap edge.

ingrowth nasally in the region of the torn hinge. The patient was taken back to the laser room and the complete cap was lifted. The bed and underside of the cap were scraped. The free cap was replaced. The patient was examined each week and no further epithelial ingrowth was noted in that area.

Over the next month, the patient developed significant epithelial ingrowth in the temporal region of the cap (Figure 42-67). The cap was again removed, the cap and bed scraped of epithelium, and the cap replaced without complications. The eye was followed closely after surgery and no further epithelial ingrowth was identified.

One year after the original procedure, the preoperative refraction had not significantly changed. LASIK was repeated in the left eye with a 200-micron plate, and this time the procedure was uncomplicated. The patient was followed for an additional 8 months. The last UCVA OS was 20/100 with an unchanged BCVA of 20/25 with refraction of -2.5 -.75 x 150=20/25, indicating some regression of the correction. Corneal topography indicated a small central island. Despite the multiple procedures and the central island, there has been no loss of BCVA. Enhancement LASIK will be performed by lifting the second successful flap rather than risking another flap complication. Enhancement LASIK was performed by lifting the second flap. She is now 6 months out with UCVA OS 20/30 and BCVA 20/25 with -.25 - .25 x 160.

In this case, the free cap could have occurred for many reasons. The corneal topography had found that the cornea was relatively flat. This increases the risk of a free cap and guarantees that the flap will be smaller with a narrower hinge. The flap may have been thin due to inadequate suction, which might explain why it detached nasally so easily. The flap may have become adherent to the microkeratome head due to a prolonged procedure or inadequate lubrication. Small flaps and free caps can be avoided in flat corneas by using a 200-micron depth plate.

Unfortunately, thin flaps are also more prone to the post-

operative problems of striae and epithelial ingrowth. Flap melts are also more common since the flap is already thin. In this case, epithelial ingrowth was removed twice. A second lamellar cut can be performed without difficulty after a previous cut, however at least 3 months should pass after the first procedure and a deeper (200 micron) plate should be used.

In the case of a free flap, it is controversial whether the refractive ablation should be performed. Since the free cap was not planned, the occurrence of this complication suggests that there was a problem during the surgery that may include a loss of suction or inappropriate technique. If the free cap is abnormal in any manner, it should be replaced without treatment. If the free cap is of an adequate size and thickness, the decision to treat can be individualized based on the surgeon's evaluation of the case.

CASE 15

Free Cap and Irregular Astigmatism with LASIK

Jonathan Woolfson, MD
Greenville, South Carolina, USA

This patient was assessed for LASIK with a refraction of -4.75 -1.25 x .25 = 20/20 OD, -5 -.5 x 165 = 20/20 OS. During LASIK OD, a free cap occurred. We elected to continue with the full refractive correction. The cap was carefully replaced making use of the corneal alignment marks to ensure that the orientation was correct. Thirty minutes later, the cap was stable and smooth. Unfortunately, in the immediate postoperative period, the patient rubbed his eye and dislodged the cap, which was identified on the patient's cheek. The patient was returned to the laser bed and the free cap was repositioned and refloated onto the stromal bed after the interface had been vigorously cleaned. The cap was repositioned and secured without the use of sutures.

On the first postoperative day, the patient had a moderate epithelial abrasion that healed over the next several days. The free cap was stable and smooth in the stromal bed. The UCVA slowly improved. By the third postoperative week, the UCVA was 20/40 with a refraction of plano, the cap was clear, and no complications were noted (Figure 42-68 and 42-69). Significant epithelial ingrowth was noted on the fifth postoperative week and was subsequently treated by lifting the cap and scraping on the base and underside of the cap.

On the third postoperative month, the UCVA was 20/60. A correction of +3.5 -2.5 x 160 improved vision to 20/25. Irregular astigmatism was evident on the corneal topography (Figure 42-70 and 42-71). Epithelial ingrowth was again identified and removed. In the immediate postoperative period, the UCVA was 20/60. Over the course of the following several weeks, the UCVA vision was 20/150.

On the fifth postoperative month, the UCVA was 20/150

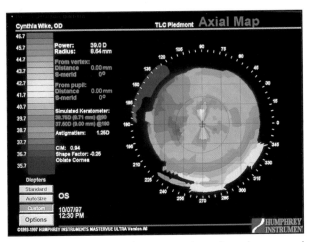

Figure 42-68. Corneal topography after the second enhancement procedure demonstrates a well-centered ablation with a small central island pattern.

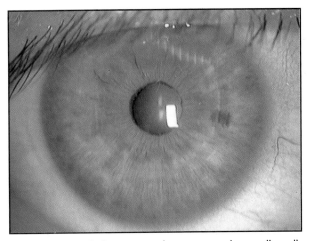

Figure 42-69. Slit lamp view demonstrates the small, well-healed free cap.

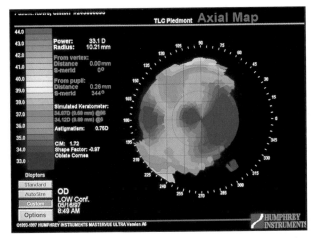

Figure 42-70. Corneal topography indicates an irregular decentered ablation.

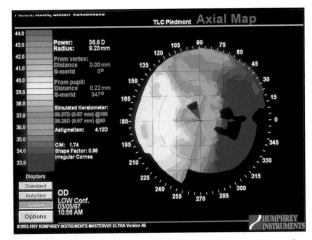

Figure 42-71. Corneal topography indicates an irregular decentered ablation.

and improved to 20/25 with pinhole and best correction. Although he could see well, the patient was not happy with the spectacle or contact lens correction. The corneal topography suggests irregular astigmatism. After one year, his UCVA is 20/70 and BCVA is 20/25.

While the free cap has remained clear, the irregular cornea has resulted in a large amount of induced astigmatism. Since the patient feels the vision is slowly improving, no immediate treatment is planned. Future considerations include topography-assisted LASIK. Similar cases may be treated with homoplastic lamellar grafts.

This case clearly demonstrates the problems that can occur following a thin, free cap. The decision to proceed with the refraction ablation with a free cap produced a very poor result. While LASIK and ALK were originally per-

formed with free caps on a routine basis, this was a planned aspect of the surgery. When an inadvertent free cap occurs during LASIK, this suggests that there has been an intraoperative problem, which could have compromised the quality of the cap. If this cap is replaced without the refractive ablation, it will sit perfectly into the stromal bed and probably heal well. If the ablation is performed, another variable has been added that may cause the already compromised cap to heal in an irregular manner. The refractive ablation should not be performed in the case of a free cap unless the surgeon is confident the cap has adequate integrity. Epithelial ingrowth seems to occur more commonly with thin flaps—possibly because of a poorly defined flap edge.

Appendix

Below is *The Options for Refractive Surgery* diagram to cut out for easy reference:

Devised by Louis E. Probst, MD, TLC Clinical Research Director

Index